Insurance Handbook for the Medical Office

MARILYN TAKAHASHI FORDNEY, CMA-AC

Instructor of Medical Insurance, Medical Terminology,
Medical Machine Transcription and Medical Office
Procedures, Ventura College, Ventura, California

With a chapter on Canadian Health Insurance by
RHODA G. FINNERON

Supervisor, Private Vocational Schools, Province of Ontario

1977

W. B. SAUNDERS COMPANY / Philadelphia / London / Toronto

W. B. Saunders Company: West Washington Square
Philadelphia, PA 19105

1 St. Anne's Road
Eastbourne, East Sussex BN21 3UN, England

1 Goldthorne Avenue
Toronto, Ontario M8Z 5T9, Canada

Library of Congress Cataloging in Publication Data

Fordney, Marilyn Takahashi.
   Insurance handbook for the medical office.

   Includes index.
   1. Insurance, Health—United States—Handbooks, manuals,
etc.   2. Medical offices—Management—Handbooks, manuals,
etc.   I. Finneron, Rhoda G.   II. Title. [DNLM: 1. Insurance, health—United States—Handbooks.   2. Insurance,
liability—United States—Handbooks. W275 AA1 F65i]

HG9396.F67   368.3'8'002461   76-22293

ISBN 0-7216-3811-2

Insurance Handbook for the Medical Office

ISBN Soft 0-7216-3812-0
ISBN Hard 0-7216-3811-2

Last digit is the print number: 9   8   7   6   5   4   3   2   1

To my parents,
Mr. and Mrs. James Takahashi,
and to my husband, Alan

PREFACE

photo by Edward Pitney

The purpose of this text is to increase the efficiency and smooth operation of that most exasperating aspect of the doctor's office routine: insurance billing. The book is at once an aid, a reference source, and a learning tool for those who are or who will be involved in the completing of medical or dental insurance claims. Although designed specifically for one-semester community college courses in the daytime and extension divisions, it can also be used for home study if no formal classes are available in the community. The lay reader not planning a career as a medical or dental office assistant will find in it many handy hints for billing his or her insurance company.

A practical approach to learning insurance billing is emphasized throughout. In the Appendix at the back of the text, patients records are presented exactly as they might appear in the doctor's files, so that the student may learn how to abstract from them to complete a claim properly and accurately. Many contain the physician's own handwritten notes. Easily removable sample forms are included at the end of the book for typing practice. You may begin these projects after reading through Chapter 3.

Behavioral Objectives are presented at the beginning of each chapter and Review Questions at the end to guide the reader over the most important points. The answers to all the review questions may be found by careful reading.

A Teacher's Guide is available for use with the text to assist in establishing a course in medical insurance or to give ideas on how to use the text as an adjunct to a medical office procedure course.

Basic medical and insurance abbreviations and terms have been explained throughout the text, to enable the student to become proficient in their meaning as she proceeds through the manual either on her own or under the instructor's guidance. Current Procedural Terminology (CPT) and Relative Value Studies (RVS), codings used nationally and in the state of California respectively, are also utilized frequently to facilitate learning the proper codes for submitting a claim or making up an itemized billing statement. Pertinent billing tips are suggested for each type of insurance covered.

Many types of insurance coverage are available in the United States and Canada. Those types most commonly used in physician's offices and clinics have been emphasized. Hospital claims processing procedures are discussed only tangentially. The following forms of insurance are considered to be most characteristic: Unemployment Compensation Disability (also known as State Disability), Workers' Compensation or

Industrial Insurance, Federal Medicare, State Medicaid (in California, Medi-Cal), Medi-Medi, group plans such as Blue Cross and Blue Shield, and CHAMPUS (Civilian Health and Medical Program, Uniformed Services). A chapter on Canadian medical office accounting and insurance form processing has been written by Rhoda Finneron, Supervisor, Private Vocational Schools, Province of Ontario.

Insurance forms are constantly changing, and insurance billing procedures are also revised frequently owing to new legislation and new regulations from insurance carriers. It is therefore essential that all medical personnel handling claims continue to update their information by reading the bulletins of state agencies and insurance carriers and speaking with their representatives, or by attending insurance workshops offered at local colleges or by local chapters of the American Association of Medical Assistants. It is hoped that this text will unravel current methods for the busy secretary; it is hoped, too, that it will become the framework upon which she hangs new knowledge as she grows in understanding and appreciation of her profession.

Marilyn T. Fordney

MARILYN T. FORDNEY, CMA-AC
Oxnard, California

ACKNOWLEDGMENTS

During my fourteen years of experience as a Medical Assistant and my eight years of teaching, I have met hundreds of students, physicians, friends, colleagues, and instructors who have contributed valuable suggestions and interesting material for this book. I wish to express my thanks to all of them, with special emphasis as follows:

Lois C. Oliver, Professor, Pierce College, Woodland Hills, California, helped me to organize my first medical insurance class in 1969 and offered assistance and encouragement throughout the preparation of the *Handbook*.

Marcia O. "Marcy" Diehl, CMA-A, Grossmont School District Health Careers Center, La Mesa, California, generously shared her knowledge, ideas, and class materials. *Gail Capolongo* of Pierce College and North Hollywood Adult School and *Barbara Speth* of Ventura College also contributed suggestions for improving the text.

Mary E. Kinn, CPS, CMA-A, Instructor in Health Technologies, Long Beach City College, Long Beach, California, provided a perceptive review of my syllabus. Without her positive endorsement this book might not have been.

I gratefully acknowledge the artists who were involved with the cover design and cartoons featured throughout the text: *Lorraine Battista*, Manager, Design Department, W. B. Saunders Company; *Diana Crawford*, Advertising Department, W. B. Saunders Company; *Debbie McKillop*, Staff Illustrator, Ventura College, Ventura, California; and *Roman Yslas*, Graphic Illustrator, Oxnard, California.

I also wish to thank Ventura College, Publications Department, Ventura, California, who printed the first California syllabus of this text.

I am indebted to many individuals on the staff of the W. B. Saunders Company for encouragement and guidance. I wish to express particular appreciation to *Marie D. Low*, Associate Medical Editor, for expert editing and coordination of the entire project. Her husband, *Erick B. Low*, Reference Librarian, Delaware School of Law, helped me to gather data for the chapters on Workers' Compensation and Medical Professional Liability. My thanks go also to *Herbert J. Powell, Jr.*, Production Manager, Medical Titles; *Kenneth Atwood*, Manager, Advertising Department; *Erika Shapiro*, Manuscript Editorial Department; and *Rita Christensen*, Secretary, Medical Department.

Lastly and most importantly, I must express overwhelming debt and enduring gratitude to *Rhoda G. Finneron*, who contributed the excellent discussion of Canadian health insurance, and to the consultants who reviewed each chapter or who provided vital information about private, state, and federal insurance programs. Without the knowledge of these advisers, the massive task of compiling an insurance text truly national in scope might never have been completed. Although the names of all those who graciously assisted me are too numerous to mention, I take great pride in listing my principal consultants on the following pages.

PRINCIPAL CONSULTANTS AND REVIEWERS

MARTHA E. ALCABES
Medicare Field Representative
Social Security Administration
Oxnard, California

HUBERT J. BARNES
Regional Program Consultant
Maternal and Child Health
Department of Health, Education, and Welfare
Regional Office IX
San Francisco, California

RAYMOND G. BENNETT
Administrator
Medical Care Services
Crippled Children Services Section
Department of Health, State of California
Sacramento, California

FRANCIENE BLACK
Subscriber Service Representative
Blue Cross of Southern California
Oxnard, California

HARVEY G. BLACKMUN
Owner and Manager
Copy Van
Santa Barbara, California

STEPHEN B. BLAIR, JR.
Acting Director
Colorado Dental Service
CHAMPUS Division
Denver, Colorado

J. J. BROSAMER
Chief, Medical Benefits
Veterans Administration
Outpatient Clinic
Los Angeles, California

ELLIOT CHAUM
Attorney
Los Angeles, California

LEON S. CONLON
Director
American Medical Association
Division of Medical Practice
Department of Professional Review
Chicago, Illinois

HARRY W. DAHL
Executive Director
International Association of Industrial
Accident Boards and Commissions
Des Moines, Iowa

LESLIE DORNFELD, M.D., F.A.C.P.
Associate Professor of Medicine
UCLA Medical Center
Los Angeles, California

RICHARD J. EALES
Assistant Director
Health Insurance Council
New York, New York

RICHARD EDWARDS
Manager
Public Affairs Department
Kaiser Permanente Medical Care Program
Oakland, California

RAYMOND C. ELLIOTT
Owner and Manager
Accounts Adjustment Bureau
Oxnard, California

RICHARD M. ELZINGA
Vice President
MedcoBill
Intellectron International, Inc.
Van Nuys, California

JOHN F. FERRIN
President
Medicount, Inc.
Long Beach, California

ASHER J. FINKEL, M.D.
American Medical Association
Chicago, Illinois

ARLENE FLOM
Information Services, Communications
Blue Cross Association
Chicago, Illinois

SUSAN FLYGARE
Senior Correspondent
Provider Service
Blue Cross and Blue Shield of Minnesota
Minneapolis, Minnesota

ROBERT W. FRASER
Director of Communications
Pennsylvania Blue Shield
Camp Hill, Pennsylvania

EMANUEL FRIEDMAN
Federal Workers' Compensation Program
Washington, D.C.

E. H. FRIEDRICHS
Field Office Manager
Employment Development Department
State Disability Insurance
Santa Barbara, California

FONDA HARRINGTON
Senior Veterans Claims Officer
Veterans Administration
Ventura, California

DANIEL K. HARRIS
Director
Computer Systems in Medicine
American Medical Association
Chicago, Illinois

GLENN JOHNSON
Director
Bureau of Medical Assistance
Commonwealth of Pennsylvania
Department of Public Welfare
Harrisburg, Pennsylvania

MICHAEL W. JONES
Staff Coordinator
Committee on Relative Value Studies
California Medical Association
San Francisco, California

WILLIAM MALDONADO
Director
Commonwealth of Puerto Rico
Department of Labor
Bureau of Employment Security
Disability Insurance Program
Hato Rey, Puerto Rico

RONALD F. MARKSON
Assistant General Manager
California Workers' Compensation Institute
San Francisco, California

PERRY MASON
Office Manager
Dental Corporation
Oxnard, California

OSCAR MELENDEZ
Claims Coordinator
State Compensation Insurance Fund
Ventura, California

MARY MONAHAN
Field Representative
Professional Relations Division
Blue Shield of California
Los Angeles, California

MOLLY NADLER
Staff Associate
Council on Dental Care Programs
American Dental Association
Chicago, Illinois

ANDREA PENDLETON
Supervisor
Ventura County Foundation for Medical Care
Ventura, California

J. ROBERT PERSONETTE
Director
Benefit Information and Development
Blue Cross–Blue Shield Federal Employee
Program
Washington, D.C.

RAYMOND E. PHILLIPS, M.D.
Acting Commissioner of Health for Orange
County
Goshen, New York

LIZZ POWER
Coordinator
Internal Professional Affairs
National Association of Blue Shield Plans
Chicago, Illinois

MICHAEL J. ROMIG
Associate Director
Economic Security, Education and Manpower
Chamber of Commerce of the United States
Washington, D.C.

CLAYTON E. SJOBLOM
Chief of Workers' Benefits
State of Washington Department of Labor and
Industries
Olympia, Washington

RICHARD SLOANE
Law Librarian and Professor of Law
Biddle Law Library
University of Pennsylvania
Philadelphia, Pennsylvania

ESMOND S. SMITH, M.D.
Chief
Crippled Children Services Section
State of California Department of Health
Sacramento, California

WILLIAM THOMPSON
Work Injury Statistics Section
Department of Industrial Relations
Division of Labor Statistics and Research
San Francisco, California

BOYD THOMPSON
Executive Director
American Association of Foundations for
Medical Care
Stockton, California

MARK E. TURK and CATHLEEN SMITH
Public Communications Representatives
Community Relations Department
Ross-Loos Medical Group
Los Angeles, California

VICKI TUTTLE
Senior Provider Representative
Santa Barbara Region
Blue Cross of Southern California
Santa Barbara, California

JAMES A. WARE
Assistant Commissioner
Income Security
State of New Jersey Department of Labor and
Industry
Trenton, New Jersey

GREG WEBER
Public Relations Assistant
Blue Cross of Greater Philadelphia
Philadelphia, Pennsylvania

KEN WITTE
Vice President and Sales Manager
National Business Systems, Inc.
ADB Systems, Inc.
Ventura, California

CONTENTS

1
Introduction to Medical Insurance

BEHAVIORAL
OBJECTIVES *The Assistant should be able to:*

1. Distinguish between the two major classes of health insurance contracts.
2. Describe in general terms the important federal, state, and private health insurance plans.
3. Define common insurance, medical, and diagnostic terms.
4. Abstract from the patient record the important information for completing an insurance claim form.
5. Handle insurance claims in the physician's or dentist's office in order to minimize their rejection by insurance carriers.

KINDS OF POLICIES

There are two ways in which a person may obtain health insurance. One is by taking out insurance through a group plan and the other is by paying the premium on an individual basis.

1. **Group contract:** Any insurance plan by which a group of employees (and their eligible dependents), or other homogeneous group, is insured under a single policy issued to their employer or leader, with individual certificates given to each insured individual or family unit. A group policy usually provides better benefits and the premiums are lower. However, the coverage for each person in the group is the same. Many physicians can obtain comprehensive group coverage through plans sponsored by the professional organizations to which they belong. Sometimes this is called a *blanket contract*.

2. **Individual contract:** Any insurance plan issued to the individual (and/or his dependents). Usually this type of policy has a higher premium and many times the benefits are less than those obtainable under a group health insurance plan. Sometimes this is called *personal insurance*.

TYPES OF INSURANCE COVERAGE

Listed below are the major forms of health insurance coverage currently in effect in the United States. Explanations of the terms used in these definitions may be found in the following section.

Accident and health insurance: Insurance under which benefits are payable in case of disease, accidental injury, or accidental death.

Aviation trip insurance: A short-term policy protecting individuals as passengers of scheduled aircraft. It is generally obtained at airports.

Blue Cross: An independent, not for profit membership corporation providing protection against the costs of hospital care, and in some policies also protection against the costs of surgical and professional care. (See Chapter 4.)

Blue Shield: An independent, not for profit membership association providing protection against the costs of surgery and other items of medical care. Some policies also offer protection against the costs of hospital care. (See Chapter 4.)

Business insurance: A policy which provides benefits principally to a business rather than to an individual. It is issued to indemnify a business for the loss of services of a key employee or partner who becomes disabled.

Catastrophic insurance: Insurance against catastrophic illness. (See definition of catastrophic illness, p. 6.)

CHAMPUS: A government-sponsored program which provides hospital and medical services for dependents of active service personnel, retired service personnel and their dependents, and dependents of deceased members who died on active duty. (See also Chapter 7.)

Coinsurance: A plan under which the insured and the insurer share hospital and medical expenses resulting from illness or injury. Sometimes seen in major medical insurance.

Comprehensive major medical insurance: A policy designed to give the protection offered by both a basic and a major medical health insurance policy.

Death insurance: See *Life insurance*.

Dental insurance: A form of insurance that provides protection against the costs of diagnostic and preventive dental care as well as oral surgery, restorative procedures, and therapeutic dental care. (See Chapter 11.)

Denti-Cal: A dental plan in California sponsored by both federal and state governments for people who are eligible for public assistance and some other low-income people. (See Chapter 11.)

Disability income insurance: A form of health insurance that provides periodic payments to replace income when the insured is unable to work as a result of illness, injury, or disease.

Dual coverage: A plan under which the insured has health insurance coverage by more than one carrier.

Family expense policy: A policy which insures both the policyholder and his immediate dependents.

Foundation for medical care: An organization of physicians, sponsored by a state or local medical association, concerned with the development and delivery of medical services and the cost of health care. (See Chapter 10.)

Franchise insurance: A form of insurance in which individual policies are issued to the employees of a common employer or the members of an association under an arrangement by which the employer or association agrees to collect the premiums and remit them to the insurer.

Fraternal insurance: A cooperative type of insurance provided by social organizations for their members.

Group health plan: See *Prepaid group practice plan*.

Health insurance: A generic term applying to all types of insurance indemnifying or reimbursing for costs of hospital and medical care or lost income arising from illness or injury. Also known as *Accident and health insurance*, or *Disability income insurance* (see p. 2).

Health Maintenance Organization (HMO): An organization that provides for a wide range of comprehensive health care services for a specified group at a fixed periodic payment. An HMO can be sponsored by the government, medical schools, hospitals, employers, labor unions, consumer groups, insurance companies, or hospital-medical plans. (See Chapter 10.)

Health Systems Agency (HSA): An organization that plans health care needs and regulates the health care industry in the United States.

Hospital expense insurance: Health insurance protection against the costs of hospital care resulting from the illness or injury of an insured person.

Hospital-medical insurance: A term used to indicate protection that provides benefits toward the cost of any or all of the numerous health care services normally covered under various health insurance plans.

Key-man health insurance: An individual or group insurance policy designed to protect an essential employee or employees of a firm against the loss of income resulting from disability. If desired, it may be written for the benefit of the employer, who usually continues to pay the salary during periods of disability.

Life insurance: Insurance which pays a specific amount to the beneficiary when the insured dies. There are various types: whole-life, term, and straight or ordinary life insurance.

Long-term disability income insurance: A provision to pay benefits to a covered disabled person as long as he or she remains disabled, up to a specified period exceeding 2 years.

Major medical expense insurance: Health insurance to finance the expense of major illnesses and injuries. Major medical policies usually include a *deductible clause*, which means that the individual or another insurer contributes toward the cost of the medical expenses. The larger the deductible, the greater the savings in premium cost. Above this initial deductible, major medical insurance is characterized by large benefit maximums, ranging up to $250,000 or even beyond. The holder is reimbursed for the major part of all charges for the hospital, the doctor, private nurse, medical appliances, and prescribed out-of-hospital treatment, drugs, and medicines.

Medicaid: A plan sponsored jointly by the federal and state governments for people eligible for public assistance and some other low-income people. Coverage and benefits vary widely from state to state. (See Chapter 5.)

Medi-Cal: The state of California's version of the nationwide program known as "Medicaid." See *Medicaid*. (See also Chapter 5.)

Medical expense insurance: A form of health insurance that provides benefits for medical care on an outpatient basis. The company may limit the amount it will pay per call or the total amount for all calls. It may also exclude the first few calls made by the physician at the beginning of an illness.

Medicare (M): The hospital insurance system and supplementary medical insurance for the aged created by the 1965 Amendments to the Social Security Act and operated under the provisions of the Act. Benefits are also extended to the totally disabled and to the blind. (See Chapter 6.)

Medicare/Medicaid (Medi-Cal): This program, also known as *Medi-Medi*, covers those persons protected under *both* the Medicare plan and the Medicaid (or Medi-Cal) plan. (See Chapter 6.)

Medigap insurance: Supplemental insurance designed to fill in some, though never all, of the gaps in Medicare's coverage.

No-Fault insurance: Automobile insurance that provides coverage against injury or other loss without the need to determine responsibility for an accident. Coverage and benefits vary widely; at present plans exist in only a few states.

Noncancellable, or noncancellable and guaranteed renewable, policy: A policy that the insured has the right to continue in force to a specified age, such as to age 65, by the timely payment of premiums. During the specified period that the policy is in force, the insurer has no right to make any unilateral change in any provision of the policy.

Nonoccupational policy: A contract that insures a person against off-the-job accident or sickness. It does not cover disability resulting from injury or sickness covered by Workers' Compensation. Group accident and sickness policies are frequently nonoccupational.

Prepaid group practice plan: A plan under which specified health services are rendered by participating physicians to an enrolled group of persons, with fixed periodic payments made in advance, by or on behalf of each person or family. If a health insurance carrier is involved, it contracts to pay in advance for the full range of health services to which the insured is entitled under the terms of the health insurance contract. Such a plan is one form of a *Health Maintenance Organization* (see p. 3).

Qualified impairment insurance: A form of substandard (see below) or special class insurance that restricts benefits to the insured's particular condition.

Regular medical expense insurance: Coverage which provides benefits toward the cost of such services as doctor fees for nonsurgical care in the hospital, at home, or in a physician's office; and x-rays or laboratory tests performed outside of the hospital.

Senior citizen policies: Contracts insuring persons 65 years of age or over. In most cases these policies supplement the coverage afforded by the government under the Medicare program.

Short-term disability income insurance: A provision to pay benefits to a covered disabled person as long as he or she remains disabled, up to a specified period not exceeding 2 years.

Special class insurance: Coverage for health insurance applicants who cannot qualify for a standard policy by reason of their health.

Special risk insurance: Coverage for risks or hazards of a special or unusual nature.

Specified disease insurance: A policy which provides benefits, usually of large amounts, toward the expense of the treatment of the disease or diseases named in the policy.

Substandard health insurance: An individual policy issued to a person who cannot meet the normal health requirements of a standard health insurance policy. Protection is given as a result of an increase in premium, through a waiver of medical condition, or under a special qualified impairment clause. See *Qualified impairment insurance.*

Surgical expense insurance: A health insurance policy that provides benefits toward the doctor's operating fees. Benefits usually consist of scheduled amounts for each surgical procedure.

Travel accident policy: A limited contract covering only accidents that occur while an insured person is traveling.

Unemployment Compensation Disability (UCD): Insurance which covers off-the-job injury or sickness and is paid for by deductions from a person's paycheck. This program is administered by a state agency and is sometimes also known as State Disability Insurance. (See Chapter 8.)

Veterans' Administration (VA) Outpatient Clinic: A clinic where medical and dental services are rendered to a veteran who has a service-related disability. (See Chapter 7.)

Workers' Compensation insurance: A contract which insures a person against on-the-job injury or illness. The employer pays the premium for his or her employees. (See Chapter 9.)

INSURANCE TERMINOLOGY

The following commonly used terms are introduced here to provide the reader with a general understanding of insurance phraseology. Additional terms will be explained in subsequent chapters.

Accident (Acc): An event or occurrence which is unforeseen and unintended.

Accidental bodily injury: Injury to the body of the insured as a result of an accident.

Accumulation: An increase in the amount of benefits provided by some policies, as a reward to the insured for continuous renewal.

Acquisition cost: The immediate cost of issuing a new policy, including cost of clerical work, agent's commission, and medical inspection fees.

Actuary: A person trained in the insurance field who determines premium rates, reserves, and dividends, and conducts various other statistical studies.

Adjuster: An individual who acts for the company or the insured in the settlement of claims. Sometimes referred to as "claim representative."

Age limits: Stipulated minimum and maximum ages, below and above which the company will not accept applications and may not renew policies.

Agent: An insurance company representative licensed by the state who solicits, negotiates, or effects contracts of insurance, and services the policyholder for the insurer.

Application: A signed statement of facts requested by the company on the basis of which the company decides whether or not to issue a policy. This then becomes part of the health insurance contract, if the policy is issued.

Assignment: The transfer of one's right to collect an amount payable under an insurance contract. Also known as *Assignment of benefits*.

Beneficiary: A person designated to receive a specified cash payment upon the policyholder's accidental or natural death.

Benefit: 1. The amount payable by the carrier toward the cost of various covered medical or dental services. 2. The medical or dental service or procedure covered by the program.

Binding receipt: A receipt given for a premium payment accompanying the application for insurance. This binds the company, if the policy is approved, to make the policy effective from the date of the receipt.

Broker: An insurance solicitor, licensed by the state, who places business with a variety of insurance companies and who represents the buyers of insurance rather than the companies, even though he or she is paid commissions by the companies.

Carrier: An insurance company that "carries" the insurance. Synonyms: *insurer, underwriter*, or *administrative agent*.

Catastrophic illness: Sickness in which hospital and other inpatient costs exceed a certain percentage of annual net income, or the amount of such income in excess of public assistance levels, whichever sum is smaller.

Certificate of insurance: A document delivered to the insured which summarizes the benefits and principal provisions of the group plan affecting the insured.

Claim: A demand for payment under an insurance contract or bond.

Comprehensive (Comp): The insuring clause of contracts can be either comprehensive or limited. Comprehensive means broader coverage on diseases or accidents and higher indemnity payments in comparison with a limited clause.

Contributory program: A method of payment for group coverage in which part of the premium is paid by the employee and part is paid by his or her employer or union.

Conversion privilege: The right of an individual covered by a group medical or dental policy to continue his or her coverage on an individual basis (paying the full premium) when he or she terminates association with the insured group. This is not common in dental contracts.

Coordination of Benefits (COB): A clause written into some health insurance policies which means that if the member has other group hospital, medical, or dental coverage with another company, the first company will take into account benefits that are payable by the other carrier in determining its own liability.

Copayment: A contract under which the insured must pay a portion toward the amount of the professional services rendered. Synonym: *coinsurance*.

Coverage: The extent of insurance benefits.

Deductible (Deduc): An amount the insured person must pay before policy benefits begin.

Deductible liability insurance: Coverage under which the insured agrees to pay up to a specified sum per claim toward the amount payable to the physician.

Dependents (D): Generally the spouse and children of a covered individual, as defined in a contract. Under some contracts, parents or other members of the family may be dependents.

Disability: A condition that renders the insured person incapable of performing one or more of the duties required by his or her regular occupation. See also *Partial Disability*, *Permanent Disability*, and *Temporary Disability*.

Dismemberment: The loss of a limb or of sight.

Dividend: A policyholder's share in the divisible surplus funds of an insurance company apportioned for distribution, which may take the form of a refund of part of the premium on the insured's policy.

Double indemnity: A policy provision usually associated with death, which doubles payment of designated benefits when certain kinds of accidents occur.

Dread disease rider (Drd dis): A clause added onto a policy which provides supplemental benefits for certain conditions.

Dual choice or dual option: Refers to federal legislation that requires employers to give their employees the option to enroll in a local health maintenance organization rather than in the conventional employer-sponsored health program.

Elective benefit: A benefit payable in lieu of another. For example, a lump sum benefit may be allowed for specified fractures or dislocations in lieu of weekly or monthly indemnity.

Elimination period: Period of time after the beginning of a *disability* for which no indemnities are payable. Not to be confused with *Excepted period* (see p. 7).

Evidence of insurability: Any statement or proof of a person's physical condition or occupation affecting his or her acceptance for insurance.

Excepted period: Time after the beginning date of a *policy* during which sickness benefits will not be payable. Also known as *Waiting period*.

Exclusions: Specified illnesses, injuries, or conditions listed in the policy for which the insurance company will not pay. Common exclusions are self-inflicted injuries, combat injuries, plastic surgery for cosmetic reasons, and on-the-job injuries covered by Workers' Compensation.

Explanation of Benefits (EOB): A recap sheet that accompanies a Medicare or Medi-Cal check, showing breakdown and explanation of payment on a claim.

Extended Benefits (EB): Coverage supplemental to either a basic hospital plan or a basic hospital–surgical–medical plan. Sometimes diagnostic x-ray and laboratory (DXL) examinations are covered on an outpatient basis.

Extended Care Facility (ECF): A medical facility for confinement of the patient after he or she is discharged from a hospital and needs further specialized care.

Fee-for-service: The method of billing by physicians or dentists in private practice, whereby the doctor or dentist charges for each professional service performed.

Fiscal intermediary or agent: An agent or insurance company that processes claims and issues payment for state or federal agencies or other insurance companies.

Grace period: A specified period after a premium payment is due, in which the policyholder may make such payment, and during which the protection of the policy continues.

Guaranteed renewable: Contracts that the insured has the right to continue in force by the timely payment of premiums for a substantial period of time, during which period the insurer has no right to make unilaterally any change in any provision of the contract while the contract is in force, other than a change in the premium rate for classes of insureds. This term is also known as "guaranteed continuable." Premiums may not be changed for an individual but only for classes of insureds, objectively determined.

Hospital benefits: Benefits provided under a policy for hospital charges incurred by an insured person because of an illness or injury.

Indemnity: A benefit paid by an insurer for a loss insured under a policy.

Individual Responsibility Program (IRP): A private medical relationship entered into by a patient and a physician. The doctor undertakes to provide the patient with the best medical services possible, and the patient assumes the responsibility of compensating the physician for his efforts.

Injury independent of all other means: An injury resulting from an accident, provided that the accident was not caused by an illness.

Inpatient (IP): A person who is a bed patient in a hospital.

Insurance: Protection by written contract against the financial hazards (in whole or in part) resulting from certain specified events.

Insurance clause: The clause which indicates the parties to a health insurance contract, sets forth the type of loss covered, and broadly defines the benefits to be paid.

Insurance company: Any corporation primarily engaged in the business of furnishing insurance protection to the public.

Lapse: Termination of a policy upon the policyholder's failure to pay the premium within the time required.

Liability: A debt; an amount owed.

Lifetime disability benefit: A payment to help replace income lost by an insured person as long as he or she is totally disabled, even for a lifetime.

Limited (Ltd): A contract which covers only certain specified diseases or accidents and restricts indemnity payments. The insuring clause of contracts can be either limited or *comprehensive* (see p. 6).

Loss of income benefits: Payments made to an insured person to help replace income lost through inability to work because of an insured disability.

Major medical: A policy especially designed to help offset heavy medical expenses resulting from catastrophic or prolonged illness or injury. (See also p. 3.)

Morbidity: Sickness.

Nonconfining sickness: An illness which prevents the insured person from working but which does not result in confinement to a hospital or to one's home.

Nondisabling injury: One which may require medical care but does not produce loss of working time or income.

Nonduplication of benefits: When a patient is covered under more than one group medical or dental program, the carrier with a nonduplication provision—as distinguished from a coordination of benefits provision—assumes no liability, frequently leaving the patient with out-of-pocket expenses.

Not-for-profit carriers: Service corporations or prepayment plans organized under state not-for-profit statutes for the purpose of providing health care coverage (for example, Delta Dental Plans, Blue Cross and Blue Shield Plans).

Outpatient (OP): A patient who receives treatment in a physician's office or in the emergency room of a hospital. The term is used whenever a patient is *not* a bed patient in a hospital.

Partial disability: An illness or injury that prevents an insured person from performing one or more of the functions of his or her regular job.

Participating physician (Member physician): A doctor who has joined a group or enrolled with the insurance company and agreed to accept its contracts.

Permanent Disability (PD): An illness or injury that prevents an insured person from performing all the functions of his or her regular job.

Physician's profile: A compilation of each doctor's charges and the payments made to him through the years for each specific professional service rendered to a patient. As charges are increased, so are payments, and the profile is then updated through the use of computer data.

Policy term: The period for which an insurance policy provides coverage.

Pre-existing condition: A physical condition that existed before the insured's policy was issued. Some companies will not cover these conditions and others will pay only after a certain waiting period.

Premium: Payment made periodically to keep an insurance policy in force.

Prepayment: Medical insurance benefits paid for in advance, generally through monthly premiums.

Prior authorization: An administrative procedure whereby a doctor or dentist submits the treatment plan to the carrier before treatment is initiated. This is common in dental contracts, the Medicaid program, and the Medi-Cal program. Synonyms: *preauthorization, precertification, predetermination, pre-estimate of cost,* and *pretreatment estimate.*

Probationary period: A specified number of days after the date of the issuance of the policy during which coverage is not afforded for sickness.

Professional Standards Review Organization (PSRO): A group of physicians working with the government to review cases for hospital admission and discharge under government guidelines. Also known as *Peer Review.* (See Chapter 10, p. 255.)

Proof of loss: Contractual right of the carrier or service corporation to request verification of services rendered by the submission of claim forms, radiographs, dental study models, and/or other diagnostic material.

Proration: An adjustment of benefits paid because of a mistake in the amount of premiums paid or the existence of other insurance covering the same accident or disability.

Provider: Supplier, physician, or one providing service to the insured (patient).

Recurring clause: A provision in some health insurance policies which specifies a period of time during which the recurrence of a condition is considered a continuation of a prior period of disability or hospital confinement.

Reinstatement: The resumption of coverage under a policy that has lapsed.

Release of information: A form which must be signed by the patient before information may be given out to an insurance company, attorney, or other third party. Also known as an *authorization form* or *consent form.* (See Chapter 14, pp. 419–421.)

Renewal: Continuance of coverage under a policy beyond its original term by the acceptance of a premium for a new policy term.

Reserve: A sum set aside by an insurance company to guarantee the fulfillment of commitments for future claims.

Rider: A legal document that modifies the protection of a policy. It may either expand or decrease the payable benefits by adding or excluding certain conditions from the policy's coverage.

Risk: Any chance of loss.

Risk, impaired or substandard: An insurance applicant whose physical condition does not meet the standards for normal health.

Service benefit: An insurance benefit that fully pays the specific hospital or medical care services rendered.

Subscriber(S): One who belongs to a group plan. Synonyms: *enrollee, certificate holder, insured,* or *policyholder.*

Superbill: An itemized billing statement furnished to the patient, giving all pertinent information so that the patient may bill the insurance company directly. (See Figs. 6–5 and 6–6, pp. 146 and 147.)

Surgical schedule: A list of cash allowances which are payable for various types of surgery, with the maximum amounts based upon the severity of the operations.

Temporary Disability (TD): An illness or injury that temporarily prevents an insured person from performing the functions of his or her regular job.

Term: Period of time for which an insurance policy is issued.

Third party payer: An insurance carrier besides the doctor or patient who intervenes to pay hospital or medical bills. Also known as *Third party carrier.*

Time limit: The period of time in which a notice of claim or proof of loss must be filed.

Total disability: An illness or injury that prevents an insured person from continuously performing every duty pertaining to his or her occupation or from engaging in any other type of work for remuneration.

Treatment Authorization Request (TAR): A form used in asking authorization to render a specific service to a patient on the Medi-Cal program.

Unallocated benefit: A policy provision providing reimbursement up to a maximum amount for the costs of all extra miscellaneous hospital services, but not specifying how much will be paid for each type of service.

Usual, Customary, and Reasonable (UCR): Refers to the charges (fees) of a physician.

Waiting period (W/p): Time which must elapse before an indemnity is paid. Also known as *Excepted period*.

Waiver: An agreement attached to a policy which exempts from coverage certain disabilities or injuries that are normally covered by the policy.

Waiver of premium: A provision included in some policies which exempts the insured person from paying premiums if he or she is disabled during the life of the contract.

Written premium: A total amount of premiums obtained in a year from all policies issued by an insurance company.

MEDICAL AND DIAGNOSTIC TERMINOLOGY

If a lay term appears on a patient record, the correct medical term should be substituted when completing an insurance claim. Some physicians write Imp (impression) or Dx (diagnosis) on the patient's record. This usually will serve as the diagnosis when completing the claim. If the diagnosis is not on the chart, and there is any doubt at all, always attach a note to the insurance form for the doctor to see before he or she signs the form. If the patient has been in the hospital, look for a carbon copy of the hospital's admitting diagnosis or impression at the end of the doctor's report.

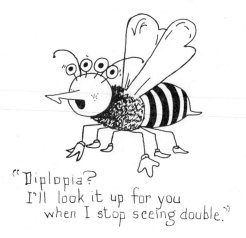

"Diplopia? I'll look it up for you when I stop seeing double."

Official American Hospital Association policy is that "abbreviations should be totally eliminated from the more vital sections of the record, such as final diagnosis, operative notes, discharge summaries, and descriptions of special procedures." Many physicians are not aware of this policy, and the final diagnosis may appear as an abbreviation on the patient record. Use your medical dictionary (most list abbreviations alphabetically with the unabbreviated words) and spell out the medical term on the insurance claim when listing the diagnosis.

An eponym (term including the name of a person) should not be used when a comparable anatomic term can be used in its place. (*Example:* "Graves' disease" is an eponym; the comparable anatomic term is "exophthalmic goiter.")

The following table of correct diagnostic, procedural, symptomatic, and treatment terms and their lay equivalents may be helpful to a person not well versed in medical terminology. Other terms commonly used to identify injuries are indicated in Figure 1–1 (regions of the abdomen) and Figures 9–4, 9–5, and 9–6 (pp. 225–228) in the chapter on Workers' Compensation. You should also be familiar with the various operational incisions (Fig. 1–2). If you would like a more thorough discussion of medical terminology, many good books are available. One is:

Chabner, Davi-Ellen: *The Language of Medicine*. Philadelphia, W.B. Saunders Company, 1976.

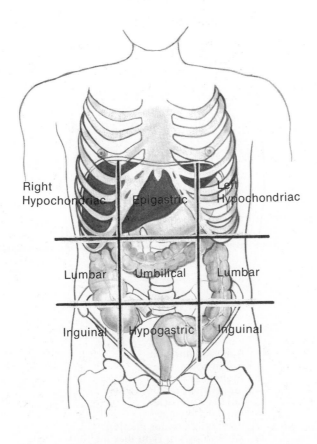

FIGURE 1–1

Regions of the abdomen. (From Anderson, P.D.: Clinical Anatomy and Physiology for Allied Health Sciences. Philadelphia, W.B. Saunders Company, 1976.)

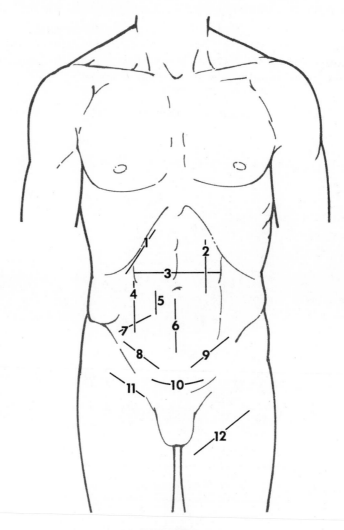

FIGURE 1–2

Operational incisions. Anterior (front) view.

1. subcostal incision
2. paramedian incision
3. transverse incision
4. upper right rectus incision
5. midrectus incision
6. midline incision
7. lower right rectus incision
8. McBurney's or right iliac incision
9. left iliac incision
10. suprapubic incision
11. hernia incision
12. femoral incision

TABLE 1–1. MEDICAL TERMINOLOGY

Lay Term	Medical Term	Pronunciation
Acute	Use the word acute when referring to a condition that runs a short but relatively severe course.	ah-KŪT
Allergy infection	Asthmatic bronchitis	az-MAT-ik-brong-KI-tis
Appetite loss	Anorexia	an″o-REK-se-ah
Athlete's foot	Pedal epidermophytosis; tinea pedis	PED-al ep″i-der″mō-fi-TŌ-sis; TIN-e-ah PED-is
Baldness	Alopecia	al″ō-PĒ-shē-ah
Bedsore	Decubitus ulcer	de-KŪ-bi-tus UL-ser
Belching	Eructation	ē-ruk-TĀ-shun
Blood poisoning	Septicemia	sep″ti-SĒ-mē-ah
Blood in stools	Melena	MEL-e-nah or me-LĒ-nah
Blood in urine	Hematuria	hēm″ah-TŪ-re-ah
Blue skin	Cyanosis	si″ah-NŌ-sis
Breathing, cessation of	Apnea	ap-NĒ-ah
Breathing, difficult	Dyspnea	DISP-nē-ah or disp-NĒ-ah
Breathing, normal	Eupnea	ūp-NĒ-ah
Breathing, rapid	Tachypnea	tak″ip-NĒ-ah
Breathing, slow	Bradypnea	brad″ip-NĒ-ah
Breathing, upright position only	Orthopnea	or″thop-NĒ-ah
Bruise or injury not involving sutures	Contusion; ecchymosis (sing), ecchymoses (pl); hematoma; extravasation	kon-TŪ-zhun; ek″i-MŌ-sis, ek″i-MŌ-sēz; hem″ah-TŌ-mah; eks-trav″ah-SĀ-shun
Bulging of eyes	Exophthalmos	ek″sof-THAL-mōs
Burning or cauterizing	Use the words "surgical removal of"	
Chafing	Intertrigo	in″ter-TRI-gō
Change of life	Menopause; climacteric	MEN-ō-pawz; kli″mak-TER-ik
Chest pain with EKG but not cardiac case	Intercostal neuritis or neurasthenia	in″ter-KOS-tal nu-RĪ-tis; nu″ras-THĒ-nē-ah
Chickenpox	Varicella; variola crystallina	var″i-SEL-ah; vah-RI-ō-lah kris″tah-LĪ-nah
Chronic	Use the word "recurrent"	
Cold	Coryza	ko-RĪ-zah
Cold with runny nose	Coryza with motor rhinitis	ri-NĪ-tis
Cold sore; fever blisters on lips	Herpes simplex	HER-pēz SIM-plex
Corn	Clavus	KLĀ-vus

Lay Term	Medical Terminology	Pronunciation
Cut	Laceration (give location, length, depth)	las″er-Ā-shun
Cutting into	Incision of	in-SIZH-un
Cutting out	Excision of	ek-SIZH-un
Dandruff	Seborrhea capitis	seb″o-RĒ-ah CAP-i-tis
Dim vision	Amblyopia	am″blē-Ō-pē-ah
Dizziness	Vertigo	VER-ti-go or ver-TI-go
Dog bite	One or more abrasions (give location)	ah-BRĀ-zhun
Double vision	Diplopia	di-PLŌ-pē-ah
Drooping eyelids	Ptosis	TŌ-sis
Ear discharge	Otorrhea	o″to-RĒ-ah
Ear procedure involving opening of ear	Myringotomy	mir″in-GOT-ō-mē
Earache	Acute otitis; otitis media; otalgia; neuralgic pain in ear (left or right)	ah-KŪT o-TĪ-tis; o-TĪ-tis MĒ-dia; o-TAL-jē-ah; nū-RAL-jik
Earwax removal	Cerumen syringed	se-ROO-men si-RINJD
Excessive eating	Polyphagia	pol″ē-FĀ-je-ah
Excessive thirst	Polydipsia	pol″ē-DIP-sē-ah
Eye exam if more than just check for eyeglasses	Refraction and eye examination	re-FRAK-shun
Fainting	Syncope	SIN-ko-pē
Fever blister	Lesion of herpes simplex	HER-pēz SIM-plex
Fit	Convulsion	kon-VUL-shun
Flat feet	Pes planus	pes PLA-nus
Flu	Influenza; la grippe	in″flu-EN-zah; lah GRIP
Freckle	Lentigo; ephelis	len-TI-go; e-FĒ-lis
Full of pus	Purulent	PU-roo-lent; PUR-u-lent
Gastrointestinal case that is not a duodenal ulcer	Gastroenteritis	gas″tro-en-ter-Ī-tis
Glands, swollen	Diffuse lymphadenitis	dif-FŪS lim-fad″e-NĪ-tis
Grippe; flu	Influenza; la grippe	in″flu-EN-zah; lah GRIP
Hangnail	Agnail	AG-nāl
Hayfever	Allergic rhinitis; rhinallergosis	ah-LER-jik ri̱-NĪ-tis; rin″al-er-GŌ-sis
Headache	Acute cephalalgia, cephalgia	ah-KŪT sef″ah-LAL-jē-ah; se-FAL-jē-ah
Heartburn	Pyrosis	pi̱-RŌ-sis

Lay Term	Medical Terminology	Pronunciation
Hives	Urticaria	ur″ti-KĀ-rē-ah
Humpback; hunchback	Kyphosis	ki-FŌ-sis
Injury	Trauma	TRAW-mah
Itching	Pruritus	proo-RĪ-tus
Jaundice	Icterus	IK-ter-us
Lockjaw	Tetanus	TET-ah-nus
Malnutrition, general ill health	Cachexia	kah-KEK-sē-ah
Measles	Rubeola	roo-BĒ-ō-lah
Measles, German	Rubella	roo-BEL-ah
Milk leg	Phlebitis	fle-BĪ-tis
Mole, moles	Nevus (sing), nevi (pl)	NĒ-vus, NĒ-vi̇
Mumps	Contagious parotitis	kon-TĀ-jus par″ō-TĪ-tis
Nosebleed	Epistaxis; rhinorrhagia	ep″i-STAK-sis; ri″nō-RĀ-jē-ah
Overweight	Exogenous obesity	eks-OJ-e-nus o-BĒS-i-tē
Piles	Hemorrhoids	HEM-o-roids
Pink eye	Acute contagious conjunctivitis	ah-KŪT kon-TĀ-jus kon-junk″ti-VĪ-tis
Pneumonia	If both lungs are involved, use bilateral pneumonitis	bi-LAT-er-al nu″mō-NĪ-tis
Poison ivy	Rhus toxicodendron sensitivity or dermatitis	rus tok″si-kō-DEN-dron sen″si-TIV-i-tē, der″mah-TĪ-tis
Postnasal drip	Catarrh	kah-TAHR
Pus	Purulent	PU-roo-lent, PUR-u-lent
Pus in urine	Pyuria	pi-Ū-rē-ah
Question of	Use "possible" or "probable"	
Residual inquiry(ies)	Sequela (sing), sequelae (pl)	se-KWE-lah, se-KWE-lē
Ringing in ears	Tinnitus	TIN-i-tus
Rule out (R/O)	Use "possible" or "probable"	
St. Vitus' dance	Chorea	kō-RĒ-ah
Scar	Cicatrix	sik-A-triks, SIK-ah-triks
Shingles	Herpes zoster	HER-pez ZOS-ter
Sleeping sickness	Encephalitis	en″sef-ah-LĪ-tis
Sore throat	Laryngitis; pharyngitis; tonsillitis; alpha hemolytic streptococcus (milder strep); beta hemolytic streptococcus (real strep throat); acute sore throat for any kind of sore throat unless it is strep	lar″in-JĪ-tis; far″in-JĪ-tis; ton″si-LĪ-tis; AL-fah hē″mō-LIT-ik strep″tō-KOK-us; BĀ-tah

Lay Term	Medical Term	Pronunciation
Speaking difficulty	Dysphonia	dis-FŌ-nē-ah
Squint	Strabismus	strah-BIZ-mus
Stiff neck; wryneck	Torticollis	tor″ti-KOL-is
Stomachache	Tonic abdominal spasm; gastritis; gastroenteritis	TON-ik ab-DOM-i-nal spazm; gas-TRĪ-tis; gas″trō-en-ter-Ī-tis
Stone, stones	Calculus (sing), calculi (pl)	KAL-kū-lus, KAL-kū-lī
Swallowing difficulty	Dysphagia	dis-FĀ-je-ah
Swayback	Lordosis	lor-DŌ-sis
Urination, excessive	Nocturia; polyuria	nok-TŪ-rē-ah; pol″ē-Ū-rē-ah
Urination, involuntary	Enuresis	en″ū-RĒ-sis
Urination, painful	Dysuria	dis-Ū-rē-ah
Urine, scanty	Oliguria	ol″i-GŪ-rē-ah
Vomiting of blood	Hematemesis	hem″ah-TEM-e-sis
Wart, warts	Verruca (sing), verrucae (pl)	ve-ROOH-kah, ve-ROO-sē
Water on the knee	Prepatellar bursitis	prē″pah-TEL-ar bur-SĪ-tis
Whooping cough	Pertussis	per-TUS-is

HANDLING INSURANCE CLAIMS

To maintain a harmonious patient-physician relationship, always be friendly and courteous when handling insurance claims. If the patient feels free to discuss personal financial problems at any time and is educated regarding the doctor's fees, collections can often be significantly improved and simplified. The value of maintaining careful records of all insurance matters cannot be overemphasized. The following handy hints will help you handle insurance claims properly.

First Visit: Patient Information Sheet

1. Obtain *complete* information on a new patient. Be *accurate*. There are two kinds of patient information sheets:
   a. A personalized record sheet developed by the physician (perhaps in conjunction with the assistant) for his or her own use. Examples of these forms can be seen on page 359 and throughout the Appendix.
   b. A form furnished the physician by a collection agency or a malpractice insurance company. An arbitration agreement is sometimes printed on this sheet. Arbitration is a legal method, provided for by statute in certain states, whereby patient and physician agree to resolve any controversy that may arise between them before an impartial panel. The advantages of arbitration are speed of settlement and reduction of expense. (See also Chapter 14.)

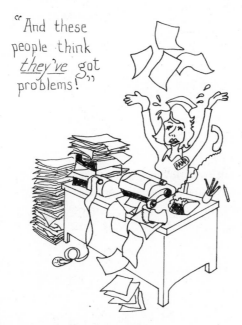

"And these people think *they've* got problems!"

2. The following facts should be recorded:
   a. Name: first, middle initial, and last.
   b. Address and telephone number.
   c. Business address, telephone number, and occupation.
   d. Date of birth. (This is now recorded on insurance forms as six digits, because many insurance forms are processed by computer. January 2, 1936, is shown as 01-02-36.)
   e. Person responsible for account or insured's name.
   f. Social Security number.
   g. Spouse's name and occupation.
   h. If patient is referred by another physician or by another patient, so indicate on the information sheet.
   i. Driver's license number.
   j. Close relative or friend (name, address, and telephone number).

3. Obtain the names and addresses of *all* insurance companies, and all policy numbers and group numbers. This is important because of the Coordination of Benefits clause (see p. 6) written into some health insurance policies.

4. Recheck insurance policy or group numbers every 6 months, since these numbers can change.

5. If the physician wishes to accept assignment, have the patient sign an "Information Release" and an "Assignment of Benefits" for each insurance company. Assignment is the transfer of one's right to collect an amount payable under an insurance contract. The assignment should be signed, dated, and preferably stamped or printed on the insurance form. If the assignment is an attachment to the insurance claim, obtain a 4-inch rubber stamp that reads "BENEFITS ASSIGNED" and stamp this in red on the front side of each form that leaves your office. Attachments to insurance forms may be lost after their arrival at the insurance company. Some assistants make two copies of the assignment, one for the insurance company and one for the doctor's office.

In reference to a Medicare patient, assignment means not only that the check will come to the physician but also that the physician will accept what Medicare will allow as a "reasonable charge." Of this charge, Medicare will pay 80 per cent and the patient will pay 20 per cent. (See Chapter 6.)

6. Date stamp *all* incoming insurance forms, whether brought in by the patient or received by mail. This will permit you to remind the patient when the form was received in the office, in the event that the patient's own records are incomplete.

Completing the Claim Form

1. File a claim form whenever you are asked to do so by the patient, even though you think there is no coverage, unless the patient accepts your tactful suggestion that he or she is not covered. An official rejection from the insurance company is the best answer to present to the patient.

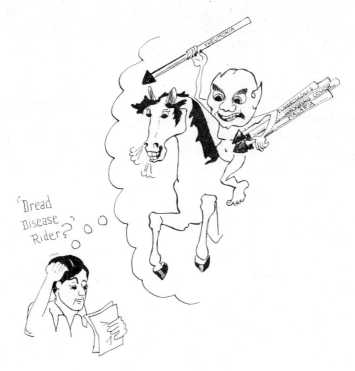

2. Use the Universal Form or Attending Physician's Statement as often as possible. The Universal Form is accepted by nearly all general insurance carriers as well as by Blue Cross, Blue Shield, and Medicare. Acceptance by Medicaid (Medi-Cal) and CHAMPUS is pending. (See Chapter 3.)

3. It is a good idea to answer all questions on an insurance form. If any are unanswerable, indicate as in item "b" below. Here are some good reasons why all blanks on insurance forms should be completed:

    a. Because of possible tampering.

    b. So that when the physician checks the form before signing it and sees that you have listed "DNA" or "DOES NOT APPLY," or "NA," "N/A" or "NOT APPLICABLE," or simply - - - - lines, he or she knows that you have gone over the form thoroughly and have not forgotten or overlooked anything.

    c. Because an insurance firm can sue a physician for incomplete records.

4. In the space marked "diagnosis," be very specific and complete. Some doctors write "IMP" (impression) or "DX" (diagnosis) on the chart. This usually suffices as an abbreviation for diagnosis. Never send in a diagnosis without the doctor's approval. Be certain the diagnosis agrees with the treatment. Use the words "possible" or "probable" instead of "rule out." Use correct medical terminology for listing the diagnosis (see pp. 10–16).

Recently, CMIT, SMRS, and ICDA coding has been developed for use on computerized billing and computerized insurance forms. Sometimes the code appears on the billing statement or claim form without terminology. This procedure is particularly useful when the physician does not wish to list the diagnosis on the claim. Three good reference books are:

International Classification of Diseases, Adapted (ICDA), Vol 2, alphabetical list, 8th ed. 1968. (Revision pending.) This can be ordered from the Superintendent of Documents, U.S. Government Printing Office, Washington, D.C. 20402, or from the American Hospital Association, 840 North Lake Shore Drive, Chicago, IL 60611.

Gordon, Burgess, M.D.: *Simplified Medical Records System* (SMRS), Publishing Sciences Group, Inc., 411 Massachusetts Avenue, Acton, MA 01720.

Current Medical Information and Terminology (CMIT), 4th ed. 1971. This can be purchased from the American Medical Association, 535 North Dearborn Street, Chicago, IL 60610.

5. Do not ditto dates for services performed.

6. To avoid confusion, it is best to list only one illness or injury and its treatment per form.

7. Office visits may be grouped if each visit resulted in the same fee. (*Example:* October 4–8, 1976 5 office visits, brief $5 ea $25.00.) However, if there is a difference in fee and several visits must be indicated on the claim, processing may be speeded up if the office visits are itemized and each charge is listed separately.

8. If more than one office visit is required per day, state times of day and justification for second visit, so that the claims clerk will know that separate procedures were done at different times and why they were performed.

9. Some insurance companies now write policies which include coverage for annual physicals. In these instances you may write "Annual physical examination" on the diagnosis portion of the form. However, if the patient comes into the office after a year's absence with a definite symptom (such as a gastrointestinal complaint or chronic headache), always ask the doctor for a specific diagnosis, even if a complete annual checkup was performed. In this way the examination may be covered, even if the patient's policy is not written to include an annual physical.

10. Itemize laboratory work separately from office calls, whether the physician is billing for work done in an outside laboratory or in his or her own laboratory.

11. When itemizing injections, state name of medication, amount of injection in cc's or gm's, and whether the injection was intramuscular (IM), intravenous (IV), subcutaneous (SC), intradermal (ID), or parenteral (parent).

12. X-rays must also be itemized separately, giving part of body filmed, number of views, and type of view: anteroposterior (AP), lateral (Lat), oblique (Obl), and so forth. If the procedure was complicated, it is a good idea to include a copy of the Radiology Report.

13. Hospital visits may be grouped if each visit resulted in the same fee. (*Example:* October 4–8, 1976   5 hospital visits, brief $10 ea $50.00.)

14. When listing a laceration, indicate length in centimeters, exact location, and whether the repair was simple, intermediate, or complex.

15. When listing a tumor, give type, number, category, size, and weight. If possible, attach a copy of the Pathology Report.

16. If a sterile surgical tray is used for office surgery, itemize and give a separate fee. The same procedure should be followed for cast materials, burn dressings, and the like.

17. For a treatment that cannot be found in the *Current Procedural Terminology* (CPT) or *Relative Value Studies* (RVS), send in a detailed report, giving the nature, extent, and need for the services. If possible, send a copy of the operative report from the hospital, the discharge summary, and any other pertinent medical reports. Be sure to use the proper RVS or CPT Code Number for unlisted services or procedures. (*Example:* Unlisted Allergy Testing Procedure 95199.) Usually the codes for unlisted services end in "99."

18. If your preprinted claim forms do not have the doctor's IRS number (also known as Employer I.D. number or Tax I.D. number) or Social Security number, you must type it in near the physician's name. Sometimes the physician's State License number or Fiscal Agent (Provider) number is also required on insurance claim forms. If the physician or supplier is employed by a Health Maintenance Organization (HMO), then he or she will be assigned an I.D. (Identifying) number.

Section 6109 of the Internal Revenue Code of 1954 requires that the IRS number be furnished. IRS Ruling 69-595, supplemented by 70-608, requires all insurance carriers to report certain payment information using Form 1099. Therefore, on certain checks that your physician receives, you will be required to type the Social Security number or the IRS number in the space immediately over the doctor's name on the face of the draft.

19. Have your physician sign the insurance claim form. There are some instances when a stamped signature is allowed, and this will be discussed in the following chapters. Always type the physician's name under the signature if the name is not preprinted. Make a red check mark where the physician should sign the claim. This will help the doctor locate the correct area, since every form has a different location for the signature.

20. To avoid confusion as to who in your office typed the insurance form, place your initials in the lower left hand corner.

21. Maintain a separate file for insurance claim copies. Do not file insurance form copy in the patient's medical chart.

Submitting and Tracing the Claim

1. Group together all the patients who have the same type of insurance and bill them all at one time. This cuts down errors and makes the job of completing the forms easier.

2. Do not bill one fee to the insurance company and a different fee to the patient.

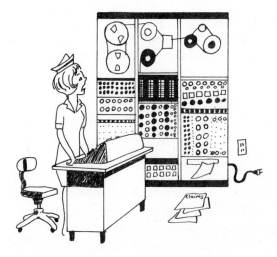

" I give up — everything I tell
you anymore just goes in one
gear and out the other! "

3. Establish a tracing file to keep track of the status of each case that has been billed.

4. Post the insurance payments on the patient's ledger card. This is a control factor for the doctor, patient, and accountant. Show the date billed, name of insurance company, amount, and name of the family member.

5. Usually claims are submitted every 30 days (monthly) after the illness or injury, but this time limit can vary with each type of insurance from 30 days to a year and a half.

For further information on following up on a claim, see Chapter 13.

Keeping up to Date

1. Make up a folder or binder of pertinent insurance information. Obtain information booklets and manuals from the local offices of the various insurance companies. Get sample copies of all the forms required for the insurance plans most used in your doctor's office.

2. Keep well informed by reading your Medicaid (Medi-Cal), Medicare, CHAMPUS, and local medical society bulletins. Maintain a chronological file on each of these bulletins for easy reference, always keeping the latest bulletin on top. This will also help you to keep this *Handbook* up to date.

3. Attend any workshops offered in your area on insurance in medical practice, since changes occur from day to day and month to month. The American Association of Medical Assistants has chapters in many states that feature educational workshops and lectures during the year. Their central headquarters is located at One East Wacker Drive, Chicago, IL 60601.

Reasons Why Claims are Rejected

1. Diagnosis is not in standard nomenclature.
2. Diagnosis is missing or incomplete.
3. Diagnosis does not correspond with the treatment rendered by the doctor.
4. Reasons for multiple visits made in one day are not stated on the claim.
5. Dates are incorrect. Make certain all dates are listed and are accurate.
6. Fee column is left blank. Be certain that the fee column is filled in if you are required to put in the doctor's fee. Total the charges.
7. Charges are not itemized.
8. The patient's insurance number is incorrect or is transposed (especially in Medicare and Medicaid [Medi-Cal] cases).
9. The patient has not answered all questions on his or her portion of the form.
10. Attachments or labels are missing on Medicaid (Medi-Cal) and Medi-Medi claims.

ABSTRACTING FROM MEDICAL RECORDS

You may be asked to abstract technical information from patient records in either of two situations:
1. When you file a health insurance claim after professional services are rendered.
2. When a patient applies for life, mortgage, or health insurance for the first time. In this instance, the insurance company may require a physical examination, or information may be requested from the patient's private physician.

Abstracting for insurance claims will be discussed in detail in subsequent chapters. In the following paragraphs, abstracting medical information for insurance applications is briefly considered.

On some application forms the release of medical information signed by the patient is printed right on the form (see Fig. 1–3). The insurance company will send a request to the attending physician along with a check. The amount of the check may vary, depending on how much information is requested. If the check is not included, the physician should request a fee based on the length of the report before sending in the completed report form. You must have the fee before completion of the form or sometimes you will not receive it.

If you are asked to abstract medical information from the patient's record, be extremely accurate. Do not guess at abbreviations on the chart. Give only the information requested. If the form has questions about high blood pressure (more than 140/90) or about kidney infection or heart problems, you can prevent a patient from obtaining life, health, or mortgage insurance if your answers are derogatory. If the urine shows albumin or sugar, a person can also be denied insurance. If a patient has had pulmonary tuberculosis, ask the doctor if there is a euphemism for it. A euphemism is a word or phrase substituted for one considered offensively explicit (*Example:* "remains" for "corpse").

Sometimes a narrative report dictated by the physician is preferable to filling in the form, especially if there are long columns to check and no space for comments. It may even be necessary to attach a copy of an operative report, pathology report, laboratory report, or x-ray report.

PHYSICIAN'S EXAMINATION REPORT

Height (In Shoes) ft.　in.	Weight (Clothed) lbs.	Males Only:			Details of "Yes" answers. (Identify item.)
		Chest (Full Inspiration) in.	Chest (Forced Expiration) in.	Abdomen, at Umbilicus in.	

Did you weigh? ☐ Yes ☐ No　　Did you measure? ☐ Yes ☐ No
Is appearance unhealthy or older than stated age?　☐ Yes ☐ No

Blood Pressure (Record ALL readings)

Systolic

Diastolic { 4th phase
5th phase

Pulse:　　　　　　　At Rest　　After Exercise　　3 Minutes Later

Rate

Irregularities per minute

Heart: Is there any:
　Enlargement　☐ Yes　☐ No　　Dyspnea　☐ Yes　☐ No
　Murmur(s)　　☐ Yes　☐ No　　Edema　　☐ Yes　☐ No
　　　(describe below — if more than one, describe separately)

Location

	Locate:
Constant ☐ ☐	apex by **X**
Inconstant ☐ ☐	
Transmitted ☐ ☐	area of murmur
Localized ☐ ☐	by outline ☐
Systolic ☐ ☐	
Presystolic ☐ ☐	point of greatest
Diastolic ☐ ☐	intensity by **O**
Soft (Gr. 1–2) ☐ ☐	
Mod. (Gr. 3–4) ☐ ☐	transmission by →
Loud (Gr. 5–6) ☐ ☐	

For comments and your impression:

After exercise:
　Increased　☐ ☐
　Absent　　☐ ☐
　Unchanged ☐ ☐
　Decreased ☐ ☐

Is there on examination any abnormality of the following:
(Circle applicable items and give details.)　　　　　　　　　　　Yes　No

(a) Eyes, ears, nose, mouth, pharynx? .... ☐ ☐
　　(If vision or hearing markedly impaired, indicate degree and correction.)
(b) Skin (incl. scars), lymph nodes, varicose veins or peripheral arteries? ...... ☐ ☐
(c) Nervous system (include reflexes, gait, paralysis)? .... ☐ ☐
(d) Respiratory system? .... ☐ ☐
(e) Abdomen (include scars)? .... ☐ ☐
(f) Genitourinary system (include prostate)? .... ☐ ☐
(g) Endocrine system (include thyroid and breasts)? .... ☐ ☐
(h) Musculoskeletal system (include spine, joints, amputations, deformities)? ☐ ☐
(i) Are there any hernias? ☐ Yes ☐ No　(j) Any hemorrhoids? .... ☐ ☐
Are you aware of additional medical history? .... ☐ ☐
　　　(A confidential report may be sent to the Medical Director)

*ANALYSIS OF URINE:

Specific Gravity	Albumin	Sugar
....	Yes ☐ No ☐	Yes ☐ No ☐

Are you sure specimen is authentic?　　　　　Yes ☐　　No ☐

Are you forwarding this specimen
　　　to the Home Office?　　　　　　　　Yes ☐　　No ☐

*With a life insurance application of $50,000 or more, health application of $1,000 or more, age 60 or over, or with history or finding of albumm or sugar, history of any urinary tract disease, or blood pressure 140/90 or over, or family history of diabetes, forward specimen to the Home Office.

Date: ....　Time: ....M.　City: ....　　　State: ....

Signature of Medical Examiner: ....M.D.

Form MD (70)a back

FIGURE 1–3

Sample of a life insurance claim form with the check to the physician included.

PART II of Application to the MASSACHUSETTS INDEMNITY AND LIFE INSURANCE COMPANY

PROPOSED INSURED OR ANNUITANT: ....

Date of Birth ....

| Mo. | Day | Year |

1. a. Name and address of your personal physician? ....
   (If none, so state)

   b. Date and reason last consulted? ....

   c. What treatment was given or medication prescribed? ....

2. Have you ever been treated for or ever had any known indication of: Yes   No
   a. Disorder of eyes, ears, nose, or throat?   ☐   ☐

   b. Dizziness, fainting, convulsions, recurrent headache, speech defect, paralysis or stroke, mental or nervous disorder?   ☐   ☐

   c. Shortness of breath, persistent hoarseness or cough, blood spitting, bronchitis, pleurisy, asthma, emphysema, tuberculosis or chronic respiratory disorder?   ☐   ☐

   d. Chest pain, palpitation, high blood pressure, rheumatic fever, heart murmur, heart attack or other disorder of the heart or blood vessels?   ☐   ☐

   e. Jaundice, intestinal bleeding, ulcer, hernia, appendicitis, colitis, diverticulitis, hemorrhoids, recurrent indigestion, or other disorder of the stomach, intestines, liver or gallbladder?   ☐   ☐

   f. Sugar, albumin, blood or pus in urine, venereal disease, stone or other disorder of kidney, bladder, prostate or reproductive organs?   ☐   ☐

   g. Diabetes, thyroid or other endocrine disorders?   ☐   ☐

   h. Neuritis, sciatica, rheumatism, arthritis, gout, or disorder of the muscles or bones, including the spine, back, or joints?   ☐   ☐

   i. Deformity, lameness or amputation?   ☐   ☐

   j. Disorder of skin, lymph glands, cyst, tumor or cancer?   ☐   ☐

   k. Allergies, anemia or other disorder of the blood?   ☐   ☐

   l. Excessive use of alcohol, tobacco, sedatives, or any habit-forming drugs?   ☐   ☐

3. Are you now under observation or taking treatment?   ☐   ☐

4. Have you had any change in weight in the past year?   ☐   ☐

5. *Other than above,* have you within the past 5 years:
   a. Had any mental or physical disorder not listed above?   ☐   ☐
   b. Had a checkup, consultation, illness, injury, surgery?   ☐   ☐
   c. Been a patient in a hospital, clinic, sanatorium, or other medical facility?   ☐   ☐
   d. Had electrocardiogram, X-ray, blood sugar, basal metabolism, other diagnostic test?   ☐   ☐
   e. Been advised to have any diagnostic test, hospitalization, or surgery which was not completed?   ☐   ☐

6. Have you ever had military service deferment, rejection or discharge because of a physical or mental condition?   ☐   ☐

7. Have you ever requested or received a pension, benefits, or payment because of an injury, sickness or disability?   ☐   ☐

8. Family History: Tuberculosis, diabetes, cancer, high blood pressure, heart or kidney disease, mental illness or suicide?   ☐   ☐

DETAILS of "Yes" answers. (IDENTIFY QUESTION NUMBER, CIRCLE APPLICABLE ITEMS: Include diagnoses, dates, duration and names and addresses of all attending physicians and medical facilities.)

	Age if Living?	Cause of Death?	Age at Death?
Father			
Mother			
Brothers and Sisters			
No. Living			
No. Dead			

(For non-medical cases only)

Height ....   Weight................

9. Females only: Yes   No

   a. Have you ever had any disorder of menstruation, pregnancy or of the female organs or breasts?   ☐   ☐

   b. To the best of your knowledge and belief are you now pregnant?   ☐   ☐

I HEREBY DECLARE that, to the best of my knowledge and belief, the statements and answers in Part II of this Application are full, complete, and true. These statements and answers are to be considered as the basis for any insurance written hereon.

Signed at: (City & State)...

Dated: ...., 19 ....

X

Signature of Witness ....

Signature of PROPOSED INSURED

Form MD (70)a

FIGURE 1–3 *(Continued)*

Place a "please read" note on the form and have the physician check over it entirely before it is signed and mailed, to make sure that the information is accurate and properly stated.

An insurance company may ask a copy service to come to your office to photocopy the patient's record. This is usually done at your convenience and an appointment should be made. Charge accordingly and quote the fee at the time of the telephone request. Remind the insurance company that you must have a Release of Medical Information form signed by the patient.

1. A person may obtain health insurance by what two types of insurance policies or contracts?_____

2. If your doctor is accepting assignment and you are attaching this to an insurance claim, what should appear on the insurance form?_____

_____

3. Name three reasons why all blanks on an insurance form should be completed.

  a._____

  b._____

  c._____

4. Match the following medical and diagnostic terms with the correct definitions. Write letters on blanks.

a bruise	_____	a. pertussis
		b. epistaxis
stone	_____	c. otitis
		d. cachexia
mole	_____	e. calculus
		f. nevus
nosebleed	_____	g. epigastrium
		h. alopecia
inflammation of ear	_____	i. ecchymosis
		j. anorexia
painful urination	_____	k. dysuria
		l. verruca
general ill health	_____	m. hypogastrium
		n. purulent
wart	_____	o. cephalgia
		p. subcostal incision
over the stomach	_____	
loss of appetite	_____	
incision below ribs	_____	
headache	_____	
pus	_____	
whooping cough	_____	
baldness	_____	

5. What is a euphemism?_____

6. If an insurance company wishes to photocopy a patient's chart, what important document must you have before it can be copied?_____

_____

7. Match the insurance terms in the first column with the definitions in the second column. Write letters on blanks.

adjuster   _____

assignment   _____

carrier   _____

coordination of benefits _____

deductible   _____

exclusions   _____

indemnity   _____

inpatient   _____

permanent disability   _____

premium   _____

subscriber   _____

time limit   _____

waiting period   _____

a. An insurance company takes into account benefits payable by another carrier in determining its own liability

b. Illness or injury that prevents an insured person from performing all functions of his or her regular job

c. Benefits paid by an insurance company to an insured person.

d. Transfer of one's right to collect an amount payable under an insurance contract

e. Time which must elapse before an indemnity is paid

f. Acts for insurance company or insured in settlement of claims

g. Periodic payment to keep insurance policy in force

h. Amount insured person must pay before policy will pay

i. Period of time in which a claim must be filed

j. Certain illnesses or injuries listed in a policy that the insurance company will not cover

k. A person who is a bed patient in a hospital

l. Insurance company that carries the insurance

m. One who belongs to a group plan

Notes:

2
Coding for Professional Services

BEHAVIORAL

OBJECTIVES The Assistant should be able to:

1. Understand the purpose of coding for professional services.
2. Explain the difference between RVS and CPT code books.
3. State the history of RVS.
4. Recognize which states utilize these code systems.
5. Understand how an RVS unit is ascertained.
6. Know basic abbreviations in the code books.
7. Learn the importance and usage of modifiers in coding.
8. Work out conversion factors mathematically for the physician's office if RVS is used in the state.
9. Code after completion of the 29 coding problems.
10. Know where to obtain an RVS or CPT code book.

CURRENT PROCEDURAL TERMINOLOGY (CPT)

Current Procedural Terminology is a dictionary of terms and codes for diagnostic and therapeutic procedures which omits the concept of "value" of the services and gives value only in the sense of reporting to the patient and/or insurance carrier. This code book is published by the American Medical Association. The second edition was published in 1970 and subsequently revised in 1973 and 1977. The current edition of CPT features two-digit numerical modifiers. Additional new code numbers in the 1977 CPT are shown with a (·) in front of the five digit code numbers.

RELATIVE VALUE STUDIES (RVS)

In 1956 the California Medical Association's Committee on Fees published the first edition of the California Relative Value Studies (CRVS). It was subsequently revised and published again in 1957, 1960, 1964, 1969, and 1974. It has become a very sophisticated system for the billing and coding of professional services. Many states have also seen the successful use of CRVS and adopted the same method of coding for professional services. Some of the specialty associations, such as the American Urological Association in Baltimore, Maryland, have published manuals for use by particular specialties. *Terminology and Relative Values of Urological Procedures* was published originally in 1963, and revised in 1968, 1971. and 1974.

Insurance companies throughout the United States use these codes to determine services rendered and appropriate payment for these services. *Since many policies actually have written into their contracts to pay on a specific edition of RVS at a certain unit value, it is important not to discard the old editions of RVS in case of need for future reference.*

The coding system used in RVS is a five-digit system with two-digit modifiers. The RVS corresponds to and does not conflict with CPT codes. However, CPT may not include all of the RVS numbers and might have numbers not included in RVS.

WHO USES RVS AND CPT?*

The following states use the California Relative Value Studies (CRVS):

Arizona	New Hampshire
Arkansas	New Jersey
California	New Mexico
Delaware	Oklahoma
Florida	Oregon
Georgia	Tennessee
Idaho	Vermont
Louisiana	Virginia
Maine	Washington
Maryland	

The following states have adopted RVS and as of this writing are using this code system in their state. Addresses for obtaining their code books are found on pages 49 and 50.

Alabama	Montana
Colorado	Nebraska
District of Columbia	North Dakota
Hawaii	South Dakota
Illinois	Utah
Michigan	Wyoming
Minnesota	

The following states use either the second or third edition of the Current Procedural Terminology (CPT) code book and in some instances also RVS:

Alabama	Colorado
Arizona	Delaware
California	District of Columbia

---

*In the latter part of 1975 the federal government filed a suit against the American Academy of Anesthesiologists, charging that its RVS restricts fees and is therefore illegal. Because of this the development and publication of a Relative Value Studies is being deferred in many states pending resolution of the present federal litigation challenging the legality of an RVS Guide.

Illinois	North Dakota
Kansas	Utah†
Minnesota	Wyoming
North Carolina	

At the present time (1976) these states are not using any code system:

Alaska	Nevada
Connecticut	Ohio
Indiana	Pennsylvania
Iowa	Puerto Rico
Kentucky	Rhode Island
Massachusetts	South Carolina
Mississippi	Texas
Missouri	West Virginia
New York	Wisconsin

PURPOSE OF RVS

The purposes of RVS are to identify services rendered by physicians, to assist doctors in determining their fees, and to help insurance carriers decide what they should pay. The code books are updated and revised about every 5 years. Revision and addition of new procedures is required by research and continually advancing technology. Without revision doctors would tend to use a single procedure number and procedure description for several services instead of for just one service. This constant revision helps physicians to receive payment on a more realistic basis. The RVS is not a fee schedule or a policing mechanism. The main difference in the two coding books is that RVS incorporates unit values for each procedure listed while CPT does not give any unit value in the entire book. However, RVS does not reflect either an individual doctor's fee or the fee of a particular locale. The RVS unit value reflects the average or common practice of physicians and the relativity of fees.

HOW THE RVS UNIT VALUE IS ASCERTAINED

The RVS unit is ascertained, after taking a poll of physicians in the state, by utilizing three sets of figures. The first is called the *mean fee*, which is the average fee or what might be called the arithmetic average. The second is called the *median fee* and is the fee charged by 50 per cent or more of the doctors submitting such charges. The third, or *modal fee*, is the fee most commonly charged by doctors in the state. These figures are then averaged and converted into a unit value. The "unit value" is not given in dollars and cents. However, there is a method, demonstrated in Table 2–1 (p. 33), which shows how the assistant can convert the unit value into a dollar and cents figure for the physician.

---

†Based on CPT, with additions as needed.

HOW TO USE THE RVS CODE BOOKS PROPERLY

These code books are divided into sections and subsections. The five main sections are: Medicine (M), Anesthesia (A), Surgery (S), Radiology (R), and Pathology (P). The subsections are divided according to anatomy and specialties. In order to use the code books properly and effectively, be sure to observe the following guidelines:

1. Read the "ground rules" (general information and instructions) in each section of the book.
2. Read the Special Services and Billing Procedures in each main section.
3. Use the index at the end of the book to find a specific item.
4. Use the descriptor as given for each procedure in the book and be careful of transposing the code numbers.
5. Always use the RVS two-digit modifiers whenever they are required, since these can either increase or decrease the physician's fee.

Modifiers

Five important reasons for modifiers are:

1. They eliminate the need for a lengthy report.
2. They give a more accurate description of services rendered.
3. They increase or decrease the fee.
4. The physician's profile is not reduced (see Chapter 1, p. 8).
5. They may indicate a component of service or adjunctive service.

Abbreviations

Following are common abbreviations and symbols used in the RVS code books:

A	Anesthesia Section	S	Surgery Section
BR	By Report	Sv	Service (See Ground Rules in each section)
M	Medicine Section		
P	Pathology Section	*	See Surgery Ground Rules in RVS
PC	Professional Component	☆	Injection procedure is included in radiographic procedure (RVS)
R	Radiology		
RNE	Relativity Not Established	△	New number in 1974 CRVS edition
RVS	Relative Value Studies		

Additional abbreviations for the Pathology Section may be found on pp. 37–39 in this chapter.

RVS Conversion Factors

Two reasons why unit values and conversion factors are important are:

1. To find out the value of a procedure that you are not used to billing in your office.

2. To look up a procedure with the same unit value for which you know the charge and charge the same amount. Remember, however, that this procedure must be in the same section.

If you wish to ascertain the conversion factor for each section of the RVS, you can do so by taking 9 or 10 procedures from a given section, listing your usual fees for each procedure, and then taking the RVS unit value and dividing it into the physician's usual fee (see Table 2–1). Total up the conversion factor column and then divide by the number of procedures to find out the middle of the range (the *median*). You may then round this figure out. The conversion factor can also help check the relativity of present fees.

Remember: Do not use the same conversion factor in all sections. Each section of the RVS must have its own conversion factor. Do not use the same conversion factors you used with the previous editions of the RVS.

TABLE 2–1. DETERMINATION OF CONVERSION FACTOR FOR 1974 CRVS MEDICINE SECTION

RVS Code No.	Procedure	Usual Fee*	RVS Unit	Conversion Factor
90050	Limited office visit	$ 7.00	5.2	$ 1.35
90000	New patient, brief office visit	8.00	5.9	1.36
90352	Skilled nursing care facility visit	9.00	6.5	1.38
90040	Brief office visit	5.00	3.5	1.43
90250	Limited hospital visit	7.50	5.2	1.44†
90605	Consultation, intermediate	20.00	13.0	1.54
90060	Intermediate office visit	10.00	6.5	1.54
93000	Electrocardiogram	12.50	8.0	1.56
90240	Brief hospital visit	6.50	3.9	1.67
				$13.27

*Dollar amounts shown are wholly fictitious and do not reflect actual data. Procedures and values are for illustrative purposes only.

†The value in the middle of the range (the median) is $1.44†. The sum of these values ($13.27) divided by the number of values (9) is $1.47 (the arithmetic mean). The physician may elect to use the median ($1.44) or the mean ($1.47), or to round out the amount to the nearest whole, such as $1.45 or $1.50.

To apply the conversion factor that you have just established to another procedure in the Medicine Section, multiply the conversion factor by the appropriate Unit Value listed in the RVS manual.

COMPREHENSIVE LISTING OF RVS MODIFIER CODES

Listed values for most procedures may be modified under certain circumstances, as listed below. The modifying circumstance should be identified by the addition of the appropriate "modifier code number" (including the hyphen) after the usual five-digit procedure code number.

Modifier Code	Explanation
-21	Test of services performed on hospital inpatients in the hospital laboratory should be identified by adding this procedure.
-22	*Unusual services:* When the services provided are greater than those usually required for the listed procedure.
-23	Used when a procedure which usually requires either no anesthesia or local anesthesia but because of unusual circumstances must be done under general anesthesia.
-24	When a service is performed by a licensed physician assistant or person other than a physician under direct supervision of a physician, but the physician renders the charge for this service, a lesser charge may be warranted.
-26	*Professional component (PC):* Under certain circumstances, the physician may wish to submit a charge for the professional component of a procedure and not for the technical component. The professional component comprises *only the professional services performed by the physician* during radiologic, laboratory, and other diagnostic procedures. These services include examination of the patient, supervision of patient examinations by other health personnel, interpretation of the results of such examinations, and consultation with referring physicians.
-27	*Technical component (TC):* Under other circumstances, a charge may be made for the technical component alone. The technical component comprises charges billed directly by the hospital, clinic, or laboratory for personnel, supplies, and the like.
-28	Debridement and/or decontamination are considered additional unit values only when appreciable amounts of devitalized or contaminated tissue are removed, as in osteomyelitis complicated by decubitus ulcer formation. Using this modifier increases the value of the procedure by 10 per cent.
-29	Used when determination of refractive state was *not* performed in the course of a diagnostic ophthalmologic examination.
-30	Anesthesia services for normal, uncomplicated anesthesia.
-32	Anesthesia procedures with a basic value of 3.0 units which become complicated by prone or difficult lateral positions, by surgical field avoidance, or by medical necessity may warrant an additional charge.
-33	Anesthesia complicated by total body hypothermia (low body temperature) above 30°C.
-35	Anesthesia complicated by extracorporeal circulation (heart pump oxygenator [bypass] or pump assist), with or without hypothermia.
-37	*Anesthesia risk:* When a nonemergency patient is an anesthetic risk because he has an incapacitating systemic disease that is a constant threat to life during the

Modifier Code	Explanation
	administration of anesthesia, an additional charge may be warranted.
-38	Anesthesia for emergency surgery on a patient with systemic disease sufficiently severe to compromise the patient's status may warrant an additional charge.
-39	Anesthesia for emergency surgery on a patient who· is near death, or who has an incapacitating systemic disease that is a constant threat to life, may warrant an additional charge.
-47	Anesthesia by surgeon.
-48	When the anesthesiologist is supervising the services of a nurse anesthetist and is involved in medical direction of the patient, including pre- and postoperative evaluation and care, but is not personally administering the anesthetic agent, he is reimbursed for the basic value of the procedure plus 1 unit per hour or part of an hour, as long as the patient is under anesthesia. The anesthesiologist must remain within sight and sound of the operating rooms under his medical direction and must extend medical direction to no more than two rooms simultaneously. He may not administer anesthesia while performing this supervisory function.
-49	*Multiple anesthesia modifiers:* Two or more modifiers may be necessary to identify the anesthesia procedure. In these instances, additional charges may be warranted. See -33 and -37.
-50	*Bilateral (secondary) procedure:* When patient care is complicated by the performance during the same operative session of two or more procedures, identify and value the first or major procedure as listed under the appropriate modifier. Then identify the secondary procedure by adding this modifier (-50) to the usual procedure number and value at 50 per cent of the listed value unless otherwise indicated. *Example:* total hysterectomy and reimplantation of ureter.
-51	*Multiple procedures:* When more than two procedures add significant time and/or complexity, and when each procedure is clearly identified and defined, the following values prevail: 100 per cent for the first or major procedure 50 per cent for the second procedure 25 per cent for the third procedure 10 per cent for the fourth procedure 5 per cent for the fifth procedure The second and each subsequent procedure should be identified by adding this modifier (-51) and valued at the appropriate percentage of its listed value. A report outlining each procedure and the clinical indications for it may be required.
-52	*Reduced values:* Used when the listed value for a procedure is reduced or eliminated because of "ground rules" (see p. 31) or common practice, or at the physician's discretion.
-53	*Primary emergency services:* When the surgical procedure is carried out by a physician who will not be providing the follow-up care, the value is 70 per cent of the listed value.

Modifier Code	Explanation
-54	*Surgical procedure only:* Used when one physician performs the surgical procedure itself and another provides the follow-up care.
-55	*Follow-up care only:* Used when one physician provides the follow-up care only and another has performed the surgery.
-58	*Asterisk (*) procedure:* When the asterisk procedure (e.g., *10000) is carried out at the time of the initial office visit, identify by adding this modifier (-58) to the usual procedure number and, instead of the usual initial visit, add an additional fee onto the surgical fee.
-62	*Two surgeons:* Used when the skills of two surgeons from different specialties may be required in the management of a specific surgical problem. The total value may be increased by 25 per cent in place of the assistant surgeon's charge. *Example:* lumbar laminectomy performed by a neurosurgeon and an orthopedic surgeon.
-64	*Cosurgeons:* When two surgeons with similar skills function simultaneously as primary surgeons performing distinct parts of a total surgical service. *Example:* complex cardiac surgical procedures.
-66	*Surgical team:* Used when highly complex procedures requiring the concurrent services of several physicians, often of different specialties, plus other highly skilled, specially trained personnel and various types of complex equipment, are carried out under the "surgical team" concept, with a single, global fee for the total service. *Example:* kidney transplant, requiring use of a vascular surgeon, urologist, anesthesiologist, nephrologist, and pathologist.
-68	*Complications:* Used when the surgical fee includes postoperative care during the listed follow-up period, but some complications requiring unusual additional services during the follow-up period may warrant additional charges on a fee-for-service basis. *Example:* appendectomy complicated by postoperative infection.
-75	Services rendered by more than one physician.
-76	Repeat procedure by same physician.
-77	Repeat procedure by another physician.
-80	*Assistant surgeon:* Valued at 20 per cent of the listed value of the surgical procedure(s).
-81	*Minimum assistant surgeon allowance:* Lesser value than -80 modifier.
-90	*Reference (outside) laboratory:* Used when lab procedures are performed by other than the billing physician.
-99	*Multiple modifiers:* Used when more than one modifier is applicable to a single procedure.

1974 CRVS LABORATORY ABBREVIATIONS

Frequently the physician orders a laboratory test, such as a complete blood count (CBC), by abbreviation only. The following list will help the assistant to locate the correct code number when only the abbreviation is given.

CODE NUMBER	ABBREVIATION	DEFINITION
85220	AcG	factor V (AcG or pro-accelerin); a factor in coagulation that converts prothrombin to thrombin
82024	ACTH	adrenocorticotrophic hormone
87015	AFB	acid-fast bacilli
82942	A/G ratio	albumin-globulin ratio
83485	AHB	alpha hydroxy butyric
85240	AHG	antihemophilic globulin; antihemolytic globulin (factor)
82135	ALA	aminolevulinic acid
82030	AMP	adenosine monophosphate
83033	APT test	aluminum precipitated toxoid test
86283	ATP	adenosine triphosphate
82293	BSP	Bromsulfonphthalein (Bromsulphalein; sodium sulfobromophthalein) test
84520	BUN	blood urea nitrogen
85022	CBC	complete blood count
88000	CNS	central nervous system
82375	CO	carbon monoxide
82531	CPB	competitive protein binding; plasma
82550	CPK	creatine phosphokinase
89051	CSF	cerebrospinal fluid
83053	D hemoglobin	Hemoglobin fractionation by electrophoresis for hemoglobin D
83596	D/A/E ratio	A/G ratio (albumin/globulin ratio)
82996	DAP	Gravindex and DAP (direct agglutination pregnancy)
83018	DEAE	diethylaminoethanol
82651	DHT	dihydrotestosterone
86225	DNA	deoxyribonucleic acid
86592	DRT	test for syphilis
85392	EACA	EACA control (epsilon-aminocaproic acid is a fibrinolysin)
82662	EMIT	enzyme immunoassay technique for drugs
86235	ENA	extractable nuclear antigen
85650	esr, ESR	erythrocyte sedimentation rate (sed rate)
85362	FDP	fibrin degradation products
82750	FIGLU	formiminoglutamic acid
82755	FRAT	free radical assay technique for drugs
83000	FSH	follicle stimulating hormone
85362	FSP	fibrin degradation (split) products
86650	FTA	fluorescent-absorbed treponema antibodies
82784	GG, Gamma G – A,D, G,M nephelometric	Gammaglobulin (immunoglobulin fractionation by electrophoresis)
82785	GG, Gamma G E, RIA	Immunization E fractionation by radioimmunoassay
86335	Gc, Gm, Inv immunoglobulin typing	Immunoglobulin typing
82980	GGT	gamma-glutamyl transpeptidase
82486, 82674	GLC	gas liquid chromatography

CODE NUMBER	ABBREVIATION	DEFINITION
83008	GMP	guanosine monophosphate
82955	G6PD	glucose-6-phosphate dehydrogenase
86285	HAA	hepatitis-associated agent (antigen)
86280	HAI	hemagglutination inhibition tests
83485	HBD	hydroxybutyrate dehydrogenase
85014	HCT	hematocrit
83020	hemoglobin, electro-phoresis (includes A_2, S, C, etc.)	letters of the alphabet used for different types or factors of hemoglobins
85050	Hgb	hemoglobin, qualitative
83003	HGH	human growth hormone
86280	HI	hemagglutination inhibition
83497	HIAA	hydroxyindoleacetic acid (urine), 25-hour specimen
86597	HLA	tissue typing
83632	HPL	human placental lactogen
83150	HVA	homovanillic acid
83002	ICSH	interstitial cell stimulating hormone
86255	IFA	intrinsic factor, antibody (fluorescent screen)
86329	IgA, IgG, IgM, IgE	immunoglobulins; quantitative by gel diffusion
83576	INH	isonicotinic acid hydrazide
83670	LAP	leucine aminopeptidase
84445	LATS	long-acting thyroid stimulating hormone
83615	LDH	lactic dehydrogenase
85545	LE Prep	lupus erythematosus cell preparation
86006, 86225, 85545	L.E. factor	antinuclear antibody
83002	LH	luteinizing hormone
83728	LSD	lysergic acid diethylamide
83661	L/S ratio	lecithin-sphingomyelin ratio
86171	MG (streptococcus)	antibody titer
87186	MIC	minimum inhibitory concentration
85550	NBT	nitro-blue tetrazolium test
83920	OCT	ornithine carbamyl transferase
82134	PAH	para-aminohippuric acid
83533	PBI	protein-bound iodine
82801	pCO_2	arterial carbon dioxide pressure (or tension)
83992	PCP	phencyclidine
85014	pcv	packed cell volume
	pH	symbol for expression of concentration of hydrogen ions (degree of acidity)
86353	PHA	phenylalanine
84030	PKU	phenylketonuria — a metabolic disease affecting mental development
82790–82817	pO_2	oxygen pressure
85618	P & P	prothrombin-proconvertin
85341	PIT	prothrombin inhibition test
85368	PPP, PPC	protamine paracoagulation
84000	PSP	phenolsulfonphthalein
85610	PT	prothrombin time
85270	PTA	plasma thromboplastin antecedent
85250	PTC	plasma thromboplastin component; phenylthiocarbamide
85341, 85730	PTT	prothrombin time; partial thromboplastin time (plasma or whole blood)

CODE NUMBER	ABBREVIATION	DEFINITION
85041	RBC, rbc	red blood cells (count)
84231	RIA	radioimmunoassay
78110	RISA	radioiodinated human serum albumin
84250	RT3U	resin triiodothyronine uptake
86592	RPR	rapid plasma reagin test
83053	S-D	strength-duration (curve)
84450	SGOT	serum glutamic oxaloacetic transaminase
84460	SGPT	serum glutamic pyruvic transaminase
86171, 86592	STS	serologic test for syphilis
83539	T_3	triiodothyronine uptake
86580, 86585, 87116–87118, 87190	TB	tubercle bacillus
84442	TBG	thyroxine-binding globulin
86357	T & B differentiation, lymphocytes	thymus-dependent lymphs and bursa-dependent lymphs; cannot tell by just normal looking—must be done by test
84442	TBG	thyroxine-binding globulin
86357	T & B differentiation, lymphocytes	thymus-dependent lymphs and bursa-dependent lymphs; cannot tell by just normal looking—must be done by test
84408	THC	tetrahydrocannabinol (marijuana)
83550	TIBC	total iron-binding capacity, chemical
84375	TLC screen	thin layer chromatography screen
84082	TRP	tubular reabsorption of phosphates
81000	UA	urinalysis
86592	VDRL	Venereal Disease Research Laboratory
84586	VMA	vanillyl mandelic acid
85048	WBC, wbc	white blood cells (count)

CODING PROBLEMS

Read over each case carefully. Use your RVS or CPT book and see if you can obtain the correct code number for each descriptor given. Full descriptors for services rendered have been omitted in some instances to give you practice in abstracting the correct descriptor from the available information. Indicate the correct modifier if necessary. These cases are only given to teach you how to use the RVS or CPT book and to familiarize you with the different sections. They are not necessarily given for billing purpose. Definitions for abbreviations may be found in the Appendix, pp. 501–505.

1. An R.N., an established patient (est. pt.), sees the doctor for an annual physical. A Pap (Papanicolaou) smear is taken and sent to an outside lab. Doctor to bill patient. Patient also has a furuncle on the right axilla at the time of visit which doctor incises and drains (I & D). Doctor always gives this patient a professional discount for annual physical, but charges usual and customary fees for laboratory and other procedures.

CODE NUMBER	DESCRIPTION
_____	Periodic physical examination
_____	Pap smear (Lab #)
_____	Collection of specimen
_____	I & D, furuncle, right axilla
_____	Sterile tray (itemized)
_____	5 cc penicillin inj IM

2. While making his rounds in the hospital during the noon hour, the doctor sees a new patient in the ER (Emergency Room) for laceration of the forehead, 5.0 cm long. Doctor does workup for possible concussion.

_____	ER care, intermediate exam
_____	_____
_____	Repair of laceration

3. The doctor sees a new patient in the office for the same problem as in the previous case, with a dressing change 2 days later by the medical assistant, and suture removal 4 days later.

_____	Initial OV, intermed exam
_____	Repair of laceration
_____	Sterile tray (itemized)
_____	Tet tox (tetanus toxoid) booster, 0.5 cc
_____	Minimal Service, dressing change (2 days) − No Charge
_____	OV, suture removal (4 days) − No Charge

4. The doctor makes a house call on Bobby Jones (est. pt.) at 11 p.m. for acute otitis media; while there she checks Bobby's sister, Mary, whom she has treated previously in the office for tonsillitis.

_____	HC (house call), limited exam (Bobby)
_____	_____
_____	5 cc penicillin inj IM (intramuscular)
_____	HC, brief exam (Mary)
_____	5 cc penicillin inj IM

5. The doctor is called to the ER at 2 a.m. Sunday to see Bobby Jones for recurrent otitis media.

_____   ER care, limited exam

_____   _____

_____   _____

_____   _____

If the doctor also performs a myringotomy on Bobby, what is the code number for this procedure?

_____   Myringotomy

6. An established male patient 55 years of age is seen in the ER on a week night at 11 p.m. for apparent congestive heart failure. A limited examination is done with telephone consultations with a cardiologist, who later sees the patient and admits him for a workup. The family physician continues to see him for diabetic management and cardiac condition. The patient responds to treatment; however, because of poor renal function, a urologist is called in to see the patient. Because of prostatic hypertrophy with obstruction, surgery is scheduled and the family physician assists. The family physician billing is as follows:

_____   ER care, limited exam

_____   _____

_____   _____

_____   Hospital visits, brief

_____   Prostatectomy, perineal, subtotal

7. The doctor sees Horace Hart, a new patient, in the office for bronchial asthma, ASHD (arteriosclerotic heart disease), and hypertension. He does an EKG (electrocardiogram) and UA (urinalysis), and takes x-rays. Seven profile (panel) tests and a CBC (complete blood count) are done by an outside laboratory. The physician is submitting the bill for the outside laboratory.

_____   Initial OV, intermed exam

_____   EKG with interpret and report

_____   UA, routine

_____   Chest x-ray, 2 views

_____ Automated multichannel tests
cholesterol, creatinine, glucose, urea nitrogen,
calcium, uric acid, albumin

_____ CBC

_____ Collection of multiple blood specimens for panel testing

8. Mr. Hart is seen again in the office on May 12. On May 25 the patient is seen at home at 2 a.m. with asthma exacerbation, possible myocardial infarct, and congestive heart failure. The doctor had to make a telephone call to consult a cardiologist. The doctor also called for arrangements for hospitalization. These services required 2½ hours to complete patient care.

_____ OV, brief exam

_____ Home visit, limited exam

_____ _____

_____ Detention time, prolonged (list time required)

9. On June 9 Horace is seen again in the hospital. The cardiologist who was called in consultation examines him and says it is necessary to perform surgery. The patient's doctor acts as assistant surgeon. The surgeon does the follow-up care.

If billing for the assistant surgeon, this is shown as:

_____ Hospital visit, brief history

_____ Pericardiotomy

If billing for the cardiologist, this is shown as:

_____ Consultation, comprehensive

_____ Pericardiotomy

10. The physician is billing for automated multichannel tests on Mrs. Gussie Gloat. Specimen is referred to an outside laboratory.

_____ Collection and handling single blood specimen for
panel testing

_____ Sodium, calcium, uric acid

11. Mrs. May I. Deliver was Grav III (pregnant for the third time). The case was worked up by Dr. Ulibarri. The patient had an uneventful pregnancy until two weeks prior to her estimated time of delivery. Lab work was done by an outside lab—billing by physician. The patient developed uterine bleeding and Dr. Ulibarri admitted her to

the hospital with a diagnosis of placenta previa. On March 2 the patient delivered a healthy boy by low cervical cesarean section. Dr. Caesar was standby at the section for the care of the newborn. Dr. Eastland was assistant surgeon at the cesarean section. Dr. Ulibarri did his own anesthesia at the cesarean. The patient was seen by Dr. Ulibarri in the office for insertion of an IUD (intrauterine device) 8 weeks following delivery.

_____   CBC, prenatal

_____   Urinalysis

_____   Total OB (obstetric) care, cesarean section

_____   Anesthesia (indicate time)

_____   IUD insertion

_____   Collection and handling of specimens

12. Bertha Hyman is seen by the doctor with a complaint of irregular bleeding of 6 months' duration. The doctor takes a Pap smear during complete exam. Pap smear reading is returned to the doctor with a diagnosis of Grade IV positive uterine CA (carcinoma). The doctor admits the patient to the hospital for a D & C (dilatation and curettage) and a cervical biopsy. Two days later Mrs. Hyman undergoes a total hysterectomy for carcinoma. (*Note:* body of uterus and part of the vagina are removed.)

_____   Examination, comprehensive

_____   Pap smear (outside lab)

_____   D & C with cervical biopsy

_____   Total hysterectomy

_____   Collection of specimen

13. Blanche Bare is seen by the doctor for irregular vaginal bleeding. The doctor diagnoses multiple cervical polyps and asks her to return in 3 days for cauterization of polyps. The doctor takes a Pap smear and a wet mount for bacterial fungi. During this initial exam, Ms. Bare asks for evaluation of possible infertility. The doctor takes tests at the time of electrocauterization of the cervix. An endometrial biopsy and injection procedure for hysterosalpingography are also done. The physician is billing for an outside lab.

_____   Initial exam, intermed

_____   Pap smear (outside lab)

_____   Wet mount for bacteria and fungi (outside lab)

_____ Culture from cervix uteri for single organism, screening only (outside lab)

_____ Electrocauterization of cervix

_____ Endometrial biopsy, suction type only

_____ *Insufflation of uterus and tubes with air and CO_2 (Rubin test)

_____ *Inj proc for hysterosalpingography

_____ Comprehensive reevaluation

_____ Collection and handling of specimen

Note: The two asterisk (*) procedures are done for infertility. Another test also performed for infertility is the Huhner test (89300).

14. On April 1 Mable Johnson, a 52-year-old established patient, was seen by Dr. Skelton for flare-up of rheumatoid arthritis and gout, with which she is badly crippled. Dr. Skelton did an exam and ordered the following tests, which were sent to an outside lab. The physician is doing the billing for the lab.

_____ Intermed exam

_____ Uric acid, blood, chemical

_____ CBC and UA

_____ Collection of single blood specimen

15. Hugh Wheeze was first seen by Dr. Coccidioides because of severe cough of 3 weeks' duration. After a CBC, sputum culture, and chest x-rays, Dr. Coccidioides diagnosed pneumonia. In regard to the sputum culture and sensitivity study, the physician is billing for the outside lab.

_____ Initial limited history and exam

_____ CBC (in doctor's office)

_____ Sputum culture for single organism

_____ Sensitivity study up to 20 discs

_____ Chest x-ray (PA and Lat views)

_____ Collection of sputum specimen

16. The physician is billing for a mixed panel where specimen(s) are referred to an outside laboratory.

_____   Collection and handling specimens with centrifuging

_____   Cholesterol, creatinine, glucose, urea nitrogen

_____   Triglycerides

_____   Lipoprotein electrophoresis

17. Virginia Lasko is seen in April for possible pregnancy. Dr. Caesar orders Gravindex (urine specimen) and DAP (blood specimen) and makes an appointment for the next month. In May Virginia returns. The uterus is now 16-week size, possibility of twins. In July x-rays are ordered to confirm twins. In August the patient is seen in ER for incomplete abortion. The doctor goes to ER at 8 p.m. and is called from outside the hospital.

_____   OV, ltd est pt

_____   Gravindex and DAP (gonadotropin, chorionic, bioassay, qualitative)

_____   X-rays for fetal position, 2 views

_____   Incomplete abortion

_____   ER care, intermed

_____   _____

_____   _____

18. Joe Lory complains of itching and also has a 0.6 cm nevus on his cheek. At the initial visit, the doctor does 7 patch tests and takes a biopsy. The patient returns in 3 days and the doctor removes the nevus. Dx (diagnosis): benign nevus right cheek.

_____   Initial visit, ltd, new patient

_____   Patch tests (5)

_____   Patch tests (2)

_____   Biopsy

_____   Removal of nevus (simple excision)

19. Dr. Skelton was called from outside the hospital to see 11-year-old Jamie Adams in the ER at 7 p.m. Jamie was in an automobile accident and had multiple

fractures and lacerations. Bilateral x-rays taken of the hip, thigh, and heel were positive. A 17.0 cm laceration on the thigh was closed by Dr. Skelton and a walking cast was applied to the left leg. The patient was seen in the doctor's office 2 weeks later.

_____ ER visit, intermed (est pt)

_____ _____

_____ _____

_____ X-ray left hip, AP (anterior posterior view)

_____ Heel x-ray

_____ Bilateral hip x-rays

_____ Laceration, simple repair

_____ Cast, long-leg (walking)

_____ OV (office visit), ltd

20. A new patient, David Ramsey, age 15, was seen by Dr. Menter for lapse of memory and frequent headaches. The doctor did an EEG (electroencephalogram) and some psychometric tests. Dr. Astro Parkinson was called in as consultant. All the tests were negative and the patient was advised to come in for weekly psychotherapy.

Dr. Menter's billing:

_____ OV, comp, new pt

_____ EEG

_____ Psychometric tests (identify test used)

_____ Psychotherapy (50 min)

Dr. Parkinson's billing:

_____ Consultation, comp

21. Danny Davis was seen for his annual visit. An EKG and step test were done. Profile tests (protein, uric acid, albumin, and calcium) were also done, as was a glucose tolerance test (4 specimens). The physician drew the blood for the laboratory work and the samples were sent to an outside lab for the results.

_____ OV

_____ EKG, interpret & report

_____   Automated multichannel tests (profile or panel tests), protein, uric acid, albumin, and calcium

_____   Glucose tolerance test

_____   _____

_____   Collection and handling fee

In handling problems 22 through 29, read over each case carefully. Select the proper RVS or CPT code number along with the description of the service they code.

22. A new patient comes into the office with a deep abrasion requiring limited H & P (history and physical), cleansing of the wound, and a tetanus booster.

_____   _____

_____   _____

_____   _____

_____   _____

23. A new adult patient is seen with acute pneumonia as an office patient. The doctor does a comprehensive H & P, including initiation of a diagnostic and treatment program. A chest x-ray is taken and he gives the patient a penicillin injection. The patient returns a week later for a limited exam.

_____   _____

_____   _____

_____   _____

_____   _____

24. A mother brings her baby into the office after a serious illness and the doctor does a comprehensive reexamination. The doctor then gives the baby a DPT (diphtheria, pertussis, tetanus) immunization and oral polio.

_____   _____

_____   _____

_____   _____

25. An established patient, a young child, is admitted to the hospital for acute asthmatic bronchitis. The doctor gives initial care after 11 p.m., performing an intermediate history and physical examination that includes initiation of diagnostic

and treatment programs and preparation of hospital records. The doctor then remains with the child an additional hour to be sure the child is out of danger.

_____   _____

_____   _____

_____   _____

26.   A new patient is seen in the hospital and undergoes a comprehensive H & P, including initiation of diagnostic and treatment program and preparation of hospital records. The physician then performs a bronchoscopy with biopsy. The results of the biopsy confirm her diagnosis, so the following day she performed a total right pneumonectomy.

_____   _____

_____   _____

_____   _____

27.   A physician assisted with the pneumonectomy on the patient in problem 26 above.

_____   _____

28.   A patient is sent to your office from a referring doctor and your employer does a consultation requiring comprehensive history and examination. He then returns the patient to the referring doctor for his recommended care.

_____   _____

29.   An established patient comes into the office for a brief examination and the doctor does a puncture aspiration of a cyst on her right breast. This requires the use of a special sterile surgical setup and tray.

_____   _____

_____   _____

_____   _____

CODE BOOK SOURCES

You may obtain RVS or CPT books from the following sources. It might also be mentioned that Blue Shield uses RVS code numbers and usually each district office can be contacted in order to obtain the Blue Shield manual. See Chapter 4.

TITLE*	SOURCE
Current Procedural Terminology 1970, 1973, and 1977 editions	American Medical Association 535 North Dearborn Street Chicago, IL 60610
Terminology and Relative Values of Urological Procedures	American Urological Association, Inc. 1120 North Charles Street Baltimore, MD 21201
	Medical Association of the State of Alabama 19 South Jackson Street Montgomery, AL 36104
California Relative Value Studies 1964, 1969, and 1974 editions	Sutter Publications, Inc. 731 Market Street San Francisco, CA 94103
	Colorado Medical Society 1601 East 19th Avenue Denver, CO 80218
	Medical Society of the District of Columbia 2007 Eye Street, Northeast Washington, D.C. 20006
	Florida Medical Association Post Office Box 2411 Jacksonville, FL 32203
Hawaii Relative Value Studies 1965 and 1970 editions	Fee Survey Committee of the Hawaii Medical Association 510 South Beretania Street Honolulu, HI 96813
	Illinois Medical Society 360 N. Michigan Avenue Chicago, IL 60601
	Kansas Medical Society 1300 Topeka Boulevard Topeka, KA 66612
	Massachusetts Medical Society 22 The Fenway Boston, MA 02215
	Michigan State Medical Society Post Office Box 950 120 West Saginaw East Lansing, MI 48823
	Minnesota State Medical Association 375 Jackson Street St. Paul, MN 55101
	Montana Medical Association 2021 11th Avenue Suite #12 Helena, MO 59601

*As of this writing, California and Hawaii are the only states to list specific titles for their code books.

TITLE	SOURCE
	Nebraska Medical Association 1902 First National Bank Building Lincoln, NE 68508
	North Carolina Medical Society 222 W. Person Street Post Office Box 27167 Raleigh, NC 27611
	North Dakota Medical Association Suite 307 M.D.U. Office Building Box 1198 Bismarck, ND 58501
	South Dakota State Medical Association 711 N. Lake Avenue Sioux Falls, SD 57104
	Utah State Medical Association 42 South 5th East Street Salt Lake City, UT 84102
	Wyoming State Medical Society 412 Randall Avenue Post Office Box 1387 Cheyenne, WY 82001

REVIEW QUESTIONS

1. When do you use the -99 RVS modifier? _____

2. What modifier is usually used when billing for an assistant surgeon? _____

What percentage is this of the listed value? _____

3. What do these abbreviations and symbols mean in the code books:

PC _____   Sv _____

BR _____   ★ _____

RNE _____   △ _____

4. When is a physician entitled to a collection and handling fee regarding laboratory tests? _____

_____

5. What does an asterisk (*) next to an RVS procedure number mean? _____

_____

6. Can you give five reasons why modifiers are used?

a. _____

b. _____

c. _____

d. _____

e. _____

7. Besides the procedure code number, what other items are necessary when listing an injection? _____

_____

8. Can you convert an RVS unit to dollars and cents for your physician's office?

_____ Would the conversion be applicable to all sections of the RVS book? _____

9. After completion of the coding problems in this chapter you should be able to decode these abbreviations:

I & D _____ EKG _____

IM _____ IUD _____

Pap _____ OB _____

ER _____ D & C _____

EEG _____ AP _____

DPT _____ OV _____

H & P _____ UA _____

10. Name the five main sections of the RVS code books.

a. _____   d. _____

b. _____   e. _____

c. _____

11. If Mrs. Vail has a fracture of the tibia, does the RVS listed value include the application and removal of the first cast?_____ Does the RVS listed value also include the subsequent replacement of a cast for follow-up care? _____

12. In billing for surgery after obtaining the correct RVS code number, what other item should be looked at in doing follow-up billing on the same patient? _____

_____

Notes:

3
The Universal
Health
Insurance
Claim Form

BEHAVIORAL
OBJECTIVES *The Assistant should be able to:*

1. Expedite the logging and processing of the Health Insurance Claim Form.
2. Define abbreviations as they appear on a Patient Record.
3. Give the history of the Universal Form.
4. State when the Universal Form may or may not be used.
5. Abstract from the patient record the necessary information for completing the Universal Form.
6. State the proper CPT or RVS coding to be used when submitting the Universal Form.
7. Minimize the number of insurance forms returned because of improper completion.
8. Know the proper information to be recorded on the patient's ledger card after submitting a claim.

HISTORY

In 1958 the Health Insurance Council (HIC) and the American Medical Association (AMA) attempted to standardize the insurance claim form by jointly developing the "Standard Form." It was not universally accepted by all third parties, and as the types of coverages became more variable, new claim forms were instituted which required more information than did the original "Standard Form." The form eventually became known as "COMB-1" or "Attending Physician's Statement." In 1968 the HIC decided to revamp the form again so that it would be more adaptable to electronic data processing.

In April 1975 the American Medical Association approved a universal claim form that can be used for both group and individual insurance claims (see Fig. 3–1). Acceptance and use of the form by governmental fiscal intermediaries and health insurance service organizations may vary from locality to locality. The National Association of Blue Shield Plans Board of Directors has adopted a motion supporting

HEALTH INSURANCE CLAIM FORM

READ INSTRUCTIONS BEFORE COMPLETING OR SIGNING THIS FORM

SAMPLE

Prudential Insurance Company
5450 Wilshire Blvd.
Woodland Hills, XY 12345

TYPE OR PRINT [ ] MEDICARE [ ] MEDICAID [ ] CHAMPUS [X] OTHER

PATIENT & INSURED (SUBSCRIBER) INFORMATION

1. PATIENT'S NAME (First name, middle initial, last name) Harry NMI Forehand	2. PATIENT'S DATE OF BIRTH 01 06 36	3. INSURED'S NAME (First name, middle initial, last name) Harry Forehand
4. PATIENT'S ADDRESS (Street, city, state, ZIP code) 1456 Main Street Woodland Hills, XY 12345	5. PATIENT'S SEX MALE [X] FEMALE 7. PATIENT'S RELATIONSHIP TO INSURED SELF [X] SPOUSE CHILD OTHER	6. INSURED'S I.D. No or **MEDICARE No.** (include any letters) 8. INSURED'S GROUP NO. (Or Group Name) GC-1117
9. OTHER HEALTH INSURANCE COVERAGE - Enter Name of Policyholder and Plan Name and Address and Policy or Medical Assistance Number DNA	10. WAS CONDITION RELATED TO: A. PATIENT'S EMPLOYMENT YES [ ] [X] NO B. AN AUTO ACCIDENT YES [ ] [X] NO	11. INSURED'S ADDRESS (Street, city, state, ZIP code) 1456 Main Street Woodland Hills, XY 12345
12. PATIENT'S OR AUTHORIZED PERSON'S SIGNATURE (Read back before signing) I Authorize the Release of any Medical Information Necessary to Process this Claim and Request Payment of MEDICARE/CHAMPUS Benefits Either to Myself or to the Party Who Accepts Assignment Below SIGNED *Harry Forehand* DATE March 3, 1976		13. I AUTHORIZE PAYMENT OF MEDICAL BENEFITS TO UNDERSIGNED PHYSICIAN OR SUPPLIER FOR SERVICE DESCRIBED BELOW SIGNED *Harry Forehand* (Insured or Authorized Person)

PHYSICIAN OR SUPPLIER INFORMATION

14. DATE OF 3-3-76	ILLNESS (FIRST SYMPTOM) OR INJURY (ACCIDENT) OR PREGNANCY (LMP)	15. DATE FIRST CONSULTED YOU FOR THIS CONDITION 3-3-76	16. HAS PATIENT EVER HAD SAME OR SIMILAR SYMPTOMS? YES [ ] [X] NO
17. DATE PATIENT ABLE TO RETURN TO WORK 3-4-76	18. DATES OF TOTAL DISABILITY FROM DNA THROUGH	DATES OF PARTIAL DISABILITY FROM DNA THROUGH
19. NAME OF REFERRING PHYSICIAN Nick E. Cutforth, M. D.		20. FOR SERVICES RELATED TO HOSPITALIZATION GIVE HOSPITALIZATION DATES ADMITTED DNA DISCHARGED
21. NAME & ADDRESS OF FACILITY WHERE SERVICES RENDERED (If other than home or office) DNA		22. WAS LABORATORY WORK PERFORMED OUTSIDE YOUR OFFICE? YES [ ] [X] NO CHARGES

23. DIAGNOSIS OR NATURE OF ILLNESS OR INJURY. RELATE DIAGNOSIS TO PROCEDURE IN COLUMN D BY REFERENCE TO NUMBERS 1, 2, 3, ETC. OR DX CODE

1. otitis media right and left ears
2.
3.
4.

24. A DATE OF SERVICE	B* PLACE OF SERVICE	C PROCEDURE CODE (IDENTIFY)	FULLY DESCRIBE PROCEDURES, MEDICAL SERVICES OR SUPPLIES FURNISHED FOR EACH DATE GIVEN (EXPLAIN UNUSUAL SERVICES OR CIRCUMSTANCES)	D DIAGNOSIS CODE	E CHARGES	F
3-3-76	0	90015	Office visit, intermed.	1	20 00	

25. SIGNATURE OF PHYSICIAN OR SUPPLIER (Read back before signing) *Concha Antrum, M.D.* SIGNED DATE 3-3-76	26. ACCEPT ASSIGNMENT (GOVERNMENT CLAIMS ONLY) (SEE BACK) YES [X] NO 30. YOUR SOCIAL SECURITY NO 000-00-0000	27. TOTAL CHARGE 20 00	28. AMOUNT PAID	29. BALANCE DUE 20 00
32. YOUR PATIENT'S ACCOUNT NO.	33. YOUR EMPLOYER I.D. NO. 95-3664021	31. PHYSICIAN'S OR SUPPLIER'S NAME, ADDRESS, ZIP CODE & TELEPHONE NO Concha Antrum, M. D. 4567 Broad Avenue Woodland Hills, XY 12345 I.D. NO. C 16021 013/486-9002		

* PLACE OF SERVICE CODES

1 — (IH) — INPATIENT HOSPITAL	4 — (H) — PATIENT'S HOME	7 — (NH) — NURSING HOME	O — (OL) — OTHER LOCATIONS
2 — (OH) — OUTPATIENT HOSPITAL	5 — DAY CARE FACILITY (PSY)	8 — (SNF) — SKILLED NURSING FACILITY	A — (IL) — INDEPENDENT LABORATORY
3 — (O) — DOCTOR'S OFFICE	6 — NIGHT CARE FACILITY (PSY)	9 — AMBULANCE	B — OTHER MEDICAL/SURGICAL FACILITY

ref initials

APPROVED BY AMA COUNCIL ON MEDICAL SERVICE 6-74

FIGURE 3–1

The Universal Health Insurance Claim Form approved by the AMA Council on Medical Service.

the concept of a uniform national claim form. However, Blue Shield Plans may not be able to immediately accept and process the Health Insurance Claim Form for their private business. Therefore, before submitting claims to these groups, it is suggested that you contact their appropriate local representatives (see Chapter 4). In California this form has been accepted by the California Medical Association Council for immediate use and has also been approved by Blue Cross of Northern and Southern California, Blue Shield of California, the Health Insurance Association, and the Bureau of Health Insurance (Medicare). Insurance carriers are working for acceptance of the form by CHAMPUS and Medicaid (Medi-Cal).

Presently many computer systems are not programmed for using this new form. Until insurance carriers (Blue Cross, Blue Shield, Medicare, CHAMPUS, Medicaid [Medi-Cal], etc.) switch to the newer programming, this fact may result in claim processing delays. In the future, widespread use of the form will save time and simplify claims processing for both physicians and carriers.

Commercial carriers and the Blue Plans will furnish forms as they become available. To purchase quantities of the Health Insurance Claim Form, write to the American Medical Association, 535 North Dearborn Street, Chicago, IL 60610.

Another standard form, an Attending Physician's Statement, was developed in California by a local county medical society (see Fig. 3–2).

For further information and booklets on health or life insurance, write to:
Health Insurance Council
750 Third Avenue
New York, N.Y. 10017

Health Insurance Institute
277 Park Avenue
New York, N.Y. 10017

PROCEDURES FOR USE OF THE UNIVERSAL HEALTH INSURANCE CLAIM FORM

1. Use the Universal Claim Form or Attending Physician's Statement as often as possible. This is accepted by nearly all general insurance carriers. Some insurance companies require answers to questions other than those included on the Universal Claim Form. In these instances you might include an additional information sheet listing the following items that may be pertinent to the case:
   a. Date your physician's services were terminated.
   b. When a nurse's (R.N.'s) services were required.
   c. Address of a referring physician, if any.
2. When a patient brings in a form from a private insurance plan, have him or her sign it as well as the Attending Physician's Statement or Universal Claim Form and fasten the two together. Make sure the patient's portion of the private insurance form is complete and accurate.
3. When the patient has group insurance through an employer, send both forms to the employer. The employer will complete his portion and forward the forms to the insurance carrier.
4. When the coverage is not group insurance, send both forms directly to the insurance company. It is not a good idea to let patients direct their own forms to insurance companies or employers.

ATTENTING PHYSICIAN'S STATEMENT

SAMPLE

To: Prudential Ins. Co. 5450 Wilshire Blvd., Woodland Hills, XY 12345 Insurance Company

Name of Insured: Harry NMI Forehand   Soc. Sec. # 123-00-4567   Policy # GC-1117

Address: 1456 Main Street, Woodland Hills, XY 12345

Name of Patient Harry NMI Forehand   Relationship to Insured: self

The following professional services were provided the above named patient as itemized, and on the dates listed below,

for the diagnosis of: otitis media right and left ears

Disability related to: ☒ Personal Illness   ☐ Personal Accident   ☐ Occupation   ☐ Pregnancy

Period of Disability: From DNA   To

DATE	RVS	SERVICE RENDERED	CHARGE
3-3-76	90015	Office visit, intermed.	20.00
		TOTAL:	20.00

ASSIGNMENT TAKEN yes
MAKE CHECKS PAYABLE TO

STATE LAW AB 1236 MAKES IT MANDATORY RATHER THAN PERMISSIVE THAT INSURANCE COMPANIES HONOR ASSIGNMENT OF BENEFITS.

Receipt of $ 5.00 will be required prior to providing additional information

DOCTOR'S SIGNATURE
Concha Antrum, M.D.,   C 16021   4567 Broad Ave.,Woodland Hills,XY 12345   013/486-9002
DOCTOR'S TYPED NAME   LIC. NO.   ADDRESS   TELEPHONE
IRS # 95-3664021

I HEREBY AUTHORIZE THE DOCTOR(S) WHOSE NAME(S) APPEARS BELOW TO FURNISH THE ABOVE INSURANCE COMPANY ALL INFORMATION WHICH SAID INSURANCE COMPANY MAY REQUEST CONCERNING MY PRESENT ILLNESS OR INJURY. I HEREBY ASSIGN TO THE DOCTOR(S) WHOSE NAME(S) APPEARS BELOW ALL MONEY TO WHICH I AM ENTITLED FOR MEDICAL AND/OR SURGICAL EXPENSE RELATIVE TO THE SERVICE REPORTED BELOW, BUT NOT TO EXCEED MY INDEBTEDNESS TO SAID PHYSICIAN AND SURGEON. IT IS UNDERSTOOD THAT ANY MONEY RECEIVED FROM THE ABOVE NAMED INSURANCE COMPANY, OVER AND ABOVE MY INDEBTEDNESS WILL BE REFUNDED TO ME WHEN MY BILL IS PAID IN FULL. I UNDERSTAND I AM FINANCIALLY RESPONSIBLE TO SAID DOCTOR(S) FOR CHARGES NOT COVERED BY THIS ASSIGNMENT.

NOTE: California law required that Insurance Code Section 556 appear on this claim form.
IT IS UNLAWFUL TO: (a) Present or cause to be presented any false or fraudulent claim for the payment of a loss under a contract of insurance.
(b) Prepare, make, or subscribe any writing, with intent to present or use the same, or allow it to be presented or used in support of any such claim.
Every person who violates any provision of this section is punishable by imprisonment in the State Prison not exceeding three years, or by fine not exceeding one thousand dollars, or by both.

X
INSURED OR GUARDIAN SIGNATURE   *Harry Forehand*   March 3, 1976
ref initials   PATIENT'S SIGNATURE   DATE

FIGURE 3-2

The standard form developed in California by a local county medical society. This form allows the doctor to indicate to the insurance company that a fee will be charged for any additional information.

5. If the patient has insurance with more than one company (sometimes called Dual Coverage), be sure to obtain assignments for both insurance companies, and bill both.

6. On an extended illness, send interim billings every 30 days, even though payment may not be made by the insurance company until the end of treatment. Type the notation "continued case" on the claim form.

7. Some policies do not allow injections on an outpatient basis. Medication is covered only when the patient is in the hospital as a bed patient. However, if the service is itemized on the claim as an office call and injection, credit can be given, since an office call for the purpose of administering an injection is covered.

8. The patient's eligibility is determined on the basis of the physician's diagnosis and the treatment rendered. The patient may be unaware of Major Medical credits accrued from nonpayment on the basic plan. It is feasible to bill for services rendered even though the patient may not think that he or she is covered.

TO THE STUDENT: Now refer to the Appendix to start completing insurance forms and coding them for billing purposes. Assignments 1, 2, and 3, pp. 507–517, pertain to this chapter.

INSTRUCTIONS FOR COMPLETION OF THE HEALTH INSURANCE CLAIM FORM (Fig. 3–1 and Assignments 1, 2, and 3, pp. 507–517)

1. Enter the name of the patient (insured or a dependent) as indicated.
2. Enter month, day, and year of patient's birth as 6 digits (Example: 01-06-76).
3. Enter name of the insured (policyholder or subscriber).
4. Furnish the patient's complete address. The top half of the space is for the patient's street address and the lower half is for the city, state, and zip code. It may also be necessary to complete the insured's address when it is different from the patient's.
5. Indicate the sex of the patient by marking an "x" in the appropriate box.
6. The full number must be filled in; be sure to include any letters.

For *Medicare* use the number on the beneficiary's red, white, and blue health insurance card.

For *Medicaid* use the Social Security number of the insured person.

For *Blue Shield* use the number on the subscriber's identification card (usually referred to as "Identification" or "Certificate" or "Contract" number).

For *private insurance companies* use the insured's policy number or other identifying number assigned by the company.

For *all others* use the number assigned by the organization or agency.

7. Check the appropriate box.
8. For third party carriers (third party payers) the "insured's group number" is the policy number assigned to the group policyholder; that is, the employer. The group name is preferred by most insurance companies.
9. Information about additional coverage is necessary to assist third parties in determining if the patient has multiple health insurance, including Medicare. The name of the policyholder (insured) should be identified.

10. *Part A:* This information is necessary so that third parties may determine the patient's eligibility for worker's compensation insurance.

Part B: This information is needed to determine the primary insurance carrier in those states with no-fault auto insurance laws.

11. Enter the insured's address if it is different from the patient's.

12. The patient's signature authorizes the provider to release medical information necessary to process the claim. It is anticipated that this simplified release of information statement will assist in limiting the release of confidential patient information. If the patient is a minor, the signature must be that of his or her parent or legal guardian. For Medicare and CHAMPUS programs, the beneficiary's signature also authorizes payment of benefits to the provider. It is important that the physician complete item 26 when filing a claim for reimbursement under these two programs.

13. This is the insured's authorization for the payment of benefits directly to the provider. Acceptance of this assignment is considered to be a contractual arrangement. If the insured desires the claim assigned, the insured's signature is necessary as a party to the contract. "Authorized person" must be the insured or a person with power of attorney on behalf of the insured.

14. a. If the patient consulted the provider as a result of illness, this block must contain the date of the first symptoms.

b. If the patient consulted the provider as a result of an accident, the block must contain the date the accident occurred.

c. If the patient consulted the provider as a result of pregnancy, the block must contain the date of the last menstrual period (LMP).

In (a), (b), or (c), the information assists third party carriers in determining patient eligibility for coverage.

15. In this space should be recorded the month, day, and year the patient first consulted the provider for the condition for which the claim is being submitted. On subsequent visits for the same condition, it may not be necessary to complete this item.

16. The provider should check "yes" or "no." If "yes" is checked, it may be necessary for the provider to attach a statement indicating when the patient had symptoms the same as or similar to those for which the present claim is being submitted. On subsequent visits for the same condition, it may not be necessary to complete item 16 if a previous claim has been filed with the same third party carrier.

17. This box should be completed only when the patient is entitled to disability benefits through insurance companies; otherwise it can be left blank.

18. This item should be completed only when the patient is entitled to disability benefits through insurance companies; otherwise it can be left blank.

19. This question must be answered for first consultations when a referring physician is involved. On subsequent visits for the same conditions it will not be necessary to complete it.

20. This should be completed only when medical service is rendered as a result of or subsequent to a related hospitalization.

21. If services are rendered in a hospital, clinic, laboratory, or any facility other than the patient's home or the physician's office, the name and address of the facility must be entered.

22. If the answer is yes, the amount of the charges is requested and the name and address of the laboratory must be entered.

23. All third party carriers require that a diagnosis or nature of the illness or injury be indicated before medical/health services will be considered covered expenses.

The diagnosis(es) should be written out, or a coding structure may be used if such code is identified and is agreeable to the carrier. (See Chapter 2.) When more than one diagnosis has been indicated on the claim, relate each diagnosis (using reference number, i.e., 1, 2, or 3, or DX code) to the appropriate procedures listed in item 24. If a procedure relates to more than one diagnosis, the primary diagnosis to which the procedure relates should be the one referred to in Column D of question 24.

24. If questions 23 and 24 are properly completed, some of the additional correspondence currently generated by third party carriers should not be necessary, and benefit payments will be made more promptly.

Column A: Enter the month, day, and year for each consultation or procedure. If "from" and "to" dates are shown here for a series of identical services, the number of these services should appear in Column C.

Column B: List the place of service utilizing the codes shown at the bottom of the form. Two coding structures have been identified. The first code is a one-position, primarily numeric code and must be used for reporting Blue Shield claims. The code shown in parentheses is a one-to-three position alphabetic code. Only one of these two coding structures should be used.

Column C: There is space for a written description of procedures and services performed as well as a box where a procedure code may be listed. If a coding structure is used, the coding structure must be identified and agreeable to the carrier. For anesthesia, show the elapsed time (hours:minutes). If "from/to" dates were entered in Column A, the number of services should be entered here.

Column D: The diagnosis reference number (i.e., 1, 2, 3, or the diagnostic code) as shown in question 23 should be filled in to relate the date of service and the procedures performed to the appropriate diagnosis more effectively.

Column E: The charge for each listed service should be entered. Describe any unusual circumstances in Column C, to avoid claims processing delays related to unexplained charges.

Column F: Blank space is provided for use by Blue Shield. Refer to your local Blue Shield instructions.

25. The physician or supplier (or his or her authorized representative) must sign. The month, day, and year that the form was signed must also be entered.

26. The physician or supplier should check one of the boxes to indicate whether or not he or she accepts assignment of benefits under government-funded programs. This does not include the Federal Employee Program.

27. Total the charges.

28. This relates to the accounting system of the physician or supplier and should be completed as deemed appropriate.

29. Enter the balance due.

30. The Social Security number should be used by all physicians in private practice or by independent suppliers.

31. This space may be completed by hand, typewriter, or rubber stamp. Some third parties or service organizations may preprint the doctor's name and number on the form.

I.D. (Identifying) No. should be used when the physician or supplier is employed by a Health Maintenance Organization that has assigned him a special number, or when he has been assigned a specific identifying number (Provider Number) by a fiscal agent. In some instances, you can place the physician's State License Number here.

32. The patient's account number, as recorded in the physician's or supplier's accounting system, may be entered for additional patient identification.

33. The Employer I.D. No. (IRS Number or Tax I.D. Number) should be completed when the physician or supplier is providing services in a group practice or is employed by a hospital or other institution and has been assigned an Employer I.D. number.

SPECIFIC REQUIREMENTS

The following sections relate specifically to the requirements of Medicare, Medicaid (Medi-Cal), CHAMPUS, Blue Shield, and insurance companies.

When Patient Is Covered by Medicare

Items that must be considered for completion: 1, 2, 4 to 6, 9, 10, 12, and 19 to 33.

Items that need not be considered for completion: 3, 7, 8, 10B, 11, 13, and 14 to 18. Additional instructions are published by the Social Security Administration (SSA). (See Chapter 6.)

When Patient Is Covered by Medicare

All items should be considered for completion as applicable for Medicaid patients, except items 17 and 18.

The Universal Health Insurance Claim Form is presently not accepted by Medi-Cal.

For additional information confer with the Medicaid intermediary in your vicinity. (See Chapter 5.)

When Patient Is Covered by CHAMPUS

Additional instructions are prepared by CHAMPUS. Consult the CHAMPUS intermediary. (See Chapter 7.)

When Patient Is Covered by Blue Shield

Check with your local Blue Shield plan concerning the use of the Universal Health Insurance Claim Form and separate instructions. (See Chapter 4.)

When Patient Is Covered by a Private Plan

All items on the form must be considered for completion when the patient is insured by third party coverage other than those mentioned above. While most items are self-explanatory as to what information is to be provided, special attention must be given to items 6, 8, 9, 10, and 13 in the Patient and Insured (Subscriber) Information section and to items 14, 17, 18, 23, and 24 in the Physician or Supplier Information section.

REVIEW QUESTIONS

1. Who developed the Standard or Uniform Form? _____

2. Who developed the Universal Health Insurance Claim Form? _____

3. Does Medicare accept the Universal Health Insurance Claim Form? _____

4. What is dual coverage? _____

_____

5. If a patient brings in a form for group insurance through his employer, where

do you send the form after completion? _____

_____

6. If the patient brings in a private insurance form that is *not* group insurance,

where do you send the form after completion? _____

_____

7. Is the Universal Health Insurance Claim Form accepted by nearly all general

insurance carriers? _____ What are the exceptions? _____

_____

8. When is the usual time for sending in an insurance form? _____

_____

9. In completing an insurance claim, the patient can be either the _____

_____ or the _____ .

10. In completing an insurance claim, the insured is also known as the

_____ or the _____ .

11. What does LMP mean on a form? _____

12. What does Dx mean on a form? _____

13. The Employer I.D. Number is also sometimes called _____ or

_____ .

After completing all the patient records in Appendix A pertinent to this chapter,
you will be able to answer the next two questions.

14. What do these abbreviations mean?

    a. PTR _____   c. HX _____

    b. TURP _____   d. IVP _____

e. c̄ _____   h. CC _____

f. Dx _____   i. UA _____

g. BP _____   j. PE _____

15. Give the abbreviations for the following terms.

a. return _____

b. cancer, carcinoma _____

c. patient _____

d. established _____

e. discharged _____

f. gallbladder _____

g. initial _____

Notes:

4

Blue Cross and
Blue Shield*

BEHAVIORAL
OBJECTIVES *The Assistant should be able to:*

1. Learn the essential features of Blue Cross and Blue Shield and explain how the plans came into existence.
2. Identify which federal and state programs the plans may administer.
3. Explain the difference between usual, customary, and reasonable fees.
4. Identify the permanent reciprocity symbol and know how to bill under this program.
5. Understand how to process claims for patients on Medicare with supplemental Blue Shield coverage.
6. Abstract from the patient's identification card(s).
7. Understand the Federal Employee Program, its benefits and nonbenefits.
8. Learn pertinent Blue Cross and Blue Shield terminology and abbreviations.
9. Complete claim forms properly.
10. Record ledger information correctly.

INTRODUCTION

Since individual Blue Cross and Blue Shield Plans vary widely, only topics of a strictly general nature are discussed in the majority of this chapter. Blue Shield coverage has been emphasized, since the medical assistant working in a private office will rarely be required to process Blue Cross (in-hospital expense) claims. One exception to this rule occurs in California, where certain Blue Cross claims are handled in the physician's office and where patients may occasionally do their own billing of claims. Essential details of the California plans are summarized at the end of the chapter.

Blue Shield Plans are unique in employing a large staff of Provider/Professional Relations Representatives for the express purpose of interpreting Blue Shield policies and procedures on a local level. These representatives make personal calls at physicians' offices, conduct seminars for doctors and medical assistants, and speak to hospital

---

*The National Association of Blue Shield Plans does not assume editorial responsibility for the accuracy of the data contained in this chapter, nor does it necessarily endorse or agree with the contents.

staffs and local medical society meetings. They also work closely with local and state components of the American Association of Medical Assistants (AAMA) on various capacities. You should get to know and keep in regular contact with the Provider/ Professional Relations Representative at the Blue Shield office in your area. He or she will be able to give you specific information about your local Plan and will keep you informed about any procedural changes.

HISTORY AND PURPOSE

Blue Cross Plans are nonprofit, community service organizations, providing health care services to their subscribers. They are called "prepayment plans" because individuals pay in advance for the health services they may need. Blue Cross was the first major health prepayment plan, and it is still the largest. The idea originated in Dallas, Texas, in 1929, when a group of teachers found the cost of hospital care a heavy load for an individual to bear. Each member agreed to pay Baylor University Hospital a small sum of money every month. In return, all members were guaranteed 21 days of hospitalization a year. The experiment worked, and soon hospitals in other cities were trying a similar arrangement. The idea took on the Blue Cross name and was adopted by the American Hospital Association as a public service. In 1972, the relationship between the Blue Cross Association (BCA) and the AHA was officially ended when the Blue Cross name and mark were turned over to BCA. Today, some Blue Cross plans provide medical and surgical benefits in addition to hospital benefits.

Blue Shield Plans are not-for-profit voluntary associations established so that subscribers may pay in advance for expenses incurred for surgery, in-hospital medical care, and in some Plans outpatient emergency services. Subscribers pay a premium to receive these benefits, and therefore this Plan, like Blue Cross, is a prepayment plan. Each local Blue Shield Plan is an autonomous corporation. The Plans are bound together by an organization known as the National Association of Blue Shield Plans (NABSP), which requires that local corporations be operated on a not-for-profit basis. That Blue Shield Plans are an important link in the doctor-patient relationship is supported by impressive statistics: 80 per cent of practicing physicians now participate in Blue Shield, and the Plans have over 73 million private subscribers.

Blue Shield Plans were introduced later than Blue Cross Plans, largely because of the traditional reluctance of physicians to support prepayment programs which might interfere with the doctor-patient relationship and restrict the quantity and quality of patient care. However, the Depression of the 1930's and the rapid advances in medical knowledge during the first half of the twentieth century underscored the need for an organized system of advance payment for medical services that the majority of American families could never afford to cover by the conventional means of cash paid for service rendered. After the American Medical Association House of Delegates endorsed the principle of voluntary health insurance in 1938, the way was paved for the formation of the first Blue Shield Plan in 1939. This Plan was started in California and was originally known as the California Physicians Service. It provided complete coverage of doctors' services to groups whose employees earned less than $3000 a year. A prepaid plan in Buffalo, New York, is credited with first using the Blue Shield name and symbol. In 1948 the name and symbol were informally adopted by the Associated Medical Care Plans, and in 1951 they were officially registered for Blue Shield Plans.

Blue Shield is not a commercial insurance company. A person becomes a member by entering into a contract with his or her local Blue Shield Plan, and by paying regular dues. He or she becomes a subscriber, not a policy-holder, and retains a certificate, not a policy, which tells him or her what to expect from the contract when medical services are required. Under a contract in which the patient has both Blue Shield and Blue Cross coverage, the Blue Cross Plan pays for hospital services and the Blue Shield Plan pays for professional services.

Blue Cross and Blue Shield may assist the federal and state governments in the administration of Medicare, Medicaid (Medi-Cal), and CHAMPUS programs. When the Blue Plans are the fiscal intermediary for Medicare, Blue Cross handles Medicare Part A and Blue Shield handles Medicare Part B. (For explanations of Medicare A and B, see Chapter 6). An estimated 12 million Americans are served by Blue Shield Plans through these government programs.

Blue Cross and Blue Shield programs across the country are currently experimenting with, and entering into, prepaid group practices, model cities health care programs, dental care programs, and prescription drug programs.

A glossary of terms commonly used in Blue Cross and Blue Shield literature and claim forms will be found beginning on page 74. Sample Blue Cross and Blue Shield identification cards are shown in Figure 4–1.

EMBOSSED PLASTIC
NATIONAL IDENTIFICATION
CARD SAMPLES

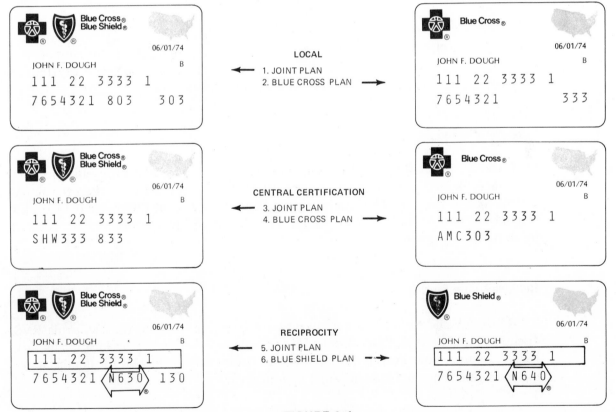

FIGURE 4–1

Typical Blue Cross and Blue Shield identification cards. Note that patients may have a single card for combined Blue Cross/Blue Shield coverage, or separate cards for Blue Cross or Blue Shield coverage only. "SHW" on the second card in the left column indicates that the patient has coverage through an employee group—in this case, Sherwin-Williams. These initials must appear on the claim form along with the group number. The boxes and arrows on the cards at the bottom of each column show that these patients are covered under Blue Shield's Permanent Reciprocity Program. For an explanation of this program, see pages 67 and 68.

SPECIAL CLAUSES AND BENEFITS

Some Blue Cross and Blue Shield contracts include a pre-existing conditions clause which requires a waiting period as outlined in the contract before benefits are payable for those conditions existing prior to the membership-effective date. The waiting period varies with the plan and with the contract.

Coverage for emergency treatment is provided under many contracts if the treatment is rendered immediately after an accident within the time specified by the contract (usually within 24 to 72 hours).

When a Blue Cross–Blue Shield member has additional coverage from a commercial insurance carrier, benefits must be coordinated. (See definition of *coordination of benefits* in Chapter 1, p. 6.)

TYPES OF BLUE SHIELD CONTRACTS

There are four basic types of Blue Shield contracts: Service Contracts, Indemnity Schedules, Relative Value Studies, and Usual, Customary and Reasonable (UCR). The UCR contracts are by far the most complicated.

Service Contract

Under a Service Contract, a participating physician agrees by signing a contract with the local Blue Shield Plan that if the family income of a patient does not exceed an amount specified within the contract, the physician accepts Blue Shield payment as payment in full. The patient must furnish proof of income.

Indemnity Schedule

Under an Indemnity Schedule, a specific payment is allocated for each procedure performed. Beneficiaries are paid on the basis of the service received, not on the actual cost of that service. The physician may bill the patient for the difference between his fee and the Blue Shield payment. About half of Blue Shield's subscribers are covered by an indemnity program.

Relative Value Studies

Relative Value Studies do not always correspond precisely to the California RVS discussed in Chapter 2. Procedure codes and nomenclature in use by local plans vary widely. Contact your Provider/Professional Relations Representative for details about the procedure codes and nomenclature in your area.

Usual, Customary and Reasonable (UCR)

Essentially, Blue Shield's UCR program means that payment is determined by (1) ascertaining the usual fee which the doctor most frequently charges to the majority of his patients for similar services; (2) considering the doctor's geographic location and specialty; and (3) interpreting medical complications or unusual circumstances. The following definitions spell out these features in greater detail:

Usual fee: That fee normally charged for a given professional service by an individual physician to his or her patients (i.e., his or her own usual fee).

Customary fee: That fee which is in the range of usual fees charged by physicians of similar training and experience for the same services within the same specific and limited socioeconomic area.

Reasonable fee: That fee which meets the two above criteria, or by responsible medical opinion is justifiable, considering special circumstances of the particular case in question.

Example:

The prevailing charge for a specific surgical procedure ranges from $300 to $350 in this geographic location. There are no special circumstances in this case except that the patient is known to have little money for payment of her bills.

The bill sent from Dr. Cutler's office is $275. Although he usually charges $325, he is giving the patient a discount.

The bill sent from Dr. Cardi's office is $350, his usual charge.

The bill sent from Dr. Parkinson's office is $375, his customary charge.

The bill sent from Dr. Ulibarri's office is $350, although he usually charges $300.

The reasonable charge for each physician is as follows:

Dr. Cutler	$275.00	Because the reasonable charge cannot exceed the actual charge.
Dr. Cardi	$350.00	Because this is his "customary" charge and is within the prevailing range.
Dr. Parkinson	$350.00	Because the physician cannot receive more than the prevailing charge.
Dr. Ulibarri	$300.00	Because the physician cannot receive more than his usual charge.

Payments Under UCR

1. The participating physician will be paid usual, customary, or reasonable fee, and will accept this amount as *payment in full* for services rendered. Various appeal mechanisms are available to the physician for fees in question. Your local Provider/Professional Relations Representative can explain these to you.

2. Participating physicians are paid directly.

3. Payments to nonparticipating physicians vary with individual plans. Again, contact your Provider/Professional Relations Representative for further information.

4. *Copayment:* Some contracts provide for percentage (75, 80, or 90 per cent) coverage of the UCR fee. The remaining 25, 20, or 10 per cent up to the UCR maximum is the responsibility of the patient. The subject of fees should be discussed by the physician and patient before a professional service is rendered.

BLUE SHIELD PERMANENT RECIPROCITY PROGRAM

The Permanent Reciprocity Program is a method by which out-of-area claims may be paid by the Blue Shield Plan where the services are rendered. The identification

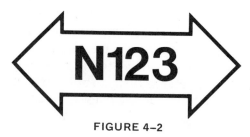

FIGURE 4–2

Blue Shield's double-end red arrow symbol: the sign of the Permanent Reciprocity Program.

cards of all patients having reciprocity coverage will show a double-end red arrow symbol containing an "N" followed by three digits (i.e., N123; see Fig. 4–2). These patients have coverage for a wide variety of services, and all data on their I.D. cards pertinent to this program are outlined in red. Physicians must bill the *local* Blue Shield Plan on the *local* Blue Shield claim form and will receive their usual, customary, or reasonable fee directly. The letter "N" and the three numbers appearing inside the red arrow must be included on the claim form, along with the identification number appearing on the Blue Shield card (i.e., N123 123-45-6789). The identification number is usually enclosed in a red box on the identification card. The numbers inside both the arrow and the box are different for each subscriber and for each Blue Shield Plan.

For those out-of-area subscribers whose cards do not bear the double-end red arrow, claims should be filed with the patient's *home plan*. (See Directory of Blue Shield Plans, pp. 82–86.) *Hospital services* rendered to out-of-state plan members should be billed to the *local Blue Cross Plan*.

Special handling is required for Medicare patients, as explained in Figure 4–3.

MEDICARE ELIGIBLE RECIPROCITY SUBSCRIBERS

Medicare recipients who are Blue Shield Reciprocity sub- scribers will carry both a red arrow card and a Medicare identi- fication card. After rendering services, include the numbers contained in the red arrow and those in the red box in the appro- priate space on the Medicare Part B Request for Payment Form.

If Your Local Blue Shield Plan IS the Medicare Part B Carrier

If the doctor accepts assignment, include the numbers in the red arrow and in the red box in the appropriate space on the Medicare Part B Request for Payment Form. Forward this form to your local Blue Shield Plan.

If Your Local Blue Shield Plan IS NOT the Medicare Part B Carrier

If the doctor accepts assignment, forward the completed Request for Payment Form to the Part B commercial insurance carrier. You and the patient will receive an Explanation of Medi- care Benefits (EOMB) from the insurance company. Either you or the patient (but not both) should file the EOMB with Blue Shield. Please include the numbers contained in the red arrow and those in the red box on the face of the patient's Blue Shield identification card when you file the claim for supplementary benefits with your local Blue Shield Plan. You will receive ap- propriate payment for both Medicare Part B and Blue Shield's covered services.

If the Doctor Does Not Accept Assignment

Please encourage your patient to file his copy of the EOMB with Blue Shield. The patient must include the numbers in the red arrow and the red box on his EOMB.

FIGURE 4–3

Special instructions for processing the claims of Medicare patients covered under the Permanent Reciprocity Program.

STANDARD BLUE SHIELD CLAIMS PROCEDURE

1. Obtain the necessary information from the patient's identification card (see Fig. 4–1):
   a. Group number.
   b. Certificate number (also known as Agreement number, Identification number, Member number, or Subscriber number). Often this is the patient's Social Security number. When the patient is a member of a federal or national group, the identification number is different. (See Federal Employee Program, p. 70, and Fig. 4–4.)
   c. Subscriber's (insured's) name and address. Sometimes this is known as member's name.

2. Blue Shield claims should be submitted no later than 30 days after the doctor's service is completed. On most contracts, Blue Shield claims received more than 1 year after service is performed are not payable. Exact time limits vary with the local plan.

3. Submit the claim on the proper Blue Shield claim form. Many Plans are now adopting the Universal or Uniform Health Insurance Claim Form (see Chapter 3). However, there will be variations on this form depending on plan area. Be sure to check with your local Blue Shield Plan office to determine the procedure in your area.

4. *Medicare and Blue Cross/Blue Shield:* Some Blue Shield or Blue Cross Plans offer a contract that supplements Medicare Part B coverage; that is, deductibles and a percentage of copay. In this instance:
   a. Bill Medicare first.
   b. Then bill Blue Shield on the Explanation of Medicare Benefits (EOMB), indicating the Blue Shield group and Subscriber Identification number on the EOMB. Submit the EOMB to the local Blue Shield plan.

FEDERAL EMPLOYEE PROGRAM (FEP)

The Commission on the Health Needs of the Nation, established by President Truman in 1951, recommended that the federal government guarantee health care insurance for its employees. In July, 1960, Blue Cross and Blue Shield founded the Federal Employee Program (FEP) for this purpose, utilizing the payroll deduction system for payment of prepaid health benefits. There are four types of plans:

1. Service Benefit Plan administered by Blue Cross and Blue Shield
2. Indemnity Benefit Plan administered by Aetna Life and Casualty Company
3. Employee Organization Plans
4. Comprehensive Medical Plans

Benefits of the Service Benefit Plan

Some of the basic benefits of this program are:

1. Inpatient hospital benefits
2. Home health care benefits in lieu of further hospitalization
3. Outpatient hospital benefits

4. In-hospital physician care during covered hospitalization, including intensive care and psychotherapy
5. Normal maternity care
6. Maternity care involving complications
7. Consultation by other than attending physician
8. Surgery and anesthesia
9. Lab, x-ray, and other diagnostic tests

Nonbenefits

These are some of the services not covered under the Federal Employee Program:

1. Annual physical or routine examination (other than initial newborn)
2. In-hospital private duty nursing
3. Dental care or treatment except that related to accidental injury
4. Hospitalization not requiring the acute facility
5. Home health care other than the intensive level
6. Charges in excess of usual, customary, and reasonable
7. Diagnostic tests unrelated to diagnosis of specific symptoms
8. Services or supplies not serving a medical purpose (primarily comfort or convenience)
9. Drugs or medications for use outside of a hospital which do not require a prescription

Claims Procedure

Persons enrolled in the FEP prior to October 1976 received a paper identification card (Fig. 4–4). Since October 1976, embossed plastic identification cards have been issued to new enrollees and as replacements for lost or stolen existing FEP cards. All federal enrollment numbers start with RO followed by eight digits. The coverage is indicated by the number 101 (which represents self only high option: only the person whose name appears on the card is covered by the contract); 102 (which means family coverage); 104 (which means self only low option); or 105 (which means family low option). This number is referred to as the enrollment code on the identification card.

Claims are submitted on a standard Blue Shield claim form. Be sure to abstract the subscriber's name, identification number, and enrollment code from the FEP card. Claims must be submitted no later than December 31 of the calendar year after the one in which the covered care or service was provided.

If the patient is receiving supplemental benefits, the Supplemental Benefits Claim Form (FSP-1) (Fig. 4–5) is completed by the patient after the annual deductible has been met. The patient attaches the physician's itemized billing statement to the FSP-1 form and sends both forms to the office of the local Blue Cross or Blue Shield Plan for processing. The FSP-1 is used for expenses that the basic plan does not cover, such as office medical care. The form must be signed by the patient, since the contract is between the Federal employee and Blue Shield. The patient should submit this form within a year of care. Payment is usually made to the subscriber. Two additional forms utilized in this program are the Private Duty Nursing Form, to report out-of-hospital nursing services, and the Mental Health Report Form, which is sent from Blue Cross or Blue Shield to a psychiatrist or psychologist to explain the patient's need for treatment of nervous and mental disorders.

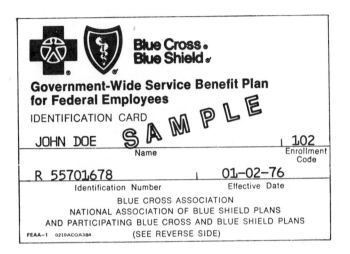

TO THE HOSPITAL OR DOCTOR
Please notify your local Blue Cross or Blue Shield Plan on its regular claim form when services are provided.

TO THE FEDERAL EMPLOYEE OR ANNUITANT
1. The Government-wide Service Benefit Plan Brochure (BRI 41-25) provides information regarding benefits of the Program and how they may be obtained.
2. Whenever you inquire about your coverage, please contact the Blue Cross or Blue Shield office serving the area where you live or work, or Blue Cross and Blue Shield Federal Employee Program, 550 12th Street, S.W., Washington, D.C. 20024. Always give your identification number and the enrollment code which appear on the face of this card.
3. Coverage normally ceases for children who marry or attain the age of 22 years. To continue protection, they should apply promptly to their local Blue Cross and Blue Shield Plan for a conversion contract.

ENROLLMENT CODES		
	HIGH OPTION	LOW OPTION
SELF ONLY	101	104
FAMILY	102	105

FIGURE 4–4

Federal Employee Program (FEP) identification card. Existing paper identification cards will continue to be valid. New enrollees will receive embossed plastic identification cards.

Blue Cross® Blue Shield®

Federal Employee Program

PLEASE TYPE OR PRINT

Supplemental Benefits Claim

FROM IDENTIFICATION CARD

ENROLLMENT CODE | IDENTIFICATION NUMBER

| 1 | 0 | 2 | | R | 5 | 5 | 7 | 0 | 1 | 6 | 7 | 8 |

1. **NAME OF PATIENT** (Last, First, and Initial)

Doe, John NMI

	Month	Day	Year	Male	Female
DATE OF BIRTH 10 | 02 | 36 SEX [X] [ ]

RELATIONSHIP OF PATIENT TO EMPLOYEE OR ANNUITANT

Self [X]   Spouse [ ]   Child [ ]   If patient's last name is different from employee's, explain relationship.

2. **DESCRIBE THE ILLNESS OR INJURY REQUIRING TREATMENT** _hypertension_

3. **WAS THE TREATMENT THE RESULT OF ACCIDENTAL INJURY**   Yes [ ]   No [X]   IF YES, GIVE DATE OF ACCIDENT   Month | Day | Year

4. **WAS ILLNESS OR INJURY IN ANYWAY WORK CONNECTED**   Yes [ ]   No [X]

5. **IS PATIENT COVERED UNDER ANY OTHER HEALTH BENEFITS PLAN HELD BY REASON OF LAW OR EMPLOYMENT (IF "YES" COMPLETE THE REMAINDER OF THIS SECTION)**   Yes [ ]   No [X]

NAME OF INSURING CO._____   ADDRESS _____

NAME OF POLICY HOLDER_____   BIRTHDATE ___ | ___ | ___   Month Day Year   SEX Male [ ] Female [ ]

RELATIONSHIP TO EMPLOYEE OR ANNUITANT   Self [ ]   Spouse [ ]   Child [ ]   TYPE OF COVERAGE (Self, Two Persons, Family, Etc.) _____

IDENTIFICATION NUMBER OF OTHER COVERAGE _____   EFFECTIVE DATE OF COVERAGE ___ | ___   Month Day Year

6. **TO BE COMPLETED REGARDLESS OF AGE OF PATIENT (SEE REVERSE SIDE FOR INSTRUCTIONS)**

IS THE PATIENT ENTITLED TO BENEFITS UNDER MEDICARE HOSPITAL INSURANCE (PART A)   Yes [ ]   EFF. ___ | ___ | ___   Month Day Year   No [X]

IS THE PATIENT ENTITLED TO BENEFITS UNDER MEDICARE MEDICAL INSURANCE (PART B)   Yes [ ]   EFF. ___ | ___ | ___   Month Day Year   No [X]

IF "YES" GIVE EFFECTIVE DATE OF ENROLLMENT FROM MEDICARE ID CARD

7. **NAME OF EMPLOYEE OR ANNUITANT** (Last, First, and Initial)

Doe, John NMI

ADDRESS (Street)

1234 South Main Street

City	State	Zip Code
Studentville,	XY	01234

I certify the above is complete and correct and that I am claiming benefits only for charges incurred by the patient named above.

Authorization is hereby given to any hospital, physician, or other provider which participated in any way in my care and treatment to release to the Blue Cross Plan or Blue Shield Plan any medical information which they in their judgment deem necessary to the adjudication of this claim.

John Doe   10-12-76

SIGNATURE OF EMPLOYEE OR ANNUITANT   DATE

WARNING - Any intentional false statement in this application or wilful misrepresentation relative thereto is a violation of the law punishable by a fine of not more than $10,000 or imprisonment of not more than 5 years, or both. (18 U.S.C. 1001.)

ITEMIZED BILLS FOR COVERED SERVICES AND SUPPLIES MUST BE ATTACHED

(See Instructions on Reverse Side)

FSP-1   0210ACOA1H4

FIGURE 4-5

Supplemental Benefits Claim Form FSP-1, used to apply for supplemental benefits from the Federal Employee Program of Blue Cross/Blue Shield.

ITEMIZED BILLS FOR COVERED SERVICES OR SUPPLIES
MUST BE ATTACHED AND THE ITEMIZED BILLS MUST CONTAIN:

NAME OF THE PERSON OR ORGANIZATION PROVIDING THE SERVICES OR SUPPLIES
NAME OF THE PATIENT RECEIVING THE SERVICES OR SUPPLIES
DATE EACH SERVICE OR SUPPLY WAS PROVIDED
CHARGE FOR EACH SERVICE OR SUPPLY
DESCRIPTION OF THE SERVICES OR SUPPLIES PROVIDED

IN ADDITION:

BILLS FOR PRIVATE DUTY NURSING SERVICE MUST SHOW THE PROFESSIONAL STATUS OF THE NURSE, SUCH AS R.N. (Registered Nurse)
BILLS FOR PRESCRIPTION DRUGS MUST SHOW THE PRESCRIPTION NUMBERS FOR EACH DRUG
BILLS FOR DRUGS & MEDICINES DISPENSED BY A PHYSICIAN MUST SHOW THE NAME OF EACH DRUG OR MEDICINE

ITEMIZED BILLS CANNOT BE RETURNED

EXAMPLE OF ITEMIZED BILL

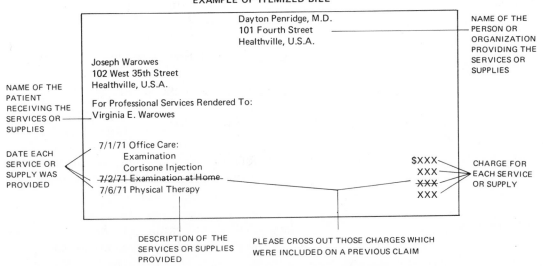

When the patient is covered under Medicare Hospital Insurance (Part A), the "Notice of Health Insurance Utilization" form furnished by the Social Security Administration (or a mechanical reproduction thereof) pertaining to charges for which benefits are claimed herein must be attached to this claim form. When the patient is covered under Medicare Medical Insurance (Part B), the "Explanation of Benefits" form furnished by the Medicare Carrier (or a mechanical reproduction thereto) pertaining to charges for which benefits are claimed herein must be attached to this claim form.

This completed form, together with itemized bills and supporting material
may be submitted to your local Blue Cross or Blue Shield Plan.

OR TO

Blue Cross and Blue Shield
Federal Employee Program
550 12th Street, S.W.
Washington, D.C. 20024
Attention: Supplemental Claims Dept.

THE GOVERNMENT WIDE SERVICE BENEFIT PLAN

CONTRACTORS: Blue Cross Association • National Association of Blue Shield Plans

FIGURE 4–5 *(Continued)*

TO THE STUDENT: Now refer to the Appendix to complete the insurance forms pertinent to this chapter. Assignments 4, 5, 6, 7, and 8, pp. 518–536, pertain to this chapter.

GLOSSARY OF BLUE CROSS AND BLUE SHIELD COMMONLY USED ABBREVIATIONS AND TERMS

AAFMC	American Association of Foundations for Medical Care (see Chapter 10)
AAMA	American Association of Medical Assistants
ACS	American College of Surgeons
ADA	American Dental Association (see Chapter 11)
Adjustments	Corrections or modifications to reflect changes in a previously submitted bill; for example, late charges.
Admitting diagnosis	The initial identification of the condition or chief complaint for which the patient is treated.
AHA	American Hospital Association
AMA	American Medical Association
AMPAC	American Medical Political Action Committee
Ancillary services	Supportive services provided by the facility other than routine hospital services.
ASIM	American Society of Internal Medicine
Assignment of benefits	An agreement signed by the insured directing the carrier to pay benefits directly to the physician.
BCA	Blue Cross Association
Beneficiary	The person named to receive benefits
BHI	Bureau of Health Insurance
Blue Shield Plan	The central office for marketing Blue Shield coverage and processing Blue Shield claims for a designated locality.

BR	By report
Carrier	An insurance company that underwrites policies which cover health care services.
CCS	Critical Care Services
CCU	Cardiovascular Care Unit
Certificate number	A number which identifies the insured.
CHAMPUS	Civilian Health and Medical Program of the Uniformed Services (see Chapter 7)
CHAP	Certified Hospital Admissions Program
CHP	Comprehensive Health Planning
Claim	A billing sent to an insurance carrier.
CLASS	Coordinated Logistic and Service Systems: credit arrangements between physicians and Blue Shield Plans which reduce paperwork and help to keep costs down.
COB	Coordination of Benefits (see Chapter 1)
Community enrollment	Special provisions that may be provided to subscribers in particular geographic areas who are not enrolled in Blue Shield through their employment groups.
Complementary benefits	Benefits designed to work together with those of another program. Medicare recipients, for example, may enroll in Blue Shield programs that pay bills not covered by Medicare.
Contract	Identifies Blue Cross or Blue Shield coverage of a patient.
Contract allowance	The maximum amount payable for a medical procedure in accordance with Blue Cross or Blue Shield coverage.
Control plan	A Blue Shield plan that negotiates and administers a contract for an organization in its area that has other employees in other states. For example, the Michigan Blue Shield Plan has a national contract for workers in the automobile industry.

CPT	Current Procedural Terminology (see Chapter 2)
CRT	Cathode Ray Tube
CRVS	California Relative Value Studies (see Chapter 2)
Daily hospital service charge	The daily charge, including room and care, nursing, meals, linen, and other commonly used services, as well as administrative costs.
dba	doing business as
Deductible	Dollar amount of covered services for which the subscriber is responsible.
DHCS	Department of Health Care Services (see Chapter 5)
Direct payment	In the context of Blue Shield, this phrase can have two meanings: (1) dues paid to a plan directly by subscribers rather than through payroll deductions; (2) payment to a physician directly by Blue Shield.
Discharge diagnosis	Description of the illness at the time of discharge.
ECF	Extended Care Facility
EDP	Electronic Data Processing
EMCRO	Experimental Medical Care Review Organization
Employment-related	An illness or injury stemming from a person's employment.
EOB	Explanation of Benefits
EOMB	Explanation of Medicare Benefits (see p. 139)
FDA	Food and Drug Administration
Fed. I.D. No.	The employer's Federal Tax Identification Number
Fee Review	See *Peer Review*

FEP	Federal Employee Program (see p. 69)
FHIP	Family Health Insurance Program
FI	Fiscal Intermediary
Financially responsible party	The person who accepts responsibility for payment of the patient's bill.
FMC	Foundation for Medical Care (see Chapter 10)
FY	Fiscal Year
HEW	Department of Health, Education and Welfare
HIAA	Health Insurance Association of America
HIBAC	Health Insurance Benefits Advisory Council
HII	Health Insurance Institute
HMO	Health Maintenance Organization (see Chapter 10)
HSA	Health Security Act
HSI	Health Service, Inc. (a wholly owned subsidiary of the Blue Cross Association)
HSMHA	Health Services and Mental Health Administration
HSO	Health Service Organization
IC	Intermediary Care
ICDA	International Classification of Diseases, adapted for use in the United States (replaced Standard Nomenclature)
ICF	Intermediate Care Facility
ICU	Intensive Care Unit
Indemnity contract	A fixed dollar amount to be applied toward the charge for specific covered services (see p. 66).
Individual consideration	A review by a committee of physicians of claims to assess special circumstances. The committee

helps to determine equitable payment and helps to protect the subscriber from additional expense.

Interim bills

Bills which are submitted while the patient is still confined.

Interplan Bank

An agreement between Blue Cross plans through which a local plan may provide benefits for any "out-of-area" Blue Cross subscriber.

Interplan transfer agreement

An agreement which permits a Blue Shield subscriber who is moving to transfer from one participating plan to another.

Itemized bill

A detailed list of all charges for services provided by a facility.

JCAH

Joint Commission on Accreditation of Hospitals

LRSP

Long Range Systems Planning: a group jointly sponsored by Blue Cross and Blue Shield and charged with development of computer systems. Its goal is to provide better service at lower cost.

LTC

Long term care

LTD

Long term disability

Medical emergency benefit

An optional benefit, available to groups, which is designed to provide coverage for treatment, on an outpatient basis, of sudden and severe medical conditions or symptoms which are or give evidence of being life-threatening. This benefit is not intended to provide coverage for office visits or routine care, but to cover care and treatment which meet the following criteria:
1. Severe symptoms occur.
2. Symptoms occur suddenly or unexpectedly.
3. Immediate care is required.
4. Immediate care is sought.

Symptoms considered to be related to Medical Emergencies include: allergic reactions, breathing difficulty or shortness of breath, chest pain, choking, coma, fainting, severe headache, hemorrhage, pain, shock, unconsciousness, severe vomiting.

Medical Record Number	A facility's internal patient identification number issued by the Medical Records Department of the hospital.
MIA	Medical Indemnity of America (a wholly owned subsidiary of the National Association of Blue Shield Plans)
MIS	Management Information System
MLHI	Maximum Liability Health Insurance
MMIS	Medical Management Information System
MPC	Medical Policy Committee
MRAD	Medical Review Administration
MSS	Medical Staff Survey
NABSP	National Association of Blue Shield Plans: a not-for-profit corporation in Chicago that acts as a national coordinating agency for local Blue Shield plans.
NAIC	National Association of Insurance Commissioners
National account	A company whose employees live in many parts of the country. Blue Shield can provide these employees with uniform coverage despite their geographic dispersion.
NCIPA	National Catastrophic Illness Protection Act
NHI	National Health Insurance
NHIPA	National Health Insurance Partnership Act
NIH	National Institutes of Health
NIMH	National Institute of Mental Health
NMA	National Medical Association
OCHAMPUS	Office of the Civilian Health and Medical Program of the Uniformed Services (see Chapter 7)
OMB	Office of Management and Budget

OSHA	Occupational Safety and Health Act (see Chapter 9)
PA	Prior Authorization
Participating physician	A physician who has agreed to accept Blue Shield's payments for services to subscribers. Eighty per cent of practicing American physicans are participating physicians.
PAT	Pre-Admission Testing
Patient Control Number	A facility's internal patient identification number issued by the Patient Accounts Office. May be the same as the Medical Record Number.
Peer Review	A review of claims or services in which local physicians participate. It is known as Fee Review when claims are questioned, and as Utilization Review when it examines possible misuse of Blue Shield benefits. Successful use of these procedures enables Blue Shield to keep down costs to subscribers.
PERS	Public Employees Retirement System
Personal charges	Charges of a nonmedical nature, such as telephone or television, incurred in the hospital.
PHP	Prepaid Health Plan (see Chapter 10)
PHS	Public Health Service
POE	Proof of Eligibility (see Chapter 5)
Primary payor	With regard to coordination of benefits, the person or insurance carrier with first-ranking responsibility for payment of a patient's bill.
Provider	One who supplies health care services
PSI	Professional Services Index
PSRO	Professional Standards Review Organization (see Chapter 10)
PUR	Plan Utilization Review (see *Peer Review*)
QAP	Quality Assurance Program (AHA's Bill)

QIT	Quality Improvement and Training
Reciprocity	Refers to Blue Shield's Permanent Reciprocity Program (see pp. 67 and 68)
RMP	Regional Medical Program
RNE	Relativity Not Established (refers to RVS units; see p. 32)
RVS codes	Relative Value Studies codes: a coding structure which may be used to identify individual services provided (see Chapter 2).
SDPH	State Department of Public Health
Secondary payor	The person or insurance carrier that pays benefits after the primary payor has discharged his obligation (see also *Coordination of Benefits* in Chapter 1).
Service Benefit Contract	A Blue Shield contract under which a participating physician agrees to accept Blue Shield's payment as payment in full for services to a subscriber whose income does not exceed a certain level. The subscriber is not required to pay any fees above Blue Shield's payment for services covered by the contract.
SMA	Schedule of Maximum Allowances
SNCFS	Skilled Nursing Care Facility Service
SNF	Skilled Nursing Facility
SSA	Social Security Administration
Subscriber	Any enrolled member of a Blue Shield or Blue Cross Plan, including: (1) the applicant or contract holder who is the person named on the membership identification card; and (2) in the case of (a) two-person coverage, (b) one adult–one child coverage, or (c) family coverage, eligible family dependents enrolled under the applicant's contract.
Summary of charges	A billing which totals detailed charges by department.
TAR	Treatment Authorization Request (see Chapter 5)

Third party payor	A carrier that has entered into an agreement with an individual or company to provide health care benefits.
TPL	Third Party Liability
UAR	Utilization, Audit and Review (see also *Peer Review*)
UCD	Unemployment Disability Compensation: a form of State Disability Insurance (SDI) which provides a daily benefit for inpatient hospitalization (see Chapter 8).
UCR	Usual, Customary and Reasonable (see pp. 66 and 67)
UR	Utilization Review (see *Peer Review*)
USPHS	United States Public Health Service
VA	Veterans' Administration
WC	Workers' Compensation (see Chapter 9)

BLUE CROSS–BLUE SHIELD DIRECTORY

National Agencies

Blue Cross Association
840 North Lake Shore Drive
Chicago, IL 60611

National Association of Blue Shield Plans
211 East Chicago Avenue
Chicago, IL 60611

Regional Blue Shield Offices

Note: Only addresses for local Blue Shield Plans are included in the following list. Except in California, the medical assistant will rarely need to file Blue Cross claims.* If she should be required to do so, she can easily obtain appropriate information from the Blue Shield Provider/Professional Relations Representative at the office in her area. Addresses in the following list are up to date as of July 1976.

---

*Blue Cross of Southern California
P.O. Box 60465
Los Angeles, CA 90060

Blue Cross of Northern California
P.O. Box 1080
Oakland, CA 94659

Alabama
Blue Cross and Blue Shield of Alabama
930 South 20th Street
Birmingham, AL 35298

Alaska
Blue Cross and Blue Shield,
   Washington-Alaska, Inc.
15700 Dayton Avenue N.
P.O. Box 327
Seattle, WA 98111 (Box);
   98133 (Street)

Arizona
Blue Shield of Arizona, Inc.
321 West Indian School Road
P.O. Box 13466
Phoenix, AZ 85002 (Box); 85013 (Street)

Arkansas
Arkansas Blue Cross and Blue Shield, Inc.
601 Gaines Street
P.O. Box 2181
Little Rock, AR 72203

California
Blue Shield of California
   (Northern California)
Two North Point
P.O. Box 3637
San Francisco, CA 94119 (Box);
   94133 (Street)

Blue Shield of California
   (Southern California)
5959 West Century Boulevard
P.O. Box 92945
Los Angeles, CA 90009 (Box);
   90045 (Street)

Colorado
Blue Shield of Colorado
(Colorado Medical Service, Inc.)
700 Broadway
Denver, CO 80203

Connecticut
Connecticut Medical Service, Inc.
Blue Shield of Connecticut
221 Whitney Avenue
New Haven, CT 06509

Delaware
Blue Cross and Blue Shield of Delaware, Inc.
201 West 14th Street
P.O. Box 1991
Wilmington, DE 19899

District of Columbia
Blue Shield Plan of the National Capital Area
(Medical Service of the District of Columbia)
550 12th Street, SW
Washington, D.C. 20024

Florida
Blue Shield of Florida, Inc.
532 Riverside Avenue
P.O. Box 1798
Jacksonville, FL 32201

Georgia
Blue Cross and Blue Shield of Georgia/
   Atlanta, Inc.
1010 West Peachtree Street, N.W.
P.O. Box 4445
Atlanta, GA 30302 (Box); 30309 (Street)

Blue Shield of Georgia/Columbus, Inc.
2357 Warm Springs Road
P.O. Box 7368
Columbus, GA 31908

Hawaii
Hawaii Medical Service Association
1504 Kapiolani Boulevard
P.O. Box 860
Honolulu, HI 96808

Idaho
Blue Shield of Idaho
(North Idaho District Medical Service
   Bureau, Inc.)
1602 21st Avenue
P.O. Box 1106
Lewiston, ID 83501

Illinois
Health Care Service Corp.
233 North Michigan Avenue
Chicago, IL 60601

Indiana
Blue Shield of Indiana
120 West Market Street
Indianapolis, IN 46204

Iowa
Blue Shield of Iowa
636 Grand Avenue
Des Moines, IA 50307

Kansas
Blue Shield of Kansas
1133 Topeka Avenue
P.O. Box 239
Topeka, KS 66601

Kentucky
Blue Shield of Kentucky
(Kentucky Physicians Mutual, Inc.)
9901 Linn Station Road
Louisville, KY 40223

Louisiana
Blue Cross of Louisiana
10225 Florida Boulevard
P.O. Box 15699
Baton Rouge, LA 70815

Maine
Maine Blue Cross and Blue Shield
110 Free Street
Portland, ME 04101

Maryland
Blue Shield of Maryland, Inc.
700 East Joppa Road
Baltimore, MD 21204

Massachusetts
Blue Shield of Massachusetts, Inc.
100 Summer Street
Boston, MA 02106

Michigan
Blue Cross and Blue Shield of Michigan
600 Lafayette East
Detroit, MI 48226

Minnesota
Blue Cross and Blue Shield of Minnesota
3535 Blue Cross Road
St. Paul, MN 55165

Mississippi
Blue Cross and Blue Shield of Mississippi, Inc.
530 East Woodrow Wilson Drive
P.O. Box 1043
Jackson, MS 39205

Missouri
Blue Shield of Kansas City
3637 Broadway
P.O. Box 169
Kansas City, MO 64141

St. Louis Blue Shield
5775 Campus Parkway
St. Louis, MO 63042

Montana
Blue Shield of Montana
(Montana Physicians' Service)
404 Fuller Avenue
P.O. Box 1677
Helena, MT 59601

Nebraska
Blue Cross and Blue Shield of Nebraska
7261 Mercy Road
P.O. Box 3248 Main Post Office Station
Omaha, NE 68180

Nevada
Nevada Blue Shield
4600 Kietzke Lane, Suite 250
P.O. Box 10330
Reno, NV 89510 (Box); 89502 (Street)

New Hampshire
New Hampshire–Vermont Physician Service
Two Pillsbury Street
Concord, NH 03301

New Jersey
Medical Surgical Plan of New Jersey
33 Washington Street
Newark, NJ 07102

New Mexico
New Mexico Blue Cross and Blue Shield, Inc.
12800 Indian School Road, N.E.
Albuquerque, NM 87112

New York
Blue Shield of Northeastern New York, Inc.
1251 New Scotland Road
Slingerlands, NY 12159
(Mailing Address) P.O. Box 8650
Albany, NY 12208

Blue Shield of Western New York, Inc.
298 Main Street
Buffalo, NY 14202

Blue Shield of Chautauqua County,
New York
(Chautauqua Region Medical Service, Inc.)
306 Spring Street
Jamestown, NY 14701

Blue Cross and Blue Shield of Greater N.Y.
622 Third Avenue
New York, NY 10017

Blue Shield of The Rochester Area
(Genesee Valley Medical Care, Inc.)
41 Chestnut Street
Rochester, NY 14647

Blue Shield of Central New York, Inc.
344 South Warren Street
Syracuse, NY 13202

Medical and Surgical Care, Inc.
5 Hopper Street
Utica, NY 13501

North Carolina
Blue Cross and Blue Shield of North Carolina
Chapel Hill–Durham Boulevard
P.O. Box 2291
Durham, NC 27702

North Dakota
Blue Shield of North Dakota
301 South 8th Street
Fargo, ND 58102

Ohio
Medical Mutual of Cleveland, Inc.
2060 East Ninth Street
Cleveland, OH 44115

Ohio Medical Indemnity, Inc.
6740 North High Street
Worthington, OH 43085

Oklahoma
Blue Cross and Blue Shield of Oklahoma
1215 South Boulder Avenue
P.O. Box 3283
Tulsa, OK 74102

Oregon
Blue Shield of Oregon
(Oregon Physicians' Service)
P.O. Box 1071
Portland, OR 97207

Pennsylvania
Pennsylvania Blue Shield
P.O. Box 62
Camp Hill, PA 17011

Puerto Rico
Seguros de Servicio de Salud de
Puerto Rico, Inc.
104 Ponce de Leon Avenue
P.O. Box "G" 3628
San Juan, PR 00936 (Box); 00919 (Street)

Rhode Island
Blue Shield of Rhode Island
444 Westminster Mall
Providence, RI 02901

South Carolina
Blue Cross and Blue Shield of South Carolina
1-20 at Alpine Road
Columbia, SC 29219

South Dakota
Blue Shield of South Dakota
(South Dakota Medical Service, Inc.)
711 North Lake Avenue
Sioux Falls, SD 57104

Tennessee
Blue Cross and Blue Shield of Tennessee
801 Pine Street
Chattanooga, TN 37402

Blue Cross and Blue Shield of Memphis
85 North Danny Thomas Boulevard
Memphis, TN 38101

Texas
Group Life and Health Insurance Company
Main at North Central Expressway
Dallas, TX 75201

Utah
Blue Shield of Utah
P.O. Box 30270
Salt Lake City, UT 84125

Vermont
New Hampshire–Vermont Physician Service
Two Pillsbury Street
Concord, NH 03301

Virginia
Blue Shield of Virginia
2015 Staples Mill Road
P.O. Box 27401
Richmond, VA 23230 (Box); 23279 (Street)

Blue Shield of Southwestern Virginia
3959 Electric Road, S.W.
P.O. Box 13047
Roanoke, VA 24045

Washington
Kitsap Physicians Service
820 Pacific Avenue
P.O. Box 339
Bremerton, WA 98310

King County Medical Blue Shield
1800 Terry Avenue
P.O. Box 21267
Seattle, WA 98111 (Box); 98101 (Street)

Washington Physicians Service
220 West Harrison Street
Seattle, WA 98119

Medical Service Corporation of Eastern
  Washington
P.O. Box 3048 Terminal Annex
Spokane, WA 99220

Pierce County Medical Bureau, Inc.
1114 Broadway
Tacoma, WA 98402

Chelan County Medical Service Corporation
517 North Mission
P.O. Box 589
Wenatchee, WA 98801

West Virginia
Surgical Service, Inc.
Commercial Bank Building
P.O. Box 131
Bluefield, WV 24701

Blue Shield of Southern West Virginia, Inc.
Commerce Square
P.O. Box 1353
Charleston, WV 25325 (Box); 25301 (Street)

Medical-Surgical Service, Inc.
Union National Bank Building
Clarksburg, WV 26301

Morgantown Medical-Surgical Service, Inc.
265 High Street
Morgantown, WV 26505

Medical-Surgical Care, Inc.
603 Union Trust Building
P.O. Box 1948
Parkersburg, WV 26101

West Virginia Medical Service, Inc.
20th at Chapline Street
P.O. Box 6246
Wheeling, WV 26003

Wisconsin
Wisconsin Physicians Service
330 East Lakeside Street
P.O. Box 1109
Madison, WI 53701

Surgical Care, The Blue Shield Plan of The
  Medical Society of Milwaukee County
756 North Milwaukee Street
Milwaukee, WI 53202

Wyoming
Blue Shield of Wyoming
4020 House Avenue
P.O. Box 2266
Cheyenne, WY 82001

AFFILIATE CANADIAN BLUE SHIELD PLANS

New Brunswick
Newfoundland
Nova Scotia
Prince Edward Island
Maritime Hospital Service Association
110 MacBeath Avenue
P.O. Box 220
Moncton, New Brunswick, Canada E1C 8L3

British Columbia
Medical Services Association
2025 West Broadway
Vancouver, British Columbia V6J 1Z6

Saskatchewan
Group Medical Services
Hamilton Plaza
1942 Hamilton Street
Regina, Saskatchewan S4P 2C6

Medical Services, Inc.
516 Second Avenue
North Saskatoon, Saskatchewan S7K 3T2

SUPPLEMENT: SPECIAL CHARACTERISTICS OF BLUE CROSS AND BLUE SHIELD IN CALIFORNIA

BLUE CROSS OF SOUTHERN CALIFORNIA

1. Members of special groups, including Trust Funds and Union Locals, must work a specified number of hours per quarter to be eligible for benefits. If in doubt about a patient's eligibility, call his or her local union office to ascertain this information.

2. Sometimes a Blue Cross member is covered under two Blue Cross contracts, a situation which is known as duplicate coverage. When this occurs, bill Blue Cross under each Coverage Code. This permits payment of the maximum amount under each coverage, up to the total amount of the fee. Notice the Coverage Code number located on the Blue Cross of Southern California membership card (Fig. 4–6).

3. *Member's Claim* (Form number 2059). Because of the vast amount of paper work in the physician's office, many insurance carriers are developing claim forms for the subscriber (insured) to complete and submit in order to obtain benefits. Blue Cross of Southern California developed the Member's Claim Form number 2059 for this purpose (see completed Figure 4–7). Part I is completed by the subscriber (insured),

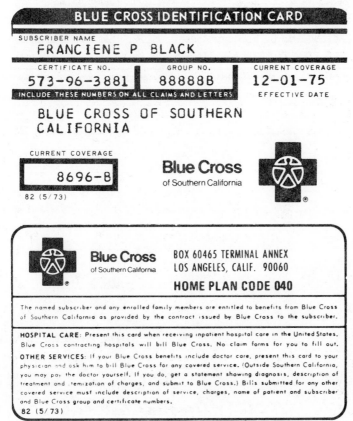

FIGURE 4–6

Sample of the Blue Cross identification card used by most Southern California Blue Cross members.

MEMBER'S CLAIM

FILL OUT A SEPARATE FORM FOR EACH BLUE CROSS MEMBER SUBMITTING BILLS FOR COVERED
SERVICES. **PLEASE PRINT OR TYPE. SEE REVERSE SIDE FOR "HOW TO USE THIS FORM."**

PART I — **IDENTIFYING INFORMATION.** Fill out completely all unshaded areas. This part identifies the patient
and/or the Subscriber. It also tells us if the patient is covered by any other company.

2 CLAIM NO.

3 GROUP NUMBER:
8 8 | 8 8 | B

4 PATIENT'S NAME: LAST	FIRST	INIT.	**5** BLUE CROSS CERTIFICATE NO.:	**6** SUBSCRIBER'S NAME AND ADDRESS: LAST	FIRST	INIT.
Black,	Franciene	P.	5 7	3 9	6 3	8 8	1	Black, Franciene		P.

7 PATIENT'S BIRTHDATE: MO. DAY YEAR	**8** PERSON NO.:	**9** S/D CODE:	**10** CORRECTED CERTIFICATE NO.:	STREET
0 1	1 8	5 4				1920 Ginger Street

11 IF INJURY, SHOW DATE: MO. DAY YEAR	PATIENT'S RELATIONSHIP TO SUBSCRIBER	X SELF ☐ SPOUSE ☐ SON ☐ DAUGHTER	CITY	STATE	ZIP
0 6 0	7 6			Oxnard	CA	93030

IS THIS ILLNESS OR INJURY EMPLOYMENT RELATED? X NO ☐ YES

13 CONTRACT CODE:

NAME OF EMPLOYER: Hi Tone Modeling Agency

DOES THE PATIENT HAVE **OTHER** HEALTH INSURANCE? ☐ NO X YES. IF YES, PLEASE COMPLETE THE FOLLOWING:

1. NAME AND ADDRESS OF OTHER HEALTH INSURANCE COMPANY Blue Cross of Southern California   2. POLICY NUMBER 570-10-6910

3. NAME OF INSURED POLICY HOLDER Dwight F. Black   4. EMPLOYER K & K Collections

IS THE PATIENT ENTITLED TO BENEFITS UNDER PART B OF MEDICARE? ☐ YES X NO

PART II — **RECORD OF HEALTH CARE SERVICES.** Use this portion to report any **covered** health service which has not already been reported
to this Blue Cross Plan by the provider of the service (the physician, clinical laboratory, ambulance company, private duty nurse,
etc.). Attach bill or a photocopy. Please be sure that duplicate bills are not submitted. (If you are covered by Medicare, please attach
the "Explanation of Medicare Benefits" which you receive from the Part B Medicare carrier.)

DATE OF SERVICE MO. DAY YR.	PROVIDER OF SERVICE (Doctor, Lab., Amb. Co., R.N., etc.)	DESCRIPTION OF SERVICES RENDERED	ILLNESS OR DIAGNOSIS	TOTAL CHARGE
06-2-76	Raymond Skelton, M. D.	Office visit	Accident-Fracture of radius	$50.00
06-2-76	Walter Radon, M. D.	X-ray rt arm	Same as above	30.00
06-2-76	Raymond Skelton, M. D.	Rt. arm cast	Same as above	20.00
06-2-76	Raymond Skelton, M. D.	crutches	Same as above	20.00
	SEE ATTACHED ITEMIZED BILLING STATEMENTS			

PART III — **RECORD OF PRESCRIPTION MEDICATIONS.** Use only if your Blue Cross coverage includes this benefit. DO **NOT** attach
pharmacy receipts.

LIST ONLY MEDICATIONS REQUIRING A WRITTEN PRESCRIPTION.

DATE OF PURCHASE MO. DAY YR.	PRESCRIBING PHYSICIAN'S NAME	NAME OF MEDICATION (PLEASE PRINT)	IDENTIFY ILLNESS FOR WHICH MEDICATION PRESCRIBED	PHARMACY CHARGES
				$
			TOTAL PRESCRIPTION CHARGES	$

I UNDERSTAND THAT I AM TO MAKE AVAILABLE UPON REQUEST THE PRESCRIPTION RECEIPTS PERTAINING TO THE ABOVE
ITEMS AND THAT THE RECEIPTS ARE TO BE RETAINED BY ME UNTIL I RECEIVE WORD THAT THIS RECORD HAS BEEN
PROCESSED BY BLUE CROSS OF SOUTHERN CALIFORNIA. I HEREBY CERTIFY THAT THE ABOVE DRUGS AND MEDICINES
WERE PRESCRIBED FOR TREATMENT OF ILLNESS OR INJURY REPORTED AND WERE PURCHASED FOR ME OR THE FAMILY
MEMBER NAMED ABOVE.

2059 9/75 170

SUBSCRIBER'S SIGNATURE ▶ *Franciene P. Black* DATE 6-16-76

FIGURE 4–7

Member's Claim. This shows a completed Member's Claim form for Southern California Blue
Cross members for use in submitting their own claims.

and Part II is completed for professional services, such as services rendered by a physician, laboratory, ambulance company, Registered Nurse, and so forth. The subscriber attaches the bill(s) from the provider(s) of service. A photocopy of the itemized billing statement should be retained by the patient. Always indicate the claim number on the retained copy. The claim number appears in red in the upper right hand corner of the form. If the patient finds it necessary to inquire about a claim, he should refer to this claim number in any correspondence with Blue Cross. If several members of a family are seen at the same time, each member must complete separate Member's Claim Forms. When the patient has Medicare and Blue Cross coverage, the patient submits the Explanation of Medicare Benefits (EOMB) with the completion of Part I of the Member's Claim Form.

Part III of the form is for prescription drugs only. Do *not* attach pharmacy receipts, but save the pharmacy receipts until the claim has been processed. The patient must always sign the completed form and date it.

4. Blue Cross of Southern California uses the Universal Claim Form. This will be found in Appendix A for the student to complete. Instructions for completion are given in Chapter 3 (pp. 57–60).

5. Obtain a current Blue Cross Manual for use in California. If the Coverage Code number is taken from the patient's identification card and the assistant looks up this number in the Manual, she will be able to ascertain some guidelines on the patient's medical coverage. However, the Coverage Code number is not necessary when completing a claim form.

BLUE SHIELD OF CALIFORNIA

Physicians may elect to become member physicians of Blue Shield of California, in which case:

1. The physician will be paid usual and customary fees and accepts these as *payment in full* for services rendered.

2. The physician will be paid directly, regardless of assignment of benefits.

3. Mandatory arbitration is written into the Blue Shield contracts to protect both physician and patient. (For an explanation of arbitration, see Chapter 14, p. 415.)

Physicians who bill Blue Shield and who are *not* member physicians fall under these guidelines:

1. The physician will be paid the reasonable fee.

2. The payment will go directly to the patient, regardless of assignment of benefits.

3. The physician must collect the entire amount of the bill directly from the patient.

Provider Number

In California a Provider Number is issued to member physicians by Blue Shield. Insurance forms are then supplied to the physician preimprinted with the name and address of the physician or supplier along with the special coding. To help you to understand the coding, an example is supplied here for R.W. Jones, M.D., in Los Angeles, California.

DEGREE	COUNTY CODE	AMA SPECIALTY	STATUS	1ST TWO DIGITS OF NAME	PROVIDER NUMBER	PROVIDER TYPE
MD	19	27	P	JO	00A88880	20

The County Code number "19" as shown above means Los Angeles County. The AMA Specialty Code number "27" means Dr. Jones is a General Practitioner. In reordering preimprinted forms the medical assistant must be certain that this coding structure is absolutely accurate before submitting any claims, or computer errors will occur in the processing of the claims. The following is the AMA Specialty List of code numbers. These classifications are used in building prevailing charge profiles. In some instances, separate specialties have been grouped together for profile purposes.

- (06) Allergy and Pediatric Allergy
- (09) Anesthesiology
- (15) Cardiovascular Disease and (66) Pediatric Cardiology
- Chiropracty
- (78) Colon and Rectal Surgery (Proctology)
- Dentistry
- (21) Dermatology
- (27) Family Practice
- (24) Gastroenterology
- (27) General Practice
- (30) General Surgery and Peripheral Vascular Disease
- (33) Internal Medicine, (12) Aviation Medicine,
  (33) Geriatrics, and (75) Preventive Medicine
- (96) Nephrology
- (36) Neurological Surgery
- (39) Neurology
- (42) Obstetrics and Gynecology
- (51) Orthopedic Surgery and (30) Hand Surgery
- (54) Otology, Laryngology, Rhinology
- (22) Pathology and (57) Pathologic Anatomy
- (60) Pediatrics
- (69) Physical Medicine and Rehabilitation
- (72) Plastic Surgery
- Podiatry
- (81) Psychiatry and (18) Child Psychiatry
- (87) Radiology, Roentgenology, and (91) Radiation Therapy
- (92) Thoracic Surgery
- (96) Urology
- (99) Miscellaneous — Physicians, Public Health Clinics,
  Public Health (Welfare) Agencies, Voluntary Health
  Agencies, and (03) Administrative Medicine

MC-163 Blue Shield of California Claim Form

There are some differences in completing the MC-163 Blue Shield claim form when submitting the claim for a standard Blue Shield case in contrast to a patient who is on the Medi-Cal program. For example, the physician's signature is *not* required on the form for a Standard Blue Shield case. See Chapter 5 for complete details on how to complete this form.

1. Name four important pieces of information to obtain from the patient's Blue Cross or Blue Shield cards.

    a. _____

    b. _____

    c. _____

    d. _____

2. What is the usual time limit for submitting a Blue Shield claim? _____

3. Blue Shield may be the fiscal agent or intermediary for what federal and state programs? _____

4. What are the four types of Blue Shield contracts?

    a. _____

    b. _____

    c. _____

    d. _____

5. If a Blue Shield subscriber from out of state comes for treatment with the double-end red arrow symbol on his card, how do you handle the bill? _____

_____

_____

6. Did Blue Shield start as a not-for-profit hospital insurance plan or as a not-for-profit physician fee plan? _____

7. What do these abbreviations mean?

    SMA _____   COB _____

    UCR _____   FEP _____

    ICDA _____   EOMB _____

8. Explain the terms usual, customary and reasonable.

a. Usual means: _____

_____

b. Customary means: _____

_____

c. Reasonable means: _____

_____

9. Where do you submit Blue Shield claims for out-of-area patients whose cards do not bear the double-end red arrow? _____

_____

10. Identify the following federal enrollment code numbers:

101 _____

102 _____

104 _____

105 _____

11. How do you identify national account numbers? _____

_____

12. Under a contract in which the patient has both Blue Shield and Blue Cross coverage, Blue Cross pays for _____ services and Blue Shield pays for _____ services.

Blue Cross–Blue Shield of California

1. If a physician is a Physician Member of Blue Shield, what fee is he or she entitled to? _____

2. If a physician is not a Physician Member of Blue Shield, what fee is he or she entitled to? _____

3. Is the signature of the physician submitting the claim required on the MC-163 form for a Standard Blue Shield claim in California? _____

4. If a patient is a union worker and has Blue Cross coverage, what is important to remember in regard to eligibility for benefits? _____

_____

Notes:

5
Medicaid and Medi-Cal

BEHAVIORAL

OBJECTIVES   *The Assistant should be able to:*

1. Understand the benefits and nonbenefits of Medicaid and Medi-Cal.
2. Know the differences among the various state Medicaid programs.
3. Develop an understanding of the terminology inherent to Medicaid and Medi-Cal programs.
4. Become familiar with two state programs and how claims are processed from a physician's office.
5. Learn who is eligible for the Medicaid program.
6. Minimize the number of insurance forms rejected because of improper completion.
7. Define Medicaid and Medi-Cal abbreviations.
8. Learn what is important information to abstract from the patient's Medicaid card.

MEDICAID

Medicaid is a plan sponsored by both federal and state governments. Coverage and benefits vary widely from state to state. To obtain up-to-date information and details on the Medicaid program in your state, write or telephone your state agency as shown on pages 97 through 104. Each state designs its own Medicaid program within federal guidelines. Individual physicians are also likely to have their own office procedures for handling Medicaid patients. Medicaid is part of the Social Security Act, Title 19. The Medical Services Administration of the Social and Rehabilitation Service of the United States Department of Health, Education and Welfare is responsible for the federal aspects of Medicaid. Medicaid is not so much an insurance program as it is an assistance program. In the State of California this program is known as Medi-Cal. Arizona is the only state that does not have this program.

ELIGIBILITY

Medicaid is for certain needy and low-income people, such as the aged (65 years or older), the blind, the disabled, members of families with dependent children, and some other children. Some states also include, at state expense, other needy and low-income people, such as those who are medically needy (MN). Funds from federal, state, and local taxes pay medical bills for eligible people. Eligibility requirements vary widely from state to state.

These 32 Medicaid programs cover people who are eligible for Aid to Families with Dependent Children (AFDC) and Supplemental Security Income (SSI), as well as some other low-income people, such as Medically Needy.

Arkansas	Kentucky	*New Hampshire	Tennessee
California	Maine	New York	*Utah
*Connecticut	Maryland	*North Carolina	Vermont
District of Columbia	Massachusetts	North Dakota	Virgin Islands
Guam	Michigan	*Oklahoma	Virginia
*Hawaii	*Minnesota	Pennsylvania	Washington
*Illinois	Montana	Puerto Rico	West Virginia
Kansas	*Nebraska	Rhode Island	Wisconsin

These 21 Medicaid programs cover only people who are eligible for Aid to Families with Dependent Children (AFDC) and Supplemental Security Income (SSI).

Alabama	Idaho	Nevada	South Dakota
Alaska	*Indiana	New Jersey	Texas
*Colorado	Iowa	New Mexico	Wyoming
Delaware	Louisiana	*Ohio	
Florida	*Mississippi	Oregon	
Georgia	*Missouri	South Carolina	

*These states do not use national Supplemental Security Income (SSI) standards for age, disability, income, and resources to determine Medicaid eligibility. They use their own standards, which are usually stricter.

BENEFITS

Medicaid pays for:

Inpatient hospital care
Outpatient hospital services
Laboratory and x-ray services
Skilled nursing facility services
Physicians' services
Screening, diagnosis, and treatment of children under 21
Home health care services
Family planning services

In some states additional services are also included, such as:

Dental care
Prescription drugs
Eyeglasses and eye refractions
Clinic services
Intermediate care facility services

Other diagnostic, screening, preventive, and rehabilitative services
Cosmetic procedures
Psychiatric services
Podiatry services
Allergy services
Dermatology services

Another benefit of the Medicaid program is the Early and Periodic Screening, Diagnosis, and Treatment (EPSDT) service. This is a program of prevention, early detection, and treatment of welfare children. The EPSDT guidlines include taking a medical history and performing a physical examination; immunization status assessment; dental, hearing, and vision screening; developmental assessment; and screening for anemia and lead absorption, tuberculosis, bacteruria, and sickle cell disease and trait.

CLAIM PROCEDURE

A Medicaid plastic or paper card (or in some states coupons) is usually issued monthly. However, under certain classifications of eligibility, identification cards are issued in some states on the first and fifteenth of each month, every two months, every three months, or every six months. When professional services are rendered, the card must show eligibility for the month of service. Some states issue cards that contain sticky labels, and a label must be used on the billing claim for payment. In other states a physician bills a fiscal intermediary, which might be an insurance company, or in some states the bill is rendered directly to the local Department of Social Services.

Many times prior authorization is required for various services, except in a bona fide emergency. Forms are usually completed to obtain authorization for a specific service or for hospitalization of a patient. If prior authorization is required immediately, a telephone call to the proper department in your locale can obtain this approval, but usually the proper form must be sent in to follow up the telephone call.

After a service has been rendered, each state has a time limit as to the submission of a claim. The time limit can vary from 2 months from the date that the service was rendered to 1 year. If a bill is submitted after the time limit, it can be rejected, unless there is some valid justification given that the state recognizes. Prescription drugs and dental services are sometimes billed to a different intermediary than services performed by an M.D., depending on the state guidelines.

STATE MEDICAID DIRECTORY

The following list gives addresses for the various single state agencies and state medical assistance units, as of September 1975. For further information regarding your state, write to the appropriate authority.

Alabama
State Health Officer
Alabama Dept. of Public Health
2500 Fairlane Drive
Montgomery, AL 36104

Director, Medical Services Admin.
Alabama Dept. of Public Health
2500 Fairlane Drive
Montgomery, AL 36104

Alaska
Commissioner,
Dept. of Health & Social Service
Pouch H
Juneau, AK 99801

Director,
Division of Medical Assistance
Dept. of Health & Social Service
Pouch H
Juneau, AK 99801

Arizona
Deputy Director
Dept. of Health Services
State Department Bldg.
1740 W. Adams Street
Phoenix, AZ 85001

Assistant Director
Dept. of Health Services
Division of Medical Assistance
State Department Bldg.
1740 W. Adams Street
Phoenix, AZ 85001

Arkansas
Commissioner
Arkansas Social Services
P.O. Box 1437
Little Rock, AR 72201

Director, Medical Care Division
Arkansas Social Services
P.O. Box 1437
Little Rock, AR 72201

California
Director, Dept. of Health
714 P Street
Office Bldg. No. 8
Sacramento, CA 95814

Acting Deputy Director
Health Care Services, Dept. of Health
714 P Street
Office Bldg. No. 8
Sacramento, CA 95814

Manager, Medi-Cal Division
Dept. of Health
714 P Street
Sacramento, CA 95814

Colorado
Executive Director
Dept. of Social Services
1575 Sherman Street
Denver, CO 80203

Director,
Division of Medical Assistance
Dept. of Social Services, Suite 1004
700 Broadway
Denver, CO 80203

Connecticut
Commissioner, State Welfare Dept.
1000 Asylum Avenue
Hartford, CT 06105

Director of Health Services
State Welfare Dept.
1000 Asylum Avenue
Hartford, CT 06105

Delaware
Secretary
Dept. of Health and Social Services
P.O. Box 309
Wilmington, DE 19899

Assistant Director
Division of Social Services
Dept. of Health and Social Services
P.O. Box 309
Wilmington, DE 19899

Chief, Medical Social Work Consultant
Division of Social Services
Dept. of Health and Social Services
P.O. Box 309
Wilmington, DE 19899

District of Columbia
Director, Dept. of Human Resources
District Bldg., Rm. 406
Washington, D.C. 20004

Director, Medical Assistance
Dept. of Human Resources
14th & E Streets, N.W.
Washington, D.C. 20004

Florida
Secretary
Dept. of Health & Rehabilitation Services
1323 Winewood Blvd.
Tallahassee, FL 32301

Director, Division of Family Services
Dept. of Health & Rehabilitation Services
P.O. Box 2050
Jacksonville, FL 32203

Chief, Bureau of Medical Services
Dept. of Health & Rehabilitation Services
P.O. Box 2050
Jacksonville, FL 32203

Georgia
Acting Commissioner
Georgia Dept. of Human Resources
State Office Bldg.
Atlanta, GA 30334

Director, Division of Benefits Payments
Georgia Dept. of Human Resources
State Office Bldg.
Atlanta, GA 30334

Guam
Director,
Dept. of Public Health & Social Service
Government of Guam
P.O. Box 2816
Agana, GU 96910

Director, Medical Care Service
Dept. of Public Health & Social Service
Government of Guam
P.O. Box 2719
Agana, GU 96910

Hawaii
Director,
Dept. of Social Service & Housing
P.O. Box 339
Honolulu, HI 96809

Medical Care Administrator
Division of Public Welfare
Dept. of Social Service & Housing
P.O. Box 339
Honolulu, HI 96809

Idaho
Administrator,
Dept. of Health & Welfare
State House
Boise, ID 83720

Director of Medical Assistance
Assistance Payments Division
Department of Health & Welfare
State House
Boise, ID 83720

Illinois
Director, Dept. of Public Aid
618 E. Washington Street
Springfield, IL 62706

Chief, Systems & Medicaid
Division of Medical Service
Dept. of Public Aid
Room 900, 209 West Jackson Blvd.
Chicago, IL 60606

Chief, Medical Admin.
Div. of Medical Service
Dept. of Public Aid
425 S. Fourth Street
Springfield, IL 62706

Indiana
Administrator
Indiana State Dept. of Public Welfare
100 N. Senate Avenue, Rm. 701
Indianapolis, IN 46204

Chief Medical Director
Indiana State Dept. of Public Welfare
100 N. Senate Avenue, Rm. 701
Indianapolis, IN 46204

Assistant Admin. for Medical Assistance
Indiana State Dept. of Public Welfare
100 N. Senate Avenue, Rm. 701
Indianapolis, IN 46204

Iowa
Commissioner
Iowa Dept. of Social Service
Lucas State Office Bldg.
Des Moines, IA 50319

Director, Bureau of Medical Services
Iowa Dept. of Social Service
Lucas State Office Bldg.
Des Moines, IA 50319

Kansas
State Director of Social Welfare
State Dept. of Social Welfare
State Office Bldg.
Topeka, KS 66612

Director, Div. of Medical Services
State Dept. of Social Welfare
State Office Bldg.
Topeka, KS 66612

Kentucky
Secretary, Dept. Human Resources
Capitol Annex
Frankfort, KY 40601

Director, Division of Disability
Determination & Medical Assistance
Dept. for Human Resources
Capitol Annex
Frankfort, KY 40601

Louisiana
Commissioner, Dept. of Public Welfare
P.O. Box 44065
Baton Rouge, LA 70804

Director, Medical Services Division
Dept. of Public Welfare
P.O. Box 44215
Baton Rouge, LA 70804

Maine
Commissioner, Dept. of Health & Welfare
State House
Augusta, ME 04330

Manager, Medical Assistance
Unit, Bureau of Social Welfare
Dept. of Health & Welfare
State House
Augusta, ME 04330

Maryland
Secretary,
Dept. of Health & Mental Hygiene
301 W. Preston Street
Baltimore, MD 21201

Director, Division of Medical Care
Programs Administration
Dept. of Health & Mental Hygiene
301 W. Preston Street
Baltimore, MD 21201

Assistant Secretary for
Medical Care Programs
Dept. of Health & Mental Hygiene
301 W. Preston Street
Baltimore, MD 21201

Massachusetts
Commissioner, Dept. of Public Welfare
600 Washington Street
Boston, MA 02111

Asst. Commissioner for
Medical Assistance
Dept. of Public Welfare
600 Washington Street
Boston, MA 02111

Commissioner
Massachusetts Commission for the Blind
39 Boylston Street
Boston, MA 02116

Michigan
Director
Michigan Dept. of Social Services
Commerce Center Bldg.
300 South Capitol Avenue
Lansing, MI 48926

Chief Deputy,
Michigan Dept. of Social Services
300 South Capitol Avenue
Lansing, MI 48926

Chief, Medical Assistance Program
Michigan Dept. of Social Services
300 South Capitol Avenue
Lansing, MI 48926

Minnesota
Commissioner, Dept. of Public Welfare
Centennial Office Bldg.
658 Cedar Street
St. Paul, MN 55101

Director, Medical Assistance
Dept. of Public Welfare
Centennial Office Bldg.
658 Cedar Street
St. Paul, MN 55101

Supervisor, Medical Assistance
Dept. of Public Welfare
Centennial Office Bldg.
658 Cedar Street
St. Paul, MN 55101

Mississippi
Acting Director
Mississippi Medicaid Commission
Room 313, Dale Bldg.
2906 N. State Street
Jackson, MS 39216
(Single State Agency and Medical
Assistance Unit are the same)

Missouri
Director, Dept. of Social Services
Broadway State Office Bldg.
Jefferson City, MO 65101

Director,
Division of Family Services
Dept. of Social Services
Broadway State Office Bldg.
Jefferson City, MO 65101

Chief, Bureau of Medical Services
Dept. of Social Services
Broadway State Office Bldg.
Jefferson City, MO 65101

Montana
Director,
Dept. of Social & Rehabilitation Services
P.O. Box 1723
Helena, MT 59601

Chief, Medical Assistance Bureau
Economic Assistance Division
Dept. of Social & Rehabilitation Service
P.O. Box 1723
Helena, MT 59601

Nebraska
Director, State Dept. of Public Welfare
1526 K Street, 4th Floor
Lincoln, NE 68508

Chief, Medical Services
State Dept. of Public Welfare
1526 K Street, 4th Floor
Lincoln, NE 68508

Nevada
Administrator, Welfare Division
Dept. of Human Resources
251 Jeanelle Drive
Carson City, NV 89701

Chief, Medical Services
Welfare Division
Dept. of Human Resources
251 Jeanelle Drive
Carson City, NV 89701

New Hampshire
Director, Division of Welfare
8 Loudon Street
Concord, NH 03301

Assistant Director for Medical Services
Division of Welfare
Dept. of Health & Welfare
State House Annex
Concord, NH 03301

New Jersey
Commissioner
Dept. of Institutions & Agencies
135 West Hanover
Trenton, NJ 08625

Director, Division of
Medical Assistance & Health Services
New Jersey Dept. of Institutions
& Agencies
324 East State Street
Trenton, NJ 08608

New Mexico
Executive Director
New Mexico Health & Social Service Dept.
P.O. Box 2348
Sante Fe, NM 87501

Director, Medical Assistance Division
New Mexico Health & Social Service Dept.
P.O. Box 2348
Santa Fe, NM 87501

New York
Commissioner
State Dept. of Social Services
1450 Western Avenue
Albany, NY 12203

Deputy Commissioner
Division of Medical Assistance
New York State Dept. of Social Services
1450 Western Avenue
Albany, NY 12203

North Carolina
Director, Division of Social Services
State Dept. of Human Resources
P.O. Box 2599
Raleigh, NC 27602

Director, Division of Medical Services
State Dept. of Human Resources
P.O. Box 2599
Raleigh, NC 27602

North Dakota
Executive Director
Social Service Board of North Dakota
State Capitol Bldg.
Bismarck, ND 58501

Director, Medical Services
Social Service Board of North Dakota
State Capitol Bldg.
Bismarck, ND 58501

Ohio
Director, Ohio Dept. of Public Welfare
408 Town Street
Columbus, OH 43215

Director, Income Maintenance
Division of Medical Assistance
Ohio Dept. of Public Welfare
30 E. Broad Street, 31st Floor
Columbus, OH 43215

Oklahoma
Director, Dept. of Institutions
Social & Rehabilitation Service
P.O. Box 25352
Oklahoma City, OK 73125

Director, Medical Services Division
Dept. of Institutions
Social & Rehabilitation Service
P.O. Box 25352
Oklahoma City, OK 73125

Oregon
Director, Dept. of Human Resources
318 Public Service Bldg.
Salem, OR 97310

Medical Director
Medical Assistance Section, Public Welfare
Division, Dept. of Human Resources
400 Public Service Bldg.
Salem, OR 97310

Pennsylvania
Secretary,
State Dept. of Public Welfare
Health & Welfare Bldg.
Harrisburg, PA 17120

Commissioner for Medical Programs
Dept. of Public Welfare
Health & Welfare Bldg.
Harrisburg, PA 17120

Director,
Bureau of Medical Assistance
Dept. of Public Welfare
Health & Welfare Bldg.
Harrisburg, PA 17120

Puerto Rico
Secretary of Health
Department of Health
P.O. Box 9342
Santurce, PR 00908

Coordinator of Medicaid Program
Department of Health
P.O. Box 10037
Caparra Heights Station
Rio Piedras, PR 00922

Director,
Medical Assistance Program
Department of Health
P.O. Box 10037
Caparra Heights Station
Rio Piedras, PR 00922

Rhode Island
Director,
Dept. of Social & Rehabilitation Service
Aime J. Forand Bldg.
600 New London Avenue
Cranston, RI 02920

Medical Director
Dept. of Social & Rehabilitation Service
Aime J. Forand Bldg.
600 New London Avenue
Cranston, RI 02920

South Carolina
Commissioner
State Dept. of Social Services
P.O. Box 1520
Columbia, SC 29202

Director, Division of Medical Assistance
State Dept. of Social Services
P.O. Box 1520
Columbia, SC 29202

South Dakota
Director, Division of Social Welfare
Dept. of Social Services
State Office Bldg. #1
Pierre, SD 57501

Senior Program Specialist, Division of
   Social Welfare, Dept. of Social Services
Dept. of Medical Services
State Office Bldg. #1
Pierre, SD 57501

Tennessee
Commissioner
State Dept. of Public Health
344 Cordell Hull Bldg.
Nashville, TN 37219

Deputy Commissioner
Bureau of Medical Care Services
State of Tennessee Dept. of Public Health
344 Cordell Hull Bldg.
Nashville, TN 37219

Texas
Commissioner
State Dept. of Public Welfare
John H. Reagan Bldg.
Austin, TX 78701

Deputy Commissioner for
   Medical Administration
Dept. of Public Welfare
John H. Reagan Bldg.
Austin, TX 78701

Utah
Executive Director
Dept. of Social Services
211 State Capitol
Salt Lake City, UT 84111

Office of Medical Services
Dept. of Social Services
211 State Capitol
Salt Lake City, UT 84111

Vermont
Commissioner
Dept. of Social Welfare
State Office Bldg.
Montpelier, VT 05602

Director of Medical Care
Dept. of Social Welfare
State Office Bldg.
Montpelier, VT 05602

Virginia
Commissioner, State Dept. of Health
109 Governor Street
Richmond, VA 23219

Director, Medical Assistance Program
State Dept. of Health
109 Governor Street
Richmond, VA 23219

Virgin Islands
Commissioner of Health
Virgin Islands Dept. of Health
Charlotte Amalie
St. Thomas, VI 00801

Director, Bureau of Health Insurance &
   Medical Assistance
Virgin Islands Dept. of Health
Franklin Bldg.
Charlotte Amalie
St. Thomas, VI 00801

Washington
Secretary
Dept. of Social & Health Service
P.O. Box 1788
Olympia, WA 98504

Chief,
Office of Personal Health Service
Health Service Division
Dept. of Social & Health Service
P.O. Box 1788
Olympia, WA 98504

West Virginia
Commissioner, Dept. of Welfare
1900 Washington Street, East
Charleston, WV 25305

Director, Division of Medical Care
Dept. of Welfare
1900 Washington Street, East
Charleston, WV 25305

Wisconsin
Secretary
Wisconsin Dept. of Health & Social Service
One West Wilson Street
Madison, WI 53702

Administrator, Income Maintenance
Wisconsin Dept. of Health & Social Service
One West Wilson Street
Madison, WI 53702

Director of Medical Services
Division of Family Service
Wisconsin Dept. of Health & Social Services
One West Wilson Street
Madison, WI 53702

Wyoming

Administrator,
Division of Health & Medical Services
Dept. of Health & Social Service
State Office Bldg.
Cheyenne, WY 82001

Director, Medical Assistance Services
Division of Health & Social Services
Dept. of Health & Social Service
State Office Bldg.
Cheyenne, WY 82001

MEDICAID—NEW YORK

To give you an idea of how a few of the Medicaid programs operate, New York and California have been chosen as examples. The following will give you the details of these plans.

ELIGIBILITY

The following groups are eligible for Medicaid in New York:

1. Persons on welfare.
2. Persons receiving Supplemental Security Income (SSI) benefits, with certain exceptions.
3. Medically needy persons who are:
   a. Under 21 years of age (or over, in some special cases).
   b. Blind or disabled.
   c. Members of families in which one or both parents are dead, absent from the home, or incapacitated, or in which the father is unemployed.
4. Persons, other than those listed above, who are stricken with catastrophic illness can be helped with hospital bills and bills for physicians' services given in hospitals when those costs exceed 25 per cent of their income. (For more on catastrophic insurance, see Chapter 1, p. 6.)

BENEFITS

The following services, care, and supplies are paid by New York Medicaid:

1. Necessary services provided by physicians, dentists, optometrists, podiatrists, chiropractors, and other professional personnel.
2. Care, treatment, maintenance, and nursing services in hospitals, nursing homes, infirmaries, or other medical institutions, including the hospital or nursing home sections of public institutions operated for the care of the mentally retarded.
3. Outpatient or clinic services.
4. Home health care services, including home nursing services and services of home health aides.
5. Drugs, sickroom supplies, eyeglasses, and prosthetic appliances.
6. In catastrophic illness, in-hospital services are covered.

IDENTIFICATION CARD

The local social service department may issue a DSS-495A "Medical Identification Card," which is effective up to a period of 6 months in certain cases (see Fig. 5–1). However, in most cases, identification cards are issued on a monthly basis. The cards show "A," "C," or "D" coverage. Cards for individuals and families receiving or eligible for public assistance show "A" coverage. Cards for all others will also show "A" coverage, except that in some cases, the parents of minor children who are fully employed will have "C" or "D" coverage. Under "A" coverage the patient is entitled to all Medicaid benefits. Under "C" and "D" coverage, inpatient services in a medical institution, such as a hospital, are available.

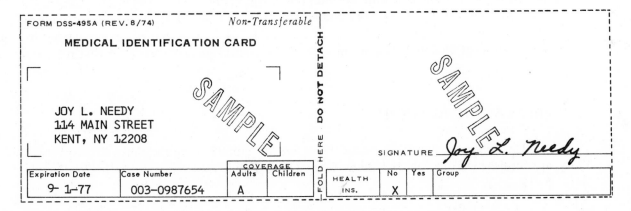

FRONT

BACK

FIGURE 5–1

Form DSS-495A. Sample of a New York Medicaid card, showing both front and back sides.

HOW TO FILE A CLAIM

There is no fiscal intermediary under New York State's Medicaid program. Physicians and providers of services may forward bills or state vouchers directly to the 58 local social services departments (see pp. 112 and 113), who in turn process the bills and execute payment directly to the physician. The provider may submit an original and one copy of Form DSS-376 Payment Request — Medical Assistance Program (see Fig. 5–2). The local social service department then files a claim with the State Department of Social Services Central Office for the federal and state portions of these expenditures.

The only exception to this process would be when billing for services rendered to Family Care patients, and in this type of case the Medical Assistant should complete the State Voucher for Public Assistance, Form DSS-196 (Fig. 5–3). If a Medicaid patient is to be admitted to the hospital under the Family Care program, the hospital is required to notify the New York State Department of Social Services within 5 days of such admission, Saturdays, Sundays, and legal holidays excluded. Form DSS-436, Notification of Hospital Admission (Fig. 5–4), should be completed for that purpose.

PRIOR AUTHORIZATION

The following specified medical services or supplies require approval before they are furnished. Complete the State Voucher for Public Assistance, Form DSS-196 (Fig. 5–3).

1. Ambulance transportation or coach service for the disabled (invalid coach service) outside New York State.

2. Prosthetic appliances, and their repair or replacement, costing more than $40 when ordered by a physician other than a qualified orthopedic physician, a qualified surgeon, or a qualified physiatrist require prior approval.

3. Tinted, case-hardened, or contact lenses; artificial eyes; orthoptic training; frames with a wholesale cost in excess of $4.

4. Nursing service provided in the home by a private practicing Registered Nurse (RN) or a Licensed Practical Nurse (LPN), except in emergencies, when the physician may order service of the nurse for no more than 2 nursing days.

5. Foot mold, balance, inlay support, or any procedure not included in the "Maximum Reimbursable Fee Schedule for Podiatrists."

6. Services provided by a qualified private practicing therapist.

7. All dental services, except those listed below, require prior approval. Requests must be accompanied by x-rays.

    a. Oral examination and oral prophylaxis.

    b. Restoration of carious permanent and primary teeth with silver amalgam, silicate cement, plastic materials, or stainless steel crowns.

    c. Pulp capping or pulpotomy; pulp therapy for single-rooted teeth. If more that one tooth requires complete pulp therapy, prior approval is required.

    d. Extraction of nonrestorable teeth. If multiple extractions are recommended and dental prosthesis is needed, prior approval is necessary.

    e. Other services required in giving emergency care or for the relief of pain or acute infection.

TO APPEAL A DECISION

If an applicant or recipient of Medicaid is dissatisfied with a decision made by his or her local department of social services, he or she may appeal to the State Department of Social Services for a review of the case. Telephone, visit, or write to the nearest office as listed below:

Albany	74 State Street Albany, NY 12201 Tel: 518/474-4142
Buffalo	125 Main Street Buffalo, NY 14203 Tel: 716/842-4377
New York City	80 Centre Street New York, NY 10013 Tel: 212/488-6550
Rochester	36 West Main Street Rochester, NY 14203 Tel: 716/454-4272
Syracuse	333 East Washington Street Syracuse, NY 13202 Tel: 315/473-8415

INSTRUCTIONS FOR COMPLETING PAYMENT REQUEST — NEW YORK MEDICAL ASSISTANCE PROGRAM FORM DDS-376 (Fig. 5–2)

Submit two copies of this completed form to the Social Security District office in your locale.

1. Give the first name, middle initial, and last name of the attending physician.
2. Enter the physician's professional license number or vendor number provided by the Social Security District.
3. State the physician's street or mailing address.
4. State the physician's city, state, and ZIP code.
5. Enter the name and address of the appropriate Social Service Department in your county (see pp. 112 and 113).
6. This form must be signed by the physician.
7. Enter the date the form was prepared.
8. Enter inclusive dates of payment request for services or supplies provided to the patient or Medicaid recipient.
9. Enter the patient's Medicaid identification card number.
10. List the name of each patient alphabetically, showing last name first. (This will not necessarily be the name that appears on the Medicaid identification card.)
11. Indicate A or B type of coverage. This indication appears on the Medicaid identification card. A means 100 per cent coverage. B means 20 per cent cost-sharing.
12. Enter the age of the patient.
13. Enter the date that each service was rendered.

FORM DSS-376 (REV. 12/74) (FACE)

PAYMENT REQUEST - MEDICAL ASSISTANCE PROGRAM

STATE OF NEW YORK   DEPARTMENT OF SOCIAL SERVICES

BILL ON THIS FORM FOR ALL MEDICAL SERVICES AND SUPPLIES EXCEPT DRUGS AND DENTAL CARE

NAME OF PROVIDER (1)	IDENTIFICATION NO. (2)

Page 1 of _____ pages

ADDRESS (3)

CITY - STATE - ZIP (4)

I certify that the care, services and supplies itemized have been furnished; the amounts listed are due and, except as noted, no part thereof has been paid, payment of fees made in accordance with established schedules is accepted as payment in full; and there has been compliance with Title VI of the Federal Civil Rights Act of 1964 without discrimination on the basis of race, color or national origin; that such records as are necessary to disclose fully the extent of care, services and supplies provided to individuals under the New York State Medicaid Program will be kept, and information will be furnished regarding any payment claimed therefore as the local social services agency or the State Department of Social Services may request; and that the vendor understands that payment and satisfaction of this claim will be from Federal, State and local public funds and that he may be prosecuted under applicable Federal and State laws for any false claims, statements, or documents or concealment of a material fact.

BILL TO:
SOCIAL SERVICES DISTRICT (5)

Signature of Provider _____ (6) _____ Date ___ (7) ___

Period covered by this Payment Request _____ (8)

PATIENT ID NUMBER	NAME OF PATIENT	C O V	AGE	DATE OF EACH SERVICE	SERVICES - SUPPLIES			FEE SCHED CODE	AMOUNT CHARGED	PAID BY INS. OR OTHER	AMOUNT BILLED S.S.D.	AGENCY USE	
					PLACE *	DIAGNOSIS	SERVICES OR SUPPLIES FURNISHED						
(9)	(10)	(11)	(12)	(13)	(14)			(15)	(16)	(17)	(18)		

* HOME = H
OFFICE = O
HOSPITAL = HSP

APPROVED BY _____

AUDITED BY _____

| PAGE TOTALS | (19) |
| GRAND TOTALS (If more than 1 page) | |

CHECK NO. _____ DATE _____

FIGURE 5–2

Form DSS-376, Payment Request—Medical Assistance Program. Used for billing the Social Security Department in New York for recipients of the Medicaid program.

14. Enter the place the service was rendered, such as H = home, 0 = office, HSP = hospital. Give the diagnosis and enter the description for the services or supplies rendered to the Medicaid recipient. If items require prior authorization, list the date of authorization.

Special directions for different types of providers:

Physicians, Podiatrists and Chiropractors: Describe diagnosis and services or supplies provided. Indicate miles traveled if over 10 one way. Indicate date(s) of visit(s) and place of service.

Optometrists: Describe services provided, if the Fee Service Code is not sufficiently descriptive; describe diagnosis and dates of service; describe items furnished as required by state fee schedule, including complete prescription, if lenses are dispensed.

Opticians: Describe items furnished as required by state fee schedule; indicate prescription number; submit copy of prescription.

Hospitals and Nursing Homes: Prepare separate requests for "inpatient" and "outpatient" services. Indicate period of hospitalization or dates of service.

Other Providers: Fully describe the service, supply, or appliance furnished; indicate name of prescribing practitioner.

15. Use the code, if any, on the state fee schedules applicable to the service billed.

16. The amount charged may not exceed applicable rates and fees in state or local schedules.

17. Indicate any payment made by, or due from, any insurance company to the practitioner or patient. Include any payment received or due from any other source.

18. Enter the actual amount for which the Social Service District is responsible for issuing payment.

19. Indicate total of page; if more than one page, indicate grand total. Do *not* write in the shaded areas of the form.

INSTRUCTIONS FOR COMPLETING NEW YORK MEDICAL ASSISTANCE PROGRAM FORM DSS-196, STATE VOUCHER FORM (Fig. 5–3)

Type four copies, sending three to:

New York State Department of Social Services
Bureau of Finance
1450 Western Avenue
Albany, NY 12243

and keeping one for the physician's files.

1. Enter the physician's name, street address, city, state, and ZIP code as it should appear on the check.

2. List the physician's federal payee – employer identification number or, if the physician or provider has never been assigned one, enter his or her Social Security number.

3. Enter the patient's last name. Be accurate, since this is essential in identifying the case for payment. If a patient has a long last name, use only the first 13 letters of the last name and the initial of the first name.

4. Enter the case number as shown on the Medicaid identification card.

5. Indicate the appropriate medical fee schedule number as outlined in the State Medical Handbook.

6. Give the diagnosis and describe the item or service provided.

7. List the date the service or item was provided to the Medicaid recipient.

8. List the amount of the service. Payment may not exceed the maximum reimbursable fees or rates as contained in the state fee or rate schedules.

9. Total the amount(s).

10. Enter discount terms, if any.

11. The physician or provider of service must sign the form.

12. Give the title of the provider, such as M.D., D.D.S., D.P.M., D.C., or D.O.

13. State the date the voucher is being submitted.

14. Enter the name of the company if the provider is supplying drugs, sickroom supplies, or prosthetic appliances.

AC-5000

FORM **DSS-196** (REV. 2/75)

Approved by State Comptroller 1/75

LEAVE BLANK
VOUCHER NO.

STATE OF NEW YORK - DEPARTMENT OF SOCIAL SERVICES
VOUCHER FOR MEDICAL ASSISTANCE

PAY TO:
PAYEE NAME: (Limit to 31 spaces)   (1)

Dept.Div.

PAYEE REFERENCE (Last Name)
LAST NAME (Limit 13 spaces)   First Initial

ADDRESS   (Limit to 29 spaces)   (1)

Audit &
Control
Use Only   1800   (3)

ADDRESS   (Limit to 29 spaces)   (1)

Payee Employer I.D. No.   Case Number

CITY AND STATE   (Limit to 24 spaces)   (1)   Zip Code

(2)   (4)

MEDICAL FEE SCHEDULE NUMBER	ITEM OR SERVICE PROVIDED	DATE OF SALE OR SERVICE	AMOUNT
(5)	(6)	(7)	(8)

TO BE COMPLETED WHEN SERVICES REQUIRE PRIOR APPROVAL

The above services as described are ☐ approved, are ☐ not approved.

AUTHORIZED SIGNATURE _____

DATE _____ TITLE _____ COUNTY _____

TOTAL   (9)

Cash Discount
_ _ _ _ _ _ %   (10)
_ _ _ _ Days

PAYEE CERTIFICATION - I certify that the above bill is true, accurate and complete; that no part thereof has been paid except as stated and that the balance is actually due and owing, and that taxes from which the State is exempt are excluded.

SIGNATURE OF PAYEE (IN INK) _____(11)_____   TITLE _____(12)_____

DATE ___(13)___   NAME OF COMPANY _____(14)_____

NET

COMPTROLLER'S PRE-AUDIT

VERIFIED

AUDITED

FIGURE 5-3

Form DSS-196, State Voucher for Public Assistance. Used for billing and/or prior authorization for Family Care patients in New York.

INSTRUCTIONS FOR COMPLETING NEW YORK MEDICAL ASSISTANCE PROGRAM FORM DSS-436, NOTIFICATION OF HOSPITAL ADMISSION (Fig. 5–4)

FORM **DSS-436** (REV. 2/75) **NOTIFICATION OF HOSPITAL ADMISSION** State of New York · Department of Social Services	PATIENT'S NAME AND ADDRESS (I)	MEDICAID NUMBER (2)
		DATE ADMITTED (3)

NAME OF ADMITTING PHYSICIAN (4)	ADMITTING DIAGNOSIS (5)
SIGNATURE (6)	HOSPITAL'S NAME AND ADDRESS (7)

L E A V E   B L A N K - - FOR DEPARTMENT OF SOCIAL SERVICES ONLY

DECISION ☐ Notification Accepted ☐ Notification Not Accepted	CHECKED BY	DATE CHECKED	DATE HOSPITAL NOTIFIED
REASON FOR REJECTION			

I N S T R U C T I O N S

1. The Department of Social Services shall be notified of hospital admissions within 5 days thereof, Saturdays, Sundays and legal holidays excluded (Social Services Law, Section 367).

2. Prepare the form in 2 copies. IT IS IMPORTANT THAT THE PATIENT'S MEDICAID NUMBER IS COPIED EXACTLY AS SHOWN ON HIS IDENTIFICATION CARD.

3. Send the original to:
   N.Y.S. Department of Social Services
   Bureau of Budgets and Accounting
   1450 Western Avenue
   Albany, New York 12243

4. The duplicate is for your files.

5. You will be advised ONLY if your Notification is NOT ACCEPTED.

FIGURE 5–4

Form DSS-436, Notification of Hospital Admission. Used by hospitals prior to the admission of a patient under the Medicaid Family Care Program in New York.

Prepare the form in two copies and keep the duplicate for the physician's files. Send the original to:

N.Y.S. Department of Social Services
Bureau of Budgets and Accounting
1450 Western Avenue
Albany, NY 12203

1. Enter the patient's first name, middle initial, and last name; complete street address, city, state, and ZIP Code.
2. List the patient's Medicaid identification number.
3. Show the admission date to the hospital facility.
4. Enter the name of the admitting physician.
5. Give the admitting diagnosis.
6. The physician must sign the form.
7. List the hospital's complete name and address.

LOCAL NEW YORK SOCIAL SERVICE DEPARTMENTS

Albany: 28 Howard Street, Albany 12207
Allegany: County Home, Angelica 14709
Broome: 119 Chenango Street, Binghamton 13901
Cattaraugus: 265 North Union Street, Olean 14760
Cayuga: County Office Bldg., 160 Genesee Street, Auburn 13021
Chautauqua: New County Office Bldg., Mayville 14757
Chemung: 203-209 William Street, Elmira 14901
Chenango: County Office Bldg., Norwich 13815
Clinton: 10 Healey Avenue, (Mail—P.O. Box 990) Plattsburgh 12901
Columbia: 610 State Street, Hudson 12534
Cortland: 133 Homer Avenue, Cortland 13045
Delaware: 126 Main Street, Delhi 13753
Dutchess: County Office Bldg., 22 Market Street, Poughkeepsie 12601
Erie: 95 Franklin Street, Buffalo 14202
Essex: Court House, Elizabethtown 12932
Franklin: Court House, Malone 12953
Fulton: County Bldg., Johnstown 12095
Genesee: 3837 West Main Road, Batavia 14020
Greene: 465 Main Street, Catskill 12414
Hamilton: Court House, Lake Pleasant 12108
Herkimer: County Office Bldg., Herkimer 13350
Jefferson: 173 Arsenal Street, Watertown 13601
Lewis: County Home, Lowville 13367
Livingston: 4223 Lakeville Road, Geneseo 14454
Madison: Wampsville 13163
Monroe: 111 Westfall Road, Rochester 14620
Montgomery: County Office Bldg., Fonda 12068
Nassau: Administration Bldg., County Seat Drive, Mineola 11501
New York City: 250 Church Street, New York 10013
Niagara: 100 Davison Road, P.O. Box 506, Lockport 14094
Oneida: County Office Bldg., 800 Park Avenue, Utica 13501
Onondaga: County Office Bldg., 600 S. State Street, Syracuse 13202
Ontario: 120 North Main Street, Canandaigua 14424
Orange: Quarry Road, Box Z, Goshen 10924
Orleans: County Home, Albion 14411
Oswego: County Office Bldg., Mexico 13114
Otsego: County Office Bldg., 197 Main Street, Cooperstown 13326
Putnam: 2 Mahopac Plaza, Mahopac 10541
Rensselaer: 133 Bloomingrove Drive, Troy 12180
Rockland: 250 West Nyack Road, West Nyack 10994
St. Lawrence: County Home, Canton 13617
Saratoga: County Complex, Bldg. A, Ballston Spa 12020
Schenectady: 487 Nott Street, Schenectady 12308
Schoharie: Professional Bldg., Schoharie 12157
Schuyler: County Office Bldg., Watkins Glen 14891
Seneca: County Road 118, Box 179, RD #3, Waterloo 13165
Steuben: County Home, Box 631, Bath 14810

Suffolk: Box 2000, 10 Oval Drive, Hauppauge 11787
Sullivan: Box 231, Liberty 12754
Tioga: Box 394, Rt. 38, RD 3, Oswego 13827
Tompkins: 108 Green Street, East, Ithaca 14850
Ulster: County Office Bldg., 244 Fair Street, Kingston 12401
Warren: Warren County Municipal Center, Lake George 12845
Washington: 6 Church Street, Granville 12832
Wayne: 16 William Street, Lyons 14489
Westchester: Room 432, County Office Bldg., 148 Martine Avenue, White Plains 10601
Wyoming: 466 North Main Street, Warsaw 14569
Yates: County Office Bldg., Court Street, Penn Yan 14527

MEDI-CAL

Medi-Cal is also known as California Medical Assistance Program; sometimes called Cal-MAP. In other states, it is known as Medicaid. Medi-Cal is administered by the State Department of Health, a department of the State Human Relations Agency. Medi-Cal became effective on March 1, 1966.

Three fiscal intermediaries are contracted by the state to receive and audit claims for payment for medical services and to make payments to providers of services. These intermediaries are:

1. Hospital Service of Southern California and Hospital Service of Northern California—Blue Cross (for hospital billing)
2. Blue Shield of California (for professional services)
3. California Dental Service (Denti-Cal for dental services) (See Chapter 11)

The state issues a paper Medi-Cal identification card (Fig. 5–5) each month to those who are eligible. The card must be valid for the month in which service is rendered. The card contains 8 sticky labels, as follows:

1. Two labels printed "MEDI" for optometry, psychology, audiology, podiatry, chiropractic services, sterilization procedures, cosmetic procedures, and physical, occupational, or speech therapy.
2. Six labels printed "POE" (Proof of Eligibility) for x-rays, laboratory tests, emergency care, inpatient hospital care, outpatient nonemergency physician's services, psychiatry, dermatology, ophthalmology, and allergy services.

A photocopy of the identification card or POE label is acceptable in lieu of a POE label. A photocopy of the MEDI label is not acceptable for use in validating the specific outpatient services as listed above.

Beneficiary Name
(maximum of 16 characters)

Beneficiary I.D. Number

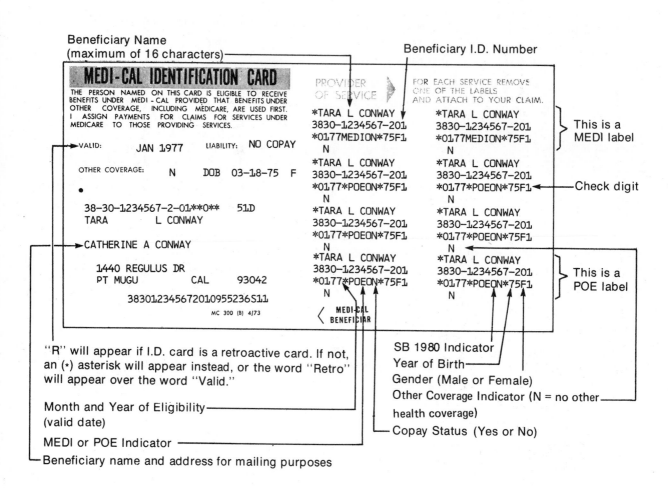

"R" will appear if I.D. card is a retroactive card. If not, an (*) asterisk will appear instead, or the word "Retro" will appear over the word "Valid."

Month and Year of Eligibility
(valid date)

MEDI or POE Indicator

Beneficiary name and address for mailing purposes

SB 1980 Indicator
Year of Birth
Gender (Male or Female)
Other Coverage Indicator (N = no other
health coverage)
Copay Status (Yes or No)

FIGURE 5–5

MC-300 Medi-Cal Identification Card showing eight adhesive peel-off labels.

STATE OF CALIFORNIA
MEDICAL ASSISTANCE PROGRAM

RECORD OF HEALTH CARE COSTS

DEPARTMENT OF HEALTH

CASE NAME - FIRST, MIDDLE, LAST

Mrs. Medically Needy

ADDRESS

1234 Main Street

CITY, STATE, ZIP

Anytown, CA 12345

EXPENSES INCURRED IN ONLY THE FOLLOWING MONTH(S) CAN BE LISTED

	MONTHLY		THREE MONTHS			
	MO	YR	MO	YR	MO	YR
FROM			1-77		THRU	3-77

COUNTY DIST: 0 1 0   COUNTY USE: 0 2 3

DATE OF ELIGIBILITY MO DAY YR: 9 - 1 - 72

DATE OF EMERGENCY MO DAY YR

AMOUNT TO BE BILLED PATIENT BEFORE BILLING MEDI-CAL: $162.00

LIST ONLY FAMILY MEMBERS WHOSE MEDICAL EXPENSES APPLY TOWARD THE AMOUNT TO BE BILLED PATIENT

CO	AID	STATE NUMBER 7 DIGIT SERIAL NO.	FBU	PERS NO.	NAME	BIRTHDATE MO DAY YR	SEX	(1) SOCIAL SEC. NO. AND (2) HEALTH INS. CLAIM NO. OR RAILROAD RETIREMENT NO.	OTHER COV. CODE
60	76	0123456	0	00	Mrs. Medically Needy	6-6-14	F	(1) 111-11-9999 (2) 222-21-3333	NO
								(1) (2)	
								(1) (2)	
								(1) (2)	
								(1) (2)	
								(1) (2)	
								(1) (2)	

DECLARATION OF PROVIDER: Each service listed below has been provided to the applicant and/or a family member for the month(s) noted above. I, the undersigned provider, hereby declare that I received payment from the applicant or will seek payment for the amount shown in the "Billed Patient" column only. I further agree that I will neither claim nor accept payment from the Medi-Cal program for the amount shown in the "Billed Patient" column. I also understand and agree that I may seek payment from the Medi-Cal program when the costs of my service exceed the amount to be billed patient (shown above). In such cases, the portion of the cost which exceeds the amount to be billed to the patient and which may be billed to the Medi-Cal program must be shown in the "Billed Medi-Cal" column. The amount shown in the "Total Bill" column is the cost of the services I rendered. I understand that if I make a claim against a third party on behalf of this patient for any service rendered to him, I will not report the service or the charge on this form, since the amount for such service may not be counted toward the amount to be billed the patient.
I am aware that financial information on this form may be subject to scrutiny by the Internal Revenue Service and/or the California State Franchise Tax Board.

PROVIDER NAME	PROVIDER NO.	DATE OF SERVICE MO DAY YR	SERVICE	PROC. CODE / PRESC. NO.	TOTAL BILL $	BILLED PATIENT $	BILLED MEDI-CAL $
Gerald Practon, M. D.	C 14021						
PATIENT NAME Mrs. Medically Needy		1 5 77	Office Visit	90040	10.00	10.00	-0-
PROVIDER SIGNATURE X Mrs Mary Smith, Billing Clerk		1 15 77	Office Visit	90040	10.00	10.00	-0-
PROVIDER NAME Fast Service Pharmacy	PROVIDER NO. A 31270						
PATIENT NAME Mrs. Medically Needy		2 4 77	Prescribed Drugs	150775	10.00	10.00	-0-
PROVIDER SIGNATURE X Thomas Fast, Reg. Pharm.		2 5 77	Prescribed Drugs	09262	10.00	10.00	-0-
PROVIDER NAME College Hospital	PROVIDER NO. 780						
PATIENT NAME Mrs. Medically Needy		2 6 77	6 days room & board				
PROVIDER SIGNATURE X		2 7 77	nursing care				
		2 8 77					
PROVIDER NAME (continued from above)	PROVIDER NO	2 10 77					
PATIENT NAME Mrs. Medically Needy		2 11 77	@ $18.98 per day		455.52	112.00	343.52
PROVIDER SIGNATURE X Betsy Foster, Billing Clerk							
PROVIDER NAME	PROVIDER NO.						
PATIENT NAME							
PROVIDER SIGNATURE X							

STATE USE ONLY			
MO	DAY	YR	REVIEWED BY:
DATE OF CERTIFICATION / VERIFICATION			

I HAVE READ THE INSTRUCTIONS ON THE BACK OF THIS FORM. I AGREE TO ASSUME FULL LEGAL RESPONSIBILITY FOR THE AMOUNTS LISTED ABOVE IN THE "BILLED PATIENT" COLUMN.

X Mrs Medically Needy   2/12/77

SIGNATURE OF APPLICANT   DATE

MC-177 (REV. 7/73) COMBINES MC-172 AND MC-177

FIGURE 5-6

Form MC-177, Record of Health Care Costs. The patient brings this form into the physician's office. After receiving service, the physician indicates the type of service rendered, date, and the amount. The doctor signs the form and gives it back to the patient.

ELIGIBILITY

The following groups are entitled to benefits under the Medi-Cal program:

1. (OAS) Californians who qualify for old age assistance benefits
2. (AFDC) Aid to families with dependent children
3. (AB) Aid to the blind ⎫
4. (ATD) Aid to the permanently disabled ⎭ on both Medicare/Medi-Cal
5. (MN) Medically Needy persons whose incomes are above the assistance level but who are unable to provide "mainstream" medical care and are eligible as medically indigent (MI). Some of these patients have a liability to meet every month. In this event, the patient will bring in a form MC-177, Record of Health Care Costs (see Fig. 5–6). After completion of the service rendered, the physician should indicate the type of service rendered, the date, and the amount on the MC-177. The physician then signs this form and gives the form to the patient, who then takes it to his social worker.

If this form shows that the patient has a liability to meet for the month and this is the first physician that the patient is seeing for treatment, be sure to obtain payment from the patient and keep a photocopy of the MC-177 form for the physician's records.

On the patient's Medi-Cal identification card is a State Coding as shown below.

	CO	AID	CASE NO.	FBU	PERS
State Coding	38	30	1234567	2	01

The first two digits indicate the county where the person resides, the second two digits indicate the aid code (see Table 5–1 for ascertaining what type of aid the person is receiving), the next seven digits indicate the case number, the next digit is the Family Budget Unit number, and the last two digits indicate the person in the family. The coding "01" might mean the father, "02" might mean the mother, and "03" might mean a child.

Additional AID codes are listed on pp. 117 and 118.

TABLE 5–1. MEDI-CAL AID CODES AND DESCRIPTION OF ELIGIBLE CATEGORIES

AID Code	Description
01	Indochinese Refugee Assistance Program (Cash or Refused Grant)
02	Indochinese Refugee Assistance (Medically Needy)
04	Aid to Adoptive Children (Indigent under 21)
06	Cuban Refugee (Medically Indigent Persons under 18 *and* Noncategorically Related Needy Person, with *or* without cost deductions for medical care)
07	Cuban Refugee (MN)
08	Cuban Refugee (Cash Grant or Refused Grant)
10	General — Old Age Security
12	Specific Substitute Payee (Aid to the Aged)
13	Long Term Non-Grant (Aid to the Aged)
14	Refused Grant (Aid to the Aged)

15	Home Over $25,000 (Aid to the Aged)
16	20% Disregard (Aid to the Aged)
17	Medically Needy (Aid to the Aged)
18	Homemaker/Chore Services (Aid to the Aged)
20	General — Aid to the Blind
22	Specific Substitute Payee (Aid to the Blind)
23	Long Term Non-Grant (Aid to the Blind)
24	Refused Grant (Aid to the Blind)
25	Home Over $25,000 (Aid to the Blind)
26	20% Disregard (Aid to the Blind)
27	Medically Needy (Aid to the Blind)
28	Homemaker/Chore Services (Aid to the Blind)
30	AFDC–FG (Aid to Families with Dependent Children–Family Group)
32	Money Management (AFDC–FG)
33	Unemployed Parent (AFDC, Money Management)
34	Refused Grant (AFDC)
35	Unemployed Parent (AFDC)
36	20% Disregard (AFDC)
37	Medically Needy (AFDC)
38	Under Age 21 and Not in School — No Grant (AFDC)
39	General Relief
40	Boarding Homes and Institutions (AFDC)
42	Boarding Homes and Institutions–Federal Participation (AFDC)
43	Boarding Homes and Institutions–Long Term Non-Grant (AFDC)
44	Boarding Homes and Institutions–Refused Grant (AFDC)
45	Children in foster care (under 21 years of age) supported in whole or part by public funds
46	Boarding Homes and Institutions — 20% Disregard (AFDC)
47	Boarding Homes and Institutions — Medically Needy (AFDC)
50	General — Potentially Self-Supporting Blind
56	20% Disregard (Potentially Self-Supporting Blind)
58	Homemaker/Chore Services (Potentially Self-Supporting Blind)
60	General — Aid to the Disabled
62	Specified Substitute Payee (Aid to the Disabled)
63	Long Term Non-Grant (Aid to the Disabled)
64	Refused Grant (Aid to the Disabled)
65	Home Over $25,000 (Aid to the Disabled)
66	20% Disregard (Aid to the Disabled)
67	Medically Needy (Aid to the Disabled)
68	Homemaker/Chore Services (Aid to the Disabled)
71	Kidney Dialysis patients eligible for dialysis coverage only, who are not otherwise eligible for Medi-Cal, and, if under 65, are not otherwise eligible for Medicare
74	Noncategorically related needy persons, age 21 through 64, determined eligible to receive Medi-Cal benefits at a county medical facility only — not paid by MI (no cost deductions for medical care)
75	Noncategorically related needy persons, age 21 through 64, determined eligible to receive Medi-Cal benefits at a county medical facility only— not paid by MI (cost deductions for medical care)
76	Medically Indigent — Not paid by MI
77	Medically Indigent — Not paid by MI
82	Indigent persons under 21 with no cost deductions for medical care
83	Indigent persons under 21 with cost deductions for medical care
84	Noncategorically related needy persons, age 21 through 64, with no cost deductions for medical care (MI)

85 Noncategorically related needy persons, age 21 through 64, with cost deductions for medical care (MN)

86 Noncategorically related needy persons, age 18 to 21 (married or not married), or ceremonially married persons under age 18 with no cost deductions for medical care (MI)

87 Noncategorically related needy persons, age 18 to 21 (married or not married), or ceremonially married persons under age 18 with cost deductions for medical care (MN)

88 Aid to the disabled — pending — with no cost deductions for medical care (MI)

89 Aid to the disabled — pending — with cost deductions for medical care (MN)

BENEFITS

The basic medical benefits provided under Medi-Cal include:

1. Physician services
2. In- or outpatient hospital services in any qualified hospital
3. Laboratory and x-ray services
4. Nursing home services
5. Home health care
6. Private duty nursing
7. Outpatient clinic services
8. Dental services (Denti-Cal)
9. Hearing aids
10. Drugs and medical supplies
11. Optometric services
12. Physical therapy and other diagnostic, preventive, or rehabilitative services.
13. Also pays the full deductible under Part A of Medicare program and "buys into" Part B of Medicare by paying the monthly premiums for those who are over 65, disabled, or blind. (These persons are called Medicare/Medi-Cal recipients; see Chapter 6).

Medi-Cal benefits are divided into two parts. They are:

1. A Uniform Basic Schedule of Benefits
2. A Uniform Supplemental Schedule of Benefits

The Basic Benefits cover the full scope of benefits available to Medi-Cal beneficiaries. The Supplemental Schedule of Benefits is limited to:

1. Outpatient physician's services
2. Prescription drugs
3. Inpatient hospital care
4. Podiatry services

These services are covered only after the same benefits available under the Basic Schedule of Benefits have been exhausted.

CLAIM PROCEDURE

The various forms used in filing Medi-Cal claims are summarized in Table 5–2.

The Service Report form (MC-163) (see Fig. 5–8) was designed to be used when submitting bills under standard Blue Shield programs as well as the Medi-Cal program and is used by physicians in submitting such claims. Medi-Cal claims must be sent in before 2 months or 60 days have elapsed since the end of the month of service, or the doctor will not receive any money for his services. The following exceptions have a 1 year time limit:

1. Retroactive eligibility
2. When patient has not informed physician that he or she is on Medi-Cal
3. Dental bills
4. Obstetric bills (usually billed at time of delivery)
5. Completion of treatment plan
6. When patient has other insurance coverage (physician may elect to bill the other insurance)

To bill a Medi-Cal claim properly, detach the correct sticky label from the patient's identification card and attach this to the upper right-hand corner of the claim above the gray area (see Fig. 5–8). Place a piece of Scotch tape over the label to secure it. Do *not* use staples, as each form is microfilmed and the microfilm machine will not accept staples. Besides attaching the label, the gray shaded area on the MC-163 form must have the identification number typed below the label. Additional labels may be placed in the bottom left portion of the form over the area which states "Special Payee Name."

TABLE 5–2. MEDI-CAL FORMS*

Form Number	Form Title	Notations	Figure Reference
MC-161	Medical Treatment Authorization Request (TAR)	Good for 120 days if no date is listed by doctor.	Fig. 5–9
MC-163	Service Report	Used for standard Blue Shield and Medi-Cal claims.	Fig. 5–8
MC-165	Medi-Cal Prescription	For prescribing nonpharmacy services.	
MC-170	Treatment Authorization for Payment Request for Nursing Home Care		
MC-173	Retroactive Authorization for Emergency Medical Services	Used when emergency services were provided prior to beneficiary application for eligibility. Must be attached to MC-163 when submitting these claims. MEDI or POE label not required.	

MC-175	Pharmacy Services Statement Form	Used by pharmacists as a billing statement.	
MC-177	Record of Health Care Services	Medically Needy expense tally form for satisfying liability. For patient's use only.	Fig. 5-6
MC-179	Visual Appliance Authorization Request	Good for 120 days.	
MC-180	Request for Extension of Stay in Hospital	Used when patient must be confined to a hospital for more than 8 days.	
SSA-1490	Request for Medicare Payment	Used for submitting claims for Medicare/Medi-Cal patients.	Fig. 6-2
MIO-204	Medi-Cal Intermediary Operations Claims Inquiry	Used for tracing claims, making corrections or adjustments, or for supplemental requests.	Fig. 5-7

*To order copies of the above preprinted forms, write to:
Blue Shield of California
Pre-Printed Form Section
P.O. Box 120
Tracy, CA 95376

The MEDI label is required for:

1. Psychology billing
2. Optometry billing
3. Audiology billing
4. Podiatry billing
5. Chiropractic services
6. Sterilization procedures
7. Cosmetic procedures
8. Physical, occupational, or speech therapy

Any unused MEDI labels from the month immediately preceding the current month of service may be used in the current month of service, but a current month's POE label must also be attached to the claim. A Treatment Authorization Request (TAR) Form MC-161 can replace a MEDI label when sending in a claim. When submitting the MC-163 claim form with a TAR attached, use a POE label affixed to the MC-163 form.

The POE label is required for:

1. Outpatient nonemergency physician services
2. Inpatient services provided by physicians (hospital inpatient)
3. Medicare/Medi-Cal outpatient claims (only one label needed for each month)
4. Dental services
5. Medical transportation
6. Emergency outpatient physician services (justification of emergency must be written at bottom of MC-163 form)

7. Drugs for both outpatients and nursing home inpatients, without restriction as to number of prescriptions per month

8. Total OB care (use POE label for month of delivery of baby). For partial OB care, use the POE label for the last month the patient was seen in the office.

9. Laboratory tests, x-rays, and radiation treatment

10. Assistive devices, durable medical equipment, and medical supplies (nondrug items)

11. Artificial limbs and braces

12. Hearing aids

13. Eyeglasses artificial eyes, and eye appliances; eye refraction by ophthalmologists

14. Durable medical equipment

15. Blood and blood derivatives

16. Chronic hemodialysis (kidney treatment)

17. Home Health Agency services

18. Skilled Nursing Facility services (nursing home)

19. Hospital inpatient care

20. Additional services available under Supplemental Schedule of Benefits

21. Screening for persons under 21

22. Intermediate care facility services

23. Family planning services

24. Psychiatry, dermatology, and allergy services

Treatment Authorization Request

A Treatment Authorization Request (TAR) Form MC-161 (Fig. 5–9) is required for prior authorization on the following services:

1. Only for outpatient extended care

2. Dental services (Denti-Cal); see Chapter 11

3. Nursing home services

4. Vision care services

5. Inpatient hospital services

6. Home health agency services

7. Chronic hemodialysis services

8. Medical transportation

9. Durable medical equipment

10. Hearing aids

11. Eyeglasses

12. Prosthetic and orthotic appliances

13. Medical supplies (nondrug items)

14. Whenever a Supplemental Service is provided from the Supplemental Schedule of Benefits (see p. 118)

The Treatment Authorization Request form is sent to the Department of Health in your area for approval. After approval this document must accompany the MC-163 billing claim with a current POE label affixed to the MC-163. However, if the TAR was obtained for the hospitalization of a patient, the original approved TAR must be sent to the hospital prior to the admission of the patient. In some cases it is not possible to obtain a TAR in advance of hospital admission or initiation of a treatment program. In those cases, a telephone authorization must be obtained. Call the local Department of

Health to receive approval, obtain the following information and then submit the TAR, showing that it was already authorized by stating the following information:

TAR Authorization by Phone

1. Complete the MC-161 TAR Form.
2. Give date authorization was given.
3. State name of person who gave authorization.
4. Indicate approximate time of day authorization was given.
5. Record log number given to you by the Department of Health.

When attaching a TAR to the MC-163 claim form, staple the two forms all the way across the top, back-to-back, and type on the face of the MC-163 that "TAR" is attached."

Medi-Screen Program

This program is an Early and Periodic Screening, Diagnosis and Treatment program (EPSDT) initiated in 1973 for Medi-Cal beneficiaries under 21 years of age. It is administered by the Department of Health and renders such services as:

Immunization and tuberculin testing
Laboratory tests
Vision tests
Hearing tests
Dental screening

For additional information on Medi-Screen and instructions for obtaining booklets and forms, see page 120.

Medi-Cal and Other Coverage

The physician should bill the other insurance and then bill Medi-Cal with an attachment showing payment received from the other insurance.

Medi-Cal and CHAMPUS

If a Medi-Cal patient also has CHAMPUS, bill CHAMPUS first. Then bill Medi-Cal and attach the Explanation of Benefits (EOB) to the claim form. See Chapter 7.

Explanation of Benefits

An Explanation of Benefits (EOB) accompanies all Medi-Cal payment checks to the physician. If there is a question concerning an item or procedure on the EOB, when making inquiry, always refer to:

1. Provider number
2. Check number
3. Beneficiary's name and Medi-Cal identification number
4. Claim number

Send the inquiry regarding the EOB data to:

Medi-Cal Provider Services
Blue Shield of California
P.O. Box 3637
San Francisco, CA 94119

NAME AND ADDRESS OF PROVIDER OF SERVICE | PROVIDER NO.

MEDI-CAL
INTERMEDIARY OPERATIONS
CLAIMS INQUIRY

PAYMENT INQUIRY — PLEASE NOTE ITEM(S) CHECKED BELOW

☐ NO PAYMENT RECEIVED   ☐ OVERPAYMENT   ☐ UNDERPAYMENT   ☐ CORRECTED BILLING ATTACHED   ☐ PAID TO WRONG PROVIDER

☐ CANNOT IDENTIFY BENEFICIARY ON EXPLANATION OF BENEFITS   ☐ LOST CHECK   ☐ OTHER (PLEASE CLARIFY UNDER REMARKS)

PATIENT INFORMATION — PLEASE FILL IN ALL PERTINENT INFORMATION REQUESTED BELOW

LAST NAME OF BENEFICIARY	FIRST NAME	INIT.	SEX	DATE OF SERVICE
			☐ M ☐ F	

MEDI-CAL I.D. NUMBER	MEDICARE MIC NUMBER	
CO. AID CASE NO. FBU PERSON		

PAYMENT INFORMATION

ADMISSION DATE	DISCHARGE DATE	DATE OF BILLING	DATE OF REMITTANCE ADVICE OR CHECK	CHECK NUMBER

AMOUNT — $	MEDICAL RECORD NUMBER	CLAIM NUMBER — PROVIDER FILL IN

REMARKS

_____   _____
SIGNATURE   DATE

FOR MIO USE ONLY

NEW I.C.N. — INTERMEDIARY USE ONLY

DISTRIBUTION: RETAIN PART 2 FOR YOUR RECORDS — SEND PARTS 1 AND 3 WITH CARBON INTACT.

BLUE CROSS OF SOUTHERN CALIFORNIA
4777 SUNSET BOULEVARD
LOS ANGELES, CALIFORNIA 90027

BLUE CROSS OF NORTHERN CALIFORNIA
1950 WEBSTER STREET
OAKLAND, CALIFORNIA 94659

BLUE SHIELD OF CALIFORNIA
P.O. BOX 7924
SAN FRANCISCO, CALIFORNIA 94120

O-204 (8/74)

FIGURE 5-7

Form MIO-204, Medi-Cal Intermediary Operations Claims Inquiry.

Incorrect Payment Refund

When a provider wishes to refund an incorrect payment, the physician should forward the refund to:

> Blue Shield of California
> Cash Receiving
> P.O. Box 7924, Rincon Annex
> San Francisco, CA 94119

To report the above inquiries, a special form has been devised: Medi-Cal Intermediary Operations Claims Inquiry Form MIO-204 (see Fig. 5–7). This form is used to trace claims, to make corrections or adjustments, and to make supplemental requests.

INSTRUCTIONS FOR COMPLETION OF THE BLUE SHIELD MC-163 CLAIM FORM (Fig. 5–8 and Assignments 9 and 10, pp. 537–544)

Note: In following instructions for completion of the Blue Shield MC-163 Claim Form, information for Standard Blue Shield patients is given in parentheses.

1. Enter the patient's last name, then the first name and middle initial.
2. Enter the patient's complete address as described, i.e., street, city, state, and ZIP Code.
3. Subscriber's Name; Subscriber's Employer: Leave these spaces blank or insert the initials "NA," meaning "not applicable." (For a Standard Blue Shield patient, insert the subscriber's name if the patient is a dependent, indicating last name, then first name and middle initial, Insert the name of the subscriber's employer.)
4. Check appropriate and applicable boxes for:
    "Condition Caused by"
    "If injury, indicate date, how and where sustained"
    "If pregnancy, Date of Commencement" (e.g., 06/10/77)
    "Is This A New Illness?"
    "Is Condition Due to Injury of Sickness Arising Out of Patient's Employment?"
    "Is This A New Patient?"
5. Check the appropriate box and indicate the name of the provider by or to whom the patient was referred.
6. Enter the name and address, if applicable, of the hospital or nursing home where the patient was treated either as an inpatient or as an outpatient. When the patient is an inpatient, show the admission date and, if applicable, the discharge date.
7. Check the appropriate box. Bill the other coverage carrier first. (For a Standard Blue Shield patient, check the appropriate box "yes" or "no" to indicate whether the patient has other coverage. If there is other coverage, indicate the name of the company or plan and give the policy number, or, if the patient is on Medicare, the health insurance claim number and letter.)
8. Enter a written diagnosis; it should be concise but complete and specific. ICDA codes may be used but must be accompanied by written diagnoses.
9. Enter the date of service by numbers (e.g., 07/13/77). Under "Procedure Number" enter the RVS (Relative Value Studies), SMA (Schedule of Maximum

NOTE: Please do not detach this stub. Detach the last copy and one carbon. 25683
Send Blue Shield of California the balance of the form with carbon insert intact. See Reverse side for billing instructions.

TAB SET

FOR BLUE SHIELD USE ONLY

SAMPLE

SERVICE REPORT
MC 163 (REV. 10/75)

PATIENT'S NAME   LAST   (1)   FIRST   MIDDLE INITIAL

1st LABEL
POE or MEDI Required

COMPLETE FOR BLUE SHIELD SUBSCRIBERS

PATIENT'S ADDRESS
STREET   (2)

CO. | AID | CASE NO. | FBU | PERS. NO.

GROUP NO.   SECTION NO.   (12)

CITY   STATE   ZIP CODE

(11)

SUBSCRIBER'S NAME (IF PATIENT IS A DEPENDENT)   LAST   (3)   FIRST   MIDDLE INITIAL

TYPE IN NUMBER

SUBSCRIBER NO.   (13)

SUBSCRIBER'S EMPLOYER   (3)

PATIENT'S RELATIONSHIP TO SUBSCRIBER
☐ SELF (14)   ☐ SPOUSE   ☐ CHILD

PATIENT'S BIRTHDATE
MONTH | DAY (15) | YR.

AGE (16)

PATIENT'S SEX
☐ MALE   ☐ FEMALE (17)   (18)

CONDITION CAUSED BY: ☐ INJURY   ☐ ILLNESS   ☐ PREGNANCY
IF INJURY: INDICATE DATE, HOW AND WHERE SUSTAINED

FOR PROVIDER'S USE ONLY

☐ AUTO ACCIDENT
☐ HOME   (4)
☐ OTHER

DATE OF INJURY
MO. | DAY | YR.

NAME AND ADDRESS OF PROVIDER OF SERVICE   PROVIDER NO.

(19)
PREPRINTED AREA. DOCTOR'S NAME AND
NUMBER MUST APPEAR THE SAME AS IT IS
ON THE MASTER PROVIDER FILE IN SAN
FRANCISCO.

IF PREGNANCY, DATE OF COMMENCEMENT

IS THIS A NEW ILLNESS?   ☐ NO   ☐ YES

IS CONDITION DUE TO INJURY OR SICKNESS ARISING OUT OF PATIENT'S EMPLOYMENT?   IS THIS A NEW PATIENT?
☐ NO   ☐ YES   ☐ NO   ☐ YES

IF PATIENT WAS REFERRED INDICATE: ☐ FROM
☐ TO   DOCTOR   (5)

DATE THIS FORM WAS PREPARED ▶ _____ (20)

IF TREATED IN HOSPITAL OR NURSING HOME
I.P. OR O.P. INDICATE NAME AND LOCATION

ADMISSION DATE
MO. | DAY | YR.

WAS LABORATORY WORK PERFORMED IN YOUR OFFICE?

☐ NO (IF NO, ENTER NAME AND ADDRESS OF LABORATORY BELOW)   ☐ YES

(6)

DISCHARGE DATE
MO. | DAY | YR.

AMOUNT CHARGED TO PHYSICIAN BY LABORATORY

OTHER GROUP HOSPITAL, MEDICAL COVERAGE INCLUDING MEDICARE.   ☐ NO   ☐ YES
NAME OF COMPANY OR PLAN   (7)   HEALTH INSURANCE CLAIM NO.   LETTER

(21) $

THIS IS TO CERTIFY THAT THE FOREGOING INFORMATION IS TRUE, ACCURATE AND COM-
PLETE. I UNDERSTAND THAT PAYMENT AND SATISFACTION OF THIS CLAIM WILL BE FROM
FEDERAL AND STATE FUNDS, AND THAT ANY FALSE CLAIMS, STATEMENTS, OR DOCUMENTS
OR CONCEALMENT OF A MATERIAL FACT, MAY BE PROSECUTED UNDER APPLICABLE
FEDERAL OR STATE LAWS.

DIAGNOSIS AND CONCURRENT CONDITIONS

LIST DIAGNOSIS, NOT SYMPTOMS
(8)

SIGNATURE OF PROVIDER OF SERVICE (REQUIRED FOR MEDI-CAL PROGRAM) ▶   (22)

PLACE OF SERVICE CODES

FAMILY PLANNING SERVICES? (MEDI-CAL)   ☐ NO   ☐ YES

1=IN-PATIENT HOSPITAL   2=OUT-PATIENT HOSPITAL   3=OFFICE   4=PATIENTS' HOME
8=NURSING HOME   9=OTHER

BLUE SHIELD USE ONLY	DATE OF SERVICE	PROCEDURE NUMBER	DESCRIBE EACH SERVICE OR APPLIANCE SEPARATELY	FOR BLUE SHIELD USE ONLY	YOUR FEE	PLACE OF SERV CODE	FOR BLUE SHIELD USE ONLY			
LINE NO.	LAST DAY	MO.	DAY	YR.	RVS NUMBER / SMA NUMBER	UNIT MODIFIER				

1 MONTH'S BILLING ON EACH

CLAIM FORM

(9)

SEE ATTACHED TAR.

2nd LABEL _____ (10) PUT ADDITIONAL LABELS ACROSS BOTTOM

CN   CO   CLM MSG   DIAG
SPECIAL PAYEE CITY, STATE   ZIP CODE

TYPE OF SERVICE | UNITS | LOC | MSG | TOTAL

D/S

CLAIM TYPE	PAY CODE	CPC	MOE	FEE	PROF.	HOSP.	MISC	QUAL	REL	PERS	ORIG EFF DATE	EXPL	DATE OF CHG OR CX
1	2	3	4	5	6	7	8	9	10				

1

FIGURE 5–8

Form MC-163, Service Report. Used for both standard Blue Shield cases and Medi-Cal claims.

Allowances), or SMR (Schedule of Maximum Reimbursement) code corresponding to the service rendered, to the left of the broken line. When two-digit modifiers are required to complete an RVS coding, they should be inserted to the right of the broken line. Do *not* use the modifier column to indicate quantities supplied or number of services provided.

Enter the description of service or appliance from the appropriate source — RVS, SMA, or SMR.

Insert your usual and customary charge for the service rendered. Insert the total of the charges at the bottom of the column in the "Total" space.

In the Place of Service Code, insert the appropriate numeric code from the listing above it, i.e.,

1. Inpatient hospital
2. Outpatient hospital
3. Office
4. Patient's home
7. This is not listed on the printed form but is to be inserted if the patient is in an intermediate care facility.
8. Nursing Home or Skilled Nursing Facility (SNF)
9. Other

If the patient has other coverage and the physician bills the other coverage carrier first, the physician must show in the "Describe Each Service. . ." column the amount paid by the carrier or the fact that the carrier denied payment. Documentation substantiating this statement must be stapled to the back of the claim form (copy of remittance advice, check, check voucher, denial form, or denial letter).

10. Extra identification POE or MEDI labels are to be affixed in this area, if necessary.

11. Enter the patient's Medi-Cal identification number in the lower part of these boxes exactly as it appears on the I.D. card and label (see Fig. 5–5).

Examples:

	COUNTY CODE	AID CODE	CASE NO.	FAMILY BUDGET UNIT	PERSON NO.
State Coding:	38	30	1234567	2	01

	COUNTY CODE	AID CODE	CONSTANT	SOCIAL SECURITY NO.
SSA Coding:	19	60	9	564194229 (disabled person)

By entering the correct and complete beneficiary I.D. number on the claim copy, the provider will be able to retain the number on his claim copy. The month of eligibility on the I.D. card must be carefully checked. The month shown on the I.D. card must be the same as the month in which the services(s) or appliance(s) was provided; if it is not, the claim will be returned to the provider.

Attach a MEDI or POE label, as required, at the top of the space so as to cover the title "Complete for Medi-Cal Program." Additional required labels should be affixed in the No. 10 space at the bottom of the claim form. Photocopies of I.D. cards or POE labels may be attached to the claim instead of the POE label itself. POE label photocopies must be attached to the front of the form with transparent tape. Photocopies of an I.D. card must be firmly stapled to the back of the form.

If the patient is a Cuban refugee or alien, so state in this gray area No. 11. (For a Standard Blue Shield patient, this gray area does not apply, so do not complete.)

12, 13, 14. Leave these spaces blank, since they are to be used only for billing Standard Blue Shield cases. (For a Standard Blue Shield patient, enter the group number from the patient's identification card. Enter the membership number, which is also known as certificate number, agreement number, identification number, or subscriber number, from the patient's identification card. Check the appropriate box to indicate the patient's relationship to the subscriber).

15. Enter the patient's birthdate (e.g., 11/02/36).

16. Enter the patient's age.

17. Indicate the patient's sex by checking the appropriate box.

18. For a "Medi-Screen Program" billing only, enter in this space a one-digit code to denote racial or ethnic origin of patient, as follows: 1 = white, 2 = black, 3 = Mexican-American, 4 = Oriental, 5 = other.

19. All MC-163 claim forms are preimprinted with the health professional's name, address, and provider number.

20. Insert the date on which this form was prepared, using numbers (e.g., 7/24/77). Type on the appropriate line, *not* in the box to the right.

21. If laboratory work was not performed at all on the patient, insert"NA" (not applicable). If laboratory work was performed, check the appropriate "Yes" or "No" box; when the "No" box is checked:

a. Enter the name and address of the laboratory which performed the tests, and

b. Enter the amount charged to the provider by the laboratory.

22. The MC-163 form must be signed in this space by the physician. Stamped signatures or initials are *not acceptable* either for the provider or any representative authorized to sign the claim form. An employee of the provider may sign the claim form when authorized to do so by the provider. A partner may sign the claim form on behalf of other partners, except that a limited partner, not subject to Medi-Cal program controls, may not sign on behalf of the other partner(s). Corporate officers with the power to sign for a corporation, and those designated employees under the direct employment and control of the corporation, may sign the claim forms. Billing firms may not sign Medi-Cal claim forms, nor may the provider sign blank claim forms for the billing service to complete. (For a Standard Blue Shield patient, the physician *does not* have to sign the claim).

INSTRUCTIONS FOR COMPLETING TREATMENT AUTHORIZATION REQUEST (TAR) — MEDI-CAL FORM MC-161 (Fig. 5–9 and Assignment 9, pp. 537–541)

1. Enter the patient's last name, first name, and middle initial. If the patient is an unnamed newborn, designate the first name as follows: "female" or "girl"; "male" or "boy."

INSTRUCTIONS

DOCTOR:— USE TYPEWRITER OR BALL POINT PEN. AFTER EXAMINATION MAIL WHITE, YELLOW AND BLUE FORMS WITH CARBONS BETWEEN TO MEDI-CAL CONSULTANT NAMED ON PATIENT'S IDENTIFICATION CARD. RETAIN PINK COPY FOR YOUR FILES.

STATE OF CALIFORNIA

MEDICAL

TREATMENT AUTHORIZATION REQUEST

DEPARTMENT OF HEALTH

FOR PROVIDER'S USE	FOR STATE USE

FOR PROVIDER'S USE

NAME AND ADDRESS OF PATIENT

(1)

AGE (2) SEX (3)

PATIENT'S IDENTIFICATION
CO. AID CASE NO. FBU PERS. NO.
(4)

NAME OF COUNTY
(5)

PLEASE PRINT YOUR NAME AND ADDRESS HERE ▶

(6)

THE ABOVE NAMED PATIENT IS IN NEED OF ADDITIONAL TREATMENT WHICH WILL EXCEED THE AMOUNT AUTHORIZED WITHOUT PRIOR APPROVAL. INITIAL DIAGNOSTIC IMPRESSIONS:

(7)

AUTHORIZATION IS REQUESTED TO CLAIM PAYMENT FOR THE FOLLOWING RECOMMENDED TREATMENT:

DESCRIPTION (BE SPECIFIC)	PROCEDURE NO.	CHARGES	AUTHORIZED		EXPLANATION
			YES	NO	
(8)			(f)		(g)

(9)
SIGNATURE   DEGREE   DATE

NOTE: AUTHORIZATION DOES NOT GUARANTEE PAYMENT. PAYMENT IS SUBJECT TO PATIENT'S ELIGIBILITY. BE SURE THE IDENTIFICATION CARD IS CURRENT BEFORE RENDERING SERVICE.

FOR STATE USE

PROVIDER: (a)

☐ YOU ARE AUTHORIZED TO CLAIM PAYMENT FOR TREATMENT AS RECOMMENDED BY YOU. AUTHORIZATION EXPIRES IN _____ DAYS. (b)

☐ REQUEST DENIED.

COMMENTS: (c)

(d)
☐ YOU ARE AUTHORIZED TO CLAIM PAYMENT FOR TREATMENT CHECKED "YES".

AUTHORIZATION EXPIRES IN __(e)__ DAYS.

MEDI-CAL CONSULTANT

BY __(h)__

DATE _____

MC - 161 (REV. 1-74)

FIGURE 5–9

Form MC-161, Medi-Cal Treatment Authorization Request.

Enter the patient's complete address, including street and number, city, state, and ZIP Code.

2. Enter the age of the patient.
3. Indicate the patient's sex by "F" for female or "M" for male.
4. Enter the patient's Medi-Cal identification number.

Example:

	CO	AID	CASE NO.	FBU	PERS
Coding:	38	30	1234567	2	01

No POE or MEDI label is required on this form. If the TAR is for retroactive authorization, a photocopy of a label is required.

5. Enter the name of the county in which the provider practices.
6. Print your physician's name and address here if the MC-161 TAR is not preimprinted.
7. Enter the reasons why the patient will need care or services, including diagnosis, severity of condition, prognosis, medical necessity for or the purpose of treatment(s), service(s), appliance(s) or equipment, or drugs. Enter number and types of services requested and anticipated frequency of specific services to be rendered. Enter operative procedure contemplated and estimated length of hospital stay.

If telephone preauthorization was given, list date of authorization, name of the person who gave the telephone authorization, time given, and log number.

8. Give a complete description of the service(s), item(s), or appliance(s) requested; RVS, SMA, or SMR procedure code number(s); and physician's usual charge.

For prescription drugs indicate drug type code(s) shown in the Medi-Cal Drug Formulary.

9. The physician must sign the TAR form, giving the date and his degree.
10. TAR data to be supplied by the state consultant:
    (a) Not generally used
    (b) The consultant's denial of all services rendered
    (c) The consultant's comments
    (d) Approval of requests. See Block (f) for specific services approved.
    (e) The expiration date of approved services
    (f) Approval or denial of requested services is shown by "yes" or "no" check marks in the authorized column
    (g) An explanation of denied or modified items
    (h) The consultant's signature and approval date

When approving retroactive requests, the consultant will, in addition to dating his or her signature, provide an effective retroactive approval date.

MEDI-CAL GLOSSARY

Cost Deduction   For the Medically Indigent person. This is the amount the patient must pay each month before he or she can be eligible for Medi-Cal assistance. Also known as *liability* or *spenddown*.

Liability   For a Medically Needy person. This is the monthly amount the patient must pay toward medical care every three months before he or she can obtain a Medi-Cal card. Also known as *Cost Deduction* or *spenddown*.

Linkage
When a person is not getting a cash grant, but is over 65, or blind, or disabled, or in a family "with a child under 21 years who is without the support of its parent because of the death, disability, unemployment, or continued absence from the home of the parent," the person is considered "linked" to one of these categories.

Maintenance Need
The amount established by the Legislature to provide the necessities of food, shelter, and so forth. It will vary with the number of members in the family.

Medi-Cal
California's name for Medicaid: the federal, state, and county program of medical assistance for needy and low-income persons of all ages.

Spenddown
The general name for a liability or cost deduction.

Note: Above information obtained from 12-75 booklet from Medi-Cal put out by State of California Department of Health.

TO THE STUDENT: In order to keep up-to-date, always read the current bulletins on the Medicaid or Medi-Cal program in your state.

You are now ready to complete the review questions at the end of this chapter. Refer to the Appendix, Assignments 9 and 10, pp. 537–544, to complete forms pertinent to the Medicaid and Medi-Cal programs by referring to the case histories.

REVIEW QUESTIONS

Medicaid

1. Medicaid is sponsored by_____ .

2. Medicaid is not an insurance program. It is a/an_____program.

3. In all other states the program is known as Medicaid but in California the program is called_____.

4. The only state that does not have this program is_____.

5. What people might be eligible for Medicaid?

a. _____

b. _____

c. _____

d. _____

e. _____

f. _____

6. The name of the program for the prevention, early detection, and treatment

of welfare children is known as _____,

It is abbreviated as _____.

7. When professional services are rendered, the Medicaid identification card must
show eligibility for: (Circle one)

a. day of service   c. month of service

b. year of service   d. week of service

8. Is prior authorization ever required in a bonafide emergency situation?

_____

9. What do these abbreviations mean?

AFDC _____

SSI _____

EPSDT _____

Medicaid—New York

10. Mark the following statements True or False (Circle T or F)

a. New York State's Medicaid program has a fiscal   T   F
    intermediary.

b. Physicians forward bills or state vouchers to a   T   F
    local social service department.

c. Prior authorization is required for hospitalizing a patient under the Family Care program.   T   F

d. Medicaid cards are issued yearly to eligible persons.   T   F

e. In-hospital services are covered for catastrophic illness.   T   F

f. Under "A" coverage the patient is not entitled to all Medicaid benefits.   T   F

Medi-Cal

11. It is July 14 and your Medi-Cal patient comes in for a routine office visit. What do you obtain from her for this visit?

_____or_____
(if she does not have first item)

12. Your Medi-Cal patient phones you August 7 and says she is out of "labels" already but she wants to be seen within the next few days as she has a terrible skin rash. You make an appointment for August 10 and then you

_____

_____

13. Your Medi-Cal patient was seen in the office late on May 1 and was scheduled for an emergency appendectomy in the wee hours of May 2. You obtained the proper

_____label when he was in the office for his office visit. What else do you need to

complete your billing to Medi-Cal?_____

_____

14. Your Medi-Cal patient also has health insurance from Pacific Mutual. She gave

you the proper label for your billing. What else do you need from her?_____

_____

15. Your Medi-Cal patient was in for an office visit and the doctor said he needed to have a cholecystectomy within the next 6 weeks to 2 months and you should schedule it when convenient. Before you schedule the surgery, what do you do?

_____ After you have completed the
above procedure, the patient was scheduled for his cholecystectomy. After the surgery

you bill Medi-Cal attaching _____ and _____ to the form.

Do you need to send any information to the hospital? _____

16. Your Medi-Cal patient also has CHAMPUS. What procedure do you follow? Be exact in your steps for a dependent of an active military man.

a. _____

b. _____

17. What is the time limit for sending in a Medi-Cal claim? _____

_____

18. What do these abbreviations mean?

POE _____   TAR _____

EOB _____   MN _____

19. Your Medi-Cal patient seen today needs chronic hemodialysis services. You phone for a TAR to get verbal approval. What four important items must you have to complete the written TAR?

a. _____   c. _____

b. _____   d. _____

20. Can a POE label be used in emergency situations? _____

_____

Notes:

Notes:

Notes:

6
Medicare and Medi-Medi

BEHAVIORAL

OBJECTIVES *The Assistant should be able to:*

1. Understand the benefits and nonbenefits of both Medicare and Medi-Medi.
2. Learn who is eligible for Medicare and Medi-Medi.
3. State how to complete the SSA-1490 claim form properly.
4. Identify a Medicare patient's card.
5. Identify a Medi-Medi patient's card.
6. Define abbreviations as they appear on a patient's record.
7. Abstract from the patient record the necessary information for completing the SSA-1490 form.
8. Know the proper CPT and RVS coding when submitting the Medicare claim.
9. Minimize the number of insurance forms rejected because of improper completion.
10. Learn how to record information on the patient's ledger after a Medicare payment has been received.

MEDICARE

Medicare is health insurance under Social Security for people over 65 who are eligible and who have filed. If a person wishes to apply for Social Security early (at age 62), the benefits are not as great as they are at age 65. Medicare is also available to the blind and to the disabled, such as disabled workers of any age, disabled widows, dependent widowers between ages 50 and 65, and adults disabled before age 22. Eligibility can be such that a person can have only Part A Medicare coverage or only Part B Medicare coverage. However, those who qualify for full eligibility will have both Part A and Part B.

I. **Part A** of Medicare is hospital insurance benefits for the aged, disabled, and blind.

    1. Funds to provide this health service come from special contributions from employees and self-employed persons, with employers paying an equal amount. These contributions are collected along with regular Social

Security contributions from wages and self-employment income earned during a person's working years.

2. A benefit period begins the day a patient enters a hospital and ends as soon as the patient has not been a bed patient in any hospital for 60 consecutive days.

3. Medicare Part A provides benefits to applicants in any of the following situations:

    a. Bed patient in a hospital up to 90 hospital days for each benefit period.

    b. Bed patient in an Extended Care Facility (ECF)* up to 100 extended care days for each benefit period.

    c. Patient at home receiving home health services for up to 100 home health visits for each benefit period up to 1 year—if the patient has been in a hospital at least 3 consecutive days and is now confined at home.

4. Cost to patient

    a. Insurance pays all hospital costs for the first 60 days after a $124 deductible is met for each benefit period. From 61 to 90 days all costs are paid except $31 a day. A one-time-only lieftime reserve of 60 days may be used—insurance then pays all except $62 per day. The lifetime reserve is never renewed and can be used after the patient has been in the hospital 90 days.

    b. Extended care facility: All costs are paid for 20 days in each benefit period; then from 21 to 100 days all costs are paid except $15.20 a day.

II. **Part B** of Medicare is supplementary medical insurance benefits for the aged, disabled, and blind.

1. Funds for this program come equally from those who sign up for it and from the federal government. Medical insurance premiums are automatically deducted from monthly checks for those who receive Social Security benefits, railroad retirement benefits, or a civil service annuity. Others pay premiums directly to the Social Security Administration.

2. Benefits to patients under Medicare Part B are:

    a. Regular medical

        (1) Sixty-dollar deductible for each year. Medicare pays 80 per cent of the "*reasonable charges*" for the rest of the year. The patient pays 20 percent of the "*reasonable charges.*"

    b. Outpatient hospital benefits: After the $60 deductible is met, Medicare pays 80 percent of the "*reasonable charges.*"

    c. Home visits: 100 visits, separate from hospital insurance visits. The agency (physical therapist, speech therapist, or similar allied health professional) makes the claim, so it never passes through the doctor's office. Medicare pays 100 per cent after the deductible has been met. A patient does not have to be hospitalized first.

3. Billing Medicare Part B

    a. *Assignment:* The physician agrees to accept payment from Medicare plus 20 per cent of "*reasonable charges*" after the $60 deductible has

*Also known as Skilled Nursing Facility.

been met. The payment goes directly to the physician. "*Reasonable charges*" means the amount that Medicare lists on the Explanation of Benefits (EOB) as a fair charge for the procedure. It may be lower than the fee the physician has listed on the claim. When a physician accepts assignment, he or she may bill the patient only 20 per cent of what Medicare considers a reasonable charge.

b. *Payment directly to patient:* The patient fills out the SSA-1490 Medicare form, attaches doctor's bills, and submits the form himself. Or the physician may give the patient an itemized statement such as Super Bill so the patient may submit his own claim (see Fig. 6–3, pp. 146 and 147.)

c. *Carry-over period:* If the patient's expenses for the covered services do not exceed $60 until the last 3 months of a year, then any expenses in the last 3 months which counted toward the $60 deductible for that year can be counted again toward the $60 for the next year.

d. *Time limit* for sending in claims is the end of the year following the year in which services were used.

e. The form that physicians and patients use to submit their claims to Medicare is SSA-1490 (see Fig. 6–5, p. 150).

f. To ascertain the mailing address for the Medicare claim form for your state or county, please refer to pages 155 to 160.

g. An Explanation of Medicare Benefits (EOMB) is received by the physician or patient (depending on who submitted the claim and whether or not assignment was taken) with the Medicare check. This occurs after the claim has been processed.

Example

Physician Accepts Assignment		Physician Does Not Accept Assignment	
Total medical bill	$115	Total medical bill	$115
Medicare reasonable charges	$100	Medicare reasonable charges	$100
Medicare pays 80%	$ 80	Medicare pays 80%	$ 80
Patient is billed for 20%	$ 20	Patient is billed for	$ 35
Check goes to physician for	$ 80	Check goes to patient for	$ 80
Write-off by physician	$ 15	No write-off by physician	

Note: If Medicare does not cover a service, the patient pays for the service whether the doctor accepts assignment or not.

4. The following list shows the kinds of doctor's services that medical insurance Part B will help pay for.

a. Medical and surgical services by a Doctor of Medicine (M.D.), Doctor of Osteopathy (D.O. or M.D.), or a Doctor of Dental Medicine or Doctor of Dental Surgery (D.D.S.).

b. Certain services by podiatrists (D.P.M.).

c. Limited services by chiropractors (D.C.), such as subluxation of the spine.

MEDICARE HEALTH INSURANCE CARD

The patient should show you his health insurance card (Fig. 6–6, p. 151) since it indicates whether the patient has both hospital and medical insurance and when each started. When a husband and wife both have Medicare, they receive separate cards and claim numbers. This card is red, white, and blue in color.

COVERAGE

Hospital

Benefits

Semiprivate room and meals
Regular nursing services
Intensive Care Unit (ICU) costs
Drugs furnished by the hospital during hospitalization
X-ray and laboratory tests
Medical supplies, such as casts, surgical dressings, and splints
Use of wheelchair, called Durable Medical Equipment (DME)
Operating Room (OR) and Recovery Room costs
Physical therapy, occupational therapy, and speech pathology services

Nonbenefits

Personal convenience items, such as television, radio, telephone
Private duty nurses
Private room
First three pints of blood

Skilled Nursing Facility

Benefits

Semiprivate room and meals
Regular nursing services
Physical, occupational, and speech therapy
Drugs furnished by the facility
Medical Supplies, such as splints and casts
Use of wheelchair, called Durable Medical Equipment (DME)

Nonbenefits

Personal convenience items, such as television, radio, telephone
Private duty nurses
Extra charge for private room, unless patient needs it for medical reasons
First three pints of blood

Medical Services

Benefits

Medical and surgical procedures
Diagnostic tests and procedures that are part of treatment

Services in the doctor's office, such as x-rays, services of doctor's office nurse, drugs that cannot be self-administered, medical supplies, physical therapy, speech pathology services, ambulance transportation, prosthetic devices, and Durable Medical Equipment (DME)

Nonbenefits

Routine physical examination

Routine foot care

Eye or hearing examinations for prescribing or fitting eyeglasses or hearing aids

Immunizations, unless required because of injury or risk of infection

Cosmetic surgery, unless needed because of injury or to improve the functioning of a malformed part of the body

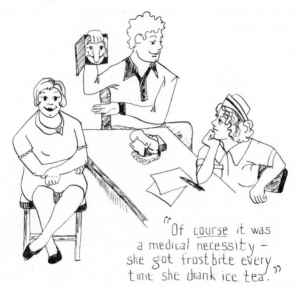

"Of course it was a medical necessity — she got frostbite every time she drank ice tea."

Home Health Services

Benefits

Part-time skilled nursing care

Physical therapy, speech therapy, and occupational therapy

Part-time services of home health aides

Medical social services

Medical supplies and equipment provided by a physical therapist, speech therapist, or occupational therapist

Nonbenefits

Full-time nursing care at home

Drugs and biologicals

Meals delivered to patient's home

Homemaker services

Medicare Does Not Cover the Following:

Acupuncture

Christian Science practitioners' services

Custodial care

Drugs and medicines with or without prescription

Eyeglasses and eye examinations

Hearing aids and hearing examinations

Homemaker services

Injections that can be self-administered (such as insulin)

Meals delivered to the patient's home

Naturopaths' services

Nursing care on a full-time basis in the patient's home

Personal convenience items, such as telephone, radio, or television at the hospital or skilled nursing facility

Physical examinations (routine)

Private duty nurses

Services performed by immediate relatives or members of the patient's household

Services which are not reasonable and necessary under Medicare guidelines or on professional medical advice by the Utilization Review Committee or by a Professional Standards Review Organization

Services payable by Workers' Compensation or another government program

Services for which neither the patient nor another party on his behalf has a legal obligation to pay

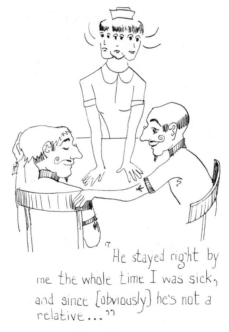

"He stayed right by me the whole time I was sick, and since [obviously] he's not a relative..."

Alien on Medicare

An alien on Medicare may have both Part A and Part B coverage, or he or she may be eligible only for Part B or only for Part A. To be eligible, the applicant must have lived in the United States as a permanent resident for 5 consecutive years. It is usually not necessary to state that the patient is an alien on the Medicare SSA-1490 form. The only exception to this is when the alien is over 65 and on Medicaid (Medi-Cal) and is not eligible for Medicare benefits at all. In this case, the Medicaid processing agent must be billed on the proper Medicaid billing form, and it is best to state on the Medicaid form that this person is "over 65 and is not eligible for Medicare benefits—ALIEN."

Medigap

The general term "Medigap" is used for Medicare supplemental insurance programs. These insurance policies help to cover the medical expenses that Medicare does not pay, such as the deductible and certain medical services. For processing the patient's supplemental insurance, the following information is required by the insurance company. (Bill Medicare first.)

A. The patient's group and policy numbers (e.g., Blue Cross requires the Group and Certificate numbers) written on the Explanation of Medicare Benefits (EOMB) attached to—

B. A copy of the original "Request for Medicare Payment" form SSA-1490 showing the diagnosis and itemization of charges

OR

C. A copy of the billing statement of the physician (or other provider of service), showing date of treatment, description of service(s) rendered, charges, and diagnosis.

MEDI-MEDI

Patients designated as Medi-Medi are those who are on both Medicare and Medicaid (Medi-Cal) simultaneously. They are usually people over 65 and entitled to Medicaid (Medi-Cal) benefits, such as those who qualify for Old Age Security (OAS) assistance benefits, the severely disabled, and the blind. In some instances they may be 62 years of age if they applied for Social Security benefits early.

BENEFITS

Medi-Medi patients have the benefits of the Medicare program as well as those of the Medicaid program. Because of this fact, the assignment on the claim form SSA-1490 must *always* be accepted. If the doctor does not accept assignment, then payment goes to the patient, and Medicaid (Medi-Cal) will not pick up the residual.

CLAIM PROCEDURE

In general, use the SSA-1490 claim form. In some states the fiscal intermediary for a Medi-Medi claim may have a different address from that used for the processing of a person who is on Medicare only. Write or call your nearest Medicare fiscal intermediary for the guidelines pertinent to your state.

The SSA-1490 claim form will automatically be processed by Medicaid (Medi-Cal) after processing is completed by Medicare. It is not necessary to submit another form. Claims should be sent in according to the time limit designated by the Medicaid program in your state. For instance, in California claims must be sent in within a 2-month period from the end of the month of service, and the case should be treated like a Medi-Cal case (see p. 145). As shown in Figure 6–1, in California a POE (Proof of Eligibility) label from the patient's Medi-Cal identification card or a photocopy of the patient's card must be included on the claim to help expedite it. The card must be valid for the month of service. Note proper placement of the POE label by looking at Figure

6–2. Any additional labels for services should be placed to the left of the first label. No Medi-Cal Treatment Authorization Request (TAR) form is required for a Medi-Medi patient treated by an M.D. The patient may be treated as often as necessary per month with only one POE label.

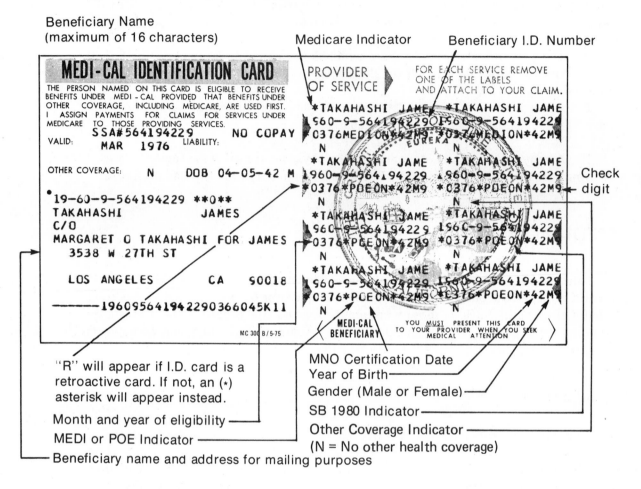

FIGURE 6–1

Medi-Medi card used in California, showing placement of sticky labels and Medicare identification number.

The letters following the Medicare number on the patient's identification card indicate the following (this is only a partial listing):

A   = wage earner
B   = husband's number (wife 62 years or older)
D   = widow
HA = disabled adult
C   = disabled child
J
K1 } = special monthly benefits, never worked under Social Security
J1
T   = uninsured and entitled only to health insurance benefits

The letters preceding the Medicare number on the patient's identification card indicate:

MA
  A with 6 digits (Example: A 000000)
WA with 6 digits   = Railroad Retirees
A with 9 digits (Example: A-000-00-0000)
WA with 9 digits

☆ U. S. GOVERNMENT PRINTING OFFICE: 1974-584-994/3

REQUEST FOR MEDICARE PAYMENT

Form Approved
OMB No.
72–RO730

MEDICAL INSURANCE BENEFITS—SOCIAL SECURITY ACT (See Instructions on Back—**Type or Print Information**)

NOTICE—Anyone who misrepresents or falsifies essential information requested by this form may upon conviction be subject to fine and imprisonment under Federal Law

PART I—PATIENT TO FILL IN ITEMS 1 THROUGH 6 ONLY

Copy from
YOUR OWN
HEALTH
INSURANCE
CARD
(See example on back)

1 Name of patient (First name, Middle initial, Last name)

2 Health insurance claim number (Include all letters)   ☐ Male   ☐ Female

3 Patient's mailing address   City, State, ZIP code   Telephone Number

4 Describe the illness or injury for which you received treatment (Always fill in this item if your doctor does not complete Part II below)

SAMPLE

Was your illness or injury connected with your employment?   ☐ Yes   ☐ No

5 If you have other health insurance or if your State medical assistance agency will pay part of your medical expenses and you want information about this claim released to the insurance company or State agency upon its request, give the following information.

Insuring organization or State agency name and address

```
1910-2192283-101
SARAH C. NILE
*0377*POE* N*F*4
```

Policy or Medical Assistance Number

6 I authorize any holder of medical or other information about me to release to the Social Security Administration or its intermediaries or carriers any information needed for this or a related Medicare claim. I permit a copy of this authorization to be used in place of the original, and request payment of medical insurance benefits either to myself or to the party who accepts assignment below.

Signature of patient (See instructions on reverse where patient is unable to sign)   Date signed

SIGN HERE ▶

PART II—PHYSICIAN OR SUPPLIER TO FILL IN 7 THROUGH 14

7	A. Date of each service	B. Place of service (*See Codes below)	C. Code surgical or medical procedures and other services or supplies furnished for each date given	D. Nature of illness or injury requiring services or supplies	E. Charges (If related to unusual circumstances explain in 7C)	Leave Blank
			Code		$	

ON CROSS OVER CLAIMS (Medi-Medi) PLACE THE IDENTIFICATION LABEL FOR THE CURRENT MONTH TO THE LEFT OF THE SPACE ENTITLED "Medi-Cal Identification Number." ADDITIONAL LABELS FOR SERVICES PERFORMED IN PREVIOUS MONTHS SHOULD BE PLACED TO THE LEFT OF THE FIRST LABEL. USE A "POE" LABEL. BE SURE TO TYPE THE NUMBER IN IF MAKING A CARBON COPY SO IT WILL BE ON YOUR FILE COPY.

8 Name and address of physician or supplier (Number and street, city, State, ZIP code)

Telephone No.

Physician or supplier code

9 Total charges $

10 Amount paid $

11 Any unpaid balance due $

12 Assignment of patient's bill
▶ ☒ I accept assignment (See reverse) ☐ I do not accept assignment.
DR. MUST ALWAYS ACCEPT ASSIGNMENT ON MEDI-MEDI CLAIM

13 Show name and address of facility where services were performed (If other than home or office visits)

14 Signature of physician or supplier (A physician's signature certifies that physician's services were personally rendered by him or under his personal direction)   Date signed
▶

*O—Doctor's Office
IL—Independent Laboratory

H—Patient's Home (If portable X-ray services, identify the supplier)
IH—Inpatient Hospital

ECF—Extended Care Facility
OH—Outpatient Hospital

OL—Other Locations
NH—Nursing Home

FORM **SSA-1490D(2)** (8-72)

Department of Health, Education, and Welfare
Social Security Administration

FIGURE 6–2

SSA-1490 D(2) claim form, showing proper placement of Medi-Cal POE sticky label.

POE Label Required For:

Outpatient care by an M.D.
Inpatient and outpatient hospital care

MEDI Label Required For:

Routine eye examinations
Physical therapist services
Chiropractic services
Optometrist services other than eye appliances
Routine foot care (podiatry services)
Nondiagnostic services billed by psychologists
Immunizations
Vaccines
Routine physical examinations

ADB SYSTEMS VEN 642 8556 OX 485 7845

Vera Cutis, M. D.
4567 Broad Avenue
Woodland Hills, XY 12345

Mr. Harry M. Bare
1200 Skin Street
Pate, XY 12345

To file your claim with your private insurance company or Medicare please complete the reverse side of this form and attach yellow copy of your statement to your claim form and mail to your insurance company according to their instructions.

PLEASE DETACH AND RETURN WITH YOUR REMITTANCE.

IRS NO. 95-2789297

DATE	DOCTOR	RVS CODE	DIAGNOSIS • DESCRIPTION	PAID ON ACCOUNT	AMOUNT
7-17-76	Dr. Cutis	90010	Neurodermatitis of groin and scrotal.		$ 25.00
8-14-76	Dr. Cutis			$25.00	
12-23-76	Dr. Cutis	90050	Eczematous dermatitis, widespread.		13.00
12-23-76	Dr. Cutis	85010	Eczematous dermatitis, widespread.		8.00
1-2-77	Dr. Cutis			21.00	
1-7-77	Dr. Cutis	90050	Neurodermatitis of groin and scrotal.		13.00
2-5-77	Dr. Cutis			13.00	
				TOTAL	-0-

THIS COPY FOR TAX PURPOSES

A

FIGURE 6–3

If the physician elects to have the patient bill Medicare directly, here is an example of Super Bill, an itemized statement containing all pertinent information, such as name and address of patient, diagnosis, dates of services, description of service, RVS or CPT codes, and charges. *A*, Front side of form. *B*, Back of form. (Courtesy of ADB Systems, Ventura, CA 93003. [Affiliated with National Business Systems, Inc.])

```
                          HEALTH INSURANCE CLAIMS

IN THE EVENT YOU HAVE INSURANCE COVERAGE OTHER THAN BLUE CROSS OR BLUE SHIELD:

    • TO FILE YOUR CLAIM WITH YOUR PRIVATE INSURANCE COMPANY OR MEDICARE, COMPLETE THE TOP PORTION ON THE REVERSE SIDE
      OF THIS FORM AND THE INFORMATION REQUIRED BELOW.

    • OBTAIN A CLAIM FORM FROM YOUR INSURANCE COMPANY REPRESENTATIVE OR MEDICAL PLAN CARRIER AND FILL IN YOUR PART OF
      THEIR FORM.

    • ATTACH THIS COPY OF YOUR STATEMENT TO YOUR CLAIM FORM AND MAIL TO YOUR INSURANCE COMPANY ACCORDING TO THEIR IN-
      STRUCTIONS. A SEPARATE CLAIM FORM AND STATEMENT ARE USUALLY REQUIRED FOR EACH FAMILY MEMBER RECEIVING SERVICES
      COVERED BY INSURANCE. STATEMENTS FROM LABORATORIES OR ANESTHESIOLOGISTS MAY ALSO BE ATTACHED TO THIS FORM.

IN THE EVENT YOU HAVE INSURANCE COVERAGE WITH BLUE CROSS OR BLUE SHIELD, THE OFFICE SHALL FILE YOUR CLAIMS.
```

Form fields: NAME OF PATIENT / DATE OF BIRTH / AGE / SEX / RELATION TO SUBSCRIBER / CONDITION CAUSED BY: INJURY, ILLNESS, PREGNANCY / IF INJURY, INDICATE DATE, HOW AND WHERE SUSTAINED — AUTO ACCIDENT, HOME, OTHER — DATE OF INJURY MO. DAY. YR. / IF PREGNANCY, DATE OF COMMENCEMENT / IS THIS A NEW ILLNESS: NO YES / IS CONDITION DUE TO INJURY OR SICKNESS ARISING OUT OF PATIENTS EMPLOYMENT? NO YES / DATE FIRST CONSULTED ANY PHYSICIAN FOR THIS CONDITION MO. DAY YR.

EVEN THOUGH YOU HAVE FILED AN INSURANCE CLAIM, YOU WILL RECEIVE A STATEMENT EACH MONTH IF YOUR ACCOUNT HAS AN OUTSTANDING BALANCE. YOU ARE RESPONSIBLE FOR PAYMENT OF YOUR ACCOUNT REGARDLESS OF INSURANCE.

RVS CODE:
1969 CALIFORNIA MEDICAL ASSOCIATION PROCEDURE CODE.   *B*

FIGURE 6–3 *(Continued)*

Hearing aid examinations
Measured eye refractions

Any of the above services provided by a physician, with the exception of eye refractions, may be authenticated for Medi-Cal payment by attachment of an approved Treatment Authorization Request (TAR) plus a POE label instead of a MEDI label.

COMMITTEE REVIEW

If the payment made by Medi-Medi is in question and you want to have the claim reviewed, send copies of any previous report of claim and all correspondence, as well as the Explanation of Benefits (EOB), to both the Public Services Committee (Department of Health) in your area and the fiscal intermediary handling Medi-Medi claims. Figure 6–4A shows a sample letter that may be used in requesting a Medicare review. Figure 6–4B shows Form SSA-1964, which may be used by the patient or by the Medical Assistant in requesting a review of Part B Medicare claims.

Hugh R. Aged, M. D.
1000 Any Street
Anytown, XY 12345
013/486-9002

January 2, 1977

Committee on Physician's Services
Medicare
Street address of fiscal intermediary
City, State, Zip Code

Re: Underpayment

Identification No.: 1910-2192283-101
Patient: Mrs. Sarah C. Nile
Type of Service: Exploratory laparotomy
Date of Service: December 1, 1976
Amount Paid: $000.00
My Fees: $000.00

Dear Sirs:

Herewith a request for a Committee Review of the above-named case,
since I consider the allowance paid very low having in mind the
location, the extent, the type, and the necessary surgical procedure
performed.

Enclosed is a photocopy of the operative report, the Medicare
Explanation of Benefits, and the Medicare SSA 1490 claim
originally submitted.

Considering these points, I hope that you will authorize additional
payment in order to bring the total fee to a more reasonable amount.

Sincerely,

Hugh R. Aged, M. D.

mf

Enclosures (3)   *A*

FIGURE 6–4

Medicare Review Request. *A*, If you wish to inquire about a disallowed procedure or about a payment which you feel should have been a larger amount, you might use the following letter, which has proven successful in a number of medical offices. It is a good idea to enclose photocopies of all original documents submitted with the claim. *B*, Request for review of Part B Medicare Claim Form SSA-1964.

Form Approved.
CMB No. 72-R0838

DEPARTMENT OF HEALTH, EDUCATION, AND WELFARE
SOCIAL SECURITY ADMINISTRATION

REQUEST FOR REVIEW OF PART B MEDICARE CLAIM
Medical Insurance Benefits — Social Security Act

Carrier's Name and Address

1 Name of Patient

2 Health Insurance Claim Number

3 I do not agree with the determination you made on my claim as described on my Explanation of Medicare

Benefits dated: or other notice dated:

4 MY REASONS ARE: *(Attach a copy of the Explanation of Medicare Benefits, or describe the service, date of service, and physician's name—NOTE.—If the date on the Notice of Benefits mentioned in item 3 is more than six months ago, include your reason for not making this request earlier.)*

5 ☐ I have additional evidence to submit. *(Attach such evidence to this form)*

☐ I do not have additional evidence.

COMPLETE ALL OF THE INFORMATION REQUESTED. SIGN AND RETURN THE FIRST 2 COPIES AND ANY ATTACHMENTS TO THE CARRIER NAMED ABOVE. IF YOU NEED HELP, TAKE THIS AND YOUR NOTICE FROM THE CARRIER TO A SOCIAL SECURITY OFFICE, OR TO THE CARRIER. KEEP THE LAST COPY OF THIS FORM FOR YOUR RECORDS.

6 SIGNATURE OF <u>EITHER</u> THE CLAIMANT <u>OR</u> HIS REPRESENTATIVE

Representative	Claimant
Address	Address
City, State, and ZIP Code	City, State, and ZIP Code
Telephone Number	Date	Telephone Number	Date

FORM SSA-1964 (2-74)   **CARRIERS COPY**   *B*

FIGURE 6–4 *(Continued)*

INSTRUCTIONS FOR COMPLETION OF THE MEDICARE
FORM SSA-1490 (See Fig. 6–5 and Assignments 11, 12, 13, 14, 15, and 16, pp. 545–565)

1. Enter the patient's name exactly as it appears on the Health Insurance Claim Card. See Figure 6–6.

2a. Enter the Health Insurance Claim Number (including the alphabetic suffix) *exactly* as it appears on the Health Insurance Card.

2b. Sex: check male or female.

FIGURE 6–5

SSA-1490 Medicare claim form with instructions on how to complete the form.

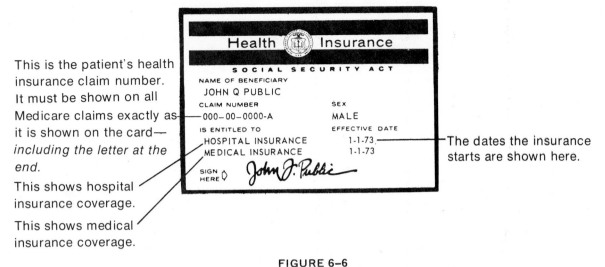

This is the patient's health insurance claim number. It must be shown on all Medicare claims exactly as it is shown on the card— *including the letter at the end.*

This shows hospital insurance coverage.

This shows medical insurance coverage.

The dates the insurance starts are shown here.

FIGURE 6–6

Medicare Health Insurance Claim Card.

3a. Enter the patient's mailing address, including zip code.

3b. Include the patient's telephone number, if available.

4a. When the patient completes this form, he describes the illness or injury in his own words or indicates the diagnosis given by the physician. If the Medical Assistant is completing the claim, she states "See 7D below."

4b. The employment-related box to the right of this block must be checked "yes" or "no."

5a. If the patient has insurance other than Medicare (such as Blue Cross or Blue Shield) for supplemental coverage, place the name of the insurance here.

5b. Indicate the policy number of such extra insurance here.

6. Signatures are required on all claims except Medi-Medi claims. Be sure the patient signs his or her name. If the patient cannot write, he should sign by mark (X) and have a witness sign his name and enter his address on this line. Or you can have the signature on file in the physician's office (see Fig. 6–7).

If the claim is filed for the patient by another person, that person should enter the patient's name and write "By," sign his or her own name and address in this space, and show relationship to the patient and why the patient cannot sign.

If the patient has died, a survivor should contact the nearest Social Security office for information on what to do. If the Medical Assistant is sending in the claim, she can sign her name as Medical Assistant and state "Unable to obtain signature, patient is deceased."

7. *Be sure to itemize the services rendered.* In Column A indicate the date of *each* service. In Column B indicate the place of service, using the codes at the bottom of the form. In Column C indicate the medical procedures and services as described in the Relative Value Studies (RVS) or Current Procedural Terminology (CPT) code books and enter the correct procedure number for each service in the "code" column. In Column D state the *diagnosis* pertinent to each procedure. In Column E indicate the physician's charge and be sure to indicate a separate charge for each service rendered.

8. Forms furnished by fiscal intermediaries sometimes are preprinted with the necessary provider or supplier information. Correct any erroneous preprinted information. If the forms are not preprinted, fill them out completely and accurately. Discard

```
                           Hugh R. Aged, M. D.
                           1000 Any Street
                           Anytown, XY 12345
                           013/486-9002



    LONG-TERM ASSIGNMENT OF BENEFITS AND INFORMATION RELEASE

    Patient's                          Patient's
    Name      Mrs. Sarah C. Nile       Account #    77-0000

    I request that payment under the MEDICAL INSURANCE PROGRAM be
    made directly to  Hugh R. Aged,      M.D. on any unpaid
    bills furnished me by that physician during the time period of

        January 2, 1977          to    December 31, 1977

    This will approve the release of necessary information to the
    MEDICAL INSURANCE PROGRAM for purposes of submitting a claim
    against my medical insurance policy.




    Signed   Sara C. Nile            Date   January 2, 1977
                 (Patient)
```

FIGURE 6-7

Long-Term Assignment of Benefits and Information Release. If unable to obtain the signature of a Medicare Patient because of confinement at home, extended care facility, or hospital, the following form may be used and kept in the patient's medical record. Attach a photocopy of this signed form to the SSA-1490 Medicare form each time a Medicare claim is submitted.

incorrect preprinted forms when new forms are received. The IRS number of the physician is also a requirement in this block if it is not preprinted. Indicate the physician's telephone number and the supplier code number (this is sometimes the state license number).

9. Indicate the total charges for this claim.

10. Enter any amount paid by the patient for services billed on this claim when the doctor has accepted assignment. If nothing has been paid, put a "0" in this space.

11. Indicate the total balance due for this claim.

12. Indicate clearly whether assignment is accepted for Medicare patients. When the beneficiary also is covered by Medicaid (Medi-Cal), assignment must always be accepted for reimbursement by Medicaid (Medi-Cal). If this block is not checked, payment will always be made to the beneficiary.

13. It is important to indicate the name and address (including zip code) of any facility where services were performed if other than office or home (such as hospital, radiology office, laboratory, and so forth).

14. When assignment is accepted, the physician's signature and degree, and the date signed, are required. A rubber stamp of the doctor's signature is acceptable on a Medicare claim. The physician can authorize a person on his staff (nurse, billing clerk, secretary) to sign his name manually or by rubber stamp in lieu of a handwritten signature.

DEPARTMENT OF HEALTH, EDUCATION, AND WELFARE
SOCIAL SECURITY ADMINISTRATION

Form Approved.
OMB No. 72-R0768

REQUEST FOR INFORMATION
MEDICARE PAYMENT FOR SERVICES TO A PATIENT NOW DECEASED

WHEN COMPLETED, SEND THIS FORM TO:	DECEASED PATIENT
	HEALTH INSURANCE CLAIM NUMBER OF DECEASED PATIENT

If bills for medical or other health services were paid by or for the deceased person, Medicare benefits may be due. We hope you will be able to help us determine who should receive payment. The person who paid the deceased's bill(s) has first right to any payment due. If the deceased or his estate paid the bill(s), benefits will be paid to the legal representative of the estate. If there is no legal representative, payment will be made to the person who stands highest in the list of relatives below. If the person who paid the bill(s) dies before being reimbursed, payment is also made to the person standing highest in the list of relatives. If there are no living relatives or legal representatives no payment will be made. Please answer the questions, sign on the reverse side and return this form in the enclosed envelope.

For Services Provided By:

PART I — (a) Who paid the deceased's bills for medical or other health services?

☐ The deceased or his estate   ☐ Yourself *(Sign on reverse*   ☐ Other person or organization
(Answer (b) below)   *side and return form)*   *(Answer Part 2 on reverse side)*

(b) Is there a legal representative of the estate?

☐ Yes *(If "Yes," give his name and address, Sign on reverse*   ☐ No *(If "No," answer (c))*
side and return form)

ALWAYS INCLUDE EVIDENCE OF PAYMENT SUCH AS A RECEIPTED BILL OR OTHER RECEIPT

NOTE: If you are the legal representative, submit a copy of your appointment papers with this form.

(c) Fill in ONLY the one block that shows the living relative that stands highest on this list:

NAME	ADDRESS
Widow or widower living in the same household as the deceased at the time of death or entitled to a monthly Social Security or Railroad Retirement benefit on the same earnings record as the deceased in the month of death.	
A child or children of the deceased entitled to monthly Social Security or Railroad Retirement benefits on the same earnings record as the deceased in the month of death. *(List the names and addresses of all entitled children of the deceased)*	
A parent or parents of the deceased entitled to monthly Social Security or Railroad Retirement benefits on the same earnings record as the deceased in the month of death.	
A widow or widower who was neither living with the deceased at the time of death nor at that time entitled on the same earnings record to a Social Security or Railroad Retirement benefit.	
A child or children of the deceased who were not entitled in the month of death to monthly Social Security or Railroad Retirement benefits on the same earnings record as the deceased. *(List the names and addresses of all such children.)*	

CONTINUED ON BACK

FORM **SSA-1660** (1-73)

A

FIGURE 6–8

Medicare Form SSA-1660, Request for Information Medicare Payment for Services to a Patient Now Deceased. *A*, Front side of form. *B*, Back of form.

A parent or parents not entitled in the month of death to monthly Social Security or Railroad Retirement benefits on the same earnings record as the deceased.

PART 2 – Give the names and addresses of persons or organizations who paid bills for medical or other health services for the deceased. If the bills were paid by more than one person or organization show the amount paid by each.

NAME	ADDRESS

I certify that if I receive the entire amount due, I will distribute it among other persons if they are legally entitled to it. Knowing that anyone making a false statement or representation of a material fact for use in determining the right to or the amount of Health Insurance benefits commits a crime punishable under Federal law, I certify that the above statements are true.

If this statement has been signed by mark (X), two witnesses who know the claimant should sign below, giving their full addresses. The signature and title of a Social Security employee will suffice in lieu of signatures of two witnesses.	SIGNATURE OF CLAIMANT (Write in ink) SIGN HERE ►
NAME	MAILING ADDRESS (Number and Street, P.O. Box or Route)
ADDRESS (Number and Street, City, State and ZIP Code)	
NAME	CITY, STATE AND ZIP CODE
ADDRESS (Number and Street, City, State and ZIP Code)	DATE (Month, Day and Year) / TELEPHONE NUMBER

If you wish assistance in completing this request, please take it to a Social Security Office. The people there will help you.

PLEASE RETURN THIS REQUEST IN THE ENCLOSED ENVELOPE

B

☆ U.S.Government Printing Office:1975—210-831/146

FIGURE 6–8 *(Continued)*

Billing for a Deceased Patient

There are two ways to submit billing for a patient who has expired. The method which will produce the quickest payment is when the doctor accepts assignment on the claim form. No signature by a family member is needed on the form, but in block number 6 where the patient's signature is required, type in "patient expired on (indicate date)." The second method is when the doctor does not accept assignment and bills Medicare. Nothing can be done about the open balance on the account until the estate is settled and then Medicare will pay. If family members of a deceased Medicare patient need to request payment for services that they have already paid for, the person(s) who paid the bill should complete Form SSA-1660, shown in Figure 6–8.

For further information, booklets, pamphlets, and the Medicare Manual, contact your nearest Social Security office.

TO THE STUDENT: Refer to the Appendix to complete the insurance forms pertinent to this chapter. Assignments 11, 12, 13 14, 15, and 16, pp. 545–565, pertain to this chapter.

MEDICARE FISCAL INTERMEDIARIES AND THEIR ADDRESSES

Insurance companies and Blue Cross and Blue Shield plans participate in the Medicare program as fiscal intermediaries for the federal government. The following list of names and addresses will help you determine to whom and where your claim should be sent.

Alabama
Medicare
Blue Cross-Blue Shield of Alabama
930 South 20th Street
Birmingham, AL 35205

Alaska
Medicare
Aetna Life & Casualty
Crown Plaza
1500 S.W. First Avenue
Portland, OR 97201

Arizona
Medicare
Aetna Life & Casualty
Medicare Claim Administration
3010 West Fairmount Avenue
Phoenix, AZ 85017

Arkansas
Medicare
Arkansas Blue Cross and Blue Shield
P.O. Box 2181
Little Rock, AR 72203

California
Counties of: Los Angeles, Orange, San Diego, Ventura, San Bernardino, Imperial, San Luis Obispo, Riverside, Santa Barbara
Medicare
*Occidental Life Insurance Co. of California
Box 54905
Terminal Annex
Los Angeles, CA 90054

*This office has Professional Relations Field Representatives (San Luis Obispo to San Diego—9 counties) for the purpose of interpreting Medicare policies and procedures. These representatives make personal calls at physician's offices, conduct seminars for doctors and medical assistants, and speak to hospital staffs and local medical society meetings.

Railroad Retirees:
Travelers Insurance Company
3600 Wilshire Boulevard
Los Angeles, CA 90010

Rest of State:
Medicare
Blue Shield of California
P.O. Box 7968, Rincon Annex
San Francisco, CA 94120

Colorado
Medicare
Colorado Medical Service, Inc.
700 Broadway
Denver, CO 80203

Connecticut
Medicare
Connecticut General Life
Insurance Co.
200 Pratt Street
Meriden, CT 06450

Delaware
Medicare
Blue Cross and Blue Shield of Delaware
201 West 14th Street
Wilmington, DE 19899

District of Columbia
Medicare
Medical Service of D.C.
550 – 12th St., S.W.
Washington, D.C. 20024

Florida
Counties of: Dade, Monroe
Medicare
Group Health, Inc.
P.O. Box 341370
Miami, FL 33134

Rest of State:
Medicare
Blue Shield of Florida, Inc.
P.O. Box 2525
Jacksonville, FL 32203

Georgia
The Prudential Insurance Co. of America
Medicare Part B
P.O. Box 95466 Executive Park Station
Atlanta, GA 30347

Hawaii
Medicare
Aetna Life & Casualty
P.O. Box 3947
Honolulu, HI 96812

Idaho
Medicare
The Equitable Life Assurance Society
P.O. Box 8048
Boise, ID 83707

Illinois
Cook County
Medicare Part B
Illinois Medical Service
P.O. Box 210
Chicago, IL 60690

Rest of State:
Medicare
CNA Insurance
Medicare Benefits Division
P.O. Box 910
Chicago, IL 60690

Indiana
Medicare Part B
120 West Market Street
Indianapolis, IN 46204

Iowa
Medicare
Blue Shield of Iowa
636 Grand Avenue
Des Moines, IA 50307

Kansas
Counties of: Johnson, Wyandotte
Medicare
Blue Shield of Kansas City
P.O. Box 169
Kansas City, MO 64141

Rest of State:
Medicare
Kansas Blue Shield
P.O. Box 239
Topeka, KA 66601

Kentucky
Medicare
Metropolitan Life Insurance Co.
1218 Harrodsburg Road
Lexington, KY 40504

Louisiana
Medicare
Pan-American Life Insurance Co.
P.O. Box 60450
New Orleans, LA 70160

Maine
Medicare
Union Mutual Life Insurance Co.
Box 4629
Portland, ME 04112

Maryland
Counties of: Montgomery, Prince George's
Medicare
Medical Service of D.C.
550 – 12th St., S.W.
Washington, D.C. 20024

Rest of State:
Maryland Blue Shield, Inc.
700 East Joppa Road
Towson, MD 21204

Massachusetts
Medicare
Blue Shield of Massachusetts, Inc.
P.O. Box 2137
Boston, MA 02106

Michigan
Medicare
Blue Shield of Michigan
P.O. Box 2201
Detroit, MI 48231

Minnesota
Counties of: Anoka, Dakota, Filmore, Goodhue, Hennepin, Houston, Olmstead, Ramsey, Wabasha, Washington, Winona
Medicare
The Travelers Insurance Company
8120 Penn Avenue, South
Bloomington, MN 55431

Rest of State:
Medicare
Blue Shield of Minnesota
P.O. Box 8899
Minneapolis, MN 55408

Mississippi
Medicare
The Travelers Insurance Co.
P.O. Box 22545
Jackson, MS 39205

Missouri
Counties of: Andrew, Atchison, Bates, Benton, Buchanan, Caldwell, Carroll, Cass, Clay, Clinton, Daviess, DeKalb, Gentry, Grundy, Harrison, Henry, Holt, Jackson, Johnson, Lafayette, Livingston, Mercer, Nodaway, Pettis, Platte, Ray, St. Clair, Saline, Vernon, Worth
Medicare
Blue Shield of Kansas City
P.O. Box 169
Kansas City, MO 64141

Rest of State:
Medicare
General American Life Insurance Co.
P.O. Box 505
St. Louis, MO 63166

Montana
Medicare
Montana Physicians' Service
P.O. Box 2510
Helena, MT 59601

Nebraska
Medicare
Mutual of Omaha Insurance Co.
P.O. Box 456, Downtown Station
Omaha, NE 68101

Nevada
Medicare
Aetna Life & Casualty
1535 Vassar Street
P.O. Box 3077
Reno, NV 89505

New Hampshire
Medicare
New Hampshire-Vermont
Physician Service
Two Pillsbury Street
Concord, NH 03301

New Jersey
Medicare
The Prudential Insurance Co. of America
P.O. Box 3000
Linwood, NJ 08221

New Mexico
Medicare
The Equitable Life Assurance Society
P.O. Box 3070, Station D
Albuquerque, NM 87110

New York
Counties of: Bronx, Columbia,
Delaware, Dutchess, Greene, Kings,
Nassau, New York, Orange, Putnam,
Richmond, Rockland, Suffolk,
Sullivan, Ulster, Westchester
Medicare
Blue Cross-Blue Shield of Greater
New York
Two Park Avenue
New York, NY 10016

County of: Queens
Medicare
Group Health, Inc.
P.O. Box 233–Midtown Station
New York, NY 10018

Counties of: Livingston, Monroe,
Ontario, Seneca, Wayne, Yates
Medicare
Genesee Valley Medical Care, Inc.
41 Chestnut Street
Rochester, NY 14647

Counties of: Allegany, Cattaraugus,
Erie, Genesee, Niagara, Orleans,
Wyoming
Medicare
Blue Shield of Western New York, Inc.
298 Main Street
Buffalo, NY 14202

Counties of: Albany, Broome,
Cayuga, Chautauqua, Chemung,
Chenango, Clinton, Cortland,
Essex, Franklin, Fulton, Hamilton,
Herkimer, Jefferson, Lewis,
Madison, Montgomery, Oneida,
Onondago, Oswego, Otsego,
Rensselaer, Saratoga, Schenectady,
Schoharie, Schuyler, Steuben,

St. Lawrence, Tioga, Tompkins,
Warren, Washington
Medicare
Metropolitan Life Insurance Co.
276 Genesee Street
P.O. Box 393
Utica, NY 13503

North Carolina
The Prudential Insurance Co. of America
Medicare B Division
P.O. Box 2126
High Point, NC 27261

North Dakota
Medicare
Blue Shield of North Dakota
301 Eighth Street, South
Fargo, ND 58102

Ohio
Medicare
Nationwide Mutual Insurance Co.
P.O. Box 57
Columbus, OH 43216

Oklahoma
Medicare
Aetna Life & Casualty
1140 N.W. 63rd Street
Oklahoma City, OK 73116

Oregon
Medicare
Aetna Life & Casualty
Crown Plaza
1500 S.W. First Avenue
Portland, OR 97201

Pennsylvania
Medicare
Pennsylvania Blue Shield
Box 65 Blue Shield Bldg.
Camp Hill, PA 17011

Rhode Island
Medicare
Blue Shield of Rhode Island
444 Westminster Mall
Providence, RI 02901

South Carolina
Medicare
Blue Shield of South Carolina
Drawer F, Forest Acres Branch
Columbia, SC 29260

South Dakota
Medicare
South Dakota Medical Service, Inc.
711 North Lake Avenue
Sioux Falls, SD 57104

Tennessee
Medicare
The Equitable Life Assurance Society
P.O. Box 1465
Nashville, TN 37202

Texas
Medicare
Group Medical and Surgical Service
P.O. Box 22147
Dallas, TX 75222

Utah
Medicare
Blue Shield of Utah
P.O. Box 270
2455 Parley's Way
Salt Lake City, UT 84110

Vermont
Medicare
New Hampshire-Vermont
Physician Service
Two Pillsbury Street
Concord, NH 03301

Virginia
Counties of: Arlington, Fairfax,
Cities of: Alexandria, Falls Church,
Fairfax
Medicare
Medical Service of D.C.
550-12th St., S.W.
Washington, D.C. 20024

Rest of State:
Medicare
The Travelers Insurance Co.
P.O. Box 26463
Richmond, VA 23261

Washington
Medicare
Washington Physicians' Service
Mail to your local
Medical Service Bureau

If you do not know which bureau
handles your claim, mail to:
Medicare Washington Physicians'
Service, 220 West Harrison,
Seattle, WA 98119

West Virginia
Medicare
Nationwide Mutual Insurance Co.
P.O. Box 57
Columbus, OH 43216

Wisconsin
County of Milwaukee
Medicare
Surgical Care—Blue Shield
P.O. Box 2049
Milwaukee, WI 53201

Rest of State:
Medicare
Wisconsin Physicians' Service
Box 1787
Madison, WI 53701

Wyoming
Medicare
The Equitable Life Assurance Society
P.O. Box 628
Cheyenne, WY 82001

Puerto Rico
Medicare
Seguros De Servicio De Salud De
Puerto Rico
P.O. Box 3628
104 Ponce de Leon Avenue
Hato Rey, PR 00936

Virgin Islands
Medicare
Seguros De Servicio De Salud De
Puerto Rico
P.O. Box 3628
104 Ponce de Leon Avenue
Hato Rey, PR 00936

American Samoa
Medicare
Hawaii Medical Service Assn.
P.O. Box 860
Honolulu, HI 96808

Guam
Medicare
Aetna Life & Casualty
P.O. Box 3947
Honolulu, HI 96812

REVIEW QUESTIONS

1. Mr. Doolittle has Medicare Part B coverage. He was well all during the past year. It is now January 1 and Mr. Doolittle is rushed to the hospital, where Dr. Input does an emergency gastric resection. Medicare is billed for $450 and the doctor agrees to accept an assignment.

Medicare allows $400 and sends you a check for $_____

The patient owes you $_____   You write off $_____

Original bill $_____   Medicare pays $_____

Medicare allowable $_____   Patient pays $_____

Difference $_____   Write off $_____

2. Mrs. James has Medicare Part B coverage. She met her deductible when she was ill in March of this year. It is now November 1 and Dr. Caesar performs a bilateral salpingo-oophorectomy, for which he bills her $300 and agrees to accept a Medicare assignment.

Medicare allows $275.

Medicare pays $_____

Mrs. James owes Dr. Caesar $_____

Dr. Caesar writes off $_____

The Assistant Surgeon charged Mrs. James $60 and does not accept an assignment. After receiving her check from Medicare, Mrs. James sends the surgeon his $60. Medicare has allowed $55 for the fee. How much of the money was from Mrs. James' private funds? $_____ . How much did Medicare pay? $_____ . How did Mrs. James let Medicare know about the Assistant Surgeon's bill?_____

_____

3. You work for Dr. Coccidioides. He does not accept assignments. He is treating Mr. Robinson for allergies. Mr. Robinson has Medicare Part A. You send in a bill to

Medicare for the $135 that Mr. Robinson owes you. What portion of the bill will

Medicare pay? _____

4. Mr. Fay was not sick until November of last year, when he had an illness resulting in $57 worth of medical bills. Since he was not eligible for any reimbursement from Medicare, he paid your bill himself. In February of the new year, he has a new illness that incurs him $89 in medical bills. He asks you to bill Medicare. Assuming that Medicare allows the entire amount of your fees, the Medicare check to the patient is

$ _____ (which comes to you). Patient's part of the bill to you is $ _____

5. What claim form was used in all of the previous billings? _____

_____

6. To whom was the form mailed? _____

7. Who is eligible for Medi-Medi? _____

_____

8. What form is used to submit a Medi-Medi claim? _____

9. What is the time limit for submitting a Medi-Medi claim? _____

10. Mrs. Davis, a Medi-Medi patient, has a cholecystectomy. In completing the

claim, the assignment portion is left blank in error. What will happen in this case? _____

_____

_____

11. A Medicare/Medi-Cal patient, Mrs. Jones, came in last month for an office visit. She had left her Medi-Cal identification card at home. She mails in a photocopy

of the card to you. Is this acceptable when submitting her claim? _____

12. Is a Medi-Cal Treatment Authorization Request (TAR) ever needed on a

Medi-Medi case? _____

13. Your Medi-Cal patient is also covered by Medicare. She comes in to your

office this month for a flu shot. What Medi-Cal label do you collect? _____ Last

month you attached a _____ label to your billing when the doctor examined her and gave her an injection for strep throat.

Notes:

7

CHAMPUS, CHAMPVA, and VA Outpatient Clinic

Behavioral

Objectives   *The Assistant should be able to:*

1. State who is eligible for CHAMPUS, CHAMPVA, and VA Outpatient Clinic.
2. Understand the benefits and nonbenefits of these government programs.
3. Be able to complete DA Form 1863-2 for professional services.
4. Identify the difference between CHAMPUS, CHAMPVA, and VA cards.
5. Identify and learn the use of other forms used with these health care programs.
6. Learn how the patient can submit his or her own claim.
7. Calculate CHAMPUS payments.
8. Define abbreviations as they appear on the patient's record.
9. Abstract from the patient record the information necessary for completing the DA Form 1863-2.
10. Learn the proper CPT and RVS coding for submission of the claim.
11. Record ledger information correctly.

CHAMPUS

CHAMPUS is the abbreviation for *Civilian Health and Medical Program of the Uniformed Services*. This is a congressionally funded comprehensive health benefits program designed to provide families of uniformed services personnel and service retirees a supplement to medical care in military and Public Health Service facilities. Beneficiaries may receive a wide range of civilian health care services, with a significant share of the cost paid for by the federal government. Usually these patients seek care from an Army or Navy hospital that is near their home. However, there are times when they can seek care through a private physician's office. We will stress delivery of care through the private physician in this chapter.

TABLE 7–1.   INPATIENT AND OUTPATIENT COST-SHARING

INPATIENT COST-SHARING

Beneficiaries	Sources of Charges	Patient's Share of Allowable Charges	CHAMPUS Share of Allowable Charges
Dependents of Active Duty Members	Hospital	First $25 or $3.90 a day, whichever is greater	100% of balance after patient's share
	Physician & Allied Health Personnel	NONE	100%
Retired Members, their Dependents & Dependents of Deceased Members	Hospital	25%	75%
	Physician & Allied Health Personnel	25%	75%

OUTPATIENT COST-SHARING

Sources of Charges	Cost-Sharing (Reasonable Charges)		
	(1) Deductible (Same for all Beneficiaries)	(2) Cost-Sharing	
		Beneficiary	CHAMPUS
All Sources of Covered Outpatient Services, to Include Physicians, Pharmacists, Hospitals, Allied Health Personnel Supply Agencies, etc.	The first $50 per patient per FISCAL YEAR (not to exceed $100 per Family) PLUS	(1) Dependent of Active Duty Members 20%	80%
		(2) Retired Members & their Dependents & the Dependents of Deceased Members 25%	75%

CIVILIAN HEALTH AND MEDICAL PROGRAM OF THE UNIFORMED SERVICES

PATIENTS	UNIFORMED SERVICES FACILITIES Hospitalization/Outpatient	Basic Program Hospitalization	Basic Program Outpatient	Program for the Handicapped
Spouse or child of active duty member	On a space-available basis	Eligible, but may need non-availability statement	Eligible	Eligible
Retired member	On a space-available basis	Eligible*	Eligible*	Not eligible
Spouse or child of retired member	On a space-available basis	Eligible*	Eligible*	Not eligible
Surviving spouse or child of deceased active duty or retired member	On a space-available basis	Eligible*	Eligible*	Not eligible
Dependent parent or parent-in-law of active duty, retired, or deceased member	On a space-available basis	Not eligible	Not eligible	Not eligible

COSTS	Uniformed Services Facilities Hospitalization	Uniformed Services Facilities Outpatient	Basic Program Hospitalization	Basic Program Outpatient	Program for the Handicapped
Spouse or child of active duty member	$3.90** per day	No charge	$3.90** per day or $25, whichever is greater	20% of allowable charges above the deductible (first $50 each fiscal year -- $100 maximum per family)	Patient's share per month depends on paygrade of sponsor -- $25 for E-1 to $250 for 0-10. CHAMPUS pays remainder up to $350 per mo.
Retired: Enlisted	No charge	No charge	25% of the allowable medical facility charges and professional fees	25% of allowable charges above the deductible (first $50 each fiscal year -- $100 maximum per family)	Not eligible
Officer	Subsistence	No charge			
Spouse or child of retired or deceased member	$3.90** per day	No charge			
Dependent parent or parent-in-law of active duty, retired, or deceased member	$3.90** per day	No charge	Not eligible	Not eligible	Not eligible

*Unless eligible at age 65 for Medicare hospital insurance

**For calendar year 1975. The amount is subject to review and change each year.

FIGURE 7-1

Chart showing inpatient and outpatient benefits of CHAMPUS, as well as eligibility and cost to patient. (From Commanders Digest, September 11, 1975, p. 6.)

ELIGIBILITY

Those who are entitled to medical benefits under the CHAMPUS program are:

1. Dependents of active service personnel.
2. Retired service personnel and dependents of retired members.
3. Dependents of service personnel who died on active duty.

BENEFITS

See Table 7–1 (p. 164) and Figure 7–1 (p. 165) for further clarification.

Spouses and children of active duty members:

For Inpatient (Hospitalized) Care: The beneficiary pays the first $25 of the hospital charge or $3.90 a day, whichever is greater, and CHAMPUS pays the remainder of the allowable charges for authorized care.

For Outpatient (Not Hospitalized) Care: The beneficiary pays the first $50 (the deductible) plus 20 per cent of the charges over the $50 deductible. A family with two or more eligible beneficiaries pays a maximum of $100 (the deductible) plus 20 per cent of the charges in excess of $100. CHAMPUS pays the remainder of the allowable charges, which is 80 per cent.

All other eligible beneficiaries (i.e., retired members, dependents of retired members, dependents of deceased members who died in active duty, and so forth):

For Inpatient (Hospitalized) Care: The beneficiary pays 25 per cent of the hospital charges and fees of professional personnel. CHAMPUS pays the remaining allowable charges for authorized care, or 75 per cent. (See Fig. 7–1 and Table 7–1.)

For Outpatient (Not Hospitalized) Care: The beneficiary pays $50 (the deductible) plus 25 per cent of the charges over the $50 deductible. A family with two or more eligible beneficiaries pays a maximum of $100 plus 25 per cent of the charges in excess of $100. CHAMPUS pays the remainder of the allowable charges for authorized care, which is 75 per cent.

CHAMPUS pays for:

1. Treatment of medical and surgical conditions.
2. Treatment of nervous, mental, and chronic conditions.
3. Treatment of contagious diseases.
4. Maternity and infant care.
5. Diagnostic tests and services (lab and x-ray).
6. Dental care as a necessary adjunct to medical or surgical treatment.
7. Drugs (including insulin) obtainable only by written prescription which are prescribed by a physician or dentist and procured from a pharmacy; also drugs furnished by a physician that are ordinarily obtained by prescription.
8. Ambulance service and home calls when medically necessary.
9. Medically necessary durable equipment, such as wheelchairs, iron lungs, and hospital beds, on a rental basis only.
10. Family planning services.

DEPENDENTS

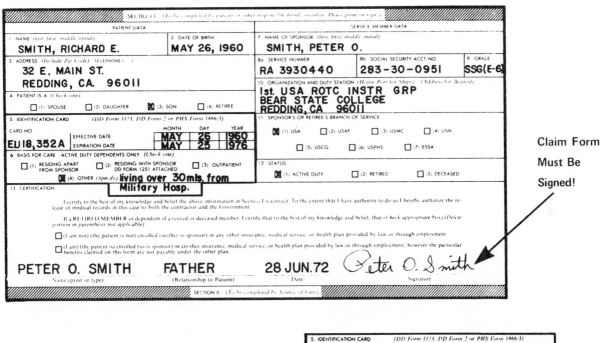

Claim Form
Must Be
Signed!

Only dependents
of active duty
complete Item 6.

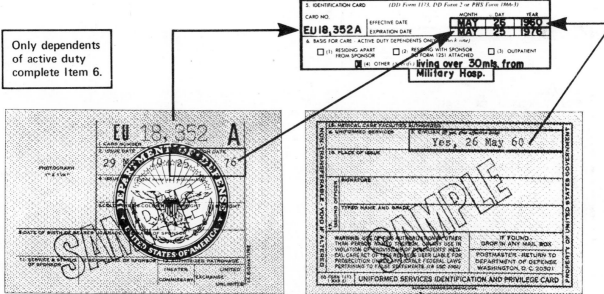

FIGURE 7–2

Dependent's I.D. card, DD Form 1173.

Depicted on these two pages are samples of the properly completed patient's portion of the CHAMPUS claim form, and Identification Cards from which essential information must be transcribed. Dependents under 10 years of age are not normally issued I.D. cards; information on their claims should be that reflected on either parent's card.

RETIREES

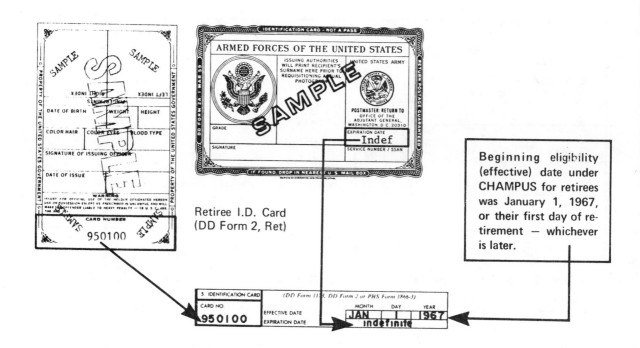

Retiree I.D. Card
(DD Form 2, Ret)

Beginning eligibility (effective) date under CHAMPUS for retirees was January 1, 1967, or their first day of retirement — whichever is later.

Claim Form Must Be Signed

FIGURE 7–3

Retiree's I.D. card, DD Form 2.

CHAMPUS does not pay for:

1. Domiciliary or custodial care.
2. Dental care (except as a necessary part of medical treatment; see Chapter 11).
3. Routine physical examinations and immunizations.
4. Well-baby care.
5. Routine refractions and eyeglasses.
6. Psychiatric treatment, except under fixed limitations.

PROVIDERS OF HEALTH CARE

The following professionals can treat a CHAMPUS patient:

1. M.D.
2. Doctor of Osteopathy
3. Doctor of Dental Surgery
4. Doctor of Dental Medicine
5. Doctor of Podiatric Medicine
6. Doctor of Optometry
7. Psychologist

CHAMPUS IDENTIFICATION CARD

All dependents 10 years of age and older are required to have a Uniformed Services Identification and Privilege card. See Figures 7–2 and 7–3 for samples of these cards and instructions for abstracting information from both the front and back sides of the card.

PRIVACY ACT OF 1974

This act, which became effective on September 27, 1975, establishes an individual's right to review records concerning himself. It covers only those acts that come under federal jurisdiction, such as the Social Security program and CHAMPUS. The Privacy Act requires that an individual from whom personal information is requested must be informed of

1. The authority for the request.
2. The principal purpose of the information requested.
3. Routine use of the information.
4. The effect on an individual not providing the information.

The Privacy Act Statements (DA Forms 1863-1-R, 1863-2-R, 1863-3-R, and 1863-4-R) were devised by CHAMPUS to be used with the corresponding CHAMPUS claim forms. Physicians are requested to furnish the appropriate Privacy Act Statement to each beneficiary at the time a CHAMPUS claim form is completed and to make a notation to this effect in item 17 on the claim form. (See Fig. 7–4.)

Another form that has evolved since the Privacy Act of 1974 is the CHAMPUS Consolidated Prescription Reimbursement Form 198 (Fig. 7–5). This is used in conjunction with DA Form 1863-2 (see Fig. 7–7) when a patient is submitting a claim to CHAMPUS and wishes to be reimbursed for prescription drugs.

DATA REQUIRED BY THE PRIVACY ACT OF 1974
(5 U.S.C. 552a)

TITLE OF FORM	PRESCRIBING DIRECTIVE
Services and/or Supplies Provided by Civilian Sources (Except Hospitals)	AR 40–121

1. AUTHORITY

10 USC 1079 and 1086; SSN: 42 USC (AR 608–14)

2. PRINCIPLE PURPOSE(S)

To collect information to evaluate eligibility for civilian health benefits authorized by 10 USC 1071–1086 and to issue checks upon establishment of eligibility and determination that health care received is authorized by statute. May include verification of certain information with the appropriate uniformed service.

3. ROUTINE USES

Compiling statistical information on number of claims for inpatient and outpatient care by category of patient, branch of service of sponsor, type of health care provided, cost by type of health care, cost in various geographical areas, and similar data. May include referral to Department of Justice for possible criminal prosecution for fraud.

4. MANDATORY OR VOLUNTARY DISCLOSURE AND EFFECT ON INDIVIDUAL NOT PROVIDING INFORMATION

Mandatory if sponsor or beneficiary desires to have a portion of the charges paid by the government. Failure to provide complete information would result in delay in payment of claim.

DA FORM 1863–2–R, Privacy Act Statement   26 Sep 75   T 1168

FIGURE 7–4

DA Form 1863-2-R, Privacy Act Statement.

DATA REQUIRED BY THE PRIVACY ACT OF 1974
(5 U.S.C. 552a)

TITLE OF FORM:

CHAMPUS Consolidated Prescription Reimbursement

PRESCRIBING DIRECTIVE:
AR 40-121

AUTHORITY: 10 USC 1079 and 1086; 42 USC

PRINCIPLE PURPOSE(S)

To provide a simple method for CHAMPUS beneficiaries to obtain reimbursement for payment of charges for authorized drugs and to identify it as being a part of a completed claims DA Form 1863-2.

ROUTINE USES

Used, in conjunction with DA Form 1863-2, by CHAMPUS Contractors to adjudicate reimbursement claims submitted by beneficiaries for cost incurred in the purchase of drugs obtainable only by prescription and to issue checks in payment therefor. May be used in compiling statistical information on pharmaceuticals by various categories. May also include referral to Department of Justice for possible criminal prosecution for fraud.

MANDATORY OR VOLUNTARY DISCLOSURE AND EFFECT ON INDIVIDUAL NOT PROVIDING INFORMATION

Disclosure of the information requested is mandatory if a sponsor or beneficiary desires to have a portion of the charges paid by the government without attaching itemized statements for drugs showing the complete name and address of the pharmacy, the prescription number, date filled and the charge for each drug. Failure to provide complete information would result in delay in payment of the claim.

CHAMPUS CONSOLIDATED PRESCRIPTION REIMBURSEMENT

1. PATIENTS' NAME

6. FISCAL ADMINISTRATOR:

2. SPONSOR'S NAME

3. SPONSOR'S SERVICE NUMBER

4. SPONSOR'S SOCIAL SECURITY NUMBER

5. PATIENTS' DIAGNOSIS (If Available)

7. CHAMPUS BENEFICIARY:

Reimbursement of your prescription claims will be expedited if you will itemize the prescription information from your pharmacy receipts or statements in order of date filled. Submit a separate list accompanied by a DA Form 1863-2 first 13 items completed, for each eligible family member. Supporting pharmacy receipts or statements must be retained a minimum of twelve months for submission if requested by the CHAMPUS Fiscal Administrator.

_____   _____
DATE   (Signature of Sponsor or eligible Family Member)

The persons signing this form are advised that the wilful making of a false or fraudulent statement herein renders them liable to prosecution under applicable Federal Laws.

8. PHARMACY NAME AND ADDRESS	9. DATE FILLED	10. PRESCRIPTION NUMBER	(If Available)		12. CHARGE
			11. DRUG NAME AND STRENGTH	QUANTITY	

CHAMPUS FORM 198
15 DEC 75

(Over, please)

FIGURE 7-5

CHAMPUS Consolidated Prescription Reimbursement Form 198, used in conjunction with DA Form 1863-2 (see Fig. 7—7) when a patient is submitting a claim to CHAMPUS for professional services rendered as well as for prescription drugs. Form 198 is to be used for drug claims only.

NONAVAILABILITY STATEMENT (DD Form 1251)

A Nonavailability Statement (DD Form 1251; see Fig. 7–6) is required for all CHAMPUS beneficiaries (dependents of active duty, retired, and deceased personnel and retired members themselves) *who live within a 40-mile radius of a uniformed services hospital* and wish to receive treatment as inpatients at a civilian hospital. The authorization for issuing Nonavailability Statements is limited to commanders of uniformed services hospitals or their designated representatives. The following are certain specific conditions under which the commander may issue a Nonavailability Statement:

1. When a maternity patient resides more than 30 miles from a uniformed services hospital.
2. When the local conditions impose an unreasonable cost or difficulty in getting to a service medical facility.
3. When hospitalization is required by a patient who has been receiving out-patient care from a civilian source, and it is medically advisable that care continue from the civilian source for the condition.
4. When there is no space available at the local service facility.
5. When the service hospital does not maintain the kind of medical facilities required.

The Nonavailability Statement must be presented to the source of care by the dependent, and this should then be attached to the claim form submitted to CHAMPUS.

A Nonavailability Statement is NOT required in the following instances:

1. In an emergency situation.
2. If a patient is residing beyond a 40-mile radius of a uniformed services hospital.
3. When the patient is hospitalized for nonadjunctive dental care.

There are other situations in which a Nonavailability Statement may not be required, but in instances other than those just mentioned it is best to check with the nearest military installation if you are in doubt.

CLAIMS PROCEDURE

1. Obtain the correct information from the patient's identification card.
2. CHAMPUS claims must be billed on Form DA 1863-2 (yellow) for professional services (see Fig. 7–7). For hospital billing the form used is Form DA 1863-1 (blue), and for the handicapped program the form is DA 1863-3 (white).
3. The CHAMPUS fiscal year is from October 1 to September 30. The time limit for submitting a claim is no later than the last day of the next calendar year.
4. *Assignment:* If the physician agrees to accept assignment, then he or she agrees to accept what CHAMPUS states are "reasonable charges," plus 20 or 25 per cent of these charges after the $50 or $100 deductible has been met. The payment goes directly to the physician. If the physician does not accept assignment, the patient fills out the top portion of Form DA 1863-2 and attaches the doctor's itemized statement, submitting the form himself. If the Medical Assistant submits the form, she can type a notation at the bottom of the form indicating that the "Doctor does not wish to

NONAVAILABILITY STATEMENT
DEPENDENTS MEDICAL CARE PROGRAM
(AR 40-121, SECNAV INST 6320.8A, AFR 160-41, PHS GEN CIR NO 6)

(This Statement is Issued for your Immediate use)

THE ISSUANCE OF THIS STATEMENT MEANS:
1. The medical care requested is not available to you at a Uniformed Services facility in this area.
2. If you receive medical care from civilian sources and such care is determined to be authorized care under the Medicare Program, it will be paid for by the Government to the extent that the program permits.
3. If you receive medical care from civilian sources and it is determined that all or part of the care is not authorized under the Medicare Program, THE GOVERNMENT WILL NOT PAY for the unauthorized care.

The determination of whether medical care you may receive from civilian sources is authorized for payment cannot be made at this time because this determination depends, among other things, upon the care you actually receive. Further, no statement regarding your condition or diagnosis made hereon will be considered in any way determinative as to whether care rendered for such condition is payable under the Medicare Program.

The use of this statement is subject to the conditions and limitations set forth in the regulation issued under the Dependents' Medical Care Act as codified in 10 U.S.C. 1071-1085.

This form must be presented with your Uniformed Services Identification and Privilege Card (DD Form 1173), identified below, when you obtain civilian medical care.

DEPENDENT, SPOUSE OR CHILD, RESIDING WITH SPONSOR

DEPENDENT'S LAST NAME - FIRST NAME - MIDDLE INITIAL

UNIFORMED SERVICES IDENTIFICATION
AND PRIVILEGE CARD (DD FORM 1173)

CARD NUMBER			EXPIRATION DATE
PREFIX	NUMERICAL	SUFFIX	

DEPENDENT'S ADDRESS *(Complete mailing address)*

SPONSOR MEMBER OF UNIFORMED SERVICES ON ACTIVE DUTY

SPONSOR'S LAST NAME - FIRST NAME - MIDDLE INITIAL

BRANCH OF SERVICE

☐ ARMY ☐ NAVY ☐ AIR FORCE

SERVICE NUMBER   GRADE OR RANK

☐ MARINE CORPS ☐ PUBLIC HEALTH

☐ COAST GUARD ☐ COAST & GEODETIC SURVEY

ORGANIZATION AND OFFICIAL DUTY STATION

REMARKS

STATION AT WHICH PERMIT ISSUED   DATE ISSUED

GRADE OR RANK, AND POSITION OF ISSUING OFFICER   SIGNATURE OF ISSUING OFFICER

Commanding Officer

DISTRIBUTION *(Three signed copies of this statement will be furnished the dependent for distribution as follows):*

DEPENDENT *(Original copy)*   ATTENDING PHYSICIAN *(Duplicate copy)*   CIVILIAN MEDICAL FACILITY *(Triplicate copy)*

FIGURE 7-6

CHAMPUS Nonavailability Statement DD Form 1251 for inpatient care rendered in a nonmilitary hospital.

SERVICES AND/OR SUPPLIES PROVIDED BY CIVILIAN SOURCES
(EXCEPT HOSPITALS)

CIVILIAN HEALTH AND MEDICAL PROGRAM OF THE UNIFORMED SERVICES (CHAMPUS)

SEE INSTRUCTIONS ON REVERSE

SECTION I (To be completed by patient or other responsible family member. Please print or type.)

SAMPLE

PATIENT DATA — SERVICE MEMBER DATA

1. NAME (last, first, middle initial): Throat, Rose E.
2. DATE OF BIRTH: 4-15-70
3. ADDRESS (Include Zip Code): 110 Vocal Avenue, Singer, CA 90001
4. PATIENT IS A (Check one): ☐ (1) SPOUSE ☒ (2) DAUGHTER ☐ (3) SON ☐ (4) RETIREE

7. NAME OF SPONSOR (last, first, middle initial): Throat, Red
8a. SERVICE NUMBER: 189 5644
8b. SOCIAL SECURITY ACCOUNT NUMBER: 234-67-4523
9. GRADE: 9
10. ORGANIZATION AND DUTY STATION (Home Port for Ships) (Address for Retired): 1st Wing Gr. Pt. Mugu, CA

5. IDENTIFICATION CARD (DD Form 1173, DD Form 2 or PHS Form 1866—3)
CARD NO.

	MONTH	DAY	YEAR
EFFECTIVE DATE	7	17	72
EXPIRATION DATE	10	30	77

11. SPONSOR'S OR RETIREE'S BRANCH OF SERVICE
☐ (1) USA ☐ (2) USAF ☐ (3) USMC ☒ (4) USN
☐ (5) USCG ☐ (6) USPHS ☐ (7) ESSA

6. BASIS FOR CARE — ACTIVE DUTY DEPENDENTS ONLY (Check one)
☐ (1) RESIDING APART FROM SPONSOR ☐ (2) RESIDING WITH SPONSOR DD FORM 1251 ATTACHED ☒ (3) OUTPATIENT
☐ (4) OTHER (Specify)

12. STATUS
☒ (1) ACTIVE DUTY ☐ (2) RETIRED ☐ (3) DECEASED

13. CERTIFICATION

I certify to the best of my knowledge and belief the above information in Section I is correct. To the extent that I have authority to do so I hereby authorize the release of medical records in this case to both the contractor and the Government.
If a RETIRED MEMBER or dependent of a retired or deceased member, I certify that to the best of my knowledge and belief, that (Check appropriate box) (Delete portion in parenthesis not applicable)

☐ (I am not) (the patient is not) enrolled (neither is sponsor) in any other insurance, medical service, or health plan provided by law or through employment.

☐ (I am) (the patient is) enrolled (so is sponsor) in another insurance, medical service, or health plan provided by law or through employment; however the particular benefits claimed on this form are not payable under the other plan.

Name (print or type): Red Throat   (Relationship to Patient): Father   Date: 6-1-77   Signature:

SECTION II (To be completed by Source of Care)

14. NAME AND ADDRESS OF SOURCE OF CARE (Include Zip Code)

56 27 P KI YYY46535Y 22
PHILLIP E. TUBES, M. D.
921 YELLOWBIRD AVENUE
SINGLE, CA 90004

a. SOURCE OF CARE LOCATION CODE

b. PROVIDER OF SERVICES
☒ (1) ATTENDING PHYSICIAN
☐ (2) OTHER (Specify)

c. PATIENT STATUS
☐ (1) INPATIENT
☒ (2) OUTPATIENT

15. NAME AND TITLE OF INDIVIDUAL ORDERING CARE

16. INCLUSIVE DATES OF CARE

	MONTH	DAY	YEAR		MONTH	DAY	YEAR
FROM	6	1	77	TO	6	10	77

17. DIAGNOSIS (Use standard nomenclature)

Severe chronic bronchial asthma

(Check when applicable) ☐ services were necessary for treatment of a bonafide medical emergency

a. INTL STAT CODE

b. 12-BREAK CODE

18. RELATED HOSPITALIZATION (If applicable)
FROM   TO

19. ENTER ESTIMATED OR ACTUAL DATE OF DELIVERY IN MATERNITY CASES. LIST BY DATE SURGICAL OPERATIONS AND/OR CARE FURNISHED INCLUDING VISITS FOR WHICH SEPARATE CHARGES ARE CLAIMED (Type or print) (Attach additional sheets if required)

DATE(S) OF SERVICE	a. ITEM OR DESCRIPTION OF SERVICE	b. CHARGES		c. PROCEDURE CODE
6-1-77	Initial office visit	$ 10	00	90010
	Bicillin inj. 2 cc IM	4	00	90730
6-2-77	Complete allergy testing (see attached report)			
	Direct bronchial mucosa testing	200	00	95070
6-4-77	Allergy serum	20	00	99070
6-8-77	Allergy Inj.	5	00	97030
6-10-77	Allergy Inj.	5	00	97030

d. TOTAL CHARGES THIS STATEMENT FOR CARE AUTHORIZED: $ 244 00
e. (PAID BY) OR (DUE FROM) PATIENT (Cross out one): $
f. DUE FROM GOVERNMENT TO SOURCE OF CARE: $
g. DUE PATIENT OR SPONSOR, REIMBURSEMENT: $ 244 00

20. CERTIFICATION BY SOURCE OF CARE

I certify that the services and/or supplies listed hereon were performed or authorized by the attending physician, dentist or other professional personnel in charge, that payment due from the Government has not been received, and that, except for the amount payable by the patient in accordance with the terms of the Civilian Health and Medical Program of the Uniformed Services, the amount paid by the Government will be accepted as payment in full for the authorized services and/or supplies listed hereon.
I further certify that I am not an intern, resident or otherwise in training status for which I am receiving compensation for services listed on this claim.

Name (print or type): Phillip E. Tubes,   Title: M. D.   Date: 6-10-77   Signature:

The persons signing this form are advised that the willful making of a false or fraudulent statement herein renders them liable to prosecution under applicable Federal Laws.

FIGURE 7-7

CHAMPUS DA Form 1863-2 (yellow), used when billing for professional services.

participate in this program." When the doctor does not accept assignment, the patient pays the deductible, 20 or 25 per cent of the charges determined to be allowable, and any amount over the allowable charge.

INSTRUCTIONS FOR COMPLETION OF CHAMPUS FORM
DA 1863-2 (Fig. 7–7 and Assignments 17, 18, and 19, pp. 566–577)

1. Enter the patient's complete name (last, first, and middle initial).
2. Enter the month, day, and year of birth; for example, 07-26-22.
3. Enter the patient's address, showing street, city, state, and ZIP Code. It is helpful to add the patient's home telephone number, including area code, in the event that information is found missing from the form.
4. The relationship of the patient to the service member must be checked.
5. Patient's identification card number:
    a. Dependent children 10 years of age and over should have their own cards (DD Form 1173).
    b. Children under age 10 years may use either parent's card.
    c. Card number can never be the same as Item 8a or 8b.
    d. For retirees, the effective date for care under CHAMPUS is 1-1-67 or their first day of retirement, whichever is later.
    e. The effective date of care under CHAMPUS for dependents is shown in Item 15b (reverse side) of their identification card (DD Form 1173). The expiration date is located on the front side of the card in block 3.
6. This item should be completed only when the service member is on active duty. Issuance of a Nonavailability Statement (DD Form 1251; see Fig. 7–6) is not necessary if the service member is residing with family more than 30 miles from a military hospital. That circumstance should be stated after "other." If emergency care is rendered, check the "other" box and state "Emergency Care."
7. Name of the service member (last, first, and middle initial).
8a. Service member's service number.
8b. Service member's Social Security number (see block 12 of dependent's card DD Form 1173).
9. Pay grade of service member should be indicated as E-6, O-5, and so forth.
10. For active duty service member, location of present duty station. Whenever this is a ship, the home port is used. For retirees and dependents of deceased members, the home address is used.
11. Check the sponsor's or retiree's branch of service.
12. Check the status of the service member, indicating whether he or she is on active duty, retired, or deceased.
13. On all claims for care provided to a retiree, his dependents, or the dependents of deceased members, one of the two boxes must be checked. The signature of the service member, or other responsible family member 18 years of age or over, should be added. A dependent spouse under age 18 may also sign.
14. If this form is not preprinted, the name, address, and provider number of the physician must be indicated. If the physician is accepting assignment, the check will be made payable to the physician. It is a good idea to include the physician's telephone number, including area code, in case any information is missing from the claim.
14a. For CHAMPUS use only.

14b. The provider of service should be checked.

14c. The patient's status (inpatient or outpatient) should be checked. (See Fig. 7–1.)

15. Name of the attending physician can be entered here, or if the claim is being submitted by a nonphysician (e.g., Allied Scientists, Medical Supplies, and so forth), the referring physician's name should be entered.

16. Show inclusive dates of care for submission of this claim.

17. The diagnosis must be noted in this space. If treatment is given for an injury, indicate the date of injury. When billing for preoperative or postoperative care, indicate the date of surgery. When billing for care relative to maternity, indicate the date of delivery or the Expected Date of Confinement (EDC). Check the box only when a bona fide medical emergency exists. Make a notation in this area also if you have given the patient a Privacy Act Statement (DA Form 1863-2-R).

18. Dates of related hospitalization and name of hospital should be entered when applicable. This information is essential because of the method used under CHAMPUS to compute charges for outpatient care related to hospitalization.

19a, b, c. Date, itemized description of service, charge, and RVS or CPT procedure code number for each service should be shown. Describe the service as completely as possible; include any special reports when indicated. Be sure the procedure number is compatible with the services described. Charge your usual fee.

19d. Total charges being billed on this claim should be shown.

19e. Payments on this claim, either by the patient or by another health plan, must be clearly shown, and the source of payment identified if payment is by another health plan.

19f. It is not necessary to complete this item, since CHAMPUS will return an Explanation of Benefits (EOB) with their check that discusses the reasonable charges and amount of payment.

19g. It is not necessary to complete this on submission of the claim, but you can explain to the patient that when the doctor accepts assignment, the patient will be responsible for 20 or 25 per cent of the balance after the reasonable charges have been given in the Explanation of Benefits (EOB).

20. This certification should never be altered on a provider-payable claim. Those claims on which an alteration to the certificate has been made or no provider's signature appears will be processed as patient-payable. If the provider does not accept assignment, which is voluntary, the provider should make this known to the patient at the outset of the service and make no entry on the claim form. The physician should simply furnish the patient with an itemized billing statement that includes the patient's name, date(s) of care, diagnosis, procedure performed or service provided, RVS or CPT code numbers, and the respective fee(s).

After completion of the claim, send it to the fiscal intermediary in your state. For a complete list of the names and addresses of CHAMPUS fiscal intermediaries, see pages 178 and 179. Two medical reviews are allowed per claim if the payment made does not meet with the satisfaction of the physician.

Source of Additional Information

The CHAMPUS program is administered by the Office for the Civilian Health and Medical Program of the Uniformed Services (OCHAMPUS), Denver, Colorado 80240. For additional information, booklets, bulletins, and pamphlets, write to this address.

CHAMPUS AND OTHER INSURANCE

If the patient has another insurance policy in addition to CHAMPUS, you must bill as follows:

1. If the patient is a dependent of an active military man, CHAMPUS is first pay and the other insurance is second pay.

2. If the patient is retired, went to work before 1965, and has other insurance, CHAMPUS pays first. (In a few exceptional instances, contracts are written on other insurance to pay first.)

3. If the patient is retired and worked from 1966, 1967, or 1968 up to and including the present year, CHAMPUS is second pay and you must bill the other insurance first.

If the patient is submitting his or her own claim to the other insurance, the procedure is:

1. Bill the other insurance carrier with the form that is supplied to you.

2. Bill CHAMPUS by completing the top Section I of the yellow Form DA 1863-2 and attach an itemized statement from your physician, listing:
    a. Dates of services
    b. Description of services
    c. Fees
    d. RVS or CPT Procedure Code numbers
    e. Diagnosis

Optional: Attach the voucher you receive back from the other insurance company or a photocopy of the voucher. This is recommended, but many CHAMPUS patients do not show that they have other coverage.

3. Send the CHAMPUS claim to the fiscal intermediary in your state.

CHAMPVA

The Veterans Health Care Expansion Act of 1973 (PL93-82) authorized a CHAMPUS-like program for the spouses and children of veterans with total, permanent, service-connected disabilities, or for the surviving spouses and children of veterans who die as a result of service-connected disabilities. People entitled to CHAMPUS benefits are excluded. The Veterans Administration (VA) elected to provide these beneficiaries with the same benefits under the same conditions and cost-sharing as dependents of retired and deceased uniformed service personnel receive under CHAMPUS. CHAMPVA became effective on September 1, 1973. The Department of Defense (DOD) and the VA have agreed to use OCHAMPUS and the CHAMPUS system of fiscal administrators and hospital contractors to receive, process, and pay CHAMPVA claims, following the same procedures currently used for CHAMPUS.

ELIGIBILITY

Determination of eligibility is the responsibility of the Veterans Administration. The prospective beneficiary goes to the nearest VA hospital or clinic and if eligible receives a VA identification card. The issuing station's number appears on the I.D. card to identify the "home station" where the beneficiary's case file is kept. The I.D. card number is the veteran's VA file number with an alpha suffix. The suffix is different for each beneficiary of a sponsor. These beneficiaries have complete freedom of choice in selecting their civilian health care providers (see Fig. 7–8).

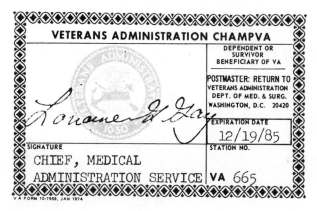

Front

Back

FIGURE 7–8

Sample of CHAMPVA card, showing both sides of the card.

BENEFITS

The benefits are the same as those authorized for CHAMPUS beneficiaries who are dependents of retired or deceased personnel. Cost-sharing is also the same as for CHAMPUS beneficiaries who are dependents of retired or deceased personnel.

CLAIMS PROCEDURE

1. CHAMPVA claims are submitted to CHAMPUS hospital contractors and fiscal administrators on forms DA 1863-1 (for hospital billing) and DA 1863-2 (for professional services).

2. Follow the instructions for completion of CHAMPUS Form DA 1863-2 (see Fig. 7–7) with these exceptions:

Block 6: Not applicable.
Block 7: Veteran's name.
Block 8a: Leave blank.
Block 8b: Veteran's VA file number (omit prefix or suffix); do not use any other former service numbers.
Block 9: Not applicable.

Block 10: Show the three-digit number of the VA station that issued the I.D. card.

Block 11: Enter "VA" added as item 8.

Block 12: Not applicable.

Block 17: The emergency item in this block is not necessary for CHAMPVA.

CHAMPUS AND CHAMPVA CLAIMS OFFICES

All beneficiaries and sources of medical care (physicians and hospitals) should use the following addresses when filing a CHAMPUS or CHAMPVA claim for services rendered in the United States, Puerto Rico, Canada, and Mexico.

1. Mutual of Omaha Insurance Company is the CHAMPUS and CHAMPVA fiscal intermediary for the states and countries listed below. The address to which claims should be sent is P.O. Box 1298, Omaha, Nebraska 68101.

Arkansas	Indiana	Minnesota	South Carolina
Canada	Iowa	Missouri	South Dakota
Florida	Kansas	Nebraska	Wisconsin
Georgia	Louisiana	North Dakota	
Illinois	Mexico	Oklahoma	

2. Blue Cross Association is the CHAMPUS and CHAMPVA fiscal intermediary for the states and Puerto Rico as listed below. The headquarters address is 840 North Lake Shore Drive, Chicago, Illinois 60611.

Alabama	Idaho	New Hampshire	Rhode Island
Alaska	Kentucky	New Jersey	Tennessee
Colorado	Maine	New York	Utah
Connecticut	Maryland	North Carolina	Vermont
Delaware	Massachusetts	Ohio	Virginia
District of	Michigan	Oregon	Washington
Columbia	Mississippi	Pennsylvania	West Virginia
Hawaii	Montana	Puerto Rico	Wyoming

3. The CHAMPUS and CHAMPVA fiscal intermediaries for the five states are listed below.

Arizona
California Physicians' Service (CPS)
CHAMPUS
P.O. Box 85019
San Diego, CA 92138

California
California Physicians' Service (CPS)
CHAMPUS
P.O. Box 85020
San Diego, CA 92138

Nevada
California Physicians' Service (CPS)
CHAMPUS
P.O. Box 85023
San Diego, CA 92138

New Mexico
California Physicians' Service (CPS)
CHAMPUS
P.O. Box 85021
San Diego CA 92138

Texas
Mutual of Omaha Insurance Company
CHAMPUS
3301 Dodge Street
Omaha, NE 68131

VETERANS ADMINISTRATION OUTPATIENT CLINIC

The Veterans Administration is authorized by law to provide a wide range of benefits to those who have served their country in the Armed Forces and to their dependents. If a service person files a claim for a service-connected disability within a year, he or she is eligible for outpatient treatment at VA expense and is issued a VA Outpatient Card (see Fig. 7–9). Usually a veteran seeks care at the nearest VA Outpatient Clinic. However, when a VA facility is not within reasonable distance, when the veteran is too ill to travel to the nearest location, or when the condition needs prompt attention, the veteran can apply for and be granted medical care through the "Home Town Care Program" and then seek care by a private physician. Payment for services rendered can be made only for a service-connected disability, and any other professional service that is not related to the service diability must be paid for by the veteran out of his own pocket. In regard to the service-connected disability, the physician must accept what the VA pays as payment in full and cannot bill the patient for any additional charges, even if there is a balance after the VA pays the claim. If the treatment is likely to cost more than $40 per month, the physician must obtain prior authorization from the nearest VA facility.

BENEFITS

1. Dental care (if the veteran files a claim within 1 year from the date that he or she was discharged from the service).
2. Professional services.
3. Hospital care in a VA Hospital.
4. Prescription drugs and medication issued by a VA Pharmacy or other participating pharmacy.
5. Emergency treatment in a hospital for a service-connected condition only.
6. Certain medical equipment, such as oxygen, prosthetics, and so forth.

EMERGENCY OUTPATIENT TREATMENT

Veterans eligible for outpatient treatment and not in the fee basis program must obtain any outpatient medical care to which they are entitled from a VA facility. The only instances in which these veterans may obtain treatment from a private physician are:

1. When treatment is emergency.
2. When the VA Outpatient Clinic is notified within 15 days of the treatment rendered.

Front

VA OUTPATIENT MEDICAL TREATMENT INFORMATION CARD

012-34-5678
Identification No.

E. Z. Slipdisk
Beneficiary's Name

DISABILITY FOR WHICH TREATMENT IS AUTHORIZED — VALID UNTIL CANCELLED BY VA

x P. O. HERNIATED NUC. PULPOSUS

VA FORM 10-1174, FEB 1971

BILLING AND REPORTS: Bill the Station of Jurisdiction monthly. Please itemize your usual statement to include (1) patient's name; (2) identification number, (3) condition treated; (4) treatment and dates rendered; and (5) your usual and customary fee. Bills for auxiliary medical services must reflect the name of the prescribing doctor of medicine or osteopathy. Submit a brief treatment report only when the cost of urgent treatment causes the $30.00 limitation to be exceeded, or when a significant clinical change in a disability occurs.

PAYMENT. Payment by the VA for services rendered is payment in full.

IMPORTANT: Direct inquiries and any change of address to the Station of Jurisdiction.

Station of Jurisdiction:

752
FOLD

VETERANS ADMINISTRATION
OUTPATIENT C 9044/136A6
425 SOUTH HILL ST.
LOS ANGELES CA 90013

Back

PLEASE READ CAREFULLY

TO VETERAN — You are authorized to obtain treatment within a reasonable distance from your permanent or temporary residence for the disability shown. When treatment is required, select a doctor of medicine or osteopathy who is licensed in the State in which treatment will be rendered. This card constitutes an agreement to provide care to you as a VA beneficiary within the limitations stated. Please alert the doctor to the instructions printed on the card and be sure he has your NAME, IDENTIFICATION NO. and the ADDRESS OF THE STATION OF JURISDICTION. If a specific therapy is authorized in lieu of listing disabilities, this card authorizes ONLY that therapy. IT MAY NOT BE USED TO OBTAIN OTHER MEDICAL SERVICES, SURGICAL PROCEDURES, PROSTHETIC APPLIANCES. Prescriptions of a recurring nature and others not needed at once should be brought or mailed to the VA station of jurisdiction. They will be filled promptly. When it is necessary to obtain medication immediately, PLEASE REQUEST THE PRIVATE PHARMACIST TO BILL THE STATION OF JURISDICTION SHOWN ON THIS CARD.

The VA may reimburse local, round trip, travel expenses between your permanent or temporary residence and the place treatment is obtained. A mileage allowance will be paid in lieu of actual and necessary expenses of travel (including lodging and subsistence). Your one-time, written request for travel expenses, when received within 30 days from the the date you first obtain medical services, will be approved to be effective with the first visit. A claim received after that 30-day period will be effective from the date received. Generally, travel expenses are paid for a 3-months period.

TO PHYSICIAN — The beneficiary named on this card is authorized OUTPATIENT TREATMENT for the disabilities shown by a doctor of medicine or osteopathy licensed in the State in which medical services are rendered. When treatment of these conditions requires eyeglasses, hearing aids, other prostheses, home nursing services and/or dental services, notify the Station of Jurisdiction. Items or services of this nature will be provided by the Veterans Administration. Please request additional medical or other information from the Station of Jurisdiction, if required.

MEDICAL SERVICES includes prescription and referral for auxiliary medical services when required. All routine treatment may not exceed a total cost of $30.00 per month without prior VA approval.

PHARMACY SERVICES: Please have Rxs filled by VA unless needed at once. Veteran may obtain stat Rx from private pharmacy if you certify, Rx, "The VA has authorized me to treat the disability for which this prescription is written."

FIGURE 7–9

Sample of VA Outpatient Clinic card, showing both sides of the card.

Form Approved
Budget Bureau No. 76-R0352

VETERANS ADMINISTRATION

CLAIM FOR PAYMENT OF COST OF
UNAUTHORIZED MEDICAL SERVICES

Each person, firm or institution claiming payments or reimbursements must complete this form. No carbon paper necessary. Please use typewriter or ball point pen, and submit both copies.

1A. VETERAN'S LAST NAME - FIRST - MIDDLE INITIAL	1B. CLAIM NO. C-	1C. SOCIAL SECURITY NO.

1D. PRESENT ADDRESS *(Include ZIP Code)*

2. NAME AND ADDRESS OF PERSON, FIRM OR INSTITUTION MAKING CLAIM *(Leave blank if same as above)*

3. STATEMENT OF CIRCUMSTANCES UNDER WHICH THE SERVICES WERE RENDERED *(Include diagnosis, symptoms, whether emergency existed, and reason VA facilities were not used)*

4. AMOUNT CLAIMED $	*Attach bills or receipts showing services furnished, dates, and charges*

5. COMPLETE A OR B, AS APPROPRIATE

A. Amount claimed does not exceed that charged the general public for similar services, and payment has not been received.	B. I certify that the amount claimed has been paid and reimbursement has not been received.
SIGNATURE AND TITLE OF PROVIDER OF SERVICE, AND DATE	SIGNATURE OF VETERAN OR REPRESENTATIVE, AND DATE

FOR VETERANS ADMINISTRATION USE ONLY

6. ACTION

☐ APPROVED $ _____   Treatment was provided in an emergency for a service-connected or adjunct disability, any disability of a veteran who has a total disability permanent in nature from a service-connected disability, or for any illness, injury, or dental condition in the case of a veteran eligible under Chapter 31 (Vocational Rehabilitation) Title 38, U.S. Code. VA facilities were not feasibly available and delay would have been hazardous.

☐ DISAPPROVED

7. SIGNATURE, CHIEF, MEDICAL ADMINISTRATION SERVICE	8. DATE	9. ADMINISTRATIVE VOUCHER NO.

VA FORM
MAY 1974 **10-583**   SUPERSEDES VA FORM 10-583, FEB 1966, AND WHICH WILL NOT BE USED.

FIGURE 7–10

VA Form 10-583, Claim for Payment of Cost of Unauthorized Medical Services.

In such cases, the treating physician must submit evidence of an emergency with his invoice to the VA Outpatient Clinic. Form 10-583, Claim for Payment of Cost of Unauthorized Medical Services (see Fig. 7–10), generally used for hospital emergency care, can also be used for professional care if the doctor is billing after the 15-day period has elapsed. The Fee Consultant Physician of the VA Outpatient Clinic makes the final decision as to whether or not an emergency existed.

CLAIM PROCEDURE

The processing of invoices from fee physicians is a somewhat lengthy procedure as required by VA regulations, and involves several steps in different VA agencies. In order to keep the delay in payment to a minimum, fee physicians are urged to bill the VA on a monthly basis. To insure prompt processing, invoices should contain the following information:

1. Patient's name as shown on the I.D. card, VA form 10-1174 (see Fig. 7–9).
2. Patient's Social Security number.
3. Condition treated must be shown on every invoice, since this is the basis for approval of payment. Diagnosis treated must be listed on the I.D. card or authorized by the statement, "for any condition."
4. Treatment given and dates rendered.
5. Physician's usual and customary fee.
6. Name and address of fee physician and his or her Social Security or Federal Taxpayer I.D. number. If the I.D. number is assigned to a group and the physician desires to be paid individually, the VA Outpatient Clinic must be so advised.

Fee physicians, as well as veterans, are urged to read the instructions on the I.D. card carefully. This is sometimes neglected and can lead to misunderstanding.

If the physician does not wish to bill the VA Outpatient Clinic, the patient can pay the physician himself and then be reimbursed, but the veteran must carefully follow the instructions given on the back of the VA Outpatient Card (see Fig. 7–9).

TO THE STUDENT: Refer to the Appendix to complete the insurance forms pertinent to this chapter. Assignments 17, 18, and 19, pp. 566–577, pertain to this chapter.

VETERANS ADMINISTRATION INSTALLATIONS

For information or assistance in applying for veteran's benefits, write, call, or visit one of the regional offices listed. Many states have toll-free telephone services to the VA from communities in the state. Consult your local directory or information assistance operator for the latest listing of these numbers. Abbreviations in the following list are explained as follows: Regional Offices (RO); other offices (O); Centers (Regional Offices and Insurance); United States Veterans Assistance Centers (USVAC); Hospitals (H); Domiciliary (D); Outpatient Clinic – independent (OC); Outpatient Clinic – physically separated from hospital (OCH); Outpatient Clinic Substation (OCS).

Alabama

Birmingham (H) 35233
700 S. 19th St.

Mobile (OCS) 36617
2451 Fillingim St.

Montgomery (H) 36109
215 Perry Hill Rd.

Montgomery (RO) 36104
474 S. Court St.

Tuscaloosa (H) 35401

Tuskegee (H) 36083

Alaska

Juneau (RO) 99802
Federal Bldg., U.S. Post
   Office & Courthouse
P.O. Box 1288
709 W. 9th St.

Anchorage (O) 99501
Rm. 214, Loussac-Sogn Bldg.
429 D St.

Arizona

Phoenix (H) 85012
7th St. & Indian School Rd.

Phoenix (RO) 85012
3225 N. Central Ave.

Prescott (H&D) 86301

Tucson (H) 85723

Arkansas

Fayetteville (H) 72701

Little Rock (RO) 72201
Federal Bldg.
700 W. Capitol Ave.

Little Rock (H) 72206
300 E. Roosevelt Rd.

California

Fresno (H) 93703
2615 E. Clinton Ave.

Livermore (H) 94550

Long Beach (H) 90801
5901 E. 7th St.

Los Angeles (RO) 90024
Federal Bldg.
11000 Wilshire Blvd.
West Los Angeles

Los Angeles (H&D) 90073
Sawtelle & Wilshire Blvd.

Los Angeles (OC) 90013
425 S. Hill St.

Martinez (H) 94553
150 Muir Rd.

Oakland (OCS) 94612
1515 Clay St.

Oakland, Phone: 893-0405

Palo Alto (H) 94304
3801 Miranda Ave.

San Diego (RO) 92101
1250 Sixth Ave.

San Diego (H) 92161
3350 LaJolla Village Dr.

San Diego (OCH) 92101
Wusaaw Medical Bldg.
2131 Third Ave.

San Francisco (RO) 94105
211 Main St.

San Francisco (H) 94121
4150 Clement St.

Sepulveda (H) 91343

Colorado

Denver (RO) 80225
Building 20
Denver Federal Center

Denver (H) 80220
1055 Clermont St.

Fort Lyon (H) 81038

Grand Junction (H) 81501

Connecticut

Hartford (RO) 06103
450 Main St.

New London, Phone: 447-0377

New Haven, Phone: 562-2113

Newington (H) 06111
555 Willard Ave.

West Haven (H) 06516
W. Spring St.

Delaware

Wilmington (RO&H) 19805
1601 Kirkwood Highway

District of Columbia
Washington (RO-VBO) 20002
941 N. Capitol St., N.E.

Washington (H) 20422
50 Irving St., N.W.

Florida
Bay Pines (H, D, & OCH) 33504

Gainesville (H) 32602
Archer Rd.

Jacksonville (O & OCS) 32201
Post Office & Courthouse Bldg.
311 W. Monroe St.

Lake City (H) 32055

Miami (H) 33125
1201 N.W. 16th St.

Miami (O) 33130
Rm. 100, 51 S.W. 1st Ave.

Orlando (OCS) 32806
83 W. Columbia St.

St. Petersburg (OCH) 33733
P.O. Box 13594

St. Petersburg (RO) 33731
P.O. Box 1437, 144 1st Ave. S.

Tampa (H) 33612
13000 N. 30th St.

Georgia
Atlanta (RO) 30308
730 Peachtree St., N.E.

Augusta (H) 30904

Decatur (H) 30033
1670 Clairmont Rd., N.E.

Dublin (H&D) 31021

Hawaii
Honolulu (RO) 96801
P.O. Box 3198 (Airmail)
680 Ala Moana Blvd.

Idaho
Boise (RO) 83724
Federal Bldg. and
   U.S. Courthouse
550 W. Fort St. Box 044

Boise (H) 83702
5th and Fort St.

Illinois
Chicago (H) 60611
333 E. Huron St. (Research)

Chicago (H) 60680
(West Side) P.O. Box 8195
820 S. Damen Ave.

Chicago (RO) 60680
P.O. Box 8136
2030 W. Taylor St.

Danville (H) 61832

Downey (H) 60064

Marion (H) 62959

Hines (H) 60141

Indiana
Evansville, Phone: 426-1403

Fort Wayne (H) 46805
1600 Randalia Dr.

Gary, Phone: 886-9184

Indianapolis (RO) 46204
575 N. Pennsylvania St.

Indianapolis (H) 46202
1481 W. 10th St.

Marion (H) 46952

Iowa
Des Moines (RO) 50309
210 Walnut St.

Des Moines (H) 50310
30th & Euclid Ave.

Iowa City (H) 52240

Knoxville (H) 50138

Kansas
Leavenworth (H&D) 66048

Topeka (H) 66622
2200 Gage Blvd.

Wichita (RO&H) 67218
5500 E. Kellogg

Kentucky
Lexington (H) 40507

Louisville (RO) 40202
600 Federal Place

Louisville (H) 40202
800 Zorn Ave.

Louisiana
Alexandria (H) 71301

New Orleans (RO) 70113
701 Loyola Ave.

New Orleans (H) 70146
1601 Perdido St.

Shreveport (H&O) 71130
510 E. Stoner Ave.

Maine
Togus (RO&H) 04330

Portland (O) 04111
76 Pearl St.

Maryland
Baltimore (RO&OCH) 21201
31 Hopkins Plaza

Baltimore (H) 21218
3900 Loch Raven Blvd.

Fort Howard (H) 21052

Perry Point (H) 21902

Massachusetts
Bedford (H) 01730
200 Spring Rd.

Boston (H) 02130
150 S. Huntington Ave.

Boston (RO) 02203
John Fitzgerald Kennedy
    Federal Bldg. Government Center

Boston (OC) 02108
17 Court St.

Brockton (H) 02401

Lowell (OCS) 01851
Old Post Office Bldg.

New Bedford (OCS) 02740
749 Purchase St.

Northampton (H) 01060

Springfield (O&OCS) 01103
1200 Main St.

West Roxbury (H) 02132
1400 VFW Parkway

Worcester (OCS) 01608
9 Walnut St.

Michigan
Allen Park (H) 48101

Ann Arbor (H) 48105
2215 Fuller Rd.

Battle Creek (H) 49016

Detroit (RO) 48232
P.O. Box 1117A
801 W. Baltimore at 3rd

Iron Mountain (H) 49801

Saginaw (H) 48602
1500 Weiss St.

Minnesota
Minneapolis (H) 55417
54th St. & 48th Ave. South

St. Cloud (H) 56301

St. Paul (C) 55111
Federal Bldg. Fort Snelling

St. Paul (OCH) 55111
Fort Snelling

Mississippi
Biloxi (H&D) 39531

Jackson (RO&H) 39216
1500 E. Woodrow Wilson Ave.

Missouri
Columbia (H) 65201
800 Stadium Road

Kansas City (O) 64106
260 Federal Office Bldg.
601 E. 12th St.

Kansas City (H) 64128
4801 Linwood Blvd.

Poplar Bluff (H) 63901

St. Louis (RO) 63103
Rm. 4705, Federal Bldg.
1520 Market St.

St. Louis (H) 63125
915 N. Grand Blvd.

Montana
Fort Harrison (RO&H) 59636

Miles City (H) 59301

Nebraska
Grand Island (H) 68801

Lincoln (RO) 68508
220 S. 17th St.

Lincoln (H) 68510
600 S. 70th St.

Omaha (H) 68105
4101 Woolworth Ave.

Nevada
Henderson (OCS) 89015
102 Lake Mead Dr.

Reno (H) 89502
1000 Locust St.

Reno (RO) 89502
1201 Terminal Way

New Hampshire
Manchester (RO) 03103
497 Silver St.

Manchester (H) 03104
718 Smyth Rd.

New Jersey
East Orange (H) 07019

Lyons (H) 07939

Newark (RO&OCH) 07102
20 Washington Pl.

Trenton, Phone: 989-8116

New Mexico
Albuquerque (RO) 87101
500 Gold Ave., S.W.

Albuquerque (H) 87108
2100 Ridgecrest Dr., S.E.

New York
Albany (H) 12208

Albany (O) 12201
Executive Park
North Stuyvesant Plaza

Batavia (H) 14020

Bath (H&D) 14810

Bronx (H) 10468
130 W. Kingsbridge Rd.

Brooklyn (H) 11209
800 Poly Place

Brooklyn (OC) 11205
35 Ryerson St.

Buffalo (RO) 14202
Federal Bldg.
111 W. Huron St.

Buffalo (H) 14215
3495 Bailey Ave.

Canandaigua (H) 14424

Castle Point (H) 12511

Montrose (H) 10548

New York City (H) 10010
1st Ave. at E. 24th St.

New York City (RO&OCH)) 10001
252 7th Ave. at 24th St.

Northport (H) 11768
Long Island

Rochester (O&OCS) 14614
100 State St.

Syracuse (O) 13202
Gateway Bldg.
809 S. Salina St.

Syracuse (H) 13210
Irving Ave. & University Pl.

North Carolina
Asheville (H) 28805

Durham (H) 27705
508 Fulton St.

Fayetteville (H) 28301
2300 Ramsey St.

Salisbury (H) 28144

Winston-Salem (RO&OCH) 27102
Wachovia Bldg.
301 N. Main St.

North Dakota
Fargo (RO&H) 58102
21st Ave. & Elm St.

Ohio
Akron, Phone: 535-3227

Brecksville (H) 44141
10000 Brecksville Rd.

Chillicothe (H) 45601

Cincinnati (H) 45220
3200 Vine St.

Cincinnati (O) 45202
Rm. 1024, Federal Off. Bldg.
550 Main St.

Cleveland (H) 44106
10701 E. Blvd.

Cleveland (RO) 44199
Federal Office Bldg.
1240 E. 9th St.

Columbus (O&OCS) 43215
360 S. Third St.

Columbus (OC) 43210
456 Clinic Drive

Dayton (H&D) 45428

Toledo, Phone: 244-5887

Oklahoma
Muskogee (H) 74401
Memorial Station
Honor Heights Dr.

Muskogee (RO) 74401
2nd & Court Sts.

Oklahoma City (O) 73102
200 N.W. 4th St.

Oklahoma City (H) 73104
921 N.E. 13th St.

Tulsa, Phone: 583-5891

Oregon
Portland (H) 97207
Sam Jackson Park

Portland (RO) 97204
426 S.W. Stark St.

Portland (OCH) 97204
426 S.W. Stark St.

Roseburg (H) 97470

White City (D) 97501

Pennsylvania
Altoona (H) 16603

Butler (H) 16001

Coatesville (H) 19320

Erie (H) 16501
135 E. 38th St. Blvd.

Harrisburg (OCS) 17108
Federal Bldg.
228 Walnut St.

Lebanon (H) 17042

Philadelphia (H) 19104
University & Woodland Aves.

Philadelphia (C) 19101
P.O. Box 8079
5000 Wissahickon Ave.

Philadelphia (OCH) 19102
1421 Cherry St.

Pittsburgh (RO & OCH) 15222
1000 Liberty Ave.

Pittsburgh (H) 15240
University Drive C

Pittsburgh (H) 15206
Leech Farm Rd.

Wilkes-Barre (O) 18701
19-27 N. Main St.

Wilkes-Barre (H) 18703
1111 E. End Blvd.

Philippines
Manila (RO) 96528
1131 Roxas Blvd.
APO San Francisco (Air Mail)

Puerto Rico
Ponce (OCS) 00731
Calle Isabel #60

San Juan (RO&H) 00936
Barrio Monacillos
Rio Piedras GPO Box 4867

Rhode Island
Providence (RO) 02903
Federal Bldg., Kennedy Plaza

Providence (H) 02908
Davis Park

South Carolina
Charleston (H) 29403
109 Bee St.

Columbia (RO) 29201
1801 Assembly St.

Columbia (H) 29201
Garners Ferry Rd.

South Dakota
Fort Meade (H) 57741

Hot Springs (H&D) 57747

Sioux Falls (RO&H) 57101
2501 W. 22nd St.

Tennessee
Chattanooga (OCS) 37411
Bldg. 6200 East Gate Center

Knoxville (OCS) 37901
Baptist Prof. Bldg.
200 Blount Ave.

Memphis (H) 38104
1030 Jefferson Ave.

Mountain Home (H&D) 37684
Johnson City

Murfreesboro (H) 37130

Nashville (RO) 37203
110 9th Ave. S.

Nashville (H) 37203
1310 24th Ave. S.

Texas
Amarillo (H) 79106
6010 Amarillo Blvd., W.

Big Spring (H) 79720

Bonham (H&D) 75418

Corpus Christi (OCS) 78404
1502 S. Brownlee Blvd.

Dallas (O) 75202
U.S. Courthouse and
  Fed. Office Bldg.
1100 Commerce St.

Dallas (H) 75216
4500 S. Lancaster Rd.

El Paso (OC) 79905
4819 Alameda Ave.

Houston (RO) 77054
2515 Murworth St.

Houston (H) 77031
2002 Holcombe Blvd.

Kerrville (H) 78028

Lubbock (O&OC) 79401
Federal Bldg.
1205 Texas Ave., Room 814

Marlin (H) 76661

McAllen (OCS) 78501
1220 Jackson Ave.

San Antonio (H) 78284
7400 Merton Minter Blvd.

San Antonio (O) 78285
410 S. Main St.

San Antonio (OC) 78285
307 Dwyer Ave.

Temple (H&D) 76501

Waco (RO) 76710
1400 N. Valley Mills Dr.

Waco (H) 76703
Memorial Drive

Waco (OCH) 76710
1400 N. Valley Mills Dr.

Utah
Salt Lake City (RO) 84138
125 S. State St.

Salt Lake City (H) 84113

Vermont
White River Junction (RO&H) 05001

Virginia
Hampton (H&D) 23667

Richmond (H) 23249
1201 Broad Rock Rd.

Roanoke (RO) 24011
211 W. Campbell Ave.

Salem (H) 24153

Washington
American Lake (H) 98493
Tacoma

Seattle (RO) 98121
6th & Lenora Bldg.

Seattle (H) 98108
4435 Beacon Ave., S.

Seattle (OCH) 98104
Smith Tower, 2nd & Yesler

Spokane (H) 99208
N. 4815 Assembly St.

Vancouver (H) 98661

Walla Walla (H) 99362
77 Wainwright Dr.

West Virginia

Beckley (H) 25801
200 Veterans Ave.

Clarksburg (H) 26301

Huntington (RO) 25701
502 8th St.

Huntington (H) 25701
1540 Spring Valley Dr.

Martinsburg (H&D) 25401

Wheeling (OCS) 26003
11th & Chapline Sts.

Wisconsin

Madison (H) 53705
2500 Overlook Terrace

Milwaukee (RO) 53202
342 N. Water St.

Tomah (H) 54660

Wood (H&D) 53193
500 W. National Ave.

Wyoming

Cheyenne (RO&H) 82001
2360 E. Pershing Blvd.

Sheridan (H) 82801

U.S. VETERANS ASSISTANCE CENTERS (USVACs)

Several Federal agencies have combined their efforts with the Veterans Administration to furnish assistance to veterans through their separate programs at U.S. Veterans Assistance Centers located at all VA regional offices except Juneau, Alaska, and Manila, Philippines; and at all VA offices except Portland, Me.; Springfield, Mass., and Shreveport, La. Additional USVACs are located in the following cities:

Compton, California, 101 South Willowbrook Avenue (90220)
East Los Angeles, California, East Los Angeles Service Center,
     929 North Bonnie Beach Place (90063)
Washington, D.C., Room 300, 25 K Street, N.E. (20002)

REVIEW QUESTIONS

1. Who are entitled to CHAMPUS medical benefits?

_____

_____

_____

2. What are the dates of the CHAMPUS fiscal year? _____

3. The CHAMPUS deductible for outpatient care is how much per patient? _____

Per family? _____

4. How much does CHAMPUS pay after the deductible has been met for dependents of active duty members? _____

For retired members or their dependents? _____

5. How much does the patient pay after CHAMPUS pays for retired members or their dependents? _____

6. When is a Nonavailability Statement needed? _____

_____

7. If a patient has other insurance besides CHAMPUS and is the dependent of an active military man, who do you bill first? _____

8. If the patient has other insurance besides CHAMPUS and is retired and went to work in 1967, who do you bill first? _____

9. If the patient has other insurance besides CHAMPUS and is retired and went to work in 1963, who do you bill first? _____

10. What is the time limit in submitting a CHAMPUS claim? _____

_____

11. Can a CHAMPUS patient go to an emergency hospital, private physician, or military hospital for medical care? _____

_____

12. A CHAMPUS patient comes in for a flu shot. Will CHAMPUS pay if the patient has met his deductible for the year? _____

13. It is October 1. Your physician sees the wife of a Navy man who is stationed at Port Hueneme, in consultation. Dr. Caesar orders her to the hospital with a suspected ectopic pregnancy. She has a laparotomy and salpingectomy. Here are her bills. Indicate what CHAMPUS will pay.

Dr. Caesar bills:	CHAMPUS		CHAMPUS
Consultation $25	_____	Assistant surgeon $60	_____
Salpingectomy $300	_____	Anesthesiologist $120	_____

Hospital bill: CHAMPUS CHAMPUS

5-day stay, drugs, lab, Oper. Rm.	$1500 _____	Patient owes you $ _____
		Patient owes hospital $ _____

14. Same situation as above, except that the patient is the wife of a retired military man.

Dr. Caesar bills: CHAMPUS

Consultation	$25 _____	Assistant surgeon	$60 _____
Salpingectomy	$300 _____	Anesthesiologist	$120 _____

Hospital bill:

5-day stay, drugs, lab, Oper. Rm.	$1500 _____	Patient owes you $ _____
		Patient owes hospital $ _____

15. An active duty dependent whose husband's port is Port Hueneme is pregnant.

She wants to go to a private physician for her care. May she?_____

Why or why not?_____

16. Your CHAMPUS patient asks you to accept an assignment on her medical care and Dr. Caesar agrees. She has not met her deductible. She is the wife of an active duty man.

Your bill:			Allowable:	
	Consultation	$ 25		$ 25
	CBC	10		10
	Urinalysis	5		5
	Blood serology and complement fixation	17		15
	PA & Lt Lat chest x-ray	15		15
	EKG	10		10
	Spirometry	100		95
	TOTAL	$182		$175

How much is your check from CHAMPUS?_____

The patient owes the doctor $_____   Doctor Caesar writes off $ _____

Notes:

Notes:

8
Unemployment Compensation Disability

BEHAVIORAL

OBJECTIVES   *The Assistant should be able to:*

1. Learn which states have a state disability insurance plan for employees.
2. Understand eligibility, benefits, and limitations of unemployment compensation disability.
3. Explain voluntary plans of disability insurance.
4. Complete a claim form if applying for benefits as a patient.
5. Complete a claim form for submission of the doctor's certificate for verification of disability.
6. Abstract from the patient record the proper information for completing the various state disability insurance forms.
7. Recognize other forms also used in processing unemployment compensation disability claims.
8. Define abbreviations as they appear on a patient's record.

Unemployment Compensation Disability (UCD) is also known as Temporary Disability Insurance (TDI) and State Disability Insurance (SDI). This form of insurance is part of an employment security program that provides temporary cash benefits for workers suffering a wage loss due to off-the-job illness or injury.

HISTORY

In 1944 Rhode Island began a state disability insurance program that proved successful. Then California became the second state to add nonindustrial disability coverage to the Social Security protection afforded to its citizens by appending Article 10 to the Unemployment Insurance Act which became law on May 21, 1946. When payment became effective on December 1, 1946, this article diverted the 1 per cent tax formerly paid by workers for Unemployment Insurance to a disability insurance fund. New York and New Jersey soon followed with similar programs. Two decades went by, and then Puerto Rico and Hawaii passed nonindustrial disability insurance laws in 1969. As of 1976, these six states are the only ones to have nonindustrial disability insurance programs. In each state the law is known by a different name:

California	California Unemployment Insurance Code
Hawaii	Temporary Disability Insurance Law
New Jersey	Temporary Disability Benefits Law
New York	Disability Benefits Law
Puerto Rico	Disability Benefits Act
Rhode Island	Temporary Disability Insurance Act

Usually a small percentage, not exceeding 1 per cent, is deducted from a worker's paycheck each month, or the employer may elect to pay all or part of the cost of the plan as a fringe benefit for employees. The money is then sent in quarterly to the state and put into a special fund.

ELIGIBILITY

As long as a person is employed part time or full time and this small percentage is deducted from his or her paycheck, or the employer is paying into the fund for the employee, the employee is entitled to the insurance. An employee who retires is no longer eligible for the insurance. Certain types of workers are not covered; examples are domestics, student employees of a school, and officers or crew members of a ship.

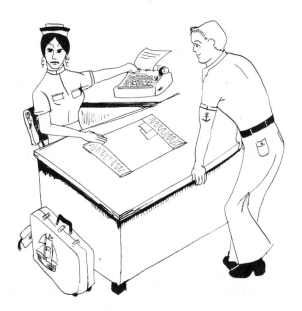

"Occupation? Er, I guess you could say I've always been kind of a *floater*."

BENEFITS

The weekly benefits are determined by the wages earned in the quarter preceding the off-the-job illness or injury. Benefits begin after the seventh consecutive day of disability. If the employee must be hospitalized, the hospital benefits are paid for 20 days, beginning with the first day of hospitalization. Some hospitals have the patient sign an assignment of benefits form so that the disability insurance benefits will be sent directly to the hospital and will help with payment of the hospital bill (see Fig. 8–7). However, costs of medical care are not included under the statutory provisions of the disability benefits law.

A claim for disability insurance should be filed within 20 days, but there is usually a grace period of 7 to 8 days before the absolute deadline. The only two states that have longer filing deadlines are Hawaii (30 days) and Puerto Rico (60 days). After the claim is approved, basic benefits become payable with the eighth day of disability or the first day of hospital confinement, whichever comes first. A person can continue to draw disability insurance for a maximum of 6 months or 26 weeks on the same illness or injury. An employee is also entitled to disability benefits 14 days after recovery from a previous disability or illness. In other words, if a patient is discharged by the physician to return to work and is on the job two weeks and then becomes ill with the same ailment, he may receive benefits again.

LIMITATIONS

There are many restrictions upon disability insurance. A few of the major situations in which a claim could possibly be denied are listed here.

1. *Pregnancy-related disability*, unless the pregnancy is complicated (as in cases where the patient has diabetes, varicose veins, ectopic pregnancy, or cesarean section). *Exceptions*: California, Hawaii, New Jersey, and Rhode Island have maternity benefits that may be applied for after the birth of a baby.

2. *Conditions covered by Workers' Compensation*, unless the rate is less than the disability insurance rate.

3. If the applicant is receiving *Unemployment Insurance benefits over a certain specified amount.* Exception: if the applicant is on Unemployment Insurance and then becomes ill or injured, he or she is put on the Temporary Disability Insurance until able to go for a job interview.

4. *Disabilities beginning during a trade dispute.* If an employee is on strike and is injured while walking a picket line, he or she is not eligible for benefits. However, if the union is on strike and an individual member remains at home and then becomes ill or injured, he or she can claim disability and will receive benefits.

5. *Confinement by court order or certification in a public or private institution* as a dipsomaniac, drug addict, or sexual psychopath; or whenever legal custody is the cause of unemployment.

6. *If the employing company has a voluntary disability plan and is not paying into a state fund.*

7. If the employee or company has a *"religious exemption certificate"* on file and is not paying into a state fund.

VOLUNTARY PLAN

Persons residing and working in states which do not feature state disability insurance programs may elect to contact a local private insurance carrier about disability insurance so they will have such coverage if necessary. If these persons become ill or disabled, they will receive a fixed weekly or monthly income, usually for about 6 months. If the disability or illness is permanent and the individual is unable to return to work at all, there is sometimes a small monthly income for the duration of the person's life. Some of the state laws provide that a "voluntary plan" may be adopted instead of the "state plan" if a majority of company employees consent to private coverage.

CLAIM PROCEDURE

If you reside in a state having Unemployment Compensation Disability, call or write the nearest office that handles the state disability insurance to obtain a claim form and insurance pamphlet. Following is a list of offices and addresses for each state.

State of California
Employment Development Department

Branch Offices:
Bakersfield: P.O. Box 1633, 93302
Chico: P.O. Box 1500, 95926
Eureka: P.O. Box 4000, 95501
Fresno: P.O. Box 2325, 93723
Glendale: P.O. Box 990, 91209
Long Beach: P.O. Box 469, 90801
Los Angeles: P.O. Box 3096, 90051
Oakland: P.O. Box 1857, 94604
Redding: P.O. Box 1898, 96001
Sacramento: P.O. Box 711, 95803
San Bernardino: P.O. Box 781, 92403
San Diego: P.O. Box 831, 92112
San Francisco: P.O. Box 3534, 94119
San Jose: P.O. Box 637, 95106
Santa Ana: P.O. Box 1466, 92702
Santa Barbara: P.O. Box 1529, 93102
Santa Monica: P.O. Box 1500, 90406
Santa Rosa: P.O. Box 700, 95402
Stockton: P.O. Box 1649, 95201
Van Nuys: P.O. Box 7708, 91409
Whittier: P.O. Box 4707, 90607

State of Hawaii
Department of Labor and Industrial Relations
Disability Compensation Division
825 Mililani
P.O. Box 3769
Honolulu, HI 96812

State of New Jersey
Department of Labor and Industry
Division of Employment Security
John Fitch Plaza
Trenton, NJ 08611

State of New York
Workmen's Compensations Board
Disability Benefits Bureau
1949 North Broadway
Albany, NY 12241

Commonwealth of Puerto Rico
Department of Labor
Bureau of Employment Security
Disability Insurance Division
414 Barbosa Avenue
Hato Rey, PR 00917

State of Rhode Island
Rhode Island Department of Employment Security
Temporary Disability Insurance Division
24 Mason Street
P.O. Box 1059
Providence, RI 02901

In some states the claim form is in three parts and must be completed by the claimant, employer, and physician; in others the form is in two parts and is completed by the claimant and physician only. In either case, the claim must be documented by a physician before the applicant can begin receiving benefits. After the claim has been completed by all parties concerned, it is submitted to the nearest local office for processing. The most important item on the claim form is the claimant's Social Security number, for without it the claim cannot be researched properly to establish wages earned in the past quarter (see Figs. 8–1 and 8–2).

Medical Examinations

The claimant may be required to submit to an examination or examinations by an independent medical examiner (IME) in order to determine any mental or physical disability. Fees for such examinations are paid by the state department handling disability insurance.

Claim Forms

To give you an idea of the different forms involved in the processing of disability insurance, California has been selected as the model state. In this way an attempt will be made to show the various forms and how they are put to use. In order to establish a claim, the First Claim for Disability Insurance Form DE 2501 (see Figs. 8–1 and 8–2) must be completed by both the patient and the attending physician. If an extension of disability is required, the Physician's Supplementary Certificate Form DE 2525X must be completed by the physician (Fig. 8–3). With the last check issued to the patient, a Notice of Final Payment Form DE 2525XX (Fig. 8–4) is included. For additional medical information that might be required, Forms DE 2547 and DE 2547A are sometimes sent to the attending physician for completion (see Figs. 8–5 and 8–6). If

Text continued on page 202

CLAIM STATEMENT OF EMPLOYEE

COMPLETE *ALL* ITEMS. IF INCOMPLETE, THIS FORM WILL BE RETURNED, CAUSING A DELAY IN BENEFIT PAYMENTS.

1. Print your full name:

Mr.	FIRST	INITIAL	LAST
Mrs.			
Miss			
Ms.			

Your mailing address:
STREET ADDRESS, P.O. OR R.F.D.   APT. NO.   CITY OR TOWN   STATE & ZIP CODE

Your home address: (if different from mailing address)
STREET ADDRESS, P.O. OR R.F.D.   APT. NO.   CITY OR TOWN   STATE & ZIP CODE

Male ☐   Female ☐   Year of birth _____

2. **IMPORTANT: Enter Your Social Security Account Number**

3. What was the first *full* day you were too sick to work even if it was a Saturday, Sunday, holiday, or normal day off?

MONTH   DATE   YEAR

4. What was the last day you worked BEFORE THIS DISABILITY?

MONTH   DATE   YEAR

5. Employer's Business Name:

Employer's Business Address: NUMBER AND STREET   CITY   STATE & ZIP CODE

FOR DEPARTMENT USE ONLY

Office: 2

6. Your occupation with this employer:

Your Badge or Payroll number:

Comp:

Were you an employer or self-employed individual?   Yes ☐   No ☐

2503 B

Did you work more than 14 days during your last period of employment which ended on the date shown in item (4) above?   Yes ☐   No ☐

Did you stop work because of sickness or injury? If "NO," please give reason: Yes ☐   No ☐

2501 H

Has your employer continued or will he continue your pay, by means of sick leave, vacation, pension, gift or other means?   Yes ☐   No ☐

5006

7. Was this disability caused by your work? If "YES," describe HOW: Yes ☐   No ☐

Are you claiming or receiving Workers' Compensation Benefits for *any* on-the-job injuries or illnesses during the period covered by this claim?   Yes ☐   No ☐

8. Have you recovered from your disability? If "YES," enter date of recovery: MONTH   DATE   YEAR   Yes ☐   No ☐

9. Have you returned to work for any day, part time or full time after the date shown in item (3) above? If "YES," please enter such dates: Yes ☐   No ☐

By

10. I hereby claim benefits and certify that for the period covered by this claim I was unemployed and disabled, that the foregoing statements including any accompanying statements are to the best of my knowledge and belief true, correct and complete. I hereby further authorize my attending physician, practitioner or hospital to furnish and disclose all facts concerning my physical condition that are within his knowledge.

Claim signed on: MONTH   DATE   YEAR

Claimant's signature: (DO NOT PRINT)

TELEPHONE NUMBER

Under Section 2101 of the California Unemployment Insurance Code, it is a misdemeanor wilfully to make a false statement or knowingly to conceal a material fact in order to obtain the payment of any benefits, such misdemeanor being punishable by imprisonment not exceeding six months or by a fine not exceeding $500 or both.

If your signature is made by mark (X) it must be attested by two witnesses with their addresses

SIGNATURE – WITNESS   SIGNATURE – WITNESS

ADDRESS   ADDRESS

If an authorized agent is filing for benefits in the claimant's behalf, a DE 2522 "Appointment of Representative for INCAPACITATED Claimant," must accompany this claim form. When a Form DE 2522 is used, the representative must complete item 10, above, by signing the claimant's name followed by the representative's signature. (Form DE 2522 is available at any department office.)

FOLD ON THIS LINE   FOLD ON THIS LINE

MOISTEN GLUE AND FOLD UP ON THIS LINE
PLEASE DO NOT STAPLE

DO NOT DETACH

FIGURE 8–1

Form DE 2501, Claim Statement of Employee. This is a two-part form and this side is completed by the claimant.

DOCTOR'S CERTIFICATE

Certification may be made by a licensed physician and surgeon, osteopath, chiropractor, dentist, podiatrist, optometrist, or an authorized medical officer of a United States Government facility. All items on this sheet must be completed.

11. I attended the patient for his present medical problem from: MONTH   DAY   YEAR   To   MONTH   DAY   YEAR   At intervals of:

12. History:

(State the nature, severity and the bodily extent of the incapacitating disease or injury.)

Findings:

Diagnosis:

13. Diagnosis confirmed by X-ray or other tests?   YES ☐   NO ☐   Findings:

14. Is this patient now pregnant or has she been pregnant since the date of treatment as reported above?   YES ☐   NO ☐   If "Yes," date pregnancy terminated or future EDC:

Is the maternity care routine?   YES ☐   NO ☐   If "No," state nature and severity of *maternal* pathology:

15. Operation: Performed ☐ (ENTER DATE)   To be performed ☐   Type of operation:

16. Has the patient at any time during your attendance for this medical problem, been incapable of performing his regular work?   YES ☐   NO ☐   If "Yes," his disability commenced on:

17. APPROXIMATE date, in your opinion, disability (if any) should end or has ended sufficiently to permit patient to resume his regular or customary work. Even if considerable question exists, make SOME "estimate". This is a requirement of the Code, and the claim will be delayed if such date is not entered. Such answers as "Indefinite" or "don't know" will not suffice.   (ENTER DATE) ☐

18. In your opinion, is this disability the result of "occupation" either as an "industrial accident" or as an "occupational disease"?   YES ☐   NO ☐   (This should include aggravation of pre-existing conditions by occupation)

19. Have you reported this OR A CONCURRENT DISABILITY to any insurance carrier as a Workers' Compensation Claim?   YES ☐   NO ☐   If "Yes," to whom? (Name of carrier or firm)

20. Further comments (if indicated):

21. In what HOSPITAL was or is patient confined as a registered bed patient?   Hospital name and address:

Zip code

22. **Date and hour** entered as a registered bed patient and discharged from such Hospital pursuant to your orders:

ENTERED		STILL CONFINED	DISCHARGED	
on , 19 , at	A.M. P.M.	on , 19	on , 19 , at	A.M. P.M.

23. I hereby certify that the above statements in my opinion truly describe the patient's disability (if any) and the estimated duration thereof, and that I am a _____ (TYPE OF DOCTOR) licensed to practice by the State of _____

_____ PRINT OR TYPE DOCTOR'S NAME   _____ SIGNATURE OF ATTENDING DOCTOR

_____ NO. AND STREET   CITY   ZIP CODE   STATE LICENSE NUMBER   TELEPHONE NO.   DATE OF SIGNING THIS FORM

FIGURE 8–2

Form DE 2501, Doctor's Certificate. This side is completed by the attending physician and submitted within 28 days of the beginning date of disability to initiate benefits. If the patient is seen by a second physician, this form is mailed to the claimant to secure the certification of a new physician or to clarify a specific claimed period of disability.

PHYSICIAN'S SUPPLEMENTARY CERTIFICATE

File_____ Patient_____ Date Issued_____

1. **To be completed by your present physician ONLY if he finds that you will be unable to work on and beyond the date entered here**_____19_____.

2. Are you still treating patient?_____ Date of last treatment_____19_____.

3. What **complications,** if any, or what **present condition** would tend to make the patient disabled **longer than normally expected** for this type of illness or injury?_____

   _____

   _____

   _____

4. Date patient recovered, or will recover sufficiently (even if under treatment) to be able to perform his regular and customary work

   _____19_____.

I hereby certify that the above statements in my opinion truly describe the claimant's condition and the estimated duration thereof.

_____19_____   _____
Date   Doctor's Signature

DE 2525X REV. 11 (3-74)

A

NOTICE TO CLAIMANT

Your claim for Disability Insurance shows that you will be able to work on the date shown in Item 1 on the reverse side of this form.

If you and your doctor believe that you will not be able to work on that date, have him complete the reverse side of this form and return it to our office.

If a Claim for Continued Disability Benefits is enclosed, it must be completed and returned for further payment.

IF UNEMPLOYED AND ABLE TO WORK — Report to the nearest office of the Employment Development Department to register for work.

STATE OF CALIFORNIA
EMPLOYMENT DEVELOPMENT DEPARTMENT

RETURN WITH YOUR CLAIM FOR CONTINUED DISABILITY BENEFITS

DE 2525X REV. 11 (3-74)
①D OSP

B

FIGURE 8–3

Physician's Supplementary Certificate Form DE 2525X. This form accompanies a check and is a notification to the claimant that benefits will cease with the next check unless the reverse side of the form is completed by the claimant's doctor, extending the duration of disability. The form is pink in color. *A*, Front side of form. *B*, Reverse side.

the patient is hospitalized, many times the hospital will have the patient sign the Hospital Verification and Assignment Transmittal Form DE 2501H (Fig. 8–7) so that the hospital benefits will be paid directly to the hospital. If this is done, credit should appear on the patient's hospital billing statement.

TO THE STUDENT: Refer to the Appendix to complete the insurance forms and work with the patient histories pertinent to this chapter. Assignments 20, 21, 22, 23, and 24, pp. 578–592, pertain to this chapter.

NOTICE OF FINAL PAYMENT

The information contained in your claim for Disability Insurance indicates that you are now able to work, therefore, this is the final check that you will receive on this claim.

IF YOU ARE STILL DISABLED: Contact your Disability Insurance office immediately for information and assistance.

IF YOU BECOME DISABLED AGAIN: File a new Disability Insurance claim form.

IF YOU ARE UNEMPLOYED AND AVAILABLE FOR WORK: Report to the nearest Unemployment Insurance office of the department for assistance in finding work and to determine your entitlement to Unemployment Insurance benefits.

STATE OF CALIFORNIA
EMPLOYMENT DEVELOPMENT DEPARTMENT

DE 2525XX REV. 7 (7-74)   — READ REVERSE SIDE —

A

This determination is final unless you file an appeal within ten (10) days from the date of mailing of this notification. You may appeal by giving a detailed statement as to why you believe the determination is in error. All communications regarding this Disability Insurance Claim should include your Social Security Account Number and be addressed to the office shown on the reverse.

OSP

B

FIGURE 8–4

Notice of Final Payment Form DE 2525XX. This form indicates that the period of disability is "closed" or terminated with the accompanying check, based on information in the claim records. The reverse side of the form contains a statement notifying the claimant of his appeal rights. This form is green in color. *A*, Front side of form. *B*, Reverse side.

STATE OF CALIFORNIA
EMPLOYMENT DEVELOPMENT DEPARTMENT

REFER TO

- Our File No.
- Your Patient
- Regular Work

REQUEST FOR ADDITIONAL
MEDICAL INFORMATION

The original basic information and estimate of duration of your patient's disability have been carefully evaluated. At the present time, the following additional information based upon the progress and present condition of this patient is requested. This will assist the Department in determining eligibility for further disability insurance benefits. Return of the completed form as soon as possible will be appreciated.

D. ALLEN TREAT, M.D., MEDICAL DIRECTOR

CLAIMS EXAMINER   **DOCTOR: PLEASE COMPLETE EITHER PART A OR B. DATE AND SIGN**

PART A   IF YOUR PATIENT HAS RECOVERED SUFFICIENTLY TO BE ABLE TO RETURN TO HIS REGULAR OR CUSTOMARY WORK LISTED ABOVE, PLEASE GIVE THE DATE_____19___.

PART B   THIS PART REFERS TO PATIENT WHO IS STILL DISABLED.

Are you still treating the patient   YES ☐   NO ☐   _____19___.
                                                           Date of last treatment.

What are the medical circumstances which continue to make your patient disabled?

_____

_____

_____

_____

_____

What is your present estimate of the date your patient will be able to perform his regular or customary work listed above?   Date_____19___

Further Comments:_____

_____

_____

_____

Date_____19___   _____
                                        Doctor's Signature

ENCLOSED IS A STAMPED PREADDRESSED ENVELOPE FOR YOUR CONVENIENCE
SE

DE 2547 REV. 13 (12-73)   △ OSP

FIGURE 8–5

Request for Additional Medical Information Form DE 2547. This form is mailed to the doctor when the normal expectancy date of the disability is reached, provided the doctor has requested a longer than normal duration without complications indicated.

STATE OF CALIFORNIA
EMPLOYMENT DEVELOPMENT DEPARTMENT

REFER TO

- Our File No.
- Your Patient   MEDICAL INQUIRY
- Regular Work

A review of the medical certificate received in conjunction with a claim
for disability insurance benefits filed by your patient, named above,
reveals that some additional information is needed in order to evaluate
the claim properly. Your cooperation in answering the question or
questions below and returning the form in the enclosed stamped and
addressed envelope will be appreciated.

D. ALLEN TREAT, M.D., MEDICAL DIRECTOR

CLAIMS EXAMINER

_____ 19 __ _____
             Date   Doctor's Signature

SE
DE 2547 A Rev. 5 (2-73)

FIGURE 8-6

Medical Inquiry Form DE 2547A. This form is mailed to the doctor at the time the first claim is
received, in the event any special questions are required or the doctor has failed to enter a prognosis
date.

SOCIAL SECURITY ACCT. NO.

HOSPITAL ENTRY DATE

HOSPITAL VERIFICATION AND ASSIGNMENT TRANSMITTAL

WE HAVE RECEIVED A CLAIM FOR DISABILITY INSURANCE FROM THE CLAIMANT IDENTIFIED BELOW WHICH INDICATES HE WAS CONFINED AS A REGISTERED BED PATIENT IN YOUR HOSPITAL ABOUT THE ABOVE DATE PURSUANT TO THE ORDER OF HIS PHYSICIAN.

CLAIMANT

PLEASE COMPLETE AND RETURN THIS FORM WITHIN TWO WORKING DAYS

TO:

DO NOT DETACH

HOSPITAL CERTIFICATION

HOSPITAL ASSIGNMENT - *I certify that we have the claimant's written assignment authorizing the payment to this hospital of benefits due covering the period identified to the right.*

ADMITTED:

DATE HOUR

DISCHARGED:

DATE HOUR

STILL CONFINED:

DATE HOUR

SIGNATURE

AMOUNT CHARGED FOR THE PERIOD OF HOSPITALIZATION $

ENTER NUMBER OF DAYS THE HOSPITAL CHARGED THE CLAIMANT A FULL DAY'S RATE:

DAYS

I certify that the claimant named above was a registered bed patient during the period indicated, and that the entries made hereon are to the best of my knowledge true, correct and complete.

SIGNATURE

TITLE

E
DE 2501H REV. 10 (1-71)

DATE

FIGURE 8-7

Hospital Verification and Assignment Transmittal Form DE 2501H. This form is sent to the hospital indicated by the doctor on the First Claim for Disability Insurance Form or by the claimant on the Continued Claim Form. If the hospital official certifies that an assignment was given, then payment is made to the hospital rather than to the claimant.

1. When is temporary disability insurance payable? _____

_____

2. Are hospital benefits paid for nonoccupational illness or injury? _____

3. Temporary disability insurance claims must be filed within how many days in your state? _____

4. For how long can a person continue to draw temporary disability insurance benefits? _____

5. After a claim begins, when do basic benefits become payable if the patient is confined at home? _____ When the patient is hospitalized? _____

_____

6. Name the usual limitations upon temporary disability insurance.

    a. _____

    b. _____

    c. _____

    d. _____

    e. _____

    f. _____

    g. _____

7. When is a Physician's Supplementary Certificate made out? _____

_____

8. If a person has recovered from a previous disability or illness and becomes ill again with the same ailment, is he or she entitled to disability benefits? _____

_____

9. If a woman has an ectopic pregnancy and is unable to work because of this complication, can she receive temporary disability benefits? _____

10. If a woman has an abnormal condition which arises out of her pregnancy, (such as diabetes or varicose veins) and is unable to work because of this condition, can she receive temporary disability benefits? _____ What four states allow for maternity benefits in normal pregnancy? _____ .

11. John S. Thatcher stubbed his toe as he was leaving work, but since the injury was only slightly uncomfortable, he thought no more about it. The next morning he found that his foot was too swollen to fit in his shoe, so he stayed home. When the swelling did not subside after 3 days, John went to the doctor. X-rays showed a broken toe, which kept John home for 2 weeks. After 1 week he applied for temporary disability benefits. Will he be paid? _____ Why? _____

_____

12. Betty T. Kraft had to stay home from her job because her 10-year-old daughter had measles. She applied for temporary disability benefits. Will she be paid?

_____ Why? _____

13. Vincent P. Michael was ill with a bad cold for 1 week. Will he receive temporary disability benefits? _____ Why? _____

_____

14. Betsy C. Palm had an emergency appendectomy and was hospitalized for 3 days. Will she receive disability benefits? _____ Why? _____

_____

15. Frank E. Thompson is a box boy at a supermarket on Saturdays and Sundays while a full-time student at college. He broke his leg while skiing so he cannot work at the market, but he is able to attend classes with his leg in a cast. Can he collect disability benefits for his Saturday and Sunday job? _____ Why? _____

_____

16. Jerry L. Slate is out of a job and is receiving unemployment insurance benefits. He is now suffering from a severe case of intestinal flu. The employment office calls him to interview for a job but he is too ill to go. Can he collect temporary disability benefits for this illness when he might have been given a job? _____

Why? _____

17. Joan T. Corman has diabetes, which sometimes makes her weak so that she has to leave work early in the afternoon. She loses pay for each hour she cannot work.

Can she collect temporary disability benefits? _____Why? _____

_____

18. While walking the picket line with other employees on strike, Gene J. Berry came down with pneumonia and was ill for 2 weeks. Can he collect temporary

disability benefits? _____Why? _____

_____Gene went back to work for 3 weeks and then developed a slight cold and cough which again was diagnosed as pneumonia. The doctor told him to stay home

from work. Would he be able to collect temporary disability benefits again? _____

Why? _____

19. A month after he retired, Roger Reagan had a gallbladder operation. Can he

receive temporary disability benefits? _____Why?_____

_____

20. Jane M. Lambert fell in the backyard of her home and fractured her left ankle. She had a nonunion fracture and was out of work for 28 weeks. For how long

will she collect temporary disability benefits?_____

Notes:

9
Workers' Compensation

BEHAVIORAL

OBJECTIVES *The Assistant should be able to:*

1. Understand who is covered under federal workers' compensation laws.
2. Understand who is covered under state workers' compensation laws.
3. Learn the difference between workers' compensation insurance and employers' liability insurance.
4. State the difference between compulsory and elective laws.
5. Describe how funding is carried out in her state.
6. Identify the exceptions to workers' compensation insurance.
7. Ascertain the purpose of workers' compensation laws.
8. Find out the waiting period in her state before benefits begin.
9. Describe the types of compensation benefits.
10. Define nondisability, temporary disability, and permanent disability claims.
11. Explain OSHA's part for those on the job.
12. Define third party subrogation.
13. Define second-injury fund.
14. Learn what a medical report should contain, how to complete forms properly, and the deadline for submitting reports.
15. Expedite billing in a workers' compensation case and know what to do about a delinquent claim.
16. Define terminology and abbreviations pertinent to workers' compensation cases.

HISTORY

Workers' Compensation Insurance is the most important of the coverages written to insure industrial accidents. Employers' Liability coverage is still used occasionally by an employer to protect himself when his employees do not come within the scope of a compensation law. Until very recently, this form of insurance was known as Workmen's Compensation. The name was changed to avoid sex connotations.

There are two kinds of statutes under Workers' Compensation: federal compensation laws and state compensation laws.

PURPOSES OF WORKERS' COMPENSATION LAWS

1. To provide the best available medical care, directed at the prompt return of the injured or ill employee to work and the achievement of maximum recovery.

2. To provide income to the injured or ill worker or to his or her dependents, regardless of fault.

3. To provide a single remedy and reduce court delays, costs, and work loads arising out of personal injury litigation.

4. To relieve public and private charities of financial drains resulting from uncompensated industrial accidents.

5. To eliminate payment of fees to attorneys and witnesses as well as time-consuming trials and appeals.

6. To encourage maximum employer interest in safety and rehabilitation through an appropriate experience-rating mechanism.

7. To promote the study of causes of accidents and reduce preventable accidents and human suffering rather then concealing the fault.

COVERAGE OF FEDERAL LAWS

A number of federal Workers' Compensation laws have been enacted. They are as follows:

1. *Workmen's Compensation Law of the District of Columbia:* This provides benefits for those working in Washington, D.C. and became effective on May 17, 1928.

2. *Federal Coal Mine Health and Safety Act:* This is sometimes referred to as the "Black Lung Benefits Act," and became effective on May 7, 1941. This act provides benefits to coal miners and is administered through the national headquarters in Washington.

3. *United States Longshoremen's and Harbor Workers' Compensation Act:* This act came into effect on March 4, 1927, and provides benefits for private or public employees engaged in maritime work nationwide. It is administered through regional offices in Boston, Chicago, Cleveland, Denver, Honolulu, Jacksonville, Kansas City, New Orleans, New York City, Philadelphia, San Francisco, Seattle, and Washington, D.C. The type of insurance provided corresponds to that available through the private insurance system. For further information contact the nearest district office, as listed on page 243.

4. *Federal Employees' Compensation Act:* This was instituted on May 30, 1908, to provide benefits for on-the-job injuries to all federal employees. The insurance is provided through an exclusive fund system. Many different claim forms are used, depending on the type of injury. For further information contact the Federal Employees' Compensation Act (FECA) by writing to the nearest office as listed on pages 244 and 245.

COVERAGE OF STATE LAWS

The state compensation laws cover those workers not protected by the federal statutes.

State compensation laws are compulsory or elective.

1. *Compulsory law:* Requires each employer to accept its provisions and provide for specified benefits.

2. *Elective law:* The employer may accept or reject the act, but if he rejects it, he loses the three common-law defenses, which are:

   a. Assumption of risk
   b. Negligence of fellow employees
   c. Contributory negligence.

In 50 states and territories, statutes require compulsory workers' compensation and employers' liability insurance. Coverage is still elective in three states; namely New Jersey, South Carolina, and Texas.

Funding. Six states require employers to insure through a monopolistic state fund. They are: Nevada, North Dakota, Ohio, Washington, West Virginia, and Wyoming. In 47 states and territories employers may qualify as self-insurers. Puerto Rico requires employers to insure through a territorial fund. Twelve states permit employers to purchase insurance from either a competitive state fund or a private insurance company. These are: Arizona, California, Colorado, Idaho, Maryland, Michigan, Montana, New York, Oklahoma, Oregon, Pennsylvania, and Utah.

Thirty-two states, the District of Columbia; and the territory of Guam permit employers to purchase insurance from a private insurance company. These states do not have competitive state funds. They are:

Alabama	Iowa	New Jersey
Alaska	Kansas	New Mexico
Arkansas	Kentucky	North Carolina
Connecticut	Louisiana	Rhode Island
District of Columbia	Maine	South Carolina
Delaware	Massachusetts	South Dakota
Florida	Minnesota	Tennessee
Georgia	Mississippi	Texas
Guam	Missouri	Vermont
Hawaii	Nebraska	Virginia
Illinois	New Hampshire	Wisconsin
Indiana		

The Workers' Compensation statutes relieve the employer of any liability for injury or illness received by an employee, and also enable the employee to be more easily and quickly compensated for loss of wages, medical expenses, and permanent disability. Before the passing of these statutes, the employer could be found legally responsible for his or her employees' injuries or illnesses, but at the same time there were frequent delays in the employee's attempt to recover damages. A physician who is incorporated is also considered as an employee under Workers' Compensation laws.

The employer pays the premium for Workers' Compensation insurance, with the amount dependent on the employee's job and the risk involved in job performance. The information that the physician must supply is usually quite comprehensive and the requirements vary from state to state. To obtain instructions and the proper forms, contact your state bureau as listed on pages 240 to 243. Also see Table 9–1.

TABLE 9–1. EMPLOYERS' AND/OR PHYSICIANS' REPORT OF ACCIDENTS*

Jurisdiction	Reporting Requirements	
	Time Limit	Injuries Covered
ALABAMA	Within 15 days	Death or disability exceeding 7 days
ALASKA	Within 10 days	Death or injury or disease or infection
ARIZONA	Immediately and as required	All injuries
ARKANSAS	Within 10 days and as required	Injury or death
CALIFORNIA	Immediately[1] (employer)	Death cases[1]
	As prescribed[1]	1 day disability or more than first aid[1]
COLORADO	Within 10 days[10]	All injuries
CONNECTICUT	1 week, or as directed	Disability of 1 day or more
DELAWARE	10 days[2]	All injuries
DISTRICT OF COLUMBIA	Within 10 days	All injuries
FLORIDA	Within 10 days and as prescribed	Injury or death
GEORGIA	Within 10 days[2]	All injuries requiring medical or surgical treatment or causing over 7 days' absence
GUAM	Within 10 days	Injury or death
HAWAII	Within 7 days[11]	1 day of absence
IDAHO	As soon as practicable but not later than 10 days after the accident[3]	Disability of 1 day or more
ILLINOIS	Within 2 working days	Death cases or serious injuries
	Between 15th & 25th of month	Disability of over 1 day
	Soon as determinable	Permanent disability
INDIANA	Within 1 week[4]	Disability of 1 day or more
IOWA	Within 48 hours	Disability of more than 7 days
KANSAS	Within 28 days	Death cases
	Within 28 days	Disability of 1 day or more
KENTUCKY	Within 1 week[3]	Disability of more than 1 day
LOUISIANA	No provision	
MAINE	Within 7 days[2]	All injuries
MARYLAND	Within 10 days	Disability of more than 3 days
MASSACHUSETTS	Within 48 hours[3]	All injuries
MICHIGAN	On 8th day[9]	All injuries
MINNESOTA	Within 48 hours	Death or serious injury
	Within 15 days	Disability of 3 days or more

TABLE 9–1. (Continued)

Jurisdiction	Reporting Requirements	
	Time Limit	Injuries Covered
MISSISSIPPI	Within 10 days	Disability of one day or working shift
MISSOURI	Within 10 days	All compensable injuries[5]
MONTANA	Within 6 days[6]	All injuries[6]
NEBRASKA	Within 48 hours of death, Within 7 days of injury	All injuries[7]
NEVADA	Within 6 working days	All injuries
NEW HAMPSHIRE	Within 48 hours	All injuries
NEW JERSEY	Immediately[8]	All injuries[8]
NEW MEXICO	Within 10 days[12]	Compensable injuries
	Within 30 days[13]	All injuries
NEW YORK	Within 10 days	Disability of 1 day or more or requiring medical care beyond two first aid treatments
	As required	All injuries
NORTH CAROLINA	Within 5 days[3]	Disability of more than 1 day
NORTH DAKOTA	Within 1 week	All injuries
OHIO	Within 1 week	All injuries causing 7 days total disability or more
OKLAHOMA	Within 10 days or a reasonable time	All injuries
OREGON	Within 5 days	All injuries
PENNSYLVANIA	Within 48 hours	Death cases
	After 7 days but not later than 10 days	Disability of 1 day or more
PUERTO RICO	Within 5 days	All injuries
RHODE ISLAND	Within 48 hours[16]	Death cases
	Within 10 days[14]	Disability of 3 days or more
SOUTH CAROLINA	Within 10 days[4]	All injuries
SOUTH DAKOTA	Within 48 hours[4]	All injuries
TENNESSEE	Within 10 days	Disability of 7 days or more
TEXAS	Within 8 days[4]	Disability of more than 1 day
UTAH	Within 1 week[15]	All injuries
VERMONT	Within 72 hours[4]	Disability of 1 day or more or requiring medical care
VIRGINIA	Within 10 days[4]	All injuries
WASHINGTON	Immediately	All injuries
WEST VIRGINIA	Within 5 days	All injuries

TABLE 9–1. (Continued)

Jurisdiction	Reporting Requirements	
	Time Limit	Injuries Covered
WISCONSIN	Within 4 days	Disability beyond 3 day waiting period
WYOMING	Within 10 days	All injuries

*In many states, except for initial reports, the insured's company relieves the *employer* of the responsibility of reporting. However, a *physician* may render progress, supplemental, and final medical reports weekly and monthly, depending on the nature of the industrial accident.

1. Insurance carrier and attending physician also required to make report (within 5 days). It should be forthwith by telephone in fatal injury cases, but this is in addition to usual report.
2. Supplemental report upon termination of disability. Occupational Safety Law requires reporting within 48 hours all deaths or serious physical injuries requiring hospitalization.
3. Supplemental report required after 60 days, or upon termination of disability.
4. Supplemental report required within 10 days after termination of compensation period.
5. Supplemental report required within 1 month for compensable injuries and injuries requiring medical aid. Missouri requires full report on prescribed form in one month; division director will collect statistics and information for OSHA.
6. Insurance carrier also required to make report.
7. Report may be made by insurance carrier or employer.
8. Uninsured employers are required to report compensable injuries only. If employer is insured, carrier is also required to make report.
9. Immediate report required if 7 days' disability or more, death, or certain injuries.
10. Immediate report in case of death.
11. Report within 48 hours if injury results in immediate death.
12. To the State Labor Commissioner.
13. To the Insurance Department of the State Corporation Commission.
14. Supplemental report upon termination of disability.
15. Copy of accident report and first medical report must be furnished employee.
16. Copies of all accident reports or statements obtained from supervising personnel shall be furnished employee and his attorney upon request, or reports are inadmissible as evidence.

Minors are covered by Workers' Compensation but in some states double compensation or added penalties are provided. In many states minors also receive special legal benefit provisions.

If a worker's occupation takes him into another state, questions may arise as to which law determines compensation payable. Most compensation laws are extra-territorial (which means they are effective outside of the state) either by specific provisions or court decision.

Several states have laws to compensate civil defense and other volunteer workers, such as firemen injured in the line of duty.

Occupational diseases usually become known soon after exposure. However, some diseases may be latent for a considerable amount of time. Some states thus have extended periods in which claims may be filed concerning certain slowly developing occupational diseases. These diseases might be silicosis, asbestosis, radiation disability, or loss of hearing.

Exceptions to State Workers' Compensation Insurance. Many states do not require Workers' Compensation Insurance for certain employees. These employees include: domestics or casual laborers, baby sitters, newspaper vendors or distributors, charity workers, and gardeners. Some states also do not require compensation insurance for farm laborers.

Waiting Periods. The laws state that a waiting period must elapse before income benefits are payable. This waiting period affects only compensation since medical and hospital care are provided immediately. To find your state's waiting period see Table 9–2 on this page.

TABLE 9–2. WAITING PERIOD FOR INCOME BENEFITS; MEDICAL BENEFITS*

Jurisdiction	Waiting Period	Jurisdiction	Waiting Period
ALABAMA	3 days	MONTANA	7 days
ALASKA	3 days	NEBRASKA	7 days
ARIZONA	7 days	NEVADA	5 days
ARKANSAS	7 days	NEW HAMPSHIRE	3 days
CALIFORNIA	3 days	NEW JERSEY	7 days
COLORADO	3 days	NEW MEXICO	7 days
CONNECTICUT	3 days	NEW YORK	7 days
DELAWARE	3 days	NORTH CAROLINA	7 days
DISTRICT OF COLUMBIA	3 days	NORTH DAKOTA	5 days
FLORIDA	7 days	OHIO	7 days
GEORGIA	7 days	OKLAHOMA	5 days
GUAM	7 days	OREGON	3 days
HAWAII	2 days	PENNSYLVANIA	7 days
IDAHO	5 days	PUERTO RICO	3 days
ILLINOIS	3 days	RHODE ISLAND	3 days
INDIANA	7 days	SOUTH CAROLINA	7 days
IOWA	7 days	SOUTH DAKOTA	7 days
KANSAS	7 days	TENNESSEE	7 days
KENTUCKY	7 days	TEXAS	7 days
LOUISIANA	7 days	UTAH	3 days
MAINE	3 days	VERMONT	3 days
MARYLAND	3 days	VIRGINIA	7 days
MASSACHUSETTS	5 days	WASHINGTON	3 days
MICHIGAN	7 days	WEST VIRGINIA	3 days
MINNESOTA	3 days	WISCONSIN	3 days
MISSISSIPPI	5 days	WYOMING	3 days
MISSOURI	3 days		

*These are statutory provisions for waiting periods. Statutes provide that a waiting period must elapse during which income benefits are not payable. This waiting period affects only compensation, since medical and hospital care are provided immediately.

TYPES OF STATE COMPENSATION BENEFITS

The four principal types of state compensation benefits which may apply in ordinary cases are:

1. *Medical treatment.* This includes hospital, medical and surgical services, medications, and prosthetic devices. Treatment may be rendered by a licensed M.D., osteopath, dentist, or chiropractor.

2. *Temporary disability indemnity.* This is in the form of weekly cash payments made directly to the injured or ill.

3. *Permanent disability indemnity.* This can be either weekly or monthly cash payments based on a rating of percentages of permanent disability, or an award made in a lump sum at one time. California has a unique system of permanent disability evaluation which requires a separate determination by the disability rating bureau in San Francisco. No other state has this system.

4. *Death benefits for survivors.* This consists of cash payments to dependents of employees who are fatally injured. In some states a burial allowance is also given.

5. *Rehabilitation benefits.* In cases of severe disabilities, this can be either medical rehabilitation or vocational rehabilitation.

TYPES OF STATE CLAIMS

There are three types of state Workers' Compensation claims.

Nondisability Claim. The first type of claim is called the *nondisability claim.* This is the simplest type of claim and it is easily adjusted. Generally speaking, a nondisability claim is considered a minor injury in which the patient is seen by the doctor but is able to continue working. The laws clearly state that the injured person must report promptly to his or her employer or immediate supervisor about the industrial injury or illness. The employer sends in an *Employer's Report of Industrial or Work Injury* form (see Fig. 9–1) to the insurance company. In different states, the time limit on submission of this form varies from "immediately" to as long as 30 days (see Table 9–1). Many states have adopted the form shown in Figure 9–1 to meet the requirements of the Federal Occupational Safety and Health Act of 1970 (OSHA) (see pp. 221 and 222) as well as for their state statistical purposes. The employer may also complete a Medical Service Order and give this to the injured employee to take to the physician's office (see Fig. 9–2). This authorizes the physician to treat the injured employee.

After the physician sees the injured person, he or she sends in a completed *Doctor's First Report of Occupational Injury or Illness* form as soon as possible (see Figs. 9–3 and 9–10, pp. 224 and 234). Since this time limit also varies from state to state, refer to Table 9–1 for the requirements of your state. Failure to file the Report can be a misdemeanor. Copies of the form, which is a legal document, go to the insurance carrier and to the state. Some physicians even send a copy to the employer. Because this is a legal document, each copy *must be signed in ink* by the physician. The insurance company waits for the doctor's report and bill, which should state that the patient has been discharged and that no further treatment is necessary. The insurance company pays the medical bill to the physician and closes the case.

State of California **EMPLOYER'S REPORT OF OCCUPATIONAL INJURY OR ILLNESS**	Please complete in triplicate. Retain one copy to your files and mail the remaining two copies to **STATE COMPENSATION INSURANCE FUND** P.O. BOX S VENTURA, CALIFORNIA 93001 Telephone: (805) 648-5311	OSHA Case or File No.

California law requires an employer to report <u>within five days</u> every industrial injury or occupational disease which: (a) Results in lost time beyond the day of injury, or (b) Requires medical treatment other than first aid.
PLEASE NOTE: If death results or if the injury or illness: (a) Requires inpatient hospitalization of more than 24 hours for other than medical observation, or (b) Results in loss of any member of the body; or (c) Produces any serious degree of permanent disfigurement, then the nearest district office of the California Division of Industrial Safety also must be notified <u>immediately</u> by telephone or telegraph. This notification is not required, however, if the injury or death results from an accident on a public street or highway.

EMPLOYER

1. FIRM NAME | DIVISION | 1A. POLICY NUMBER | PLEASE DO NOT USE THIS COLUMN

2. MAILING ADDRESS (PLEASE INCLUDE CITY, ZIP) | 2A. PHONE NUMBER | CASE NO.

3. LOCATION, IF DIFFERENT FROM MAIL ADDRESS | EMPLOYER NO.

4. NATURE OF BUSINESS (E.G., SHOE MANUFACTURER, CABINET WORKS) | 5. STATE UNEMPLOYMENT INSURANCE ACCT. NUMBER | INDUSTRY

EMPLOYEE

6. NAME | 7. SOCIAL SECURITY NUMBER

8. HOME ADDRESS (NUMBER AND STREET, CITY, ZIP) | 8A. PHONE NUMBER | SEX

9. SEX ☐ MALE ☐ FEMALE | 10. OCCUPATION (REGULAR JOB TITLE, NOT SPECIFIC ACTIVITY AT TIME OF INJURY) | 11. DATE OF BIRTH __/__/__ MONTH DAY YEAR | AGE

12. DEPARTMENT IN WHICH REGULARLY EMPLOYED | 12A. DATE OF HIRE __/__/__ MONTH DAY YEAR | OCCUPATION

13. WAGES $_____ PER WEEK | 13A. IS EMPLOYEE PAID ON COMMISSION OR PIECE WORK BASIS, OR PAID BOARD OR LODGING ALLOWANCE? ☐ YES ☐ NO | 13B. UNDER WHAT CLASS CODE OF YOUR POLICY WERE WAGES ASSIGNED? | WEEKLY WAGE

INJURY OR ILLNESS

14. WHERE DID ACCIDENT OR EXPOSURE OCCUR? (ADDRESS, CITY AND COUNTY) | 15. ON EMPLOYER'S PREMISES? ☐ YES ☐ NO | COUNTY

16. WHAT WAS EMPLOYEE DOING WHEN INJURED? (PLEASE BE SPECIFIC. IDENTIFY TOOLS, EQUIPMENT OR MATERIAL THE EMPLOYEE WAS USING) | ACCIDENT TYPE / AGENCY

17. HOW DID THE ACCIDENT OR EXPOSURE OCCUR? (PLEASE DESCRIBE FULLY THE EVENTS THAT RESULTED IN INJURY OR OCCUPATIONAL DISEASE. TELL WHAT HAPPENED AND HOW IT HAPPENED. PLEASE USE SEPARATE SHEET IF NECESSARY) | AGENCY PART / SUPPLEMENTAL AGENCY / NATURE OF INJURY

18. OBJECT OR SUBSTANCE THAT DIRECTLY INJURED EMPLOYEE (E.G., THE MACHINE EMPLOYEE STRUCK AGAINST OR WHICH STRUCK HIM; THE VAPOR OR POISON INHALED OR SWALLOWED; THE CHEMICAL THAT IRRITATED HIS SKIN; IN CASES OF STRAINS, THE THING HE WAS LIFTING, PULLING, ETC.) | PART OF BODY / INJURY DATE

19. NATURE OF INJURY OR ILLNESS AND PART OF BODY AFFECTED

20. NAME AND ADDRESS OF PHYSICIAN | 21. IF HOSPITALIZED, NAME AND ADDRESS OF HOSPITAL | EXTENT OF INJURY

22. DATE OF INJURY OR ILLNESS __/__/__ MONTH DAY YEAR | 23. TIME OF DAY _____ A.M. _____ P.M. | 24. WAS EMPLOYEE UNABLE TO WORK ON ANY DAY AFTER INJURY? ☐ YES, DATE LAST WORKED _____ ☐ NO | INSURANCE CARRIER

25. HAS EMPLOYEE RETURNED TO WORK? ☐ YES, DATE RETURNED _____ ☐ NO, STILL OFF WORK | 26. DID EMPLOYEE DIE? ☐ YES, DATE _____ ☐ NO | REPORT LAG

27. WAS ANOTHER PERSON RESPONSIBLE? ☐ YES ☐ NO

28. WAS INJURED AN EXECUTIVE OFFICER? ☐ YES ☐ NO | CODED BY

COMPLETED BY (TYPE OR PRINT)	SIGNATURE	TITLE	DATE

SCIF FORM 67 (REV. 4-74) | FILING OF THIS REPORT IS NOT AN ADMISSION OF LIABILITY | 34465-218 6-75 50M T OSP

FIGURE 9–1

Employer's Report of Occupational Injury or Illness. This form complies with OSHA requirements as well as California State Workers' Compensation laws.

```
┌─────────────────────────────────────────────────────────────┐
│            STATE COMPENSATION INSURANCE FUND                  │
│              P.O. Box S, Ventura, California 93001            │
│                                                               │
│                   Medical Service Order                       │
│                                                               │
│  Dr./Clinic   Max Gluteus, M. D.                              │
│                                                               │
│  Address      4567 Broad Avenue, Woodland Hills, XY 12345     │
│                                                               │
│  We are sending Mrs. Ima Hurt                                 │
│         to you for treatment in accordance with the terms     │
│         of the Workers' Com-                                  │
│         pensation Laws. Please submit your report to the      │
│         State Compensation                                    │
│         Insurance Fund at once. Compensation cannot be paid   │
│         without complete                                      │
│         medical information.                                  │
│                                                               │
│  Employer    The Conk Out Company                             │
│                                                               │
│  Signature    U.R. Wright          Date 4-3-77                │
│         If patient is able to return to work today or         │
│         tomorrow, please show date                            │
│         and time below—sign and give to patient to return     │
│         to employer. If there                                 │
│         are any work restrictions indicate on the back of     │
│         this form. Please submit                              │
│         your usual first report in any case.                  │
│                                                               │
│  Date/Time_____By_____           │
│  SCIF FORM 358 (REV. 3-75)        13      32053-218 3-75 50M ① ◊ OSP │
└─────────────────────────────────────────────────────────────┘
```

FIGURE 9–2

Medical Service Order. A form similar to the one shown here may be brought to the physician's office by the patient requesting treatment under Workers' Compensation. The form will be completed and signed by the patient's employer. Make a photocopy of the form for the physician's files and then attach the original to the "Doctor's First Report of Occupational Injury or Illness" (preliminary report) which you are sending to the address listed on the form. An employer may also write the service order on his business letterhead, billhead, or a piece of scratch paper.

Temporary Disability Claim. The second type of claim involves cases in which *temporary disability* (TD) is present. In California the law states that there must be a three-day waiting period before temporary disability (salary replacement) can begin (see Table 9–2). The insurance adjuster's most important function in adjusting the claim is to put up the proper reserves. In other words, the adjuster must predict in advance how much money will be needed during the course of the claim, and calculate as accurate a reserve as possible. This is frequently a difficult task, since a seemingly minor back strain may ultimately require fusion, or a small cut may become gangrenous and lead to an amputation. The insurance carrier wants to provide the best possible medical care for the patient and if a specialist is required on a case, the patient will be immediately referred to the specialist.

Compensation benefits are not subject to income tax. Usually Workers' Compensation weekly temporary disability payments are based upon the employee's earnings at the time of the injury.

Normally when a private patient seeks care by a physician and agrees to treatment, the contract exists between the patient and the physician. In Workers' Compensation cases, the contract exists between the physician and the insurance carrier. In a temporary disability case, after two to four weeks of treatment a *supplemental report* is sent to the insurance carrier to give information on the current status of the patient.

If there is a significant change in the prognosis, a detailed progress report (sometimes called a *re-examination report*) is sent to the insurance carrier. Temporary disability (TD) is ended when the doctor tells the insurance carrier that the patient is able to return to work. Usually these cases involve no permanent disability (PD). Sometimes the report which is required at the time of discharge is called the *Doctor's Final Report*. When the patient resumes work, the insurance carrier closes the case and the temporary disability benefits cease.

Permanent Disability Claim. The third type of claim is a case in which there is *permanent disability* (PD). In this type of claim the patient or injured party is usually on temporary disability benefits for a time and then is unable to return to his or her former occupation. The physician states in the report that the patient has residual disability which will hamper his or her opportunity to compete in the open job market. Examples of residual disability include loss of a hand, loss of an eye, loss of a leg, neurologic problems, and so forth. The permanent disability rating depends on the severity of the injury, the age of the injured person, and the patient's occupation at the time of the injury. The older the person, the greater the permanent disability benefit will be. One might think that a younger person deserves higher compensation because he will be disabled for a longer portion of his working career. However, the Workers' Compensation laws assume that a young person has a better chance of being rehabilitated into another occupation.

In a permanent disability claim, the physician's final report must include the words *"permanent and stationary"* (P and S). This phrase means that the doctor is unable to do anything more for the patient and that the patient will be hampered by the disability to some extent for the rest of his or her life. The case is rated for permanent disability, and a settlement is made which is called a *compromise and release* (C and R). This is an agreement upon a total sum between the injured and the insurance company. The case can then be closed. If an injured person is dissatisfied with the rating after the case has been declared permanent and stationary, he may appeal the case to the Workers' Compensation Appeals Board or to the Industrial Accident Commission.

In rating a case, *subrosa films* are sometimes shown to document the extent of the patient's permanent disability. (Subrosa means "under the rose." In ancient times the rose was a symbol of silence or secrecy.) These films are made without the knowledge of the patient.

A *deposition* is sometimes taken in permanent disability cases. This is testimony of the patient, physician(s), and witnesses made under oath but not in open court. It is written down to be used when the case comes to trial.

OCCUPATIONAL SAFETY AND HEALTH ADMINISTRATION (OSHA) ACT OF 1970

Congress has established an office, known as the Occupational Safety and Health Administration (OSHA), to protect employees against on-the-job health and safety hazards. This program includes tougher health and safety standards and a sensible complaint procedure enabling individual workers to trigger enforcement measures. The work standards are designed to minimize exposure to on-the-job hazards such as faulty machinery, noise, dust, and toxic chemical fumes. Employers are required by law to meet these health and safety standards. Failure to do so can subject the employer to fines that could run into thousands of dollars. The law applies to almost all businesses, large or small. It applies to heavy industries, light industries, service industries, and retailers. Employees of state and local governments are also covered. Federal employees and household domestic workers are *not* covered. To file a complaint, the proper form is obtained from the federal Division of Industrial Safety and completed by the employee. An inspector may be sent to the place of employment, and the employer may be cited for specific violations of the law.

SPECIAL CIRCUMSTANCES

Third Party Subrogation

The legal term *subrogation* means "to substitute" one person for another. When applied to Workers' Compensation cases, it means a transfer of the claims and rights of the original creditor. In a Compensation case involving third party subrogation, the participants are the patient, the insurance carrier, and a third party responsible for the injury.

Imagine, for example, that a secretary is going to the bank to deposit some money for her employer. While she is on the errand, her car is rear-ended by another automobile and she is injured. In such a case there is no question of fault and no question of cause. The secretary was hurt during the performance of her work and the Workers' Compensation insurance carrier is liable. The carrier must adjust the claim, provide all medical treatment, and pay all temporary disability benefits and all permanent disability benefits.

However, the insurance carrier does have legal recourse. It may send a representative to visit with the secretary, explain to her that she has a good subrogation case, and encourage her to seek the advice of an attorney and sue the third party in civil court.* If the secretary agrees to sue, the insurance carrier puts in a demand for repayment of all the money that it has paid out.† If an award is made to the secretary when the case is settled, the insurance carrier is first reimbursed for all that it has paid and the secretary then receives the balance.

In some states, such as California, the patient is legally prevented from collecting twice. If the patient's attorney should call the doctor's office for information, it is only ethical and legal to ask permission from the insurance carrier before giving out any medical information because, as stated before, the contract exists between the physician and the insurance carrier, not between the physician and the patient.

Second-Injury Fund (Subsequent Injury Fund)

This fund was established to meet problems arising when an employee has a pre-existing injury or condition and is subsequently injured at work. The pre-existing injury combines with the second injury to produce disability that is greater than that caused by the latter alone.

---

*This is sometimes referred to as *litigation*, which is the process of carrying on a lawsuit.
†In legal language, this is called a *lien*.

Two functions of the fund are:
1. To encourage hiring of the physically handicapped
2. To allocate more equitably the costs of providing benefits to such employees. "Second-injury" employers pay compensation related primarily to the disability caused by the second injury, even though the employee receives benefits relating to his combined disability; the difference is made up from the Second-Injury Fund, also known as the Subsequent Injury Fund.

Unemployment Compensation Disability and Workers' Compensation

As mentioned in Chapter 8 there are six states that have State Disability Insurance (Unemployment Compensation Disability Insurance); namely, California, Hawaii, New Jersey, New York, Puerto Rico, and Rhode Island. If a recipient is collecting benefits from a Workers' Compensation insurance carrier and the amount that the compensation carrier pays is less than that allowed by the Unemployment Compensation Disability Insurance program, then the state disability program will pay the balance.

Reasons That Delay Closing a Workers' Compensation Case

1. Unanswered questions
2. Incomplete answers
3. Vague terminology
4. Omitted signatures from forms or written reports
5. Incorrect billing
6. Inadequate progress reports

MEDICAL REPORTS

In most states, the first report of an industrial injury submitted by the employer and by the physician is a requirement of the law (see Figs. 9–1, 9–3, and 9–10). However, subsequent progress or supplemental reports may be narrative and are not necessarily completed on the special forms which are available in most states (see Figs. 9–11, 9–12, and 9–13). The insurance carrier authorizing the examination should be furnished with the report in triplicate or quadruplicate, depending on its needs. A copy should always be retained for the physician's files. To become familiar with some of the medical terminology used in industrial injury cases, see Figures 9–4, 9–5, and 9–6. If the physician prefers to submit a narrative letter, the medical report should include the following:

1. Complete *history* of the accident, injury, or illness. The physician should state whether there is a causal connection between the accident and conditions that may appear subsequently but are not obvious sequelae.

2. The patient's *present complaints*; sometimes given as *subjective* complaints.

3. The patient's *past history* and whether the employee has a pre-existing defect which might entitle him or her to benefits from the Subsequent Injury Fund or represent the actual cause of the present condition.

4. Complete *medical findings* on examination; sometimes given as *objective* findings.

NEBRASKA WORKMEN'S COMPENSATION COURT
First Treatment Medical Report
(Must be filed with Compensation Court & Employer within 14 days of first treatment)

TYPE OR PRINT

PATIENT & INSURED (SUBSCRIBER) INFORMATION

1. PATIENT'S NAME (First name, middle initial, last name)

2. PATIENT'S DATE OF BIRTH

3. INSURED'S NAME (EMPLOYER)

4. PATIENT'S ADDRESS (Street, city, state, ZIP code)

5. PATIENT'S SEX

MALE ☐ FEMALE ☐

6. INSURED'S I.D. No. (include any letters)

7. PATIENT'S RELATIONSHIP TO INSURED
SELF ☐ SPOUSE ☐ CHILD ☐ OTHER ☐

8. INSURED'S GROUP NO. (Or Group Name)

9. OTHER HEALTH INSURANCE COVERAGE - Enter Name of Policyholder and Plan Name and Address and Policy or Medical Assistance Number

10. WAS CONDITION RELATED TO:

A. PATIENT'S EMPLOYMENT
YES ☐ NO

B. AN AUTO ACCIDENT
YES ☐ NO

11. INSURED'S ADDRESS (Street, city, state, ZIP code)

12. PATIENT'S OR AUTHORIZED PERSON'S SIGNATURE
I Authorize the Release of any Medical Information Necessary to Process this Claim

SIGNED _____ DATE _____

13. I AUTHORIZE PAYMENT OF MEDICAL BENEFITS TO UNDERSIGNED PHYSICIAN OR SUPPLIER FOR SERVICE DESCRIBED BELOW

SIGNED (Insured or Authorized Person) _____

PHYSICIAN OR SUPPLIER INFORMATION

14. DATE OF:
ILLNESS (FIRST SYMPTOM) OR INJURY (ACCIDENT)

15. DATE FIRST CONSULTED YOU FOR THIS CONDITION

16. HAS PATIENT EVER HAD SAME OR SIMILAR SYMPTOMS?
YES ☐ NO

17. DATE PATIENT ABLE TO RETURN TO WORK

18. DATES OF TOTAL DISABILITY
FROM _____ THROUGH _____

DATES OF PARTIAL DISABILITY
FROM _____ THROUGH _____

19. NAME OF REFERRING PHYSICIAN

20. FOR SERVICES RELATED TO HOSPITALIZATION GIVE HOSPITALIZATION DATES
ADMITTED _____ DISCHARGED _____

21. NAME & ADDRESS OF FACILITY WHERE SERVICES RENDERED (If other than home or office)

22. WAS LABORATORY WORK PERFORMED OUTSIDE YOUR OFFICE?
YES ☐ NO CHARGES:

23. DIAGNOSIS OR NATURE OF ILLNESS OR INJURY. RELATE DIAGNOSIS TO PROCEDURE IN COLUMN D BY REFERENCE TO NUMBERS 1, 2, 3, ETC. OR DX CODE

1.
2.
3.
4.

24 A DATE OF SERVICE	B* PLACE OF SERVICE	C FULLY DESCRIBE PROCEDURES, MEDICAL SERVICES OR SUPPLIES FURNISHED FOR EACH DATE GIVEN PROCEDURE CODE (IDENTIFY:) (EXPLAIN UNUSUAL SERVICES OR CIRCUMSTANCES)	D DIAGNOSIS CODE	E CHARGES	F

24.A. HISTORY. GIVE BRIEF DESCRIPTION OF WHAT OCCURRED. PATIENT'S ACCOUNT OF ACCIDENT.

25. SIGNATURE OF PHYSICIAN OR SUPPLIER (Read back before signing)

SIGNED _____ DATE _____

26. ACCEPT ASSIGNMENT (GOVERNMENT CLAIMS ONLY) (SEE BACK)
YES ☐ NO ☐

27. TOTAL CHARGE

28. AMOUNT PAID

29. BALANCE DUE

30. YOUR SOCIAL SECURITY NO.

31. PHYSICIAN'S OR SUPPLIER'S NAME, ADDRESS, ZIP CODE & TELEPHONE NO.

32. YOUR PATIENT'S ACCOUNT NO.

33. YOUR EMPLOYER I.D. NO.

I.D. NO.

*PLACE OF SERVICE CODES

1 – (IH) – INPATIENT HOSPITAL	4 – (H) – PATIENT'S HOME	7 – (NH) – NURSING HOME	O – (OL) – OTHER LOCATIONS
2 – (OH) – OUTPATIENT HOSPITAL	5 – DAY CARE FACILITY (PSY)	8 – (SNF) – SKILLED NURSING FACILITY	A – (IL) – INDEPENDENT LABORATORY
3 – (O) – DOCTOR'S OFFICE	6 – NIGHT CARE FACILITY (PSY)	9 – AMBULANCE	B – OTHER MEDICAL/SURGICAL FACILITY

NWCC FORM 45

FIGURE 9–3

First Treatment Medical Report form used in the state of Nebraska. This form follows the format of the Universal or Standard Form developed by the American Medical Association Council on Medical Service (see Chapter 3).

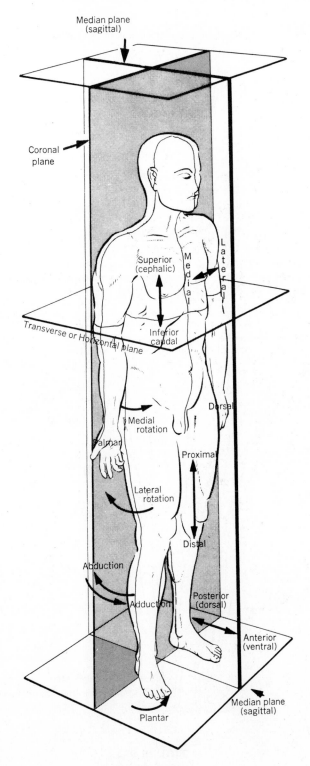

FIGURE 9–4

Directional terminology used in Workers' Compensation reports. This is a diagram illustrating the use of some anatomic terms referring to position and movement. (From *Radiography: A Tool of Medical Science*. GAF Corporation, 1970, p. 5.)

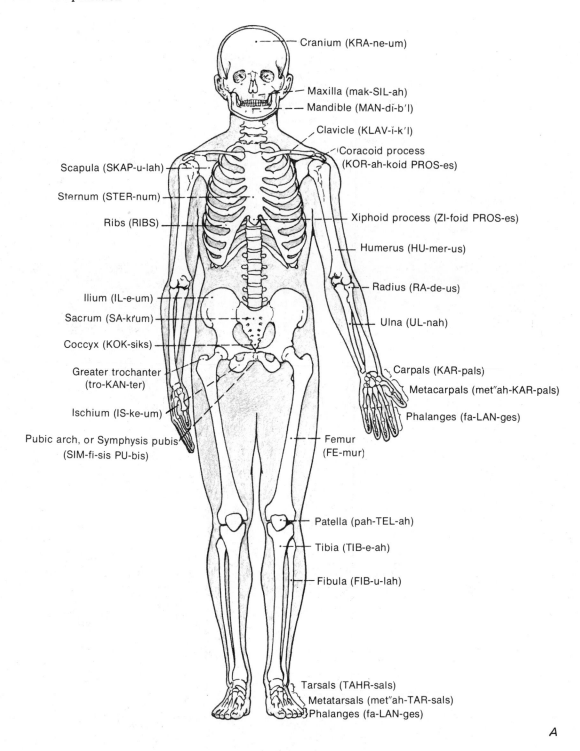

Cranium (KRA-ne-um)

Maxilla (mak-SIL-ah)
Mandible (MAN-dĭ-b'l)

Clavicle (KLAV-ĭ-k'l)

Coracoid process
(KOR-ah-koid PROS-es)

Scapula (SKAP-u-lah)

Sternum (STER-num)

Ribs (RIBS)

Xiphoid process (ZI-foid PROS-es)

Humerus (HU-mer-us)

Radius (RA-de-us)

Ilium (IL-e-um)

Sacrum (SA-krum)

Ulna (UL-nah)

Coccyx (KOK-siks)

Greater trochanter
(tro-KAN-ter)

Carpals (KAR-pals)

Metacarpals (met"ah-KAR-pals)

Ischium (IS-ke-um)

Phalanges (fa-LAN-ges)

Pubic arch, or Symphysis pubis
(SIM-fi-sis PU-bis)

Femur
(FE-mur)

Patella (pah-TEL-ah)

Tibia (TIB-e-ah)

Fibula (FIB-u-lah)

Tarsals (TAHR-sals)

Metatarsals (met"ah-TAR-sals)

Phalanges (fa-LAN-ges)

A

FIGURE 9–5

Terminology pertinent to the skeletal anatomy, indicating the common medical terms seen in reports on injury cases. (From Jacob and Francone: *Structure and Function in Man*, 3rd ed. Philadelphia, W.B. Saunders Company, 1974, pp. 83, 84.)

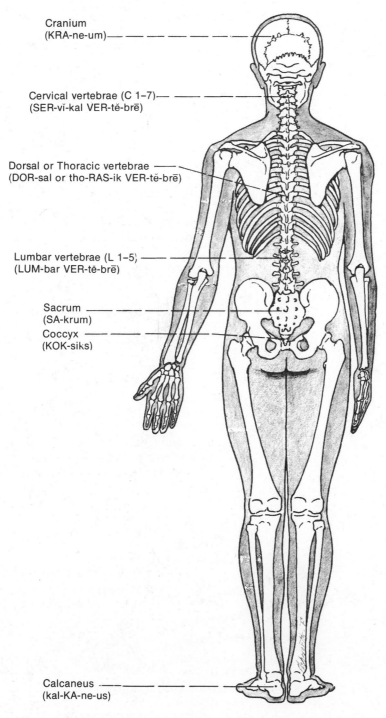

Cranium
(KRA-ne-um)

Cervical vertebrae (C 1–7)
(SER-vĭ-kal VER-tĕ-brē)

Dorsal or Thoracic vertebrae
(DOR-sal or tho-RAS-ik VER-tĕ-brē)

Lumbar vertebrae (L 1–5)
(LUM-bar VER-tĕ-brē)

Sacrum
(SA-krum)

Coccyx
(KOK-siks)

Calcaneus
(kal-KA-ne-us)

B

FIGURE 9–5 *(Continued)*

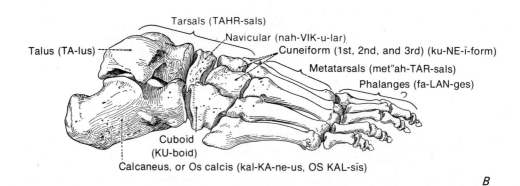

(D) Distal phalanx (DIS-tal FA-lanks)
(M) Middle phalanx (MID-I FA-lanks)
(P) Proximal phalanx (PROK-si-mal FA-lanks)

Metacarpal (met"ah-KAR-pal)
Lesser multangular
Greater multangular } (mul-TANG-gu-lar)
Capitate (KAP-i-tāt)
Navicular (nah-VIK-u-lar)
Lunate (LU-nāt)

Hamate (HAM-at)
Pisiform (PI-si-form)
Triangular or Cuneiform
(Triquetrum)
(tri-ANG-gu-lar
ku-NE-i-form
tri-KWE-trum)

Radius (RA-de-us)

Ulna (UL-nah)

Lateral condyle of humerus
(LAT-er-al KON-dīl of HU-mer-us)
Olecranon (o-LEK-rah-non)

A

Tarsals (TAHR-sals)
Navicular (nah-VIK-u-lar)
Cuneiform (1st, 2nd, and 3rd) (ku-NE-i-form)
Talus (TA-lus)
Metatarsals (met"ah-TAR-sals)
Phalanges (fa-LAN-ges)

Cuboid
(KU-boid)
Calcaneus, or Os calcis (kal-KA-ne-us, OS KAL-sis)

B

FIGURE 9–6

Terminology pertinent to (*A*) the hand and (*B*) the foot, indicating the common medical terms seen in reports on injury cases. (*A* redrawn from Marble, H.C.: *The Hand*; *B* from Hauser, E.D.W.: *Diseases of the Foot*.)

5. Report of *laboratory or x-ray* findings.

6. Complete *diagnosis*.

7. Opinion as to *relationship*, if any, between the injury or disease and the condition diagnosed.

8. The planned scope, course, and duration of recommended *treatment*.

9. The patient's *disability and prognosis*, giving:

    a. Period that the patient has been unable to work because of the injury or illness.

    b. Opinion as to probable further temporary disability, and a statement as to when the patient will be able to return to work or has returned to work.

    c. Statement indicating whether the condition is currently permanent and stationary, or the probability of future permanent disability.

An evaluation of subjective factors should be given. Subjective disability can best be evaluated by:

1. A description of the activity which produces the disability.

2. The duration of the disability.

3. The activities which are precluded by, and those which can be performed with, the disability.

4. The means necessary for relief.

The following definitions were developed as examples of interpretations of *subjective* complaints.

1. A *severe pain* would preclude the activity causing the pain.

2. A *moderate pain* could be tolerated, but would cause marked handicap in the performance of the activity precipitating the pain.

3. A *slight pain* could be tolerated, but would cause some handicap in the performance of the activity precipitating the pain.

4. A *minimal or mild pain* would constitute an annoyance, but would cause no handicap in the performance of the particular activity. It would be considered a nonratable permanent disability.

Information to be Included in Detailed Progress or Re-Examination Reports

1. Date of most recent examination
2. Present condition and progress since last report
3. Measurements of function
4. X-ray or laboratory report since last examination
5. Treatment (give type and duration)
6. Work status (patient working or estimated date of return to work)
7. Permanent disability to be anticipated

FEES

In those states that have adopted the Relative Value Studies (see Chapter 2), an Official Minimum Medical Fee Schedule book is usually available for Workers' Compensation billing purposes. In some states the fee schedule may go back many years, utilizing 4-digit coding. In using 5-digit updated RVS coding systems, the Workers' Compensation insurance carriers may convert the 5-digit code number to a 4-digit code number. Some states have already adopted the 1974 editions of RVS that utilize 5-digit coding. In these states a different conversion factor of so many dollars and cents is used for each of the five sections of the RVS code books.

Example:

1974 California Relative Value Studies

$3.50/unit — Medicine Section
$18.00/unit — Anesthesia Section
$80.00/unit — Surgery Section
.65/unit — Pathology Section
$7.00/unit — Radiology Section (total unit value column)
.85/unit — Radiology Section (professional component unit value column)

Handy Hints for Billing

1. Use appropraite 4-digit or 5-digit code numbers to insure prompt and accurate payment for services rendered.

2. Any charges in excess of the Fee Schedule should be clearly defined by the physician. Attach any x-ray reports, operative reports, discharge summaries, pathology reports, and so forth to clarify such excess charges.

3. Drugs and dressings furnished by the physician should be itemized in detail and charged at cost.

4. If you have a question regarding the fee, call the insurance carrier and talk with the adjuster who is familiar with the patient's case.

5. If the case becomes delinquent, send one of the appropriate letters as shown in Figures 9–7, 9–8, or 9–9.

INSTRUCTIONS FOR COMPLETION OF THE DOCTOR'S FIRST REPORT OF OCCUPATIONAL INJURY OR ILLNESS (Fig. 9–10 and Assignments 25 and 26, pp. 593–600)

Type an original and four or five copies. This form must be submitted anywhere from "immediately" to "within 5 days" after the patient has been seen by the physician, depending upon state law. Distribute copies as follows:

One copy to the state
Original and one or two copies to the insurance carrier
One copy to the patient's employer
One copy retained for the physician's files

A. Enter the insurance carrier's complete name, street address, city, state, and ZIP Code.

1. List the employer's full name. If the policy number is known, list it also on this line, since some insurance carriers file by employer and then by policy number. Sometimes the employer's telephone number is required on this line.

2. Give the employer's street address, city, state, and ZIP Code.

3. List the type of business the company is involved in, such as manufacturing shoes, building construction, retailing men's clothes, and so forth.

```
                    Max Gluteus, M. D.
                    4567 Broad Avenue
                  Woodland Hills, XY 12345
                      013/486-9002


June 1, 1977


Best Insurance Company
1100 Fine Street
Happiness, XY 12345

Re: Case No.:        0000000
    Injured:         Mrs. Ima Hurt
    Date of Injury:  April 3, 1977
    Employer:        The Conk Out Company
    Amount:          $100.00

Gentlemen:

Our records indicate that our final statement for the above
case dated April 16, 1977  remains unpaid.

Your cooperation in furnishing us the present status of this
statement will be appreciated.  A notation on the bottom of
this letter will be sufficient.

Thank you.

Very truly yours,



_____, M. D.

ref initials

------------------------------------------------------------------

_____No Employer's Report on file
_____No Doctor's First Report on file
_____Did not receive itemized billing statement
_____Payment was made.  Check No._____Date_____
_____Other reason(s)_____
```

FIGURE 9–7

If a Workers' Compensation claim becomes 45 days delinquent, the Medical Assistant should send this letter to the insurance carrier.

```
                        Max Gluteus, M. D.
                         4567 Broad Avenue
                      Woodland Hills, XY 12345
                          013/486-9002



June 15, 1977



The Conk Out Company
3300 Debilitated Street
Repair, XY 12345

Re:  Case No.:       0000000
     Injured:        Mrs. Ima Hurt
     Date of Injury: April 3, 1977

Gentlemen:

I  have been informed by your workers' compensation insurance
carrier that they have not as yet received the employer's
report in regard to the above injured person.

Unless you have already done so, may I  ask your cooperation
in completing and sending this report so that the case may
be closed.

Should you have any questions or if I  can be of assistance to
you in any way, please do not hesitate to call on me.

Very truly yours,



_____, M. D.

ref initials
```

FIGURE 9–8

If the insurance company notifies the physician's office that the employer's preliminary report of injury has not been received, then send this letter to the employer.

```
                        Max Gluteus, M. D.
                         4567 Broad Avenue
                     Woodland Hills, XY 12345
                          013/486-9002




July 15, 1977



Division of Industrial Accidents
Los Angeles State Office Building
107 South Broadway, Room 4107
Los Angeles, CA 90012

Re:  Failure of employer to follow Section #3760

Gentlemen:

Your office is being solicited to help secure an Employer's
Report of Work Injury from the employer listed below.

                Case No.:          0000000
                Name of Employer:  The Conk Out Company
                     Address:      3300 Debilitated Street
                                   Repair, XY 12345
                Name of Injured:   Mrs. Ima Hurt
                     Address:      23 Broke Street
                                   Fractured, XY 12345
                Date of Injury:    April 3, 1977
                Name of Insurance Carrier:  Best Insurance Co.
                Amount of Unpaid Bill:      $100.00

Your cooperation in this matter will be greatly appreciated.  If
you need further information, please feel free to contact my
office.

Sincerely yours,



_____, M. D.

ref initials
```

FIGURE 9–9

If the employer does not respond to your letter requesting the Employer's Report of Work Injury after 30 days' lapse of time from the date of the letter, send this letter to the Workmen's Compensation Board or Industrial Accident Commission in your state.

DOCTOR'S FIRST REPORT
OF
OCCUPATIONAL INJURY OR ILLNESS

STATE OF CALIFORNIA
AGRICULTURE AND SERVICES AGENCY
DEPARTMENT OF INDUSTRIAL RELATIONS
DIVISION OF LABOR STATISTICS AND RESEARCH
P. O. Box 965, San Francisco, Calif. 94101

Immediately after first examination mail one copy **directly** to the Division of Labor Statistics and Research. Failure to file a report with the Division is a misdemeanor. (Labor Code Section 6413.5) Answer all questions fully.

☛ **A. INSURANCE CARRIER** Best Insurance Company, 1100 Fine St., Happiness, XY 12345

	Do not write in this space

1. **EMPLOYER** The Conk Out Company
2. Address (No., St. & City) 3300 Debilitated Street, Repair, XY 12345
3. Business (Manufacturing shoes, building construction, retailing men's clothes, etc.) repair plumbing

4. **EMPLOYEE** (First name, middle initial, last name) Mrs. Ima Hurt   Soc. Sec. No. 023-45-6789
5. Address (No., St. & City) 3300 Broke Street, Fractured, XY 12345
6. Occupation clerk typist   Age 23   Sex F
7. Date injured 04-03-77   Hour 2 P. M. Date last worked 04-03-77
8. Injured at (No., St. & City) 3300 Debilitated Street, Repair, XY 12345   County Humboldt
9. Date of your first examination   Hour   M. Who engaged your services? employer
10. Name other doctors who treated employee for this injury   none

11. **ACCIDENT OR EXPOSURE:** Did employee notify employer of this injury? Yes   Employee's statement of cause of injury or illness:

    Patient states, "lifted corner of typewriter to dust desk, temporarily lost control, and typewriter came down on my left little finger."

12. **NATURE AND EXTENT OF INJURY OR DISEASE** (Include all objective findings, subjective complaints, and diagnoses. If occupational disease state date of onset, occupational history, and exposures.)

    Pain and some slight swelling of left little finger.

    Diagnosis: Fracture of distal interphalangeal joint of 5th phalanx.

13. X-rays: By whom taken? (State if none) Max Gluteus, M. D.
    Findings: AP and lat. films taken of left hand reveal hairline fracture of distal interphalangeal joint of 5th phalanx.

14. Treatment: Examination, x-rays, applied splint to left hand, advised restricted use of left hand and return in one week for recheck.

15. Kind of case (Office, home or hospital) office   If hospitalized, date   Estimated stay
    Name and address of hospital
16. Further treatment (Estimated frequency and duration) To be seen every 2 weeks
17. Estimated period of disability for: Regular work about 6 weeks   Modified work
18. Describe any permanent disability or disfigurement expected (State if none) none anticipated

19. If death ensued, give date

20. **REMARKS** (Note any pre-existing injuries or diseases, need for special examination or laboratory tests, other pertinent information.)

Name Max Gluteus   Degree M. D. [PERSONAL SIGNATURE OF DOCTOR] *Max Gluteus, M. D.*
(Type or print)

Date of report 4-4-77   Address (No., St. & City) 4567 Broad Avenue, Woodland Hills, XY 12345

FORM 5021 (REV. 1)   *Use reverse side if more space required*   D OSP

ref initials

FIGURE 9–10

Doctor's First Report of Occupational Injury or Illness form, used in the state of California.

4. State the patient's complete first name, middle initial, and last name. Give the patient's Social Security number. Some insurance carriers use the Social Security number as the industrial case number.

5. List the patient's street address, city, state, ZIP Code, and telephone number.

6. Give the title of the patient's occupation. It is important to be accurate in listing the occupation so that the insurance carrier can be certain the patient was doing the job for which he or she was insured. List the patient's age and sex.

7. Enter the date the patient was injured and give the exact or approximate time of the injury. State the date the patient last worked. It is important to list this so that the insurance carrier will know whether the patient is still working or has been disabled and cannot return to work.

8. The exact location where the patient was injured should be given. Many times this may occur off the premises of the company or factory, depending on the type of job at which the employee was working. List the county where the patient was injured.

9. Enter the date of the doctor's first examination. It is important for the insurance carrier to know how soon after the accident the patient sought medical attention. List as nearly as possible the time the physician saw the patient. Regarding the question "who engaged your services?": Usually the employer or insurance carrier calls the physician's office to make the initial request for examination and treatment for the patient. Occasionally a patient may call the physician directly. When this occurs, the insurance carrier must be informed or the patient may be responsible for the complete medical bill. In some states, the employee may select his attending physician after a certain lapse of time after the injury.

10. Give the name of any other physician or first aid assistant who administered to the patient prior to your physician's examination and treatment, such as the company nurse, or an ambulance attendant. Indicate the nature of this treatment as precisely as possible.

11, 12, 13, 14. These answers are found in the patient's medical record, or the physician may dictate the information to the secretary.

15. If the patient is first seen in the hospital, then list hospital as the type of case. If the patient is seen first in the home, then list home. If the patient is seen in the office, list office.

16. It is very important for the insurance company to anticipate how much future treatment will be required so that money can be set aside for temporary disability benefits, medical benefits, and if necessary permanent disability benefits.

17. It is important to give the date or number of days of absence from work. If this should change at all after the form is submitted, then a supplemental report or progress note should be sent to the insurance carrier to change the date of the disability by extending or shortening it.

18. If there is any possibility of a permanent disability or disfigurement, then it should be so stated. If none is anticipated, state "none."

19. If the patient's injury is such that death ensues, then the date of death should be listed.

20. It is always a good policy to list again in the "Remarks" space the date the patient is resuming regular work if it is known at the time the Doctor's First Report of Occupational Injury or Illness form is submitted. The insurance adjuster appreciates this as it stands out and the date will not be overlooked.

At the bottom of the form type in the physician's name, degree (i.e., M.D., D.C., etc.), and the date this report is submitted. Indicate the doctor's complete address. It is

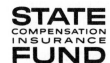

STATE
COMPENSATION
INSURANCE
FUND

470 EAST THOMPSON BLVD. · VENTURA, CALIFORNIA
TELEPHONE (805) 648-5311

IN REPLY REFER TO:

Case No.:
Injured:
Injury date:

DOCTOR'S SUPPLEMENTAL REPORT

The information requested in this report is necessary to establish eligibility for further benefits.
You may make your notations on this form (including reverse side if more space required) or, if more convenient, forward
a brief report containing the necessary information.

1. Have you discharged patient?_____If so, when?_____
   (if answer to above is yes and you expect *no* permanent residuals, you may disregard remainder of form, sign and
   return)

2. Date of last examination_____

3. Present condition and prognosis (indicate if diagnosis changed since last report)_____
   _____
   _____
   _____

4. Treatment required by injury in question (type, length and frequency)_____
   _____
   _____
   _____

5. Date injured was or will be able to return to work_____
6. When do you expect full recovery from injury in question?_____
   _____

_____   _____
(Doctor's Signature)   (Date)

| If you wish to discuss this case in greater detail, please contact our Claims Department at the above |
| address. Arrangements can be made for discussion with our Medical Department if you so desire. |

FORM C-9

MAIL ADDRESS: BOX S · VENTURA, CALIFORNIA 93001

FIGURE 9–11

Doctor's Supplemental Report form.

STATE COMPENSATION INSURANCE FUND

470 EAST THOMPSON BOULEVARD, VENTURA, CALIFORNIA 93001

DOCTOR'S FINAL (OR MONTHLY) REPORT AND BILL

Monthly itemized bills required on all cases under continuing treatment.
Services beginning late in month and extending into succeeding month may be itemized on one statement.

CASE No.

EMPLOYEE

DATE OF INJURY

EMPLOYER

SERVICES FOR MONTH OF 19

Patient refused treatment 19   Patient able to return to work 19

Patient stopped treatment   Patient discharged as cured 19
    without orders 19   Condition at time of last visit

Patient entered hospital 19

Further treatment anticipated?
                                (Yes)   (No)

Any other charges authorized such as Drugs? .... Hospital?
                                (Check)   (Check)

Code: O—Office; V—Home Visit; H—Hospital Visit; N—Night Visit; S—Operation; X—X-ray.

Month	1	2	3	4	5	6	7	8	9	10	11	12	13	14	15	16	17	18	19	20	21	22	22	24	25	26	27	28	29	30	31

TOTALS

First aid treatment (describe) .... $

Office Visits .... $
Home Visits .... $
Hospital Visits .... $
Operations .... $
MATERIAL (Itemize at cost) .... $

Any charges shown above which are in excess of the scheduled fee must
be explained regarding nature of such services, indicating the date rendered.   TOTAL $

Make check payable to:

Doctor

Signature

Address

Date

(Street)

(City)   (ZIP)

Internal Revenue Service Employer Identification
Number or Social Security Number

LEAVE BLANK

APPROVED

BY

(Dollars)   (Cents)

DATE

IMPORTANT.—
Bills Must Be Submitted in Duplicate

MAIL ADDRESS: P.O. BOX S, VENTURA, CALIFORNIA 93001

SCIF FORM 60 (REV. 8-72)
25091-218 7-74 35M △ OSP

FIGURE 9–12

Doctor's Final or Monthly Report and Bill form.

REPORT OF DENTAL INJURY

STATE COMPENSATION INSURANCE FUND

- Authorization should be obtained for all treatment other than ordinary first aid or emergency care.
- Under the Workmen's Compensation Laws employers are only liable for repair or replacement of teeth actually damaged or lost due to occupational injuries.
- Mail report immediately after seeing patient for first time.

Claim No.

ALSO, Immediately after first examination mail one copy directly to the Division of Labor Statistics and Research, P. O. Box 965, San Francisco 94101. Failure to file a report with the Division is a misdemeanor. (Labor Code, Sections 6407-6413.)

1. **EMPLOYER**
2. Address

3. **EMPLOYEE** (First name, middle initial, last name)
4. Address (No. and Street)   (City or Town)   Social Security No.   Zip
5. Date injured   Hour   M. Date of your first examination

6. **ACCIDENT OR EXPOSURE:** Did employee notify employer of this injury?   Employee's statement of cause of injury or illness?

7. **PRIOR HISTORY:**

Briefly comment on condition of oral cavity prior to present injury. Include comments on oral hygiene, periodontal disease, teeth missing, dental caries, and teeth filled, crowned, or replaced by bridges or plates.

8. **NATURE AND EXTENT OF INJURY:**

Give nature and extent of present injury. Include all objective findings, subjective complaints and diagnoses, outline on dental chart injuries caused by present occupational injury.

9. **REPAIR, REPLACEMENT OR TREATMENT REQUIRED:**

Indicate the types of materials to be used in fillings, crowns, partial and full dentures. Name the teeth to be replaced and those to be clasped in partial dentures. Name the type of prosthetic appliances to be used on abutment teeth, the type of pontics, and name the teeth being replaced by the bridges.

Note: Payment will be made only for care required because of the industrial injury.

RIGHT 1 2 3 4 5 6 7 8 9 10 11 12 13 14 15 16 LEFT

32 31 30 29 28 27 26 25 24 23 22 21 20 19 18 17

10. **COST:** (Applicable fees may be determined from V.A. fee schedule)

Total $

11. This report will be considered a request for authorization to undertake the described dental repair at the cost specified. You are requested to obtain authorization for all elective procedures. Submit an itemized bill, IN DUPLICATE, when work is completed.

Name   Degree   { PERSONAL SIGNATURE }
(Type or print)

Date of report   Address   Tel. No.

SCIF FORM 71 (REV 9-68)   21   *Use reverse side if more space required*

FIGURE 9–13

Report of Dental Injury form.

always wise to include the physician's telephone number after the address. The Assistant should type reference initials in the lower left hand corner of the form. This form *must be signed in ink* by the physician. Each carbon copy must also be signed in ink. A stamped signature will *not* be accepted if the case goes into litigation or is presented for a permanent disability rating. Only those documents considered as original medical records are acceptable, and this means a handwritten signature by the attending physician.

TO THE STUDENT: Refer to the Appendix to complete the insurance forms pertinent to this chapter. Assignments 25, 26, and 27, pp. 593–605, pertain to this chapter.

DELINQUENT CLAIMS

If a Workers' Compensation claim becomes delinquent, a letter should be directed to the insurance carrier (see Fig. 9–7). After receiving a response from the insurance carrier, it may be necessary to send subsequent letters to the employer. See Figures 9–8 and 9–9 for how these letters might be worded.

GLOSSARY OF WORKERS' COMPENSATION ABBREVIATIONS

CAL/OSHA	California Occupational Safety and Health Administration
CIRB	California Inspection Rating Bureau
CMA	California Medical Association
C & R	Compromise and release
CWCI	California Workers' Compensation Institute
DIA	Division of Industrial Accidents
FECA	Federal Employees' Compensation Act
IAIABC	International Association of Industrial Accident Boards and Commission
OFEC	Office of Federal Employees' Compensation
OSHA	Occupational Safety and Health Administration
OWCP	Office of Workers' Compensation Programs
PD	Permanent disability
P & S	Permanent and stationary
RVS	Relative Value Studies

SDIA	State Division of Industrial Accidents
SS#	Social Security number
TD	Temporary disability
UCR	Usual, customary, and reasonable (fees)
WC	Workers' Compensation
WCAB	Workers' Compensation Appeals Board
WCB	Workers' Compensation Board

WORKERS' COMPENSATION DIRECTORY

State Plan Offices

Alabama
Department of Industrial Relations
Industrial Relations Building
Montgomery, AL 36104

Alaska
Department of Labor
P.O. Box 1149
Juneau, AK 99801

Arizona
Industrial Commission
1601 West Jefferson
P.O. Box 19072
Phoenix, AZ 85005

State Compensation Fund
1616 West Adams
Phoenix, AZ 85007

Arkansas
Workmen's Compensation Commission
Justice Building
State Capitol Grounds
Little Rock, AR 72201

California
Division of Industrial Accidents
455 Golden Gate Avenue
P.O. Box 603
San Francisco, CA 94102

Workmen's Compensation Appeals Board
455 Golden Gate Avenue
San Francisco, CA 94102

State of California
Human Relations Agency
Department of Industrial Relations
Division of Labor Statistics and Research
P.O. Box 965
San Francisco, CA 94101

Division of Industrial Accidents
Los Angeles State Office Building
107 South Broadway, Room 4107
Los Angeles, CA 90012

Colorado
Department of Labor and Employment
200 East 9th Avenue
Denver, CO 80203

Connecticut
Workmen's Compensation Commission
110 Broadway, Box 1025
Norwich, CT 06360

Delaware
Industrial Accident Board
618 North Union Street
Wilmington, DE 19801

District of Columbia
Deputy Commissioner
Office of Workers' Compensation
1717 K Street, N.W., Room 802
Washington D.C. 20211

Benefits Review Board
1111 20th Street, N.W.
Washington, D.C. 20210

Florida
Industrial Relations Commission
Ashley Building
1321 Executive Center Drive East
Tallahassee, FL 32301

Georgia
Board of Workmen's Compensation
499 Labor Building
254 Washington Street, S.W.
Atlanta, GA 30334

Hawaii
Workmen's Compensation Division
Department of Labor and Industrial
    Relations
825 Mililani Street
Honolulu, HI 96813

Labor and Industrial Relations Appeals
    Board
888 Mililani Street
Honolulu, HI 96813

Idaho
Industrial Commission
State House
Boise, ID 83720

Illinois
Industrial Commission
160 North LaSalle Street
Chicago, IL 60601

Indiana
Industrial Board
601 State Office Building
100 North Senate Avenue
Indianapolis, IN 46204

Iowa
Industrial Commissioner
State Capitol Complex
610 Des Moines Street
Des Moines, IA 50319

Kansas
Office of Workmen's Compensation
535 Kansas Avenue, 6th Floor
Topeka, KS 66603

Kentucky
Workmen's Compensation Board
Department of Labor
Frankfort, KY 40601

Louisiana
Department of Labor
1045 State Land & Natural
    Resources Building
Box 44063
Baton Rouge, LA 70804

Maine
Industrial Accident Commission
97 Exchange Street
Portland, ME 04111

Maryland
Workmen's Compensation Commission
108 East Lexington Street
Baltimore, MD 21202

Massachusetts
Industrial Accidents Board
Leverett Saltonstall Office Building
100 Cambridge Street
Boston, MA 02202

Michigan
Bureau of Workmen's Compensation
Department of Labor
300 East Michigan Avenue
Lansing, MI 48926

Minnesota
Department of Labor and Industry
444 LaFayette Road
St. Paul, MN 55101

Mississippi
Workmen's Compensation Commission
1404 Walter Sillers State Office Building
P.O. Box 987
Jackson, MS 39205

Missouri
Division of Workmen's Compensation
Department of Labor and Industrial
    Relations
P.O. Box 58
Jefferson City, MO 65101

Montana
Workmen's Compensation Division
815 Front Street
Helena, MT 59601

Nebraska
Workmen's Compensation Court
State Capitol
Lincoln, NE 68509

Nevada
Industrial Commission
515 East Musser Street
Carson City, NV 89701

New Hampshire
Department of Labor
1 Pillsbury Street
Concord, NH 03301

New Jersey
Department of Labor and Industry
John Fitch Plaza
Trenton, NJ 08625

New Mexico
Labor and Industrial Commission
137 East DeVargas Street
Santa Fe, NM 87501

New York
Workmen's Compensation Board
Two World Trade Center
New York, NY 10047

North Carolina
Industrial Commission
Eastgate Office Center
4000 Old Wake Forest Road
Raleigh, NC 27611

North Dakota
Workmen's Compensation Bureau
State Capitol Building
Bismarck, ND 58501

Ohio
Industrial Commission
Ohio Department Building
Columbus, OH 43215

Bureau of Workmen's Compensation
Ohio Department Building
Columbus, OH 43215

Oklahoma
State Industrial Court
Jim Thorpe Building
P.O. Box 53038
Oklahoma City, OK 73105

Oregon
Workmen's Compensation Board
Labor and Industries Building
Salem, OR 97310

State Accident Insurance Fund
400 High Street Southeast
Salem, OR 97310

Pennsylvania
Bureau of Workmen's Compensation and
    Disease Compensation
Department of Labor and Industry
Labor and Industry Building
Harrisburg, PA 17120

Puerto Rico
Industrial Commission
G.P.O. Box 4466
San Juan, PR 00936

Rhode Island
Workmen's Compensation Commission
25 Canal Street
Providence, RI 02903

South Carolina
Industrial Commission
1026 Sumter Street
Columbia, SC 29201

South Dakota
Department of Labor and Management
Office Building No. 2
Pierre, SD 57501

Tennessee
Workmen's Compensation Division
Department of Labor
C1-130 Cordell Hull Building
Nashville, TN 37203

Texas
Industrial Accident Board
Box 12757, Capitol Station
Austin, TX 78701

Utah
Industrial Commission
350 East 500 South
Salt Lake City, UT 84111

Vermont
Department of Labor and Industry
Montpelier, VT 05602

Virginia
Industrial Commission
Blanton Building
Richmond, VA 23214

Washington
Department of Labor and Industries
General Administration Building
Olympia, WA 98504

Board of Industrial Insurance Appeals
1601 Second Avenue Building, 4th Floor
Seattle, WA 98101

West Virginia
Workmen's Compensation Fund
112 California Avenue
Charleston, WV 25305

Wisconsin
Department of Industry, Labor and
    Human Relations
201 East Washington Avenue, Box 2209
Madison, WI 53701

Wyoming
Workers' Compensation Division
2305 Carey Avenue
Cheyenne, WY 82001

Longshoremen's and Harbor Workers' Act District Offices

District No. 1
Office of Workers' Compensation
147 Milk Street
Boston, MA 02109

District No. 2
Office of Workers' Compensation
1515 Broadway (@ West 44th)
New York, NY 10036

District No. 3
Office of Workers' Compensation
Gateway Building
Room 15440
3535 Market Street
Philadelphia, PA 19104

District No. 4
Office of Workers' Compensation
Federal Building, Room 1026
Charles Center South
31 Hopkins Plaza
Baltimore, MD 21201

District No. 5
Office of Workers' Compensation
Stanwick Building, Room 101
3661 Virginia Beach Boulevard, East
Norfolk, VA 23502

District No. 6
Office of Workers' Compensation
400 West Bay Street, Box 35049
Jacksonville, FL 32202

District No. 7
Office of Workers' Compensation
600 South Street, Room 1048
Federal Office Building, South
New Orleans, LA 70130

District No. 8
Office of Workers' Compensation
2320 La Branch Street, Room 2108
Houston, TX 77004

District No. 9
Office of Workers' Compensation
1240 East 9th Street, Room 879
Cleveland, OH 44199

District No. 10
Office of Workers' Compensation
230 South Dearborn Street, 8th Floor
Chicago, IL 60604

District No. 13
Office of Workers' Compensation
450 Golden Gate Avenue
Box 36066
San Francisco, CA 94102

District No. 14
Office of Workers' Compensation
4010 Federal Office Building
909 First Avenue
Seattle, WA 98174

District No. 15
Office of Workers' Compensation
1833 Kalakaua Avenue, Room 610
Honolulu, HI 96815

Federal Employees' Compensation Act (FECA) Offices:

Geographical Boundaries	Address
Arizona California Nevada	450 Golden Gate Avenue, Box 36022 San Francisco, CA 94102
Colorado Montana North Dakota South Dakota Utah Wyoming	Rio Grande Building, Room 303 1531 Stout Street Denver, CO 80202
Delaware Maryland Pennsylvania Virginia Washington, D.C. West Virginia	McLachlen Building, Room 405 666 — 11th Street, N.W. Washington, D.C. 20211
Alabama Florida Georgia Kentucky Mississippi North Carolina South Carolina Tennessee	400 West Bay Street, Box 35049 Jacksonville, FL 32202
Hawaii	1833 Kalakaua Avenue, Room 610 Honolulu, HI 96815
Illinois Minnesota Wisconsin	230 South Dearborn Street, 8th Floor Chicago, IL 60604
Arkansas Louisiana New Mexico Oklahoma Texas	Federal Office Building, South 600 South Street New Orleans, LA 70130
Connecticut Maine Massachusetts New Hampshire Rhode Island Vermont	147 Milk Street Boston, MA 02109
Iowa Kansas Missouri Nebraska	1910 Federal Office Building 911 Walnut Street Kansas City, MO 64106

Geographical Boundaries	*Address*
New Jersey New York Puerto Rico Virgin Islands	1515 Broadway (at West 44th) New York, NY 10036
Indiana Michigan Ohio	1240 East 9th Street, Room 879 Cleveland, OH 44199
Alaska Idaho Oregon Washington	Arcade Building, Room M-17 1319 Second Avenue Seattle, WA 98101

When in doubt about Federal benefits write to the:

Office of Federal Employees' Compensation
Washington, D.C. 20211

REVIEW QUESTIONS

1. What are the two kinds of statutes under Workers' Compensation?

    a. _____

    b. _____

2. What four classifications of employees fall under federal statutes?

    a. _____

    b. _____

    c. _____

    d. _____

3. Fifty states have _____ Workers' Compensation and Employers' Liability Insurance.

4. Three states have _____ Workers' Compensation and Employers' Liability Insurance.

5. Workers' Compensation funding can occur through what five methods?

    a. _____

b. _____

c. _____

d. _____

e. _____

6. How does funding occur in your state? _____

7. What jobs sometimes are not covered by Workers' Compensation insurance?

a. _____ d. _____

b. _____ e. _____

c. _____ f. _____

8. Briefly state the seven purposes of Workers' Compensation laws.

a. _____

_____

b. _____

_____

c. _____

_____

d. _____

_____

e. _____

_____

f. _____

_____

g. _____

_____

9. What is the waiting period in your state that must elapse before Workers' Compensation income benefits become payable? _____

10. Name the five types of compensation benefits.

a. _____

b. _____

c. _____

d. _____

e. _____

11. What are the three types of Workers' Compensation claims?

a. _____

b. _____

c. _____

12. What does the employer submit in your state? _____

_____

13. What do these abbreviations mean?

a. TD _____ c. P & S _____

b. PD _____ d. C & R _____

14. Explain a *nondisability* claim: _____

_____

15. Explain a *temporary disability* claim: _____

_____

16. Explain a *permanent disability* claim: _____

_____

17. Can an injured person appeal his case if he is not satisfied with the rating? _____ If so, to whom does he appeal? _____ or _____

18. What is the name of the report the physician completes? _____

What is the time limit on submitting this report in your state? _____

19. Where does the physician send the report? _____

20. What is the first thing an employee should do after he or she is injured? _____

21. Weekly temporary disability payments are based on what? _____

22. In Workers' Compensation cases the contract exists between _____

_____ and _____

23. Under OSHA employers are requested by law to meet what standards? _____

_____ and _____

24. A man takes his girlfriend to a roofing job and she is injured. Is she covered under Workers' Compensation insurance? _____

25. If the physician feels the injured employee can return to work after having been on temporary disability, what does the physician do? _____

26. Can a person receiving permanent disability benefits still work in another occupation? _____

27. Explain third party subrogation _____

_____

_____

28. What is litigation? _____

29. Can the Medical Assistant stamp the physician's signature on the Doctor's First Report of Work Injury? _____

_____

30. When do you submit the bill in a Workers' Compensation case? _____

_____

31. Who can treat an industrial injury? _____

_____

32. Who pays the Workers' Compensation insurance premiums? _____

33. What is a Medical Service Order? _____

_____

34. What is the Second-Injury Fund (Subsequent Injury Fund)? _____

_____

_____

35. Who selects the attending physician for an industrial accident or illness? _____

_____

_____

Notes:

10
Special Plans

BEHAVIORAL

OBJECTIVES   *The Assistant should be able to:*

1. Define a prepaid health plan (PHP).
2. Identify the types of prepaid health plans in existence.
3. Understand the two different operations of foundations.
4. Define the Health Maintenance Organization Act of 1973.
5. Explain the Health Maintenance Organization benefits and eligibility.
6. Define Peer Review.
7. Explain an optometric service plan and its benefits.

INTRODUCTION

This chapter will define some of the various types of prepaid group practice plans. Generally speaking, a prepaid health plan is a plan or program under which specified health services are rendered by participating physicians to an enrolled group of persons, with fixed periodic payment made in advance by or on behalf of each person or family. If a health insurance carrier is involved, it contracts to pay in advance for the full range of health services to which the insured is entitled under the terms of the health insurance contract. Such a plan is one form of what is known as a *Health Maintenance Organization* (HMO). Other plans in existence are the Ross-Loos Medical Group, the Kaiser Permanente Medical Care Program, and Foundations for Medical Care. The following is a brief description of what these programs are all about.

PREPAID GROUP PRACTICE HEALTH PLANS

The *Ross-Loos Medical Group* in Los Angeles, California, is America's oldest privately owned, prepaid medical group. It was founded in 1929 by Dr. Donald E. Ross and Dr. H. Clifford Loos and exists only in Southern California, where it has expanded to 17 medical group locations. Most Ross-Loos patients are served under a prepayment group plan, but several thousand others are private, and treated on a fee-for-service basis. A patient pays a monthly premium and receives hospital, surgical, and professional benefits from a Ross-Loos staff physician or Ross-Loos Medical Center. In the case of an emergency when the patient is outside the area of a Ross-Loos Medical Center, he or she may seek professional or hospital benefits in other facilities, but Ross-Loos must be notified. A dental plan and Medicare supplemental plan are also available through Ross-Loos. In 1975 the Ross-Loos Medical Group formed a corporation and received a federal grant to develop a health care system under the federal Health Maintenance Organization Act of 1973 (Public Law 93-222). A Health Maintenance Organization (HMO) provides a wide range of basic and supplemental health care services under federally mandated standards to an enrolled patient population for a prepaid, fixed fee that does not vary with the volume of services provided.

Another pioneer of the prepaid concept is the *Kaiser Permanente Medical Care Program*. Its history began in 1933 when Dr. Sidney R. Garfield and a few doctors working for him gave combined industrial accident and personal medical care to about 5000 workers building a fresh-water aqueduct across the California desert to Los Angeles. Dr. Garfield charged the insurance carriers $1.50 per man per month and the workers an equal sum, a nickel a day. In return he provided comprehensive care. Then in 1938 Henry J. Kaiser and his son, Edgar, started a joint venture to complete the Grand Coulee Dam in Washington and invited Dr. Garfield to form a medical group to furnish care to the workers for seven cents a day prepaid by the employer. The group expanded to include the workers' wives and children. Kaiser Permanente now has centers in Northern California, Southern California, Oregon, Hawaii, Ohio, and Colorado. Patients are served under a prepayment group plan and receive hospital, surgical, and professional benefits from physicians located at the Kaiser Permanente Medical Care Centers. Kaiser does not provide care on a fee-for-service basis or a cost reimbursement basis. In emergency situations when patients are out of reach of a Kaiser Center, they may seek the services of outside facilities or physicians. The Kaiser Permanente Medical Plan is a *closed panel program*, which means it limits the patient's choice of personal physicians to those practicing in one of the six multispecialty medical groups—one in each geographic region.

FOUNDATIONS FOR MEDICAL CARE

A *Foundation for Medical Care (FMC)* is an organization of physicians, sponsored by a state or local medical association, concerned with the development and delivery of medical services and the cost of health care. The first Foundation for Medical Care was established in 1954 in Stockton, California. Foundations have sprung up across the United States, and some comprehensive Foundations have assumed a portion of the underwriting risk for a defined population and have provided comprehensive health services for a fixed yearly sum on a capitation basis, thereby qualifying as Health Maintenance Organizations (HMO's). There are basically two different types of Foundations for Medical Care operations:

1. A *comprehensive* type, which designs and sponsors prepaid health programs or sets minimum benefits of coverage.

2. A *claims-review* type, which provides Peer Review by physicians to the numerous fiscal intermediaries involved in its area, including the ones processing Medicare and Medicaid. *Peer Review* is an evaluation of the quality and efficiency of services rendered by a practicing physician or physicians within the specialty group. This is done for an insurance claim or for services rendered to the patient that exceed local community guidelines for the fee and/or service.

A key feature of the Foundation is its dedication to an incentive reimbursement system for participating physicians, in which income is received in direct proportion to the number of medical services delivered (i.e., fee-for-service). In some areas Foundation physicians agree to accept the Foundation allowance as payment in full for covered services. The patient is *not* billed for the balance. However, the patient is billed for nonbenefit items and deductible coinsurance. The patient may select any physician he or she wishes, whether the physician is a Foundation physician or a non-Foundation physician. Member physicians agree to bill the Foundation directly, and a nonmember physician may wish to collect his fee directly from the patient (see Fig. 10–1). The Foundation movement now has a national society, the American Association of Foundations for Medical Care at 540 East Market Street, Stockton, CA 95201. For further information contact the foundation or foundations in your state that are a member of this society (see pp. 257–260).

HEALTH MAINTENANCE ORGANIZATION ACT OF 1973

The Health Maintenance Organization (HMO) Act of 1973 (Public Law 93-222) is an amendment to the Social Security laws that established legislation to provide a wide range of comprehensive health care services for both prepaid group practice and foundations for medical care at a fixed periodic payment. Basically an HMO is a prepaid group practice which can be sponsored and operated by the government, medical schools, clinics, foundations, hospitals, employers, labor unions, community or consumer groups, insurance companies, the "Blue" plans, hospital-medical plans, or the Veterans' Administration.

Benefits

Benefits fall under two categories: basic and supplemental health services.

1. *Basic Health Services:*
   a. Physicians' services, consultant or referral services
   b. Inpatient and outpatient hospital services
   c. Emergency health services
   d. Short-term (not to exceed 20 visits) ambulatory, evaluative, and crisis intervention mental health services
   e. Alcohol, drug abuse, and addiction medical treatment
   f. Diagnostic laboratory and x-ray services
   g. Home health services
   h. Preventive health services
   i. Family planning and infertility services
   j. Preventive dental services for children under age 12
   k. Health education and medical social services
2. *Supplemental Health Services:*
   a. Intermediate and long-term care facilities' services
   b. Vision care, dental care, and mental health services not included in basic benefits
   c. Long-term physical medicine and rehabilitative services, such as physical therapy
   d. Prescription drugs

PATIENT'S NAME	LAST		FIRST		MIDDLE INITIAL	GROUP NO.			PATIENT'S RELATIONSHIP TO SUBSCRIBER

PATIENT'S NAME LAST / FIRST / MIDDLE INITIAL

PATIENT'S ADDRESS STREET

CITY · STATE · ZIP

PATIENT'S BIRTHDATE MONTH / DAY / YEAR · **AGE** · **PATIENT'S SEX** · ☐ MALE ☐ FEMALE

INSURED'S NAME LAST / FIRST / MIDDLE INITIAL

INSURED'S BIRTHDATE MONTH / DAY / YEAR · **INSURED'S SOCIAL SECURITY NUMBER**

INSURED'S EMPLOYER

CONDITION CAUSED BY: ☐ INJURY ☐ ILLNESS ☐ PREGNANCY

IF INJURY: INDICATE DATE, HOW AND WHERE SUSTAINED · **DATE OF INJURY**
☐ AUTO ACCIDENT ☐ HOME ☐ OTHER · MO / DAY / YR

DATE PATIENT FIRST CONSULTED YOU FOR THIS CONDITION. / /

PATIENT EVER HAD SAME OR SIMILAR CONDITION? YES ☐ NO ☐
IF "YES" WHEN AND DESCRIBE

PATIENT STILL UNDER YOUR CARE FOR THIS CONDITION? YES ☐ NO ☐

PATIENT WAS CONTINUOUSLY TOTALLY DISABLED: (UNABLE TO WORK) FROM · THRU

IF PREGNANCY, DATE OF COMMENCEMENT.

IS CONDITION DUE TO INJURY OR SICKNESS ARISING OUT OF PATIENT'S EMPLOYMENT? YES ☐ NO ☐ · **IS THIS A NEW PATIENT?** YES ☐ NO ☐

IF PATIENT WAS REFERRED INDICATE → ☐ FROM ☐ TO · DOCTOR

DIAGNOSIS AND CONCURRENT CONDITIONS

GROUP NO. · **PATIENT'S RELATIONSHIP TO SUBSCRIBER** ☐ SELF ☐ SPOUSE ☐ CHILD

WAS LABORATORY WORK PERFORMED IN YOUR OFFICE?
☐ NO (IF NO, ENTER NAME AND ADDRESS OF LABORATORY BELOW) ☐ YES
AMOUNT CHARGED TO PHYSICIAN BY LABORATORY $_____

NAME AND ADDRESS OF PROVIDER OF SERVICE · **IRS, EMP, OR PROVIDER NO.**

DATE THIS FORM WAS PREPARED ▶
THIS IS TO CERTIFY THAT THE FOREGOING INFORMATION IS TRUE, ACCURATE AND COMPLETE.

SIGNATURE OF PROVIDER OF SERVICE ▶

IF TREATED IN HOSPITAL OR NURSING HOME **I.P. OR O.P. INDICATE NAME AND LOCATION** · **ADMISSION DATE** Mo / Day / Yr · **DISCHARGE DATE** Mo / Day / Yr

OTHER GROUP HOSPITAL, MEDICAL COVERAGE INCLUDING MEDICARE NAME OF COMPANY OR PLAN AND IDENTIFICATION NO · ☐ YES ☐ NO

IS SPOUSE EMPLOYED? WHERE? · ☐ YES ☐ NO

PLACE OF SERV. CODE	DATE OF SERVICE MO / DAY / YR	PROCEDURE NUMBER RVS NUMBER ◄ SMA NUMBER ► Unit Modifier	DESCRIBE EACH SERVICE OR APPLIANCE SEPARATELY	YOUR FEE
			TOTAL	

SPONSORED BY VENTURA COUNTY MEDICAL SOCIETY

MAIL COMPLETED FORM TO

VENTURA COUNTY FOUNDATION FOR MEDICAL CARE
2981 LOMA VISTA ROAD   VENTURA, CA. 93003
(805) 648-5971

PLACE OF SERVICE CODES

†0 – Doctor's Office	IH – Inpatient Hospital	NH – Nursing Home
H – Patient's Home	OH – Outpatient Hospital	OL – Other Locations

I/We jointly certify that the above information is true and correct. I/We hereby authorize all doctors, pharmacists, hospitals, or other institutions rendering care and treatment to furnish the Ventura Foundation for Medical Care with full information regarding treatment rendered (including copies of their records.) I/We also authorize any Union, Trust Fund, Employer or Insurance Carrier to furnish the Ventura Foundation for Medical Care with information regarding benefits to which I/We may be entitled. (If claim for spouse, spouse also must sign.) A photostatic copy of this authorization shall be considered as effective and valid as the original.

I hereby authorize payment to the above physician.

DATE ____/____/____

FORM FORM 001 FM (11-73) · SPOUSE'S SIGNATURE · EMPLOYEE'S SIGNATURE

FIGURE 10–1

Sample of a form used by a foundation, Ventura County Foundation for Medical Care.

Eligibility

Eligible persons are those who have voluntarily enrolled in the plan from a specific geographic area, or who are covered by an employer who has paid an established sum per person to be covered by the plan. Medicare and Medicaid beneficiaries may also join. The federal government reimburses the HMO's on a per-capita basis, depending on the size of the enrollment. This means that a fixed amount is paid per month per patient, for which the patient is entitled to receive the prescribed benefits.

To qualify as an HMO, an organization must present proof of its ability to provide comprehensive health care. To retain eligibility, an HMO must render periodic performance reports to the offices of the Department of Health, Education, and Welfare (HEW). Thus, accurate and complete medical records are imperative to the survival and cost control of an HMO.

Peer Review

Practitioners in the HMO program may come under a Peer Review to determine the quality and operation of health care. Peer Review (also known as Professional Standards Review Organization [PSRO]) means that one or more physicians working with the federal government under federal guidelines evaluate another physician in regard to the quality of professional care, to settle disputes on fees, or to examine evidence for admission and discharge of a patient to and from a hospital. The law states that an employer employing 25 or more persons may offer the services of an HMO clinic as an alternative health treatment plan for employees.

The operation of an HMO, like that of the Kaiser Permanente Plan, is under the *closed panel structure*, which means that it limits the patient's choice of personal physicians to those doctors practicing in the HMO group practice within the geographical location and/or facility.

OPTOMETRIC SERVICE PLANS

Some states have service plans which are not considered health insurance but are very specialized in the area of optometric care. There is no national program and no standardization of forms or procedures. Member doctors are given a detailed instruction manual on processing and claims procedure. This form of prepaid group vision care program is available to group health and welfare trust funds as well as to businesses having a certain number of full-time employees. The cost of the plan is paid by the employer as a fringe benefit. Some plans cover both the employee and his or her dependents; others are limited and cover only members or employees. This type of coverage provides for a yearly eye examination and corrective glasses if necessary. Certain costs of frames may be included, as may contact lenses for certain conditions. Some plans may even cover vision therapy. In some instances, there may be a small deductible to meet before the plan is effective. For further information contact:

The American Optometric Association
Division of Public Information
7000 Chippewa Street
St. Louis, MO 63119

CRIPPLED CHILDREN'S SERVICES (CCS)

All states and certain other jurisdictions, including territories and the District of Columbia (56 programs total) operate Crippled Children's Services with federal grant support under Title V of the Social Security Act. The state agency tries to locate crippled children under 21 years of age or those who may have conditions leading to crippling, to see that their conditions are diagnosed, and then to insure that each child gets the medical and other health-related care, hospitalization, and continuing follow-up that he or she needs. After a child is examined at a crippled children's clinic and a diagnosis is made, the parents are advised about the treatment that will benefit the child and the agency helps them to locate this care. If care of a handicapped child is a financial burden greater than the parents can afford, the agency assists the parents with financial planning and may assume part or all of the cost of treatment, depending on the child's condition and the family's resources.

ELIGIBILITY

Each agency operates under a law passed by the state legislature. The state law either defines the crippling conditions to be included or directs the crippled children's agency to define them. All states include children who have some kind of handicap that needs orthopedic or plastic treatment. A few add other conditions as well. A list of both types of conditions follows:

1. Cleft lip
2. Cleft palate
3. Club foot
4. Chronic conditions affecting bones and joints
5. Paralyzed muscles
6. Cerebral palsy
*7. Rheumatic and congenital heart disease
*8. Epilepsy
*9. Cystic fibrosis
*10. Vision problems requiring surgery
*11. Hearing problems
*12. Mental retardation
*13. Multiple handicaps

*Indicates that only some states include this item in their crippled children's program.

Claims Procedure

Each jurisdiction operates its own crippled children's program with its own unique administrative characteristics. Thus, each has its own system and forms for billing and related procedures. The official plans and documents are retained in the individual state offices and are not available on either a regional or national office basis. For specific information about your state's policies, write to the state agency listed on pages 261 to 263.

AMERICAN ASSOCIATION OF FOUNDATIONS FOR MEDICAL CARE

Arizona
Maricopa FMC
2025 N. Central Avenue
Phoenix, AZ 85004

Pima FMC
2343 E. Broadway — #204
Tucson, AZ 85719

Arkansas
Arkansas FMC
214 N. 12th Street — P.O. Box 1208
Fort Smith, AR 72901

California
Butte-Glen FMC
813 E. Fifth Avenue
Chico, CA 95926

Fresno FMC
3425 N. First Street
Fresno, CA 93719

Health Care Foundation for
  San Mateo County, Inc.
3080 La Selva, Suite 5
San Mateo, CA 94403

Humboldt–Del Norte Foundation
P.O. Box 1395
Eureka, CA 95501

Kern FMC
2603 G Street
Bakersfield, CA 93301

Marin FMC
4460 Redwood Highway
San Rafael, CA 94903

Mendocino-Lake Foundation
P.O. Box 73
Ukiah, CA 95482

Monterey FMC
P.O. Box 308
Salinas, CA 93901

Orange County FMC
300 S. Flower Street
Orange, CA 92668

Riverside FMC
6833 Indiana Avenue
Riverside, CA 92506

Sacramento Medical Care Foundation
650 University Avenue
Sacramento, CA 95825

San Bernardino FMC
666 Fairway Drive
San Bernardino, CA 92408

San Diego FMC
3702 Ruffin Road — P.O. Box 23015
San Diego, CA 92123

San Francisco Medical Society
  Health Plan, Inc.
250 Masonic Avenue
San Francisco, CA 94118

San Joaquin FMC
540 E. Market Street — P.O. Box 230
Stockton, CA 95201

Santa Clara FMC
700 Empey Way
San Jose, CA 95128

Sonoma FMC
2466 Mendocino Avenue
Santa Rosa, CA 95407

Stanislaus FMC
2030 Coffee Road, Suite A-6
Modesto, CA 95354

Tulare FMC
1821 W. Meadow Lane
Visalia, CA 93277

Ventura County FMC
3212 Loma Vista Road
Ventura, CA 93003

Colorado
Colorado FMC
1601 E. 19th Avenue
Denver, CO 80218

Rocky Mountains HMO
2525 N. 7th Street
Grand Junction, CO 80501

Connecticut
Greater Bridgeport Medical
  Foundation, Inc.
60 Katona Drive
Fairfield, CT 06430

Hartford County Health Care Plan
40 Woodland Street
Hartford, CT 06105

New Haven County FMC, Inc.
270 Amity Road – Suite 126
Woodbridge, CT 06525

Florida
Big Bend FMC
P.O. Box 3094
Tallahassee, FL 32303

Dade County FMC
444 Brickell Avenue, Suite M-100
Miami, FL 33131

Duval County FMC
515 Lomax Street
Jacksonville, FL 32204

Georgia
Georgia Medical Care Foundation, Inc.
1100 Spring Street, N.W., Suite 450
Atlanta, GA 30309

Metro-Atlanta FMC
875 W. Peachtree Street, N.E.
Atlanta, GA 30309

Hawaii
Hawaii FMC
510 S. Beretania Street
Honolulu, HI 96813

Idaho
Idaho FMC
427 N. Curtis
Boise, ID 83704

Illinois
Central Illinois FMC
One Horace Mann Plaza
Springfield, IL 62715

Champaign County FMC
407 S. Fourth Street
Champaign, IL 61820

Chicago FMC
310 S. Michigan Avenue
Chicago, IL 60604

Illinois State Foundation
55 E. Monroe Street, Suite 3510
Chicago, IL 60603

Northern Illinois FMC
310 N. Wyman Street
Rockford, IL 61101

Quad River FMC
3033 W. Jefferson #220
Joilet, IL 60435

Western Illinois FMC
1118 Broadway
Quincy, IL 62301

Indiana
Calumet Area FMC
2825 Jewett Street
Highland, IN 46322

Iowa
Iowa FMC
1001 Grand Avenue
West Des Moines, IA 50265

Kansas
Kansas FMC
1300 Topeka Avenue
Topeka, KS 66612

Sedgwick County FMC
1102 S. Hillside
Wichita, KS 67211

Kentucky
Medical Society Health Plan, Inc.
1169 Eastern Parkway – P.O. Box 17145
Louisville, KY 40217

Maryland
Delmarva FMC
108 N. Harrison Street
Easton, MD 21601

Maryland Foundation for Health Care
1211 Cathedral Street
Baltimore, MD 21201

Montgomery County Medical
  Care Foundation, Inc.
11141 Georgia Avenue #510
Wheaton, MD 20902

Prince George's FMC
5801 Annapolis Road, Suite 302
Hyattsville, MD 20784

Massachusetts
Bay State Health Care Foundation
100 Charles River Plaza
Boston, MA 02214

Commonwealth Institute of Medicine
100 Charles River Plaza
Boston, MA 02214

Health Care Foundation of Western
  Massachusetts
103 Van Deene Avenue
West Springfield, MA 01089

Pilgrim FMC
P.O. Box 676, Route 28
Middleboro, MA 02346

Michigan
Genesee Medical Corporation
700 Metropolitan Bldg.
432 N. Saginaw Street
Flint, MI 48502

Minnesota
Foundation for Health Care Evaluation
1535 Medical Arts Bldg.
Minneapolis, MN 55402

Mississippi
Mississippi State FMC
735 Riverside Drive
Jackson, MS 39216

Montana
Montana FMC
2717 Airport Way – P.O. Box 191
Helena, MO 59601

New Hampshire
New Hampshire FMC
Pettee Brook Offices
Durham, NH 03824

New Jersey
Bergen County Medical Society
210 River Street
Hackensack, NJ 07601

New Jersey Foundation for Health
  Care Evaluation
315 W. State Street
Trenton, NJ 08618

New Mexico
New Mexico State Foundation
2650 Yale Blvd., S.E.
Albuquerque, NM 87106

New York
Adirondack FMC
66 Park Street
Glens Falls, NY 12801

Bronx FMC
684 Britton Street
Bronx, NY 10467

Monroe Plan for Medical Care
11 N. Goodman
Rochester, NY 14610

Nassau County FMC
1200 Stewart Avenue
Garden City, NY 11530

N.Y. Institute for Research and Develop-
  ment in Health Care, Inc.
P.O. Box 720, Times Square Station
New York, NY 10036

Onondaga FMC
244 Harrison Street
Syracuse, NY 13202

Suffolk Medical Services Foundation
850 Veterans Memorial Highway
Hauppauge, L.I., NY 11787

Westchester Health Care Foundation
Westchester Academy of Medicine
Purchase, NY 10577

Ohio
Midwest FMC
206 Lytle Towers
Cincinnati, OH 45202

Western Ohio FMC
1030 Fidelity Medical Bldg.
Dayton, OH 45402

Oregon
Multnomah FMC
5201 S.W. Westgate Drive, Suite 24
Portland, OR 97221

Oregon FMC
2164 S.W. Park Place
Portland, OR 97205

Pacific Hospital Association
2350 Oakmont, Suite 101
Eugene, OR 97401

Physicians Service of Clackamas
   County, Inc.
18600 S.E. McLoughlin Blvd.
P.O. Box 286
Gladstone, OR 97027

Portland Metro Health Care
   Foundation
5201 S.W. Westgate Drive, Suite 111
Portland, OR 97221

Pennsylvania
Pennsylvania Medical Care Foundation
20 Erford Road
Lemoyne, PA 17043

South Carolina
South Carolina FMC
P.O. Box 1118 – Capitol Station
Columbia, SC 92901

Tennessee
Davidson County FMC
Executive Plaza Bldg.
3200 West End Avenue, Suite 305
Nashville, TN 37203

Tennessee FMC
Continental Plaza, Suite 300
4301 Hillsboro Road
Nashville, TN 37215

Texas
Bexar County Medical Foundation
P.O. Box 12635
San Antonio, TX 78212

Texas Medical Care Foundation
7800 Shool Creek, Suite 390 W
Austin, TX 78757

Utah
Utah Professional Review Organization
555 E. 2nd South
Salt Lake City, UT 84102

Washington
Kitsap Physicians Service
820 Pacific Avenue
Bremerton, WA 98310

Wisconsin
Milwaukee County Medical Society
756 N. Milwaukee Street
Milwaukee, WI 53202

Wisconsin Health Care Review, Inc.
P.O. Box 1109
Madison, WI 53701

Wyoming
Wyoming Health Service
2727 O'Neil Avenue, P.O. Drawer 4009
Cheyenne, WY 82001

Associate Members

American Academy of Family Practice
1740 W. 92nd Street
Kansas City, MO 64114

American College of Radiology
20 N. Wacker Drive
Chicago, IL 60606

American Society of Internal Medicine
535 Central Tower Bldg.
3rd & Market Streets
San Francisco, CA 94103

Arapahoe Medical Foundation
690 E. Girard Avenue
Englewood, CO 80110

Broome, Delaware & Otsego
   Counties Medical Society
4550 Old Vestal Road
Binghamton, NY 13902

College of American Pathologists
7400 N. Skokie Blvd.
Skokie, IL 60074

Joint Council of Socio Economics
   of Allergy
950 Lee Street, Suite 102
Des Plaines, IA 60016

Long Beach FMC
c/o Bauer Hospital
1050 Linden Avenue
Long Beach, CA 90801

Queens County Medical Society
112-25 Queens Blvd.
Forest Hills, NY 11375

STATE AGENCIES ADMINISTERING SERVICES FOR CRIPPLED CHILDREN

Alabama
State Department of Education
Crippled Children's Services
Montgomery, AL 36104

Alaska
State Department of Health and Welfare
Division of Public Health
Branch of Child Health
Juneau, AK 99801

Arizona
State of Arizona
Crippled Children's Services
Phoenix, AZ 85006

Arkansas
State Department of Social
and Rehabilitative Services
Crippled Children's Division
Little Rock, AR 72201

California
State Department of Public Health
Bureau of Crippled Children Services
Berkeley, CA 94704

Colorado
Colorado Department of Health
Child Health Services Division
Crippled Children Section
Denver, CO 80220

Connecticut
State Department of Health
Crippled Children Section
Hartford, CT 06106

Delaware
Department of Health and Social Service
Crippled Children's Services
Dover, DE 19901

District of Columbia
D.C. Health Services Administration
Bureau of Maternal and Child Health
Washington, D.C. 20001

Florida
Department of Health and Rehabilitative
Services
Bureau of Crippled Children
Tallahassee, FL 32304

Georgia
State Department of Public Health
Crippled Children's Service
Atlanta, GA 30303

Guam
Department of Public Health
and Social Services
Crippled Children's Services
Agana, GU 96910

Hawaii
State Department of Health, Children's
Health Services Division
Crippled Children Branch
Honolulu, HI 96801

Idaho
State Department of Health, Child
Health Division
Crippled Children's Services
Boise, ID 83707

Illinois
University of Illinois
Division of Services for Crippled Children
Springfield, IL 62703

Indiana
State Department of Public Welfare
Division of Services for Crippled Children
Indianapolis, IN 46207

Iowa
University of Iowa
State Services for Crippled Children
Iowa City, IA 52241

Kansas
Crippled Children's Commission
Wichita, KS 67202

Kentucky
Commission for Handicapped Children
Louisville, KY 40217

Louisiana
State Department of Health
Section of Crippled Children's Services
New Orleans, LA 70160

Maine
State Department of Health and Welfare
Division of Child Health and Crippled
 Children's Services
Augusta, ME 04330

Marianas Islands
Trust Territory
Department of Medical Services
Trust Territory of the Pacific Islands
Saipan, Marianas Islands 96950

Maryland
State Department of Health
Division of Crippled Children and Heart
 Disease Control
Baltimore, MD 21201

Massachusetts
State Department of Public Health
Bureau of Handicapped Children's Services
Boston, MA 02133

Michigan
State Department of Public Health
Bureau of Maternal and Child Health
Lansing, MI 48913

Minnesota
Department of Public Welfare
Crippled Children's Service
St. Paul, MN 55101

Mississippi
State Board of Health
Crippled Children's Service
Jackson, MS 39205

Missouri
University of Missouri
Crippled Children's Services
Columbia, MO 65201

Montana
State Department of Health
Child Health Services Division,
 Crippled Children
Helena, MT 59601

Nebraska
State Department of Public Welfare
Services for Crippled Children
Lincoln, NB 68502

Nevada
Department of Health, Welfare, and
 Rehabilitation
Bureau of Maternal, Child, and
 School Health
Carson City, NV 89701

New Hampshire
State Department of Health and Welfare
Division of Public Health
Crippled Children's Services
Concord, NH 03301

New Jersey
State Department of Health
Crippled Children's Program
Trenton, NJ 08625

New Mexico
State Department of Health and Social
 Services
Crippled Children's Section
Santa Fe, NM 87501

New York
State Department of Health
Bureau of Medical Rehabilitation
Albany, NY 12206

North Carolina
State Board of Health
Crippled Children's Section
Raleigh, NC 27602

North Dakota
Public Welfare Board of North Dakota
Division for Children and Youth
Crippled Children's Services
Bismarck, ND 58501

Ohio
State Department of Public Welfare
Division of Social Administration
Bureau of Crippled Children Services
Columbus, OH 43215

Oklahoma
Department of Institutions
Social and Rehabilitative Services
Crippled Children's Unit
Oklahoma City, OK 73105

Oregon
University of Oregon Medical School
Crippled Children's Division
Portland, OR 97201

Pennsylvania
State Department of Health
Division of Maternal and Child Health
    and Crippled Children's Services
Harrisburg, PA 17120

Puerto Rico
Department of Health
Bureau of Health
Division of Maternal and Child Health
San Juan, PR 00908

Rhode Island
State Department of Health
Division of Child Health and
    Crippled Children's Services
Providence, RI 02903

Samoa
LBJ Tropical Medical Center
Government of American Samoa
Pago Pago, American Samoa 96920

South Carolina
State Board of Health
Crippled Children's Care
Columbia, SC 27201

South Dakota
State Department of Health
Division of Maternal and Child Health
Pierre, SD 57501

Tennessee
State Department of Public Health
Crippled Children's Services
Nashville, TN 37219

Texas
State Department of Health
Crippled Children's Service
Austin, TX 78756

Utah
State Department of Social Services
Division of Health
Crippled Children's Services
Salt Lake City, UT 84113

Vermont
State Department of Health
Crippled Children's Services
Burlington, VT 05401

Virginia
State Department of Health
Bureau of Crippled Children's Services
Richmond, VA 23219

Virgin Islands
Department of Health
Services for Crippled Children
Charlotte Amalie, St. Thomas, VI 00802

Washington
State Department of Social and Health
    Services
Crippled Children's Services
Olympia, WA 98502

West Virginia
Department of Welfare
Division of Crippled Children's Services
Charleston, WV 25305

Wisconsin
State Department of Public Instruction
Bureau for Handicapped Children
Crippled Children Division
Madison, WI 53702

Wyoming
State Department of Public Health
Division of Maternal and Child Health
    and Crippled Children
Cheyenne, WY 82001

REVIEW
QUESTIONS

1. What is a prepaid health plan? _____

_____

_____

_____

2. Name some of the prepaid health plans in existence.

a. _____

b. _____

c. _____

d. _____

3. What does the phrase "closed panel program" mean? _____

_____

_____

4. What is a Foundation for Medical Care? _____

_____

_____

5. Name the two types of operations of Foundations for Medical Care and explain the main features of each.

a. _____

_____

_____

b. _____

_____

_____

6. Mark the following statements True or False — circle T or F

   a. An HMO can be sponsored and operated by a Foundation   T   F

   b. Peer Review determines the quality and operation of health
care   T   F

   c. An employer may offer the services of an HMO clinic if he
has five employees or more   T   F

   d. Medicare and Medicaid beneficiaries may not join an HMO   T   F

   e. An optometric service plan is considered a form of prepaid
group vision care program   T   F

7. CCS means _____ and covers the following

age group: _____

_____

Notes:

11
Dental Insurance

INTRODUCTION

Because dental insurance has grown to such large proportions, many plans discussed at other points in the text now include it. The practicing dental assistant and the student wishing to enter this field should consult the following chapters for more comprehensive information and handy hints:

PREPAID DENTAL INSURANCE

One of the fastest growing health care benefits is prepaid dental insurance. Increasing numbers of labor contracts are including provisions for some type of prepaid dental care. And many employers are voluntarily offering such protection to their employees. The Delta Dental Plans are the dental society–sponsored and approved service corporations organized by the profession in most states to provide prepaid dental care coverage to the public on a group basis. Most states now have these plans and operate on a nonprofit system. Sometimes these programs are referred to as "blue tooth" programs because they operate similarly to the Blue Shield/Blue Cross prepaid medical care programs. They can be identified by the Delta Dental Plan symbol (Fig. 11–1).

In some instances the plan may be administered for the dental society by an insurance company. Payment is made to the participating dentist on the basis of his usual, customary, and reasonable (UCR) fee (see Chapter 4, pp. 66–67. Dentists who provide services under a UCR plan may be required to list their UCR fees (dentist's profile) with the insurance carrier. This is similar to the physician's profile, except that the dentist updates this himself when necessary. For further information and booklets, contact your nearest Delta Dental Plan Office. A comprehensive address list is found on pages 300 to 303.

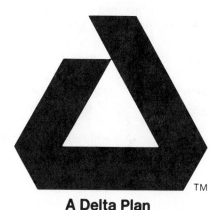

A Delta Plan

FIGURE 11–1

Symbol of the Delta Dental Plans. (Courtesy of Delta Dental Plans Association, Chicago, Illinois.)

Types of Coverage

Dental insurance policies vary widely. Some pay a fixed sum for each procedure; others set a dollar limit on reimbursement for each year's bills. Some policies have a deductible the patient has to meet.

There are two types of coverage:

1. *Comprehensive coverage:* Insurance pays about 70 per cent of the routine dental care and about 50 per cent of orthodontic or periodontal treatment. The subscriber is responsible for payment of the balance as a copayment.

2. *Incentive copayment*: Insurance pays for an increasing percentage of the employee's dental bills if the employee has regular preventive dental care.

To give you an idea of how the incentive program works, a description of the California Dental Service (CDS)—one of the Delta Dental Plans—is given here. The dentist is paid directly. If the full amount of the bill is not covered, the insured is billed for the excess.

CDS Incentive Plan

In the first year of eligibility CDS will pay 70 per cent of the dentist's fees. During the second year, if the insured meets the requirement of the yearly visit with all prescribed treatment performed, CDS increases its payment to 80 per cent. CDS's portion goes up to 90 per cent during the third year and 100 per cent during the fourth and all subsequent years, provided the basic checkup requirements continue to be met. However, if the subscriber fails to go to the dentist at least once a year, the portion of his or her bill that CDS will pay simply drops back by a 10 per cent reduction until it reaches the 70 per cent level.

Benefits

Benefits vary from contract to contract, but the following are some of the basic benefits on most group contracts.

1.	Diagnostic	Procedures to assist the dentist in evaluating the existing conditions to determine the required dental treatment.
2.	Preventive	Prophylaxis once every 6 months. Topical application of fluoride solutions. Space maintainers.
3.	Oral surgery	Procedures for extractions and other oral surgery, including pre- and postoperative care.
4.	General anesthesia	When administered for a covered oral surgery procedure performed by a dentist.
5.	Restorative	Provides amalgam, synthetic porcelain, and plastic restorations for treatment of carious lesions. Gold restorations, crowns, and jackets will be provided when teeth cannot be restored with the above materials.
6.	Endodontic	Procedures for pulpal therapy and root canal filling for treatment of nonvital teeth.
7.	Periodontic	Procedures for treatment of the tissues supporting the teeth.

Identification Card

Many dental insurance companies do not issue an identification card to the policy holder. The patient may bring in a booklet or pamphlet which shows the group number to which he or she belongs. Blue Cross of Southern California does issue an identification card (Fig. 11–2).

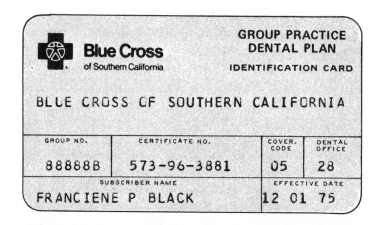

FIGURE 11–2

Blue Cross of Southern California Group Practice Dental Plan Identification Card.

Prior Authorization

Most dentists find it desirable to submit the claim form in advance of providing services. However, when the amount of the claim is under $100, prior authorization is not required by most plans. The advantages of prior authorization are:

1. Clearance of eligibility as member of the group.
2. Description of available benefits when work to be completed is over $100.
3. Calculation of insurance payment to be made to the dentist on behalf of the patient. This way the patient can then be told what he or she will have to pay.

How Eligibility is Shown

When a prior authorization claim is returned, the period of eligibility for completion of treatment may be indicated in one of two ways:

1. For manually processed groups, by the date entered in the "From and Thru" spaces in the upper left corner of the prestatement of costs (see Fig. 11–6, p. 288, *arrow*).

2. For computer processed groups, by a nine-digit number stamped in red (see Fig. 11–7, p. 289), the first four numbers of which are based upon the numbered days of the year, and which can be interpreted as shown in the following example:

If the stamped number is 7160 29811:

7 = the year 1977.
160 = the 160th day of 1977 (June 9). (See the Julian Calendar, Table 11–1.)
29811 = an index number used by California Dental Service to identify the specific treatment form in process. In a continuous attempt to improve processing, more groups are being converted to computer processing.

The eligibility period is extended for 60 days beyond the date represented by the first four digits (to August 9 in the example shown). If treatment cannot be completed within this period, eligibility should be reconfirmed with the insurance company.

TABLE 11–1
Perpetual Julian Calendar

JAN	FEB	MAR	APR	MAY	JUN	JUL	AUG	SEPT	OCT	NOV	DEC
001	032	060	091	121	152	182	213	244	274	305	335
031	059	090	120	151	181	212	243	273	304	334	365

Leap Year Julian Calendar

JAN	FEB	MAR	APR	MAY	JUN	JUL	AUG	SEPT	OCT	NOV	DEC
001	032	061	092	122	153	183	214	245	275	306	336
031	060	091	121	152	182	213	244	274	305	335	366

Fee Basis

There are two ways in which treatment or claim forms are computed to the dentist's filed fees:

1. *Usual, Customary, and Reasonable Fees:* Payment to the participating member dentists for services provided to an eligible patient under the group benefit is calculated against the currently filed fee information.
2. *Table of Allowances* (see sample of table on pp. 279–280): Payment to all dentists for services provided an eligible patient is calculated against amount specified in the Table of Allowances. The patient is responsible for the difference between the amount listed in the Table of Allowances and the dentist's usual and customary fees.

Groups purchasing dental benefits for their employees or members select a fee basis best suited to their requirements. The numbers listed in the Table of Allowances are *not* fees. They are simply amounts of which the insurance company will pay a portion, when one or both of the following conditions are present:

1. The patient's group contract states that the Table of Allowances fee basis is used in computing treatment of claims.

2. The dentist is not a member physician of the insurance company in question.

Under the Table of Allowances approach, the dentist enters his usual fees on the claim form, just as he would under the Usual and Customary approach, for comparison with the currently filed fee information. The insurance company will then compute the difference between the dentist's usual and customary fees and the amount listed in the table, taking into consideration the percentage of the coverage. The remaining amount is payable by the patient.

Example:

Fee Basis:	Usual and Customary
Coverage:	80% Basic Services 80% Prosthetic Services
Total Fee Charged:	$360.00
Insurance Company Pays:	$288.00 (80% of total Usual and Customary Fee)
Patient Pays:	$72.00

Fee Basis:	Table of Allowances
Coverage:	90% Basic Services 90% Prosthetic Services
Total Fee Charged:	$360.00
Total Table of Allowance:	$245.00
Insurance Company Pays:	$220.50 (90% of total Table of Allowance)
Patient Pays:	$139.50

Code on Dental Procedures and Nomenclature

The Uniform Code on Dental Procedures and Nomenclature was developed by the American Dental Association as an attempt to identify and categorize the most usual dental service procedures covered under prepaid, insured, and other third party group purchase programs. The code is sometimes referred to as *ADA procedure numbers*. It is a five-digit system of procedure identification (see pp. 274–278).

1. The first digit is a zero throughout the code, and it identifies all procedures as being dental rather than medical, hospital, or surgical services.

2. The second digit designates the category of dental service. See Table 11–2 for the 10 categories.

3. The third digit indicates the class of service within the dental category.

4. The fourth digit designates the subclass of specific procedure within a given category.

5. The fifth digit allows for further expansion of the code when necessary.

Example:

Using this code system, the number 02120 would indicate a two-surface amalgam restoration on a deciduous tooth.

TABLE 11-2. DENTAL SERVICE CATEGORIES OF THE ADA UNIFORM
CODE ON DENTAL PROCEDURES AND NOMENCLATURE*

	Category of Service	Code Series
I	Diagnostic	00100–00999
II	Preventive	01000–01999
III	Restorative	02000–02999
IV	Endodontics	03000–03999
V	Periodontics	04000–04999
VI	Prosthodontics, removable	05000–05999
VII	Prosthodontics, fixed	06000–06999
VIII	Oral surgery	07000–07999
IX	Orthodontics	08000–08999
X	Adjunctive general services	09000–09999

*From Reports of Councils and Bureaus. JADA, 92:647–652, March, 1976.

The first digit, 0, indicates a dental procedure.
The second digit, 2, indicates a restorative service.
The third digit, 1, indicates an amalgam restoration.
The fourth digit, 2, indicates a deciduous tooth and
the number of surfaces involved.
The fifth digit at the present time is usually 0.

To properly code the insurance claim, see pages 274 to 278 of this chapter. Blue Cross uses the ADA procedure code numbers.

Many of the dental insurance plans have their own three-digit coding system so it is best to obtain the specific code for the specific plan. An example is the California Dental Service Table of Allowances procedure codes, included in this chapter (pp. 279–280).

Dual Coverage

If a patient is covered under two group policies originating from the same insurance carrier, submit only one treatment form. A coordination of benefits clause is usually written into such policies.

If a patient is covered under two group policies originating from different insurance carriers and one program does not contain a nonduplication (coordination of benefits) provision, that Plan must pay its benefits before the Plan which has such a clause. When two or more programs contain a nonduplication clause, coordination of payment benefits is necessary.

There are some variables to be considered in dual coverage cases:

1. Excluded or limited benefits are not subject to dual coverage.

2. Certain group contracts specify that if husband and wife are both employees within the same group, they shall *not* have dual coverage.

3. If husband and wife are covered by two separate groups with employee-only coverage, there is no dual coverage.

ADA PROCEDURE NUMBERS

00100-00999 **I. Diagnostic**

00100 **Clinical Oral Examinations**
00110 Initial oral examination
00120 Periodic oral examination
00130 Emergency oral examination

00200 **Radiographs**
00210 Intraoral—complete series (including bitewings)
00220 Intraoral periapical—single, first film
00230 Intraoral periapical—each additional film
00240 Intraoral—occlusal, film
00250 Extraoral—single, first film
00260 Extraoral—each additional film
00270 Bitewing—single film
00272 Bitewings—two films
00273 Bitewings—three films
00274 Bitewings—four films
00290 Posteroanterior and lateral skull and facial bone, survey film
00310 Sialography
00321 Temporomandibular joint, film
00330 Panoramic—maxilla and mandible, film
00340 Cephalometric film

00400 **Tests and Laboratory Examinations**
00410 Bacteriologic cultures for determination of pathologic agents
00420 Caries susceptibility tests
00450 Histopathologic examination
00460 Pulp vitality tests
00470 Diagnostic casts
00471 Diagnostic photographs

01000-01999 **II. Preventive**

01100 **Dental Prophylaxis**
01110 Adults
01120 Children

01200 **Fluoride Treatments**
01210 Topical application of sodium fluoride—four treatments (excluding prophylaxis)
01211 Topical application of sodium fluoride—four treatments (including prophylaxis)
01220 Topical application of stannous fluoride—one treatment (excluding prophylaxis)
01221 Topical application of stannous fluoride—one treatment (including prophylaxis)
01230 Topical application of acid fluoride phosphate—one treatment (excluding prophylaxis)
01231 Topical application of acid fluoride phosphate—one treatment (including prophylaxis)

01300 **Other Preventive Services**
01310 Dietary planning for the control of dental caries
01330 Oral hygiene instruction
01340 Training in preventive dental care
01350 Topical application of sealants—per quadrant

01500 **Space Management Therapy**
01510 Fixed—unilateral type
01515 Fixed—bilateral type
01520 Removable unilateral type
01525 Removable bilateral type
01550 Recementation of space maintainer

02000-02999 **III. Restorative**

Diagnostic Procedures—see Section I

02100 **Amalgam Restorations** (including polishing)
02110 Amalgam—one surface, deciduous
02120 Amalgam—two surfaces. deciduous
02130 Amalgam—three surfaces, deciduous
02131 Amalgam—four surfaces, deciduous
02140 Amalgam—one surface, permanent
02150 Amalgam—two surfaces, permanent
02160 Amalgam—three surfaces, permanent
02161 Amalgam—four or more surfaces, permanent
02190 Pin retention—exclusive of amalgam

02200 **Silicate Restorations**
02210 Silicate cement per restoration

02300 **Acrylic or Plastic Restorations**
02310 Acrylic or plastic
02330 Composite resin—one surface
02331 Composite resin—two surfaces
02332 Composite resin—three surfaces
02334 Pin retention—exclusive of composite resin
02335 Composite resin (involving incisal angle)
02340 Acid etch for restorations

02400 **Gold Foil Restorations**
02410 Gold foil—one surface
02420 Gold foil—two surfaces
02430 Gold foil—three surfaces

02500 **Gold Inlay Restorations**
02510 Inlay—gold, one surface
02520 Inlay—gold, two surfaces
02530 Inlay—gold, three surfaces
02540 Onlay—per tooth (in addition to above)

02600 **Porcelain Restorations**
02610 Inlay—porcelain

02700-02899 **Crowns—Single Restorations Only**
02710 Plastic (acrylic)
02711 Plastic—prefabricated
02720 Plastic with gold
02721 Plastic with nonprecious metal
02722 Plastic with semiprecious metal
02740 Porcelain
02750 Porcelain with gold
02751 Porcelain with nonprecious metal
02752 Porcelain with semiprecious metal
02790 Gold (full cast)
02791 Nonprecious metal (full cast)
02792 Semiprecious metal (full cast)
C2810 Gold (¾ cast)
02830 Stainless steel
02840 Temporary (fractured tooth)
02891 Cast post and core in addition to crown
02892 Steel post and composite or amalgam in addition to crown

02900 **Other Restorative Services**
02910 Recement inlays
02920 Recement crowns
02940 Fillings (sedative)
02950 Crown buildups—pin retained

03000-03999 **IV. Endodontics**

Diagnostic Procedures—see Section I

03100 **Pulp Capping**
03110 Pulp cap—direct (excluding final restoration)
03120 Pulp cap—indirect (excluding final restoration)

A

03200 **Pulpotomy** (excluding final restoration)
03220 Vital pulpotomy

03300 **Root Canal Therapy** (includes treatment plan, clinical procedures, and follow-up care)
03310 Anterior (excludes final restoration)
03320 Bicuspid (excludes final restoration)
03330 Molar (excludes final restoration)
03350 Apexification (treatment may extend over period of 6 to 18 months)

03400 **Periapical Services**
03410 Apicoectomy—performed as separate surgical procedure (per root)
03420 Apicoectomy—performed in conjunction with endodontic procedure (per root)
03430 Retrograde filling
03440 Apical curettage
03450 Root resection
03460 Endodontic implants

03900 **Other Endodontic Procedures**
03910 Surgical procedure for isolation of tooth with rubber dam
03920 Hemisection
03940 Recalcification of perforations
03950 Canal preparation and fitting of preformed dowel or post
03960 Bleaching of nonvital discolored tooth

04000–04999 **V. Periodontics**

Diagnostic Procedures—see Section I

04200 **Surgical Services** (including usual postoperative services)
04210 Gingivectomy or gingivoplasty—per quadrant
04220 Gingival curettage and root planing
04240 Gingival flap procedure
04250 Mucogingival surgery—per quadrant
04260 Osseous surgery (including flap entry and closure)—per quadrant
04261 Osseous graft—single site (including flap entry, closure, and donor site)
04262 Osseous grafts—multiple sites (including flap entry, closure, and donor site)
04270 Pedicle soft tissue grafts
04271 Free soft tissue grafts (including donor site)
04272 Vestibuloplasty
04280 Periodontal pulpal procedures

04300 **Adjunctive Periodontal Services**
04320 Provisional splinting—intracoronal
04321 Provisional splinting—extracoronal
04330 Occlusal adjustment (limited)
04331 Occlusal adjustment (complete)
04340 Periodontal scaling (entire mouth)
04341 Periodontal scaling (fewer than 12 teeth)
04350 Tooth movement for periodontal purposes (by report)
04360 Special periodontal appliances (including occlusal guards) (by report)
04370 Case pattern modifiers (by report)

CASE PATTERN SECTION
(Includes all necessary diagnostic, surgical, and adjunctive services)

04500 TYPE I—**Gingivitis**—shallow pockets, no bone loss

Treatment:
1. All necessary diagnostic procedures
2. Training in personal preventive dental care
3. Mouth preparation procedures
4. Routine finishing procedures
5. Posttreatment evaluation

04600 TYPE II—**Early Periodontitis**—moderate pockets, minor to moderate bone loss, satisfactory topography

Treatment:
1. All necessary diagnostic procedures
2. Training in personal preventive dental care
3. Mouth preparation procedures
4. Occlusal adjustment (if necessary)
5. Surgical procedures usually involving curettage and/or gingivectomy
6. Routine finishing procedures
7. Posttreatment evaluation

04700 TYPE III—**Moderate Periodontitis**—moderate to deep pockets, moderate to severe bone loss, unsatisfactory topography

Treatment:
1. All necessary diagnostic procedures
2. Training in personal preventive dental care
3. Mouth preparation procedures
4. Occlusal adjustment
5. Surgical procedures usually involving flap entry and osseous procedures
6. Routine finishing procedures
7. Posttreatment evaluation

04800 TYPE IV—**Advanced Periodontitis**—deep pockets, severe bone loss, advanced mobility patterns (usually cases involving missing teeth and reconstruction)

Treatment:
1. All necessary diagnostic procedures
2. Training in personal preventive dental care
3. Mouth preparation procedures
4. Occlusal adjustment
5. Surgical procedures usually involving complex techniques
6. Routine finishing procedures
7. Posttreatment evaluation

04900 **Other Periodontic Services**
04910 Preventive periodontal procedures (periodontal prophylaxis)
04920 Unscheduled dressing change (by other than treating dentist)

05000–05999 **VI. Prosthodontics, Removable**

Diagnostic Procedures—see Section I

05100 **Complete Dentures**—including six months' postdelivery care
05110 Complete upper
05120 Complete lower
05130 Immediate upper
05140 Immediate lower

05200 **Partial Dentures**—including six months postdelivery care
05211 Upper—without clasps, acrylic base
05212 Lower—without clasps, acrylic base
05215 Upper—with two gold clasps with rests, acrylic base
05216 Upper—with two chrome clasps with rests, acrylic base

A (Continued)

05217 Lower—with two gold clasps with rests, acrylic base
05218 Lower—with chrome clasps with rests, acrylic base
05230 Lower—with gold lingual bar and two clasps, acrylic base
05231 Lower—with chrome lingual bar and two clasps, acrylic base
05240 Lower—with gold lingual bar and two clasps, cast base
05241 Lower—with chrome lingual bar and two clasps, cast base
05250 Upper—with gold palatal bar and two clasps, acrylic base
05251 Upper—with chrome palatal bar and two clasps, acrylic base
05260 Upper—with gold palatal bar and two clasps, cast base
05261 Upper—with chrome palatal bar and two clasps, cast base
05280 Removable unilateral partial denture—one-piece gold casting, clasp attachments, per unit including pontics
05281 Removable unilateral partial denture—one-piece chrome casting, clasp attachments, per unit including pontics
05291 Full cast partial—with two gold clasps (upper)
05292 Full cast partial—with two chrome clasps (upper)
05293 Full cast partial—with two gold clasps (lower)
05294 Full cast partial—with two chrome clasps (lower)

05300 Additional Units for Partial Dentures
05310 Each additional clasp with rest
05320 Each tooth (applies to 05291—05294 only)

05400 Adjustments to Dentures
05410 Complete denture
05421 Partial denture (upper)
05422 Partial denture (lower)

05600 Repairs to Dentures
05610 Repair broken complete or partial denture—no teeth damaged
05620 Repair broken complete or partial denture—replace one broken tooth
05630 Replace additional teeth—each tooth
05640 Replace broken tooth on denture—no other repairs
05650 Adding tooth to partial denture to replace extracted tooth—each tooth (not involving clasp or abutment tooth)
05660 Adding tooth to partial denture to replace extracted tooth—each tooth (involving clasp or abutment tooth)
05670 Reattaching damaged clasp on denture
05680 Replacing broken clasp with new clasp on denture
05690 Each additional clasp with rest

05700 Denture Duplication
05710 Duplicate upper or lower complete denture
05720 Duplicate upper or lower partial denture

Denture Relining
05730 Relining upper or lower complete denture (office reline)
05740 Relining upper or lower partial denture (office reline)
05750 Relining upper or lower complete denture (laboratory)
05760 Relining upper or lower partial denture (laboratory)

05800 Other Prosthetic Services
05810 Denture—temporary (complete) upper

05811 Denture—temporary (complete) lower
05820 Denture—temporary (partial-stayplate), upper
05821 Denture—temporary (partial-stayplate), lower
05830 Obturator for surgically excised palatal tissue
05840 Obturator for deficient velopharyngeal function (cleft palate)
05850 Tissue conditioning
05860 Overdenture complete (by report)
05861 Overdenture partial (by report)

06000–06999 **VII. Prosthodontics, Fixed**

Fixed Bridges (each abutment and each pontic constitutes a unit in a bridge)

06200 **Bridge Pontics**
06210 Cast gold
06211 Cast nonprecious
06212 Cast semiprecious
06220 Slotted facing
06230 Slotted pontic
06235 Pin facing
06240 Porcelain fused to gold
06241 Porcelain fused to nonprecious metal
06242 Porcelain fused to semiprecious metal
06250 Plastic processed to gold
06251 Plastic processed to nonprecious metal
06252 Plastic processed to semiprecious metal

06500 **Retainers**
06520 Gold inlay—two surfaces
06530 Gold inlay—three or more surfaces
06540 Gold inlay (onlaying cusps)

06600 **Repairs**
06610 Replace broken pin facing with slotted or other facing
06620 Replace broken facing where post is intact
06630 Replace broken facing where post backing is broken
06640 Replace broken facing with acrylic
06650 Replace broken pontic

06700 **Crowns**
06710 Plastic (acrylic)
06720 Plastic processed to gold
06721 Plastic processed to nonprecious metal
06722 Plastic processed to semiprecious metal
06740 Porcelain
06750 Porcelain fused to gold
06751 Porcelain fused to nonprecious metal
06752 Porcelain fused to semiprecious metal
06760 Reverse pin facing and metal
06780 Gold (¾ cast)
06790 Gold (full cast)
06791 Nonprecious metal (full cast)
06792 Semiprecious metal (full cast)

06900 **Other Prosthetic Services**
06930 Recement bridge
06940 Stress breaker
06950 Precision attachment
06960 Dowel pin—metal

07000–07999 **VIII. Oral Surgery**

Diagnostic Procedures—see Section I

A (Continued)

07100 **Extractions**—includes local anesthesia and routine postoperative care
07110 Single tooth
07120 Each additional tooth

07200 **Surgical Extractions**—includes local anesthesia and routine postoperative care
07210 Extraction of tooth—erupted
07220 Impaction that requires incision of overlying soft tissue and the removal of the tooth
07230 Impaction that requires incision of overlying soft tissue, elevation of a flap, removal of bone, and the removal of the tooth
07240 Impaction that requires incision of overlying soft tissue, elevation of a flap, removal of bone, and sectioning of the tooth for removal
07241 Impaction that requires incision of overlying soft tissue, elevation of a flap, removal of bone, sectioning of the tooth for removal, and/or presents unusual difficulties and circumstances
07250 Root recovery (surgical removal of residual root)
07260 Oral antral fistula closure (and/or antral root recovery)

Other Surgical Procedures
07270 Tooth replantation
07271 Tooth implantation
07272 Tooth transplantation
07280 Surgical exposure of impacted or unerupted tooth for orthodontic reasons—including wire attachment when indicated
07281 Surgical exposure of impacted or unerupted tooth to aid eruption
07285 Biopsy of oral tissue (hard)
07286 Biopsy of oral tissue (soft)
07290 Surgical repositioning of teeth

07300 **Alveoloplasty** (surgical preparation of ridge for dentures)
07310 Per quadrant—in conjunction with extractions
07320 Per quadrant—not in conjunction with extractions

Stomatoplasty—including revision of soft tissue on ridges, muscle reattachment, tongue, palate, and other oral soft tissues
07340 Per arch—uncomplicated
07350 Per arch—complicated—including ridge extension, soft tissue grafts, and management of hypertrophied and hyperplastic tissue

07400 **Surgical Excision**—excision of reactive inflammatory lesions (scar tissue or localized congenital lesions)
07410 Radical excision—lesion diameter up to 1.25 cm
07420 Radical excision—lesion diameter over 1.25 cm
07425 Excision pericoronal gingiva

Excision of Tumors
07430 Excision of benign tumor—lesion diameter up to 1.25 cm
07431 Excision of benign tumor—lesion diameter over 1.25 cm
07440 Excision of malignant tumor—lesion diameter up to 1.25 cm
07441 Excision of malignant tumor—lesion diameter over 1.25 cm

Removal of Cysts and Neoplasms
07450 Removal of odontogenic cyst or tumor—up to 1.25 cm in diameter
07451 Removal of odontogenic cyst or tumor—over 1.25 cm in diameter
07460 Removal of nonodontogenic cyst or tumor—up to 1.25 cm in diameter

07461 Removal of nonodontogenic cyst or tumor—over 1.25 in cm diameter
07465 Destruction of lesions by physical methods: electrosurgery, chemotherapy, cryotherapy

Excision of Bone Tissue
07470 Removal of exostosis—maxilla or mandible
07480 Partial ostectomy (guttering or saucerization)
07490 Radical resection of mandible with bone graft

07500 **Surgical Incision**
07510 Incision and drainage of abscess—intraoral
07520 Incision and drainage of abscess—extraoral
07530 Removal of foreign body, skin, or subcutaneous areolar tissue
07540 Removal of reaction-producing foreign bodies—musculoskeletal system
07550 Sequestrectomy for osteomyelitis
07560 Maxillary sinusotomy for removal of tooth fragment or foreign body

07600 **Treatment of Fractures**—simple
07610 Maxilla—open reduction, teeth immobilized (if present)
07620 Maxilla—closed reduction, teeth immoblized (if present)
07630 Mandible—open reduction, teeth immobilized (if present)
07640 Mandible—closed reduction, teeth immobilized (if present)
07650 Malar and/or zygomatic arch—open reduction
07660 Malar and/or zygomatic arch—closed reduction
07670 Alveolus—stabilization of teeth, open reduction splinting
07680 Facial bones—complicated reduction with fixation and multiple surgical approaches

07700 **Treatment of Fractures**—compound
07710 Maxilla—open reduction
07720 Maxilla—closed reduction
07730 Mandible—open reduction
07740 Mandible—closed reduction
07750 Malar and/or zygomatic arch—open reduction
07760 Malar and/or zygomatic arch—closed reduction
07770 Alveolus—stabilization of teeth—open reduction splinting
07780 Facial bones—complicated reduction with fixation and multiple surgical approaches

07800 **Reduction of Dislocation and Management of Other Temporomandibular Joint Dysfunctions**
07810 Open reduction of dislocation
07820 Closed reduction of dislocation
07830 Manipulation under anesthesia
07840 Condylectomy
07850 Meniscectomy
07860 Arthrotomy
07870 Arthrocentesis

07900 **Other Oral Surgery**

Repair of Traumatic Wounds
07910 Suture of recent small wounds up to 5 cm

Complicated Suturing (reconstruction requiring delicate handling of tissues, wide undermining for meticulous closure)
07911 Up to 5 cm
07912 Over 5 cm
07920 Skin grafts (identify defect covered, location, and type of graft)

A (Continued)

Other Repair Procedures
07930 Injection of trigeminal nerve branches for destruction
07931 Avulsion of trigeminal nerve branches
07940 Osteoplasty (that is, for orthognathic deformities)
07950 Osseous, osteoperiosteal, periosteal, or cartilage graft of the mandible—autogenous or nonautogenous
07955 Repair of maxillofacial soft and hard tissue defects
07960 Frenulectomy—separate procedure (frenectomy or frenotomy)
07970 Excision of hyperplastic tissue—per arch
07980 Sialolithotomy
07981 Excision of salivary gland
07982 Sialodochoplasty
07983 Closure of salivary fistula
07990 Emergency tracheotomy

08000–08999 **IX. Orthodontics**

Diagnostic Procedures—see Section I

Preventive Treatment Procedures

08100 **Minor Treatment for Tooth Guidance**
08110 Removable appliance therapy
08120 Fixed or cemented appliance therapy

08200 **Minor Treatment to Control Harmful Habits**
08210 Removable appliance therapy
08220 Fixed or cemented appliance therapy

08350 **Interceptive Orthodontic Treatment**
08360 Removable appliance therapy
08370 Fixed appliance therapy

Comprehensive Orthodontic Treatment

08450 **Treatment of the Transitional Dentition**
08460 Class I malocclusion
08470 Class II malocclusion
08480 Class III malocclusion

08550 **Treatment of the Permanent Dentition**
08560 Class I malocclusion
08570 Class II malocclusion
08580 Class III malocclusion

08650 **Treatment of the Atypical or Extended Skeletal Case**

08750 **Posttreatment Stabilization**

09000–09999 **X. Adjunctive General Services**

Unclassified Treatment
09110 Palliative (emergency) treatment of dental pain, minor procedures

09200 **Anesthesia**
09210 Local (not in conjunction with operative or surgical procedures)
09211 Regional block anesthesia
09212 Trigeminal division block
09220 General
09230 Analgesia

09300 **Professional Consultation**—(diagnostic service provided by physician or dentist other than practitioner providing treatment)
09310 Consultation—per session

09400 **Professional Visits**
09410 House calls
09420 Hospital calls
09430 Office visit—during regularly scheduled office hours (no operative services performed)
09440 Office visit—after regularly scheduled office hours (no operative services performed)

09600 **Drugs**
09610 Therapeutic drug injection (by report)
09630 Other drugs and/or medicaments (by report)

09900 **Miscellaneous Services**
09910 Application of desensitizing medicaments
09930 Complications (postsurgical—unusual circumstances) (by report)
09950 Occlusion analysis (mounted case)
09960 Completion of claim form
09999 Unspecified (by report to be described by statement of attending dentist)

A (Concluded)

TABLE OF ALLOWANCES   APPENDIX B

This is not a fee schedule. The amounts listed in this Table are allowances which are made toward usual and customary fees. Usual and customary fees vary with individual dental practices.

Proc. No.	Procedures (B/R means By Report)	Allowance
VISITS AND DIAGNOSTIC (020-199)		
020	Office visit for treatment and observation of injuries to teeth and supporting structure, other than for routine operative procedures (Regular office hours)	4.00
030	Professional visits after hours (Dentist may elect payment on basis of services rendered or visits whichever is greater)	10.00
040	Special consultation (by specialist for case presentation when diagnostic procedures have been performed by general dentist)	10.00
049	Prophylaxis – children to age 14	6.00
050	Prophylaxis – to include scaling and polishing	9.00
061	Topical application of sodium fluoride (one treatment including prophylaxis under age 4)	12.00
062	Topical application of stannous fluoride (one treatment including prophylaxis – payment limited to once each year to age 18)	14.00
080	Emergency treatment – palliative per visit	5.00

Film allowances include exam and diagnosis

110	Single film	4.00
111	Additional, up to 12 films, each	1.00
112	Entire denture series, including examination consisting of at least 14 films (bite wings if necessary)	17.00
113	Intra-oral, occlusal view, maxillary or mandibular, each	4.00
114	Superior or inferior maxillary, extra oral, one film	10.00
115	Superior or inferior maxillary, extra oral, two films	15.00
116	Bite wing films, including examination	
	2 films	5.00
	4 films	7.00
	Additional films, each	1.00
150	Biopsy of oral tissue	8.00
160	Microscopic examination	15.00

ORAL SURGERY (200-299)

***All hospital costs are the responsibility of the patient. CDS will allow for the procedures listed in this schedule. Additional fees charged by the dentist for performing procedures in the hospital are the responsibility of the patient.

***CDS allowances for General Anesthesia . . . . See Procedure #400
Any further charges for anesthetics, anesthetists, or anesthesiologists are the responsibility of the patient.

***Allowances for procedures not listed in this schedule will be paid at the rate listed in the Relative Value Study as approved by the American Society of Oral Surgeons. Consultation (by specialist for case presentation when diagnostic procedures have been performed by general dentist) . . . . See Procedure #040

EXTRACTIONS:

200	Uncomplicated single, including routine post operative visits	8.00
201	Each additional tooth, including routine post operative visits	6.00
202	Surgical removal of erupted teeth	B/R
220	Post-operative visit (sutures and complications)	3.00

IMPACTED TEETH (enclose film):

230	Removal of tooth (soft tissue)	17.00
231	Removal of tooth (partially bony)	25.00
232	Removal of tooth (completely bony)	40.00 or B/R

ALVEOLAR OR GINGIVAL RECONSTRUCTION:

250	Alveolectomy (edentulous) per quadrant	25.00
252	Alveolectomy (in addition to removal of teeth) per quadrant	10.00
256	Alveoplasty with ridge extension, per arch	42.00
257	Removal of palatal torus	35.00 or B/R
258	Removal of mandibular tori per quadrant	35.00
259	Excision of hyper plastic tissue per arch	32.00

Proc. No.	Procedures (B/R means By Report)	Allowance
CYSTS AND NEOPLASMS:		
260	Intra-oral incision and drainage of abscess	10.00
261	Extra-oral incision and drainage of abscess	15.00 or B/R
262	Excision pericoronal gingiva	10.00
263	Sialolithotomy: removal of salivary calculus, intra-orally	33.00
264	Sialolithotomy: removal of salivary calculus, extra-orally	100.00
265	Closure of salivary fistula	60.00
266	Dilation of salivary duct	17.00
270	Resection of benign tumor of soft tissue (2.5 cm or larger)	25.00
271	Resection of malignant tumor	B/R
275	Transplantation of tooth or tooth bud	70.00
276	Removal of foreign body from bone (independent procedure)	B/R
277	Radical resection of bone for tumor with bone graft	B/R
278	Maxillary sinusotomy for removal of tooth fragment or foreign body	65.00 or B/R
279	Closure of oral fistula of maxillary sinus	40.00 or B/R
280	Excision of cyst, small	25.00 or B/R
281	Excision of cyst, large (2.5 cm or larger)	75.00 or B/R
282	Sequestrectomy for osteomyelitis or bone abscess superficial	20.00 or B/R
285	Condylectomy of temporomandibular joint	300.00
289	Meniscectomy of temporomandibular joint	250.00

MISCELLANEOUS:

290	Incision and removal of foreign body from soft tissue	10.00 or B/R
291	Frenectomy	25.00
292	Suture of soft tissue wound or injury	B/R
293	Crown exposure for orthodontia	15.00
294	Injection of sclerosing agent into temporomandibular joint	30.00
295	Treatment trigeminal neuralgia by injection into second and third divisions	34.00

DRUGS (300-399)

300	Drugs administered by dentist – based on cost	B/R

ANESTHESIA (400-449)

400	Anesthesia: General	15.00

PERIODONTICS (450-499)

Special consultation (by specialist for case presentation when preliminary diagnostic procedures (films, models, etc.) have been performed by general dentist) . . . . see Procedure #040

Prophylaxis (includes scaling and polishing) . . . See Procedure #050

451	Emergency treatment (periodontal abscess, acute periodontitis, etc.)	10.00
452	Subgingival curretage, root planing per quadrant (not prophylaxis)	12.00
453	Correction of occlusion per quadrant	12.00
472	Gingivectomy per quadrant (including post surgical visits)	50.00
473	Gingivectomy, osseous or muco-gingival surgery per quadrant (includes post surgical visits)	60.00
474	Gingivectomy, treatment per tooth (fewer than six teeth)	10.00

ENDODONTICS (500-599)

Special consultation (by specialist for case presentation when diagnostic procedures have been performed by general dentist) . . . . see Procedure #040

500	Pulp capping	6.00
501	Therapeutic pulpotomy (in addition to restoration, per treatment)	6.00
502	Vital pulpotomy	12.00
503	Remineralization (Caoh, temporary restoration) per tooth	10.00

ROOT CANALS:

510	Culturing canal	7.00
511	Single rooted canal tooth therapy	45.00
512	Bi-rooted tooth canal therapy	60.00
513	Tri-rooted tooth canal therapy	75.00
530	Apicoectomy (including filling of root canal)	50.00

Proc. No.	Procedures	(B/R means By Report) Allowance
531	Apicoectomy (separate procedure)	35.00
	Allowances do not include final restoration or necessary roentgenograms.	

RESTORATIVE DENTISTRY (600-679)

AMALGAM RESTORATIONS PRIMARY TEETH:

600	Cavities involving one tooth surface	6.00
601	Cavities involving two tooth surfaces	9.00
602	Cavities involving three or more tooth surfaces ...	12.00

AMALGAM RESTORATIONS PERMANENT TEETH:

611	Cavities involving one tooth surface	8.00
612	Cavities involving two tooth surfaces	11.00
613	Cavities involving three or more tooth surfaces ...	15.00

GOLD RESTORATIONS:

635	One tooth surface	35.00
636	Two tooth surfaces	40.00
637	Three or more tooth surfaces	50.00
638	Onlays extra per tooth	10.00

SILICATE, ACRYLIC, PLASTIC RESTORATIONS:

640	Silicate cement filling	9.00
645	Acrylic or plastic filling	11.00

RESTORATIVE DENTISTRY UNDER GENERAL ANESTHESIA
(Special cases only) (Handicapped Patients)

649	Long term operative cases performed under General Anesthesia on hourly basis:*	
	— One hour duration from beginning to end	75.00
	— Two and one half hours, maximum	150.00
	— Three and one half hours, maximum	175.00
	— Four or more hours	200.00
	The above includes all operative procedures, extractions, pulpotomies, necessary treatments, stannous fluoride and oral prophylaxis. Fees for anesthesiologists must be paid by patient.	

CROWNS:

650	Acrylic...........................	60.00
651	Acrylic with metal	75.00
652	Porcelain.........................	75.00
653	Porcelain with metal	100.00
660	Gold (full)........................	65.00
663	¾ Gold	60.00
670	Stainless Steel (primary)	17.00
671	Stainless Steel (permanent)	20.00
672	Gold dowel pin	10.00
	CDS does not pay for facings on crowns, posterior to 2nd bicuspids (if placed, fees must be paid by patient).	

PROSTHETICS (680-799) (Includes Fixed Bridges)

PONTICS:

680	Cast gold (sanitary)	40.00
681	Steele's facing	45.00
682	Tru-Pontic Type	55.00
692	Porcelain baked to gold	80.00
693	Plastic processed to gold	55.00

REMOVABLE (UNILATERAL BRIDGES):

683	One piece casting, chrome cobalt alloy clasp attachment (all types) per unit — including pontics	20.00

RECEMENTATION:

685	Inlay	5.00
686	Crown	5.00
687	Bridge	10.00

REPAIRS, CROWN AND BRIDGES:

690	Repairs — based on time and laboratory charges ..	B/R

DENTURES:

Dentures, partial dentures and reline allowances include adjustments for six month period following installation. Fees for specialized techniques involving precision dentures, personalization or characterization must be paid by patient.

700	Complete maxillary denture	155.00
701	Complete mandibular denture	155.00
702	Partial acrylic upper or lower with gold or chrome cobalt alloy clasps — base	75.00
712	Teeth and clasps — extra per unit	5.00
703	Partial lower or upper with chrome cobalt alloy lingual or palatal bar and acrylic saddles — base .	150.00
704	Teeth and clasps — extra per unit	5.00
705	Simple stress breakers — extra	14.00
706	Stayplate — base	30.00
716	Teeth and clasps — extra per unit	3.00
720	Denture adjustment...................	4.00
721	Office reline — cold cure — acrylic	15.00
722	Denture reline	35.00
723	Special tissue conditioning, per denture, in addition to reline — maximum 2 per denture	15.00
724	Denture duplication (jump case) per denture	55.00

REPAIRS, DENTURES, ACRYLIC:

790	Broken denture, repairing (no teeth involved) ...	12.00
	Replacing missing or broken teeth, each additional	3.00
	Adding teeth to partial denture to replace extracted natural teeth:	
793	First tooth	25.00
794	First tooth with clasp	30.00
795	Each additional tooth and clasp	5.00
796	Partial denture repairs — based on time and laboratory charges	B/R

SPACE MAINTAINERS (800-899)

Allowances include all adjustments within six months following installation.

800	Fixed space maintainer (band type)	35.00

REMOVABLE ACRYLIC SPACE MAINTAINERS:

801	With stainless steel round wire rest only	40.00
802	Stainless steel clasps and/or activating wires, in addition per wire or clasp	5.00
803	Study models	5.00
810	Removable inhibiting appliance to correct thumbsucking	40.00
832	Fixed or cemented inhibiting appliance to correct thumbsucking	40.00
	Office visit for observation, adjustment and activation per visit	4.00

FRACTURES AND DISLOCATIONS (900-999)

900	Treatment of simple fracture of the maxilla, open reduction	200.00
901	Treatment of simple fracture of the maxilla, closed reduction	125.00
902	Treatment of simple fracture of the mandible, open reduction	230.00
903	Treatment of simple fracture of the mandible, closed reduction	125.00
904	Treatment of compound or comminuted fracture of the maxilla, closed reduction	200.00
905	Treatment of compound or comminuted fracture of the maxilla, open reduction	300.00
906	Treatment of compound or comminuted fracture of the mandible, closed reduction	200.00
907	Treatment of compound or comminuted fracture of the mandible, open reduction	300.00
910	Treatment of luxation (dislocation) of the mandible (uncomplicated)	8.00
911	Treatment of condylar fracture, open reduction ..	350.00
912	Treatment of condylar fracture, closed reduction .	150.00
913	Reduction of dislocation of temporomandibular joint	35.00
915	Treatment of malar fracture, simple, closed reduction	100.00
916	Treatment of malar fracture, simple or compound depressed, open reduction	200.00

B (Concluded)

Other Forms

California Dental Service has developed an Inquiry Form 495 (Fig. 11–3). This is used for group contract claims and also for the Denti-Cal program (see p. 282). Another new innovation is their Short Form (Fig. 11–4), which is an abbreviated version of their standard Attending Dentist's Statement. It is designed to save the Assistant valuable time when completing paperwork for patients who receive limited treatment during their visits. As you will notice, different procedure code numbers are preimprinted on the Short Form, with space to add in the last digit of the three-digit coding. The tooth chart has been eliminated. The Short Form can be used only for group contract payment requests and cannot be used for the Denti-Cal program. Figure 11–4 shows how the Short Form looks when completed.

STATE AND/OR FEDERAL GOVERNMENT–SPONSORED DENTAL PROGRAMS

Medicaid, authorized by Title XIX of the Social Security Act, is a federal-state grant-in-aid program designed to share the cost of providing health care to certain low-income persons. Each state has different guidelines regarding eligibility of recipients (see Chapter 5). It is important that children receive regular and periodic dental care from early childhood through their teens. Thus under Medicaid was established the Early and Periodic Screening, Diagnosis, and Treatment Program (EPSDT), which includes benefits for dental care. In California this program is called Denti-Cal and is administered by the California Dental Service (CDS). EPSDT benefits consist of:

1. Emergency services and operative procedures to control bleeding and pain, eliminate acute infection, prevent pulpal death, and treat injuries to the teeth and surrounding structures.
2. *Preventive Services:*
    a. Oral hygiene instruction
    b. Oral prophylaxis (cleaning of teeth)
3. *Therapeutic Services:*
    a. Pulp therapy
    b. Restoration of carious teeth
    c. Scaling and curettage
    d. Maintenance of space for posterior primary teeth lost prematurely
    e. Prosthetic appliances for impaired masticatory function

Information on state-sponsored dental programs is available from the Division or Bureau of Dental Health, care of your State Health Department.

Denti-Cal

Benefits

1. Prophylaxis for adults and prophy-fluoride for children age 6 to 18 years, limited to one treatment in each full 12-month period.
2. Relines
    a. Cold cure relines, limited to one per appliance in a full 12-month period.

△ **CDS INQUIRY FORM**

TO: **CALIFORNIA DENTAL SERVICE**
P. O. BOX 7736
SAN FRANCISCO, CALIFORNIA 94120

DATE _____

ATTN: Benefit Services Department

☐ CHECK HERE FOR DENTI-CAL OR VA

We would like to inquire regarding the treatment plan submitted for the patient indicated below.

PATIENT NAME	DENTI-CAL ID #
EMPLOYEE	SOCIAL SECURITY #

CDS GROUP #	UNION LOCAL	EMPLOYER NAME

AMOUNT OF CLAIM	DATE SUBMITTED	
$		☐ AUTH. ☐ PYMT.

DENTIST'S NAME	LICENSE #

CHECK APPROPRIATE NUMBERS:

☐ 1. Dual Coverage Case (list second coverage information): CARRIER NAME _____
   EMP. _____ S.S. # _____ GR. # _____

☐ 2. Payment not received.

☐ 3. Authorization not received.

☐ 4. Amount of CDS payment does not appear correct. PAYMENT # _____

☐ 5. Cannot identify patient in this office. CHECK # _____ PAYMENT # _____

☐ 6. Verify deductible, previously satisfied. PAYMENT # _____

☐ 7. Verify maximum for _____ (YEAR) ; patient believes not yet reached.

☐ 8. Dentist's fees appear to have been adjusted in error. (Latest fee revisions accepted on _____)
   PRO. # _____ TOOTH # _____

☐ 9. Patient advises he is eligible for denied services in month(s) of _____

☐ 10. CDS authorization time for this case has expired. Please grant extension of eligibility for month of _____
   (Not applicable to Denti-Cal).

☐ 11. Other: _____
   _____

EXPLANATION AND/OR COMMENTS: _____
_____
_____
_____

PLEASE RESPOND TO:

CDS WILL RESPOND ON REVERSE SIDE OF THIS FORM

NAME

STREET ADDRESS

LICENSE # (IF APPLICABLE)
PHONE #
AREA CODE
/ —

CITY, STATE   _ZIP CODE_

CDS FORM #495

A

FIGURE 11–3

California Dental Service Inquiry Form 495, used for both group and Denti-Cal follow-up inquiries.

NOTE: THIS SIDE WILL BE COMPLETED BY CALIFORNIA DENTAL SERVICE TO ANSWER YOUR INQUIRY

IN REPLY TO YOUR INQUIRY, PLEASE REFER TO ITEM CIRCLED:

1. The treatment planning form for this patient was authorized and returned to your office for signature and/or dates of service. If you have not received the original authorization, please advise and we will send you a duplicate.

2. Our check #_____ issued _____ included payment for services provided this patient.

3. Payment for services provided this patient will be issued on _____ .

4. Dual Coverage is involved in this case and CDS is secondary carrier. We are unable to make payment until _____ _____ as primary carrier, has made payment. If you have information as to the amount paid by the primary carrier, please advise immediately.

5. Under the provisions of the contractual agreement, treatment planning forms received for patient(s) covered by this group are computed on the _____ Table of Allowances.

6. Patient's name on check # _____ is _____ , Social Security # _____ , Denti-Cal Identification # _____ .

7. Under the provisions of the contractual agreement with this group, for covered benefits, CDS will pay _____ % of the CDS Table of Allowances. In addition to this portion of the Table, the patient is also responsible for the difference between the dentist's usual fees and the Table amounts, any optional services plus the deductible and excess of maximum if applicable.

8. Supplemental payment in the amount of $ _____ will be made. We apologize for an error made by CDS in computation.

9. A brief description of this patient's dental coverage is: Fee Basis _____ ; Co-payment, Basic _____ %; Prosthodontic _____ %; Deductible _____ (_____); Maximum _____ per calendar year.

10. Under the provisions of the contractual agreement with this group, CDS agrees to pay _____ % for basic and _____ % for prosthodontic services based upon the usual and customary fees for CDS participating member dentists. Our records indicate that Dr. _____ is not a participating member dentist; therefore, payment for the services performed is based upon the CDS Table of Allowances. A copy of the treatment planning form is enclosed.

11. Under the provisions of the contractual agreement with this group, there is an initial/annual $ _____ deductible. (Services were provided in two calendar years; two separate deductibles have been taken to satisfy each year.)

12. The total amount of the treatment plan has been credited toward the patient's deductible.

13. The claim is being held pending verification of eligibility from the Trust/School District/Employer.

14. CDS records indicate this patient did not become eligible for dental benefits under this group until _____ _____ . Any service provided prior to that time is the responsibility of the patient.

15. Under the provisions of the contractual agreement with this group, no payment for services performed for this patient can be made, as benefits terminate as of age _____ .

16. Under the provisions of the DENTI-CAL Contractual Agreement, payment for Procedure # _____ , performed for this patient, cannot be made, as benefits terminate as of age _____ .

17. This DENTI-CAL patient reached the age of 18 on _____ , after which date services were computed on the "Adult Table of Allowances".

18. Group # _____ terminated coverage with CDS on _____ . Please send inquiries concerning dental claims to _____ .

19. Payment was made according to dates of service indicated on the attached copy of the treatment form. If the services completed are different from those paid by CDS, please submit a new form with appropriate dates of service. Be sure to obtain the necessary signatures.

20. CDS has no record of receiving a treatment form for this patient. Please submit a new form marked "Duplicate". Be sure to indicate dates of service and obtain the necessary signatures.

21. Authorization time has been extended through _____ , 197____ . PLEASE ATTACH THIS NOTICE OF EXTENSION TO YOUR ORIGINAL WHITE COPY WHEN SUBMITTING FOR PAYMENT.

22. _____
_____
_____
_____

B   **FIGURE 11–3** *(Continued)*

FIGURE 11-4

California Dental Service Form 105-A Short Form 500M, showing proper completion.

b. Laboratory-processed relines, limited to one per appliance in a full 12-month period.
c. Tissue conditioning, limited to two per appliance for a full 12-month period.

3. Dentures

Prior authorization may be granted for full dentures, removable partial dentures that are necessary for the balance of a complete artificial denture, stayplates, and reconstructions of removable dentures only in the following circumstances:

a. The beneficiary cannot be employed without such prostheses and the need is documented by certification of the Department of Rehabilitation; or

b. The dentures are necessary to prevent a significant disability. "Significant disability" must be documented by certification from both the treating dentist and the beneficiary's physician, with authorization or approval by a Medi-Cal consultant, showing that dentures are essential to masticate foods that the beneficiary requires in the treatment of a specific medical condition for which the patient is currently under medical care. Prior authorization for the dentures must be obtained before extraction of the teeth, unless the case is an emergency.

Prior authorization is required for the following:

1. Space maintainer (but not for extraction).
2. When more than one pulpotomy must be done.
3. When more than one steel crown is needed.

Claims Procedure

See Figure 11–6 for proper location of Proof of Eligibility (POE) label for month of service. See Instructions for Completion of the Attending Dentist's Statement (pp. 286–292).

Health Maintenance Organizations

If the dentist is a member of a Health Maintenance Organization (HMO), the doctor is paid a fixed monthly or annual sum per patient. This cost is paid in part by the subscriber and in part by the employer or by the government. The dentist is expected to provide all the basic dental care necessary to keep the patient healthy (see Chapter 10).

CHAMPUS and CHAMPVA

Refer to Chapter 7 for eligibility, description of the program, and other pertinent information.

Dental Benefits

1. Care for accidental injury to teeth or supporting structures, or oral surgery.
2. Care for pregnant women with dental problems related to the pregnancy.
3. Orthodontic care for severe malocclusion may be covered under the CHAMPUS Program for the Handicapped.

Claims Procedure in California

1. Use the California Dental Service (CDS) Treatment Form No. 105 (Attending Dentist's Statement) and attach the CHAMPUS Form 1863-2 (see Chapter 7, Fig. 7–7.)
2. Send the claim to the fiscal intermediary (see Chapter 7).

Veterans Administration Dental Program

The veteran-patient will supply the dentist with a special VA treatment form and instruction sheet from his VA office. The dentist's examination finding and treatment recommendations are entered on this claim, using the proper procedure numbers and the dentist's usual and customary fees. Mail the completed treatment form and x-rays to the appropriate VA office. See Chapter 7 for information on eligibility, description of program, and list of VA offices.

Eligibility and benefits will be established and authorized by the VA. In California the forms are then transmitted to California Dental Service (CDS), where payment is made by CDS based on usual, customary, and reasonable fees for CDS-participating member dentists. For all other dentists payment is based on customary fees.

The amount payable shown on the approved treatment form is the maximum amount allowable for the service authorized, and in no event may the veteran-patient be asked to pay an additional fee for an authorized service.

Approval by the VA is required prior to payment of any case for which charges involve an additional cost in excess of $130. Both the veteran-patient and dentist must sign the treatment form. Submit the case for payment within 90 days after treatment. If the veteran-patient does not report for treatment within 60 days after authorization is given, then return the form to the VA or in California to CDS.

UNIVERSAL CLAIM FORM – ATTENDING DENTIST'S STATEMENT

In 1973 the American Dental Association took steps to develop a universal claim form that would be acceptable to all prepayment carriers. The task force was composed of representatives from the Delta Dental Plans Association, the National Association of Blue Shield Plans, the Blue Cross Association, and the Health Insurance Association of American (HIAA). In April of 1975 the Council on Dental Care Programs of the American Dental Association approved the first ADA-sponsored Universal Claim Form (Fig. 11–5).

When a patient brings in a form provided by a third party carrier, the section completed by the patient and/or dentist is always the same. Other areas on the form, such as at the very top and bottom, are open to individual use by different carriers. The location of signature blocks also varies with the discretion of the carrier. Various company forms may look different by virtue of color, coding, shading, or use of the open areas, but the sections of concern to the dentist are uniform (compare Figs. 11–5 and 11–6). The statement, "Form Approved by the Council on Dental Care Programs of the ADA 1975," appears on all claim forms that maintain the ADA-standardized format.

Use of an ADA-approved carrier form brought in by the patient will speed handling and reduce office costs. Printed at the very bottom of the ADA-approved form are logos for the Delta Dental Plans Association and HIAA (see Fig. 11–5). Exceptions to use of the uniform form are state and federal Medicaid programs. However, California Dental Service (CDS), the fiscal intermediary for the Denti-Cal program, features a form which is based on the universal claim form and is used for both group contracts and the Denti-Cal program (see Figs. 11–6 and 11–7).

TO THE STUDENT: For further information on insurance terminology, refer to Chapter 1.

Instructions for Completion of the Attending Dentist's Statement (Fig. 11–5 and Assignments 28 and 29, pp. 606–610)

Note: In the following instructions for completion of the Universal Claim Form, information for Denti-Cal patients is given in parentheses.

1. *Patient Name:* Enter the first name, middle initial, and last name. Give surname if it is different, as for foster child. If the patient is the employee (same as Item 6), no entry is needed in Item 1 and "self" should be marked in Item 2. (For a Denti-Cal patient, Items 1 and 6 should be the same. A Denti-Cal patient is always considered the employee.)

ATTENDING DENTIST'S STATEMENT

CHECK ONE:

☐ DENTIST'S PRE-TREATMENT ESTIMATE
☐ DENTIST'S STATEMENT OF ACTUAL SERVICES

CARRIER-NAME AND ADDRESS

PATIENT SECTION

1. PATIENT NAME
2. RELATIONSHIP TO EMPLOYEE   SELF   SPOUSE   CHILD   OTHER   3. SEX   M   F   4. PATIENT BIRTHDATE   MO.   DAY   YEAR   5. IF FULL TIME STUDENT   SCHOOL   CITY

6. EMPLOYEE/SUBSCRIBER NAME   FIRST   MIDDLE   LAST
7. EMPLOYEE/SUBSCRIBER SOCIAL SECURITY NO.
9. NAME OF GROUP DENTAL PROGRAM

8. EMPLOYEE/SUBSCRIBER MAILING ADDRESS
CITY, STATE, ZIP
10. EMPLOYER (COMPANY) NAME AND ADDRESS

11. GROUP NUMBER   12. LOCATION (LOCAL)   13. ARE OTHER FAMILY MEMBERS EMPLOYED?   EMPLOYEE NAME   SOC. SEC. NO.   14. NAME AND ADDRESS OF EMPLOYER IN ITEM 13

15. IS PATIENT COVERED BY ANOTHER DENTAL PLAN?   DENTAL PLAN NAME   UNION LOCAL   GROUP NO.   NAME AND ADDRESS OF CARRIER

I HAVE REVIEWED THE FOLLOWING TREATMENT PLAN. I AUTHORIZE RELEASE OF ANY INFORMATION RELATING TO THIS CLAIM.

▶

SIGNED (PATIENT, OR PARENT IF MINOR)   DATE

I HEREBY AUTHORIZE PAYMENT DIRECTLY TO THE BELOW-NAMED DENTIST OF THE GROUP INSURANCE BENEFITS OTHERWISE PAYABLE TO ME.

▶

SIGNED (INSURED PERSON)   DATE

DENTIST SECTION

16. DENTIST NAME
24. IS TREATMENT RESULT OF OCCUPATIONAL ILLNESS OR INJURY?   NO   YES   IF YES, ENTER BRIEF DESCRIPTION AND DATES

17. MAILING ADDRESS
25. IS TREATMENT RESULT OF AUTO ACCIDENT?
26. OTHER ACCIDENT?

CITY, STATE, ZIP
27. ARE ANY SERVICES COVERED BY ANOTHER PLAN?

18. DENTIST SOC. SEC. OR T.I.N.   19. DENTIST LICENSE NO.   20. DENTIST PHONE NO.
28. IF PROSTHESIS, IS THIS INITIAL PLACEMENT?   (IF NO, REASON FOR REPLACEMENT)   29. DATE OF PRIOR PLACEMENT

21. FIRST VISIT DATE CURRENT SERIES   22. PLACE OF TREATMENT   OFFICE   HOSP   ECF   OTHER   23. RADIOGRAPHS OR MODELS ENCLOSED?   NO   YES   HOW MANY?   30. IS TREATMENT FOR ORTHODONTICS?   IF SERVICES ALREADY COMMENCED, ENTER   DATE APPLIANCES PLACED   MOS. TREATMENT REMAINING

IDENTIFY MISSING TEETH WITH "X"   31. EXAMINATION AND TREATMENT PLAN - LIST IN ORDER FROM TOOTH NO. 1 THROUGH TOOTH NO. 32 - USE CHARTING SYSTEM SHOWN.   FOR ADMINISTRATIVE USE ONLY

FACIAL

RIGHT   LEFT   UPPER   PERMANENT   PRIMARY   LINGUAL   LOWER

FACIAL

32. REMARKS FOR UNUSUAL SERVICES

TOOTH # OR LETTER	SURFACE	DESCRIPTION OF SERVICE (INCLUDING X-RAYS, PROPHYLAXIS, MATERIALS USED, ETC.) LINE NO.	DATE SERVICE PERFORMED MO. DAY YEAR	PROCEDURE NUMBER	FEE

SEE REVERSE SIDE FOR ORDER INFORMATION

I HEREBY CERTIFY THAT THE PROCEDURES AS INDICATED BY DATE HAVE BEEN COMPLETED.

▶

SIGNED (DENTIST)   DATE

TOTAL FEE CHARGED	
MAX. ALLOWABLE	
DEDUCTIBLE	
CARRIER %	
CARRIER PAYS	
PATIENT PAYS	

Delta Dental Plans Assoc.

Form Approved by the Council on Dental Care Programs of the A.D.A. 1975

ADS (75)

FIGURE 11-5

Attending Dentist's Statement (ADS 75) Universal Claim Form, approved by the Council on Dental Care Programs of the American Dental Association in 1975.

RETAIN LAST COPY FOR YOUR FILES. MAIL ALL OTHER COPIES TO PLAN.
* IF PREDETERMINATION, PLAN WILL COMPLETE DATES FROM AND THRU IMMEDIATELY BELOW
IF SERVICE WILL EXTEND BEYOND THRU DATE YOU MUST INQUIRE TO PLAN FOR CONFIRMATION OF CONTINUED ELIGIBILITY (SEE DENTISTS HANDBOOK)

STAPLE X RAYS (NOT REQUIRED FOR AMALGAMS, PLASTICS, SILICATES, EXCEPT FOR DENTI-CAL PATIENTS) TO TOP RIGHT CORNER OF FORMS.

TYPE OR PRINT YOU ARE PREPARING MULTIPLE COPIES

CHECK HERE IF DENTI-CAL CLAIM ☒
AFFIX BELOW A MEDI-CAL PROOF OF ELIGIBILITY LABEL FOR EACH MONTH SERVICES WERE PROVIDED.

342349
SHADED AREA FOR CDS USE ONLY.

ATTENDING DENTIST'S STATEMENT SIGN BELOW FOR PREDETERMINATION * OR PAYMENT **

APPROVED BY w.f 4/8/75
FROM 3/14/75
THRU 5/8/75
MANUAL ELIGIBILITY ESTABLISHED

USE THIS NUMBER FOR INQUIRY

CALIFORNIA DENTAL SERVICE
P. O. BOX 7736
SAN FRANCISCO, CALIFORNIA 94120
A DELTA PLAN

1. PATIENT NAME	2. RELATIONSHIP TO EMPLOYEE	3. SEX	4. PATIENT BIRTHDATE	5. IF FULL TIME STUDENT
Roger B. Middleton	SELF X SPOUSE CHILD OTHER	M X F	MO 11 DAY 01 YEAR 27	SCHOOL / CITY

6. EMPLOYEE/SUBSCRIBER NAME — FIRST MIDDLE LAST
Roger B. Middleton
7. EMPLOYEE SOCIAL SECURITY NUMBER 422-14-4977
9. NAME OF GROUP DENTAL PROGRAM
POE Label for 3-77

JAN.	FEB.	JAN.	FEB.
MAR.	APR.	MAR.	APR.
MAY.	JUN.	MAY.	JUN.
JUL.	AUG.	JUL.	AUG.
SEP.	OCT.	SEP.	OCT.
NOV.	DEC.	NOV.	DEC.

8. EMPLOYEE MAILING ADDRESS
6767 Best Street
CITY, STATE, ZIP
Woodland Hills, CA 91364
10. EMPLOYER (COMPANY) NAME AND ADDRESS

11. GROUP NUMBER | 12. LOCATION (LOCAL) | 13. ARE OTHER FAMILY MEMBERS EMPLOYED? EMPLOYEE NAME SOC. SEC. NO. | 14. NAME AND ADDRESS OF EMPLOYER, ITEM 13

15. IS PATIENT COVERED BY ANOTHER DENTAL PLAN? No
DENTAL PLAN NAME | UNION LOCAL | GROUP NO. | NAME AND ADDRESS OF CARRIER

16. DENTIST NAME
Stanley Porter, DDS   8053
17. MAILING ADDRESS
4567 Broad Avenue   213/486-9002
CITY, STATE, ZIP
Woodland Hills, CA 91364

	NO	YES	IF YES, ENTER BRIEF DESCRIPTION AND DATES
24. IS TREATMENT RESULT OF OCCUPATIONAL ILLNESS OR INJURY?	X		
25. IS TREATMENT RESULT OF AUTO ACCIDENT?	X		
26. OTHER ACCIDENT?			
27. ARE ANY SERVICES COVERED BY ANOTHER PLAN?	X		

18. DENTIST SOC. SEC. NO. OR T.I.N. 62-9565990
19. DENTIST LICENSE NO. 8053
20. DENTIST PHONE NO. 213/486-9002
28. IF PROSTHESIS, IS THIS INITIAL PLACEMENT? IF NO, ENTER REASON FOR REPLACEMENT. X
29. DATE OF PRIOR PLACEMENT

21. FIRST VISIT DATE CURRENT SERIES 3-14-77
22. PLACE OF TREATMENT OFFICE X HOSP ECF OTHER
23. RADIOGRAPHS OR MODELS ENCLOSED? NO ☐ YES ☒ HOW MANY? 3
30. IS TREATMENT FOR ORTHODONTICS? NO X YES
IF SERVICES ALREADY COMMENCED ENTER → DATE APPLIANCES PLACED | MOS. TREATMENT REMAINING

IDENTIFY MISSING TEETH WITH "X"

31. EXAMINATION AND TREATMENT RECORD - LIST IN ORDER FROM TOOTH NO. 1 THROUGH TOOTH NO. 32. USE CHARTING SYSTEM SHOWN.

TOOTH # OR LETTER	SURFACES	DESCRIPTION OF SERVICE (INCLUDING X-RAYS, PROPHYLAXIS, MATERIALS USED, ETC.)	DATE SERVICE PERFORMED MO DAY YEAR	PROCEDURE NUMBER	FEE	USUAL AND CUSTOMARY ALLOWANCE
		<u>INCORRECT</u> Listing of Procedures				
		Three x-rays and exam	3 14 77	110	6 00	
		<u>CORRECT</u> Listing of Procedures				
		First x-ray	3 14 77	110	4 00	
		Two additional x-rays	3 14 77	111	2 00	
		Handy Hint: When listing additional x-rays it might be a good idea to indicate area filmed.				

32. REMARKS FOR UNUSUAL SERVICES

I ACCEPT THIS ATTENDING DENTIST'S STATEMENT AND AUTHORIZE RELEASE OF INFORMATION RELATING HERETO. I CERTIFY THE TRUTH OF ALL PERSONAL INFORMATION CONTAINED ABOVE. I AGREE TO BE RESPONSIBLE FOR PAYMENT FOR SERVICES PROVIDED DURING ANY INELIGIBLE PERIOD.

PATIENT (PARENT OR EMPLOYEE) SIGNATURE x Roger B. Middleton

! IMPORTANT !
WE HAVE REVIEWED AND APPROVED THIS ATTENDING DENTIST'S STATEMENT. THE COMPUTATIONS AND ANY ADJUSTMENTS MADE BY C.D.S.
x RBM   SP
PATIENT (EMPLOYEE)   DENTIST

* (PREDETERMINATION OF COST)
THE TREATMENT LISTED IS NECESSARY IN MY PROFESSIONAL JUDGMENT AND I REQUEST AUTHORIZATION IN ACCORDANCE WITH C.D.S. PARTICIPATING DENTIST RULES AND/OR DENTI-CAL RULES (See Reverse side of Page 4)

DENTIST SIGNATURE   DATE

** (TREATMENT COMPLETED - PAYMENT REQUESTED)
THE TREATMENT LISTED WAS COMPLETED AND WAS NECESSARY IN MY PROFESSIONAL JUDGMENT. I REQUEST PAYMENT IN ACCORDANCE WITH C.D.S. PARTICIPATING DENTIST RULES AND/OR DENTI-CAL RULES (See Reverse Side of Page 4)

DENTIST SIGNATURE Stanley Porter DDS   DATE 3/15/77

TOTAL FEE CHARGED	
PATIENT PAYS	
PLAN PAYS	
AMOUNT APPLIED TO DEDUCTIBLE	

PAYMENT OF ABOVE BALANCE SUBJECT TO PERCENT WITHHOLD AS APPROVED BY PLAN BOARD OF DIRECTORS

MARKED NUMBERS BELOW REFER TO ADJUSTMENTS AS EXPLAINED ON REVERSE SIDE OF PAGES 1, 2 & 3.

| 1 | 2 | 3 | 4 | 5 | 6 | 7 | 8 | 9 | 10 | 11 | 12 | 13 | 14 | 15 | 16 | 17 | 18 | 19 | 20 | 21 | 22 | 23 | 24 | 25 | 26 | 27 | 28 | 29 | 30 | 31 | 32 | 33 | 34 | 35 |
| 36 | 37 | 38 | 39 | 40 | 41 | 42 | 43 | 44 | 45 | 46 | 47 | 48 | 49 | 50 | 51 | 52 | 53 | 54 | 55 | 56 | 57 | 58 | 59 | 60 | 61 | 62 | 63 | 64 | 65 | 66 | 67 | 68 | 69 | 70 |

1. (SUBMIT TO CDS) - WHITE
2. (SUBMIT TO CDS) - GREEN
3. (SUBMIT TO CDS) - YELLOW
4. (RETAIN FOR YOUR FILES) - GOLDENROD

A SEPARATE FORM (CDS-505) LISTS DENTI-CAL PROCESSING POLICIES. CDS AND DENTI-CAL PARTICIPATION RULES ARE ON REVERSE SIDE OF PAGE 4 OF THIS FORM (CDS-105).

CDS 105 Rev. 9/75 ℗s   FORM APPROVED BY THE COUNCIL ON DENTAL CARE PROGRAMS OF THE A.D.A. 1975   1

IMPORTANT - WHEN PAYMENT IS MADE BY CDS, THE PATIENT WILL RECEIVE THIS FORM AS A NOTICE OF PAYMENT.

FIGURE 11-6

California Dental Service Form 105—Attending Dentist's Statement—showing incorrect and correct completion of the claim form as well as how manual eligibility is shown. Also shows correct placement of Proof of Eligibility (POE) Denti-Cal label.

RETAIN LAST COPY FOR YOUR FILES. MAIL ALL OTHER COPIES TO PLAN.

* IF PREDETERMINATION, PLAN WILL COMPLETE DATES FROM AND THRU IMMEDIATELY BELOW
IF SERVICE WILL EXTEND BEYOND THRU DATE YOU MUST INQUIRE TO PLAN FOR CONFIRMATION OF CONTINUED ELIGIBILITY (SEE DENTISTS HANDBOOK.)

STAPLE X-RAYS (NOT REQUIRED FOR AMALGAMS, PLASTICS, SILICATES, EXCEPT FOR DENTI-CAL PATIENTS) TO TOP RIGHT CORNER OF FORMS.

TYPE OR PRINT
YOU ARE PREPARING MULTIPLE COPIES

CHECK HERE IF DENTI-CAL CLAIM. ☐
AFFIX BELOW A MEDI-CAL PROOF OF ELIGIBILITY LABEL FOR EACH MONTH SERVICES WERE PROVIDED. SHADED AREA FOR CDS USE ONLY.

342348

ATTENDING DENTIST'S STATEMENT
SIGN BELOW FOR PREDETERMINATION * OR PAYMENT **

APPROVED BY
FROM
THRU

USE THIS NUMBER FOR INQUIRY
COMPUTER ELIGIBILITY ESTABLISHED
→ 7160 29811

CALIFORNIA DENTAL SERVICE
P. O. BOX 7736
SAN FRANCISCO, CALIFORNIA 94120
A DELTA PLAN

1. PATIENT NAME	Jane K. Freeman
2. RELATIONSHIP TO EMPLOYEE	SELF SPOUSE X / CHILD / OTHER
3. SEX	M / F X
4. PATIENT BIRTHDATE	MO. 10 DAY 10 YEAR 25
5. IF FULL TIME STUDENT SCHOOL / CITY	
6. EMPLOYEE/SUBSCRIBER NAME (FIRST MIDDLE LAST)	Robert M. Freeman
7. EMPLOYEE SOCIAL SECURITY NUMBER	
9. NAME OF GROUP DENTAL PROGRAM	Aerojet
8. EMPLOYEE MAILING ADDRESS	1234 Blank Street
CITY, STATE, ZIP	Sacramento, CA 95823
10. EMPLOYER (COMPANY) NAME AND ADDRESS	Aerojet — 20 Main St., Sacramento, CA
11. GROUP NUMBER	45
12. LOCATION (LOCAL)	Sacramento
13. ARE OTHER FAMILY MEMBERS EMPLOYED?	No
15. IS PATIENT COVERED BY ANOTHER DENTAL PLAN?	No

(Months grid: JAN. FEB. JAN. FEB. / MAR. APR. MAR. APR. / MAY. JUN. MAY. JUN. / JUL. AUG. JUL. AUG. / SEP. OCT. SEP. OCT. / NOV. DEC. NOV. DEC.)

16. DENTIST NAME	John Doe, DDS 13568
17. MAILING ADDRESS	4321 "K" Street 023/532-4124
CITY, STATE, ZIP	Sacramento, CA 95823
18. DENTIST SOC. SEC. NO. OR T.I.N.	222-28-3523
19. DENTIST LICENSE NO.	13568
20. DENTIST PHONE NO.	023/532-4124
21. FIRST VISIT DATE CURRENT SERIES	6-1-77
22. PLACE OF TREATMENT	OFFICE X HOSP ECF OTHER
23. RADIOGRAPHS OR MODELS ENCLOSED?	NO X YES

Question	NO	YES	IF YES, ENTER BRIEF DESCRIPTION AND DATES
24. IS TREATMENT RESULT OF OCCUPATIONAL ILLNESS OR INJURY?	X		
25. IS TREATMENT RESULT OF AUTO ACCIDENT?	X		
26. OTHER ACCIDENT?			
27. ARE ANY SERVICES COVERED BY ANOTHER PLAN?	X		
28. IF PROSTHESIS, IS THIS INITIAL PLACEMENT? IF NO, ENTER REASON FOR REPLACEMENT.	X		
30. IS TREATMENT FOR ORTHODONTICS?	X		

29. DATE OF PRIOR PLACEMENT
IF SERVICES ALREADY COMMENCED ENTER → DATE APPLIANCES PLACED / MOS. TREATMENT REMAINING

31. EXAMINATION AND TREATMENT RECORD - LIST IN ORDER FROM TOOTH NO. 1 THROUGH TOOTH NO. 32. USE CHARTING SYSTEM SHOWN.

TOOTH FOR LETTER	SURFACES	DESCRIPTION OF SERVICE (INCLUDING X-RAYS, PROPHYLAXIS, MATERIALS USED, ETC.)	DATE SERVICE PERFORMED MO. DAY YEAR	PROCEDURE NUMBER	FEE	USUAL AND CUSTOMARY ALLOWANCE
		INCORRECT Listing of Procedures				
28		Ceramco Crown Veneer		653		
29		Ceramco Pontic		692	245 00	
30		Gold Crown		660		
		or				
28						
29		Ceramco Bridge			245 00	
30						
		CORRECT Listing of Procedures				
28		Ceramco Crown		653	100 00	
29		Ceramco Pontic		692	80 00	
30		Gold Crown		660	65 00	

32. REMARKS FOR UNUSUAL SERVICES

I ACCEPT THIS ATTENDING DENTIST'S STATEMENT AND AUTHORIZE RELEASE OF INFORMATION RELATING HERETO. I CERTIFY THE TRUTH OF ALL PERSONAL INFORMATION CONTAINED ABOVE. I AGREE TO BE RESPONSIBLE FOR PAYMENT FOR SERVICES PROVIDED DURING ANY INELIGIBLE PERIOD.

PATIENT (PARENT OR EMPLOYEE) SIGNATURE   x Jane K. Freeman

! IMPORTANT !
WE HAVE REVIEWED AND APPROVED THIS ATTENDING DENTIST'S STATEMENT. THE COMPUTATIONS AND ANY ADJUSTMENTS MADE BY C.D.S.

x J.F. (PATIENT (EMPLOYEE))   J Doe (DENTIST)

TOTAL FEE CHARGED	
PATIENT PAYS	
PLAN PAYS	
AMOUNT APPLIED TO DEDUCTIBLE	

* **(PREDETERMINATION OF COST)**
THE TREATMENT LISTED IS NECESSARY IN MY PROFESSIONAL JUDGMENT AND I REQUEST AUTHORIZATION IN ACCORDANCE WITH C.D.S. PARTICIPATING DENTIST RULES AND/OR DENTI-CAL RULES (See Reverse side of Page 4)

DENTIST SIGNATURE   John Doe DDS   DATE 6/1/77

** **(TREATMENT COMPLETED - PAYMENT REQUESTED)**
THE TREATMENT LISTED WAS COMPLETED AND WAS NECESSARY IN MY PROFESSIONAL JUDGMENT. I REQUEST PAYMENT IN ACCORDANCE WITH C.D.S. PARTICIPATING DENTIST RULES AND/OR DENTI-CAL RULES (See Reverse Side of Page 4)

DENTIST SIGNATURE   John Doe, DDS   DATE 6/15/77

PAYMENT OF ABOVE BALANCE SUBJECT TO PERCENT WITHHOLD AS APPROVED BY PLAN BOARD OF DIRECTORS.

MARKED NUMBERS BELOW REFER TO ADJUSTMENTS AS EXPLAINED ON REVERSE SIDE OF PAGES 1, 2 & 3.

1 2 3 4 5 6 7 8 9 10 11 12 13 14 15 16 17 18 19 20 21 22 23 24 25 26 27 28 29 30 31 32 33 34 35
36 37 38 39 40 41 42 43 44 45 46 47 48 49 50 51 52 53 54 55 56 57 58 59 60 61 62 63 64 65 66 67 68 69 70

1. (SUBMIT TO CDS) - WHITE
2. (SUBMIT TO CDS) - GREEN
3. (SUBMIT TO CDS) - YELLOW
4. (RETAIN FOR YOUR FILES) - GOLDENROD

A SEPARATE FORM (CDS-505) LISTS DENTI-CAL PROCESSING POLICIES. CDS AND DENTI-CAL PARTICIPATION RULES ARE ON REVERSE SIDE OF PAGE 4 OF THIS FORM (CDS-105).

CDS 105 Rev. 9/75   FORM APPROVED BY THE COUNCIL ON DENTAL CARE PROGRAMS OF THE A.D.A. 1975
®s

1

Left margin (vertical): IMPORTANT - WHEN PAYMENT IS MADE BY CDS, THE PATIENT WILL RECEIVE THIS FORM AS A NOTICE OF PAYMENT.

IDENTIFY MISSING TEETH WITH "X"

FIGURE 11–7

California Dental Service Form 105—Attending Dentist's Statement—showing incorrect and correct completion of the claim form as well as how computer eligibility is shown.

2. *Relationship to Employee:* Check appropriate box for spouse or dependent child; "other" is used for stepchild, foster child, and so forth. Be sure to enter the legal relationship. This relationship sometimes affects the patient's eligibility as well as the level of benefits available. (For a Denti-Cal patient, either leave this section blank or mark "self".)

3. *Sex:* Mark appropriate box "M" for male or "F" for female. This is requested for identification purposes as well as for statistical analysis.

4. *Patient Birthdate:* Enter the patient's birthdate. This is necessary to verify eligibility. Benefits for certain groups are modified as to age for students, restricted for orthodontics, and so forth.

5. *If Full-Time Student:* For dependent children who are full-time students, enter the name of the school attended and the city where it is located. (Not applicable for Denti-Cal.) Eligibility of the patient may be affected if the patient is over a certain age and is still a full-time student.

6. *Employee/Subscriber Name:* This refers to the insured person and is not necessarily the patient. Enter first name, middle name or initial, and last name. (This is not applicable to Denti-Cal patients.)

7. *Employee/Subscriber Social Security Number:* This is for the employee named in Item 6; not the patient, unless the patient is the employee. This number is commonly used for computer and manual filing. (Denti-Cal requires only the patient's Social Security number, if available; if not, Denti-Cal will assign a "dummy" Social Security number.)

8. *Employee/Subscriber Mailing Address:* Enter employee's mailing address as shown in the patient's records. Be sure to include city and ZIP Code, since many times the insurance company will send a Notice of Payment to the employee after the Attending Dentist's Statement has been processed for payment. (For Denti-Cal patients enter the home address.)

9. *Name of Group Dental Program:* Enter the name of the employer, union, or trade designation which represents a group of employees or negotiated entities; such as United Auto Workers, John Doe School District, Plumbers Union, Aerojet-General, and so forth. (For Denti-Cal check the Denti-Cal box located on the top tab of the form and attach POE label(s) in this area.) (See Fig. 11–6.)

10. *Employer (Company) Name and Address:* List place of employment or name of association, if it is not identical to name of Group Dental Program in Item 9; for example, Ford Motor Company. (Not applicable for Denti-Cal.)

11. *Group Number:* The patient should provide this number at the time of his or her first visit. It refers to the master contract policy number or the complete number appearing on an identification card or in the employee's group brochure or letter. The omission of this number will cause delays and may result in the form being returned to the physician's office for additional identification. (Not applicable for Denti-Cal.)

12. *Location (Local):* This refers to the union local number or specific site where the insured employee works. (Not applicable for Denti-Cal.)

13. *Are Other Family Members Employed?* This refers to any other family member—such as wife, son, or daughter—who is employed elsewhere and who may have dental coverage. This helps in coordinating benefits with the dual coverage. Enter the family member's name and Social Security number.

14. *Name and Address of Employer in Item 13:* Enter the place of employment, name of group dental program, or association through which other family member (employee) has dental coverage.

15. *Is Patient Covered by Another Dental Plan;* Enter "yes" or "no." If "yes," give name of dental plan, union local, group number, and name and address of carrier. Like questions 13 and 14, this question indicates whether the patient is covered by other dental plans. The information contained in items 13, 14, and 15 is very important in determining which other carriers, if any, have primary liability for the treatment rendered. (If a Denti-Cal patient has dual coverage, Denti-Cal is always considered the secondary carrier.)

Patient Signature Block: Make sure the patient signs the appropriate signature block.

Insured Person's Signature Block: This block must be signed if the patient and/or dentist wish to have benefits paid directly to the provider. These signature blocks are optional in placement on the form and may appear elsewhere on third party forms.

*16. *Dentist Name:* Enter the dentist's name as recorded on his or her state license.

*17. *Mailing Address:* Enter the dentist's street address, city, state, and ZIP Code.

*18. *Dentist Social Security or Taxpayer Identification Number (TIN):* Enter the dentist's Social Security number or Taxpayer Identification number. If the dental office is incorporated, use the individual dentist license number rather than the incorporation number.

*19. *Dentist License Number:* Sometimes the license number is the key to the dentist's name and address in the insurance company's computer files, and to proper payment of the claim.

*20. *Dentist Phone Number:* Enter the dentist's phone number. It is helpful if the area code is also provided.

21. *First Visit Date Current Series:* This date is very important in determining what services are covered when a patient becomes eligible in the middle of an active treatment plan. *Do not leave blank.*

22. *Place of Treatment:* Check office, hospital, extended care facility (ECF), or other. When "other" applies, use entire space to identify location.

23. *Radiographs or Models Enclosed?* Check "yes" or "no" and indicate how many are enclosed. If other supporting materials are provided, identify these also. X-rays and models submitted should be properly labeled with the name and Social Security number (employee) of the patient and the dentist's name and license number. Staple the envelope containing *mounted* and *labeled* x-rays to the upper right corner of the form. If you forget to include the x-rays, *do not* submit them separately but wait until they are requested. X-rays may be required for inlays, onlays, individual crowns, fixed bridges, surgical extractions, impactions, and endodontic services. (Most Denti-Cal procedures require x-rays.)

24. *Is Treatment Result of Occupational Illness or Injury?* This refers to the possible application of Workers' Compensation, which would alter the coverage available and the carrier involved. This information is important for prompt and accurate claims processing and reimbursement.

25. *Is Treatment Result of Auto Accident?* This will affect reimbursement in no-fault auto insurance cases and also indicates whether another party may be responsible for reimbursement.

26. *Other Accident?* This is similar to items 24 and 25 in that it permits more accurate determination of appropriate coverage and liability.

---

*16, 17, 18, 19, 20: This information is sometimes preprinted on Attending Dentist's Statements.

27. *Are Any Services Covered by Another Plan?* This is asked as a means of double-checking information supplied by the patient in items 13, 14, and 15. The answer may also evolve from independent knowledge of the dentist.

28. *If Prosthesis, Is This Initial Placement?:* Most dental contracts have specific limitations on replacement of dentures, and this information is necessary to determine eligibility and liability.

29. *Date of Prior Placement:* Contracts specify time limitations or requirements concerning the placement or replacement of dentures.

30. *Is Treatment for Orthodontics?:* When such services are covered, dates and months of treatment remaining will affect the prorated monthly reimbursement made to the dentist. Not all commercial programs cover orthodontic treatment.

31. *Examination and Treatment Plan:* Indicate the tooth number or letter by using the diagram on the form. Indicate the tooth surface, such as mesial occlusal (MO). Describe the service rendered and date service will be or was performed. Using the insurance company booklet or confidential fee listing, indicate the procedure code number, which might be either three digit or five digit. Indicate the fee separately for each procedure code number and description of service. (If this is a Denti-Cal patient and you cannot determine what procedure code number to use for a specific procedure, use 999.)

32. *Remarks for Unusual Services:* Use this section for additional comments or more elaborate explanation of specific services resulting from complications or difficult cases. This may increase the fee, so proper justification must be given. If necessary supplementary material will not fit in this space, indicate "By Report" and attach a separate sheet to the claim.

Dentist Signature Block: The dentist signature block usually appears below the dentist treatment section. However, it may appear in different locations on third party forms. In some instances there may be two dentist signature blocks. One is for predetermination of cost and the other is signed when treatment has been completed and payment is requested.

Total Fee Charged: The columns under Total Fee Charged will be completed by the carrier and are optional in nature. They may vary somewhat from carrier to carrier. It is not necessary to indicate the Total Fee Charged by adding up the amounts on the claim. This will be completed by the carrier.

TOOTH CHART

On the Attending Dentist's Statement (see Figs. 11–5, 11–6, and 11–7) you will notice a picture on the lower left-hand side of the form that shows the primary (deciduous) teeth and the secondary (permanent) teeth. In the standard system of numbering and lettering teeth, the primary (deciduous) teeth are indicated by capital letters (e.g., the upper right second primary molar becomes tooth A, with the lower left second primary molar becoming tooth K) and the secondary (permanent) teeth are indicated by numbers. There are many different methods of charting (see Figs. 11–8 and 11–9). To look at another method of charting, see the patient dental history on page 609. If a tooth is going to be extracted, it might be marked out on the chart with an "X," or if it is a cavity which needs filling, it may be colored in (Fig. 11–9). To help you understand the chart on the insurance claim form, an enlarged tooth from the lower jaw has been abstracted from the form and is shown in Figure 11–10. This will explain the various tooth surfaces.

Sample method of entering coded information on jotting chart*

TOOTH NUMBER:

1. To be extracted = X
2. Linguo-occlusal inlay = LO
3. Mesio-occlusal cavity = MO
4. Disto-occlusal cavity = DO
5. Mesio-occlusal-distal amalgam = MOD
6. Full crown veneer, labial facing = FVC
7. Mesial, composite = M comp.
8. Distal, silicate = D sili
9. Labial or facial gingival cavity = CL V lab
10. Pontic-cantilever bridge = P
11. ¾ gold crown = ¾ GC
12.
13. Occlusal = O
14.
15. Disto-occlusal (distal pit) = DO pit
16. Missing = □
17. Missing = □
18. Occlusal = O
19. Mesio-occlusal-distal = MOD
20. Mesio-occlusal = MO
21. Disto-occlusal cavity = DO
22. Distal cavity = D
23.
24. Mesial cavity = M
25. Distal cavity = D
26. Mesial cavity = M
27. Distal cavity amalgam = D
28. Occlusal inlay = O
29. Occlusal amalgam = O
30. Disto-occlusal inlay = DO
31.

32. To be extracted = X

Record conditions on jotting chart using double ended colored pencil.

Restorations present (amalgam, gold or others). Mark on chart in *blue*.

Defect in restoration, needs replacement—outline in *red*.

Caries mark in *red* (solid).

A JOTTING CHART (Adult or child)

L R		U R
LOWER RIGHT		UPPER RIGHT
32	X	1*
31	LO	2
30		3
E 29		4 E
D 28		5 D
C 27		6 C
B 26		7 B
A 25		8 A
A 24		9 A
B 23		10 B
C 22		11 C
D 21		12 D
E 20		13 E
19		14
18		15
17		16
L L		U L
LOWER LEFT		UPPER LEFT

*NOTE: The dental office will have indicated the preferred manner of coding the teeth by numbers, i.e., the Palmer method, 1-8, quadrants, or the ADA Standardized system of numbering, 1-32, or a combination of numbers and letters, or the International, Federation Dentaire system of charting.

FIGURE 11-8

Streamlined charting—a system for recording conditions of the oral cavity during the clinical examination. (From J.A.D.A., March, 1971. Reprinted from *The Dental Assistant*, with permission from the American Dental Assistants Association.)

HELPFUL HINTS FOR FILING INSURANCE FORMS IN THE DENTAL OFFICE

1. Establish chronological tickler files for pending insurance claims. These should have tabs for each day of the month and master tabs for the 12 months of the year. Forms submitted for payment or prior authorization should be filed in the tickler file until payment is received or the authorized treatment form is returned to the dentist's office. The dental assistant should establish one chronological file folder for prior authorization and one for payment. Alphabetize within each date by the employee's last name. In this way all information needed to make an inquiry will be readily available if it is necessary to call the patient or follow up on a claim.

2. When a prior authorization claim is returned by the insurance company, remove the office copy from the tickler file and attach the authorized copies to the front of the office copy. Place them in the patient's file for completion of the services.

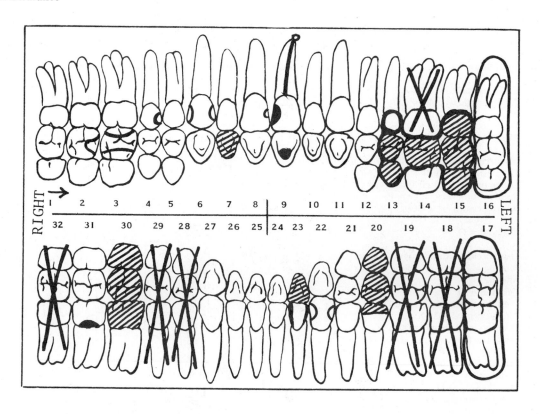

FIGURE 11-9

A clinical dental chart with conditions and restorations present.

Tooth number 1—erupted-mesial position; 2—MO caries; 3—MOD caries; 4—mesial caries; 6—distal and mesial caries; 7—ceramic jacket crown; 8—mesial caries; 9—completed root canal treatment, lingual-amalgam restoration; 13—full veneer gold crown; 14—missing-replaced with pontic; 15—full gold crown; (13, 14 and 15 are 3 unit fixed bridge); 16—impacted; 17—impacted; 18—missing; 19—missing; 20—gold onlay; 22—distal and mesial caries; 23—3/4 veneer gold crown; 28—missing; 29—missing; 30—full gold crown; 31—facial (gingival) foil restoration (Class V); 32—missing.

Alternate method of charting. Tooth number 14—to be extracted; 16—missing; 17—missing; 18—to be extracted; 19—to be extracted; 28—to be extracted; 29—to be extracted; 32—to be extracted.

Note: Missing dentition on the lower arch to be restored with a removable prosthetic appliance (removable partial denture). The authors realize there are many systems of charting human dentition; these samples represent only two of the systems. The chairside assistant must learn the charting symbols and method approved by the individual dentist.)

(From Torres and Ehrlich: *Modern Dental Assisting.* Philadelphia, W.B. Saunders Company, 1976, p. 488.)

When services have been completed, mail in the proper copy(ies) to the insurance company and place an office copy in the *payment tickler file* on the date the form for payment is submitted. When a check has been received from the insurance company, remove the office copy from the chronological file, indicate the date and amount paid, and place the form back in the patient's regular file. In this way, the dental assistant will never misplace a form or forget it is outstanding, because only those treatment forms that have received prior authorization and are awaiting the patient's visit, or those that have been completed and paid by the insurance company, will be in the patient's record file.

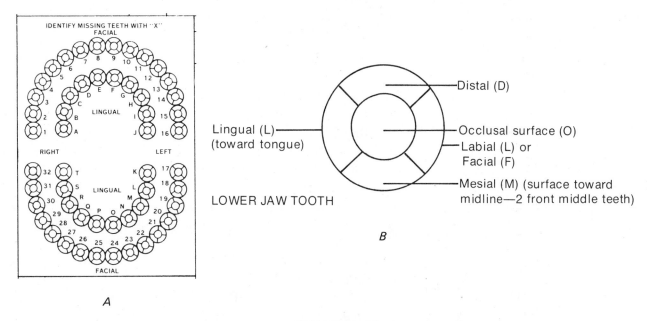

FIGURE 11–10

A, Tooth chart abstracted from the Attending Dentist's Statement (Form ADS 75). *B*, Enlarged picture of one tooth from the tooth chart to give proper terminology and abbreviations.

3. Check each tickler file on a daily basis.

4. Claim forms mailed for payment should be checked after 35 days have elapsed. If there is no response, send an inquiry to the insurance company indicating the employee name, Social Security number, group number, patient name, amount of the claim, and whether there is dual coverage. When writing to the California Dental Service (CDS), use Inquiry Form 495 (see Fig. 11–3). This form can be used for group, government, or state treatment plans.

5. To keep up to date and well informed, make sure the dentist is receiving any newsletters, bulletins, booklets, or handbooks available from the various insurance carriers. Some companies, such as CDS, put out both a monthly newsletter and a Dentist's Handbook that is revised from time to time.

TO THE STUDENT: Refer to the Appendix, Assignments 28 and 29, pp. 606–610, to complete the insurance forms and work with the patient histories pertinent to this chapter.

DENTAL ABBREVIATIONS AND SYMBOLS

Abbreviations

A/C	Adapt and cement (refers to bands)
ADA	American Dental Association
Adj NC	Adjustment No Charge when dentures are finished

amal	Amalgam (silver filling)
appl	Appliance
appt	Appointment
AW	Arch wire
B	Buccal; bicuspid (premolar)
BA	Broken appointment
bicusp	Bicuspid (premolar)
Bite appt	Appointment to check fit of patient's preliminary denture after confirming that it matches the impression
BO	Bucco-occlusal
Br	Bridge (replacement for missing teeth held by attachments to restored [abutment] teeth and usually not removable)
BW	Bitewing
BWX	Bitewing x-ray
C	Canine; crown
CAOH	Calcium hydroxide (alloy adaptic)
cap	Jacket
CDS	California Dental Service
Ceramco	Porcelain with metal
ChA	Chairside Assistant
CiA	Circulating Assistant
Cons	Consultation of the diagnosis
CR, CRN	Crown (fixed restoration covering natural tooth)
CRN (Cap)	Gold or stainless steel capping of tooth
CRN Cem	Crown is cemented in place
CRN Del	Crown delivery appointment; too th is restored back to chewing capacity and should feel very good.
Cr Prep	Crown preparation
d or D	Distal (back side of tooth away from lips)
DB	Debanding
DDS	Doctor of Dental Surgery
DEF rate	Decayed, Extracted, Filled rate
Dent Del	Dentures delivered or inserted
DI	Distoincisal
Diag	Diagnose
DL	Distolingual
DMD	Doctor of Dental Medicine
DMF rate	Decayed, Missing, Filled rate
DO	Disto-occlusal (back part and center) surface
Dr Ch	Dressing change for dry socket
D Socket	Dry socket (caused from lack of bleeding at time of extraction or other causes)
E	Exterior surface
Ed	Edentulous (toothless)
EPL	Esthetic profile
Ex	Examination

Ext	Extraction
F or Fac	Facial (surface)
F1 or F1$_2$	Fluoride (topical application to prevent caries)
FMX or FMXR	Full mouth x-rays
Fo	Foil
Full Mand Dent	Full lower denture
Full Max Dent	Full maxillary denture
G	Gold
G or Ging	Gingiva(e), gingival, the gums
Hbt	Habit
HG	Headgear
I	Interior (surface)
i	Incisor (deciduous), incisal ⎞ anterior tooth with
I	Incisor (permanent) ⎠ cutting edge
ICPMM	Incisors, Canines, Premolars, Molars
Imp	A co-alginate impression is taken of the patient's mouth and from there a true impression of the individual patient is made
Imp Appt	Appointment at which impressions are taken for a crown partial denture, or full denture
Impr	Impressions are made from which the gold crown is cast and at a later appointment cemented in the mouth
Impr Appt	Impression appointment for partial denture. Tooth and shade selection follows
In	Inlay (porcelain or gold dental restoration)
Inc	Incisal
L or Lab	Labial (toward the lips)
L	Lingual (toward the tongue)
L Dis	Lower discrepancy
LFD	See *Mand FD*
LL Part	Partial denture for lower left side of mouth
LO	Linguo-occlusal
LPD	See *Mand PD*
M	Molar (one of 12 posterior teeth, 6 on each side)
M	Mesial (toward center of mouth)
Mand FD	Mandibular Full Denture; also known as LFD
Mand PD	Mandibular Partial Denture; also known as LPD
max & mand	For full upper and lower dentures discussed at a consultation appointment
MC	Metacortilone
MFD	Maxillary full denture; also known as UFD
MI	Mesioincisal
MID	Mesioincisodistal
MIL	Mesiolinguodistal
ML	Mesiolingual
MO	Mesio-occlusal (2-surface cavity), middle and center

MOB	Mesio-occlusobuccal
MOD	Mesial, Occlusal, and Distal (3-surface cavity), front, middle, and back
MODBL	Mesio-occlusodistobuccolingual
MOFD	Mesial, Occlusal, Facial, and Distal surfaces
MPD	Maxillary Partial Denture; also known as UPD
N$_2$	Novocaine
NC	No Charge for brief adjustment
NS	No Show (regarding appointment)
O	Occlusal (part of tooth [center] or biting surface of opposing teeth)
OB	Overbite
Occ exp	Occlusion exposure
Onlay	Small gold replacement for silver
p	Pin, dowel
Pa #4	Single film
Pan	Panorex x-ray
Part Mand or Part Max	For a partial denture, also known as an appliance
PC	Pulp cap (capping exposed nerve with medicated substance before filling)
periap	Periapical (area of tooth around apex [tip] of the root)
Perio tr #1, #2, #3	Periodontia treatment (scaling of calculus from teeth to correct the condition)
PI	Porcelain inlay
PJC	Porcelain jacket crown
Pmt	Payment
pontic	Artificial tooth on fixed partial denture
PO	Pulpotomy (removal of the nerve)
Post op	Postoperative visit for suture removal (generally no charge)
Pres	Presentation of the diagnosis
Prob	Problems—mostly requiring examination appointment
Prophy	Prophylaxis (cleaning teeth through removal of calculus or tartar by scaling and polishing)
Pulp Cap	Pulpotomy or root canal
Quad only	Quadrant only (only a quarter of the mouth is done at one time when the procedure is involved, as it is quite painful to some)
R	Resin
RC	Root canal or pulpotomy
RCT or RC Therap	Root canal therapy (treatment of tooth with damaged pulp)
RDH	Registered Dental Hygienist
Reg Appt	See *Bite appt*
rest	Restoration: filling, inlay, crown, bridge, dentures, etc.
Ret	Retention or retainer
Rt C	Root canal
Rx	Prescription (antibiotic or other medication for infection, gum condition, etc.)

SC	Steel crown
Sel of teeth	Selection of the correct teeth and the shade the patient wishes to have them made in
Set	Appointment for set of crown, 2 weeks following impression; sometimes includes tooth number
Sili	Silicate
SM	Space maintainer; study models
SSCr	Stainless steel crown
St	Stitch or suture
Syn	Synthetic
TA	Toothache (with or without swelling)
TE	Tooth extraction
TM	Temporomandibular joint
Topical F1$_2$	Topical application of stannous fluoride
Tray Imp	Appointment at which an impression of the patient's arch is made from the tray that fits his or her mouth
Try In	Try in of actual teeth selected, set in pink wax only
TT	Tongue thrust
U & L	For full upper and lower dentures; discussed at a consultation appointment
U Dis	Upper discrepancy
UFD	Maxillary full denture; also known as MFD
UPD	Maxillary partial denture; also known as MPD
UR Partial	Upper right partial denture
W/F1$_2$	With fluoride
XB	Crossbite

Symbols

/ or M	Missing
X	Extraction

Symbols for Primary Teeth*

⌐A	Upper left A tooth
⌐B	Upper left B tooth
⌐C	Upper left C tooth
⌐D	Upper left D tooth
⌐E	Upper left E tooth
⌊A	Lower left A tooth
⌊B	Lower left B tooth
⌊C	Lower left C tooth
⌊D	Lower left D tooth
⌊E	Lower left E tooth
A⌐	Upper right A tooth

*These symbols correspond to Figure 11–9 on page 294. However, the tooth chart in Assignment 29 shows the left and right sides reversed from the way they are shown in this Figure, so keep in mind that symbols are variable in dental offices.

B⏌	Upper right B tooth
C⏌	Upper right C tooth
D⏌	Upper right D tooth
E⏌	Upper right E tooth
A⏋	Lower right A tooth
B⏋	Lower right B tooth
C⏋	Lower right C tooth
D⏋	Lower right D tooth
E⏋	Lower right E tooth

DENTAL INSURANCE ADDRESS LIST

National Dental Organizations

American Academy of Pedodontics
211 East Chicago Avenue, Suite 1235
Chicago, IL 60611

American Dental Association
211 East Chicago Avenue
Chicago, IL 60611

American Society of Dentistry for Children
211 East Chicago Avenue
Chicago, IL 60611

National Dental Association
P.O. Box 197
Charlottesville, VA 22902

State Dental Societies

The assistant may contact the local society by checking in the phone book under the state name, such as Alabama Dental Association, California Dental Association, Iowa Dental Association, and so forth.

Active Dental Service Corporations

Alabama
Delta Dental Plan of Alabama
P.O. Box 1572
Montgomery, AL 36102

Alaska
Delta Dental Plan of Alaska
P.O. Box 3-726
Anchorage, AK 99501

Arizona
Arizona Dental Service
4425 West Olive Avenue
Glendale, AZ 85302

California
California Dental Service
P.O. Box 7736
San Francisco, CA 94120

Colorado
Colorado Dental Service
1600 Downing Street
Denver, CO 80218

Florida
Florida Dental Services, Inc.
P.O. Box 5037
Jacksonville, FL 32207

Georgia
Delta Dental Plan of Georgia
22 Perimeter Center East, N.E.
Atlanta, GA 30346

Hawaii
Hawaii Dental Service
700 Bishop Street
Honolulu, HI 96813

Idaho
Delta Dental Plan of Idaho
903 Warren Street
Boise, ID 83706

Illinois
Illinois Dental Service
211 East Chicago Avenue
Chicago, IL 60611

Iowa
Delta Dental Plan of Iowa
636 Grand Avenue, Ruan Building
Des Moines, IA 50307

Kansas
Delta Dental Plan of Kansas
410 Petroleum Building
Wichita, KS 67202

Kentucky
Delta Dental Plan of Kentucky
3101 Bardstown Road
Louisville, KY 40205

Louisiana
Louisiana Dental Care Corporation
2100 St. Charles Avenue, Suite 1
New Orleans, LA 70130

Maine
Maine Dental Service Corporation
776 Main Street
Westbrook, ME 04092

Maryland
Maryland Dental Service Corporation
26 West Pennsylvania Avenue
Towson, MD 21204

Massachusetts
Massachusetts Dental Service
100 Summer Street
Boston, MA 02106

Michigan
Delta Dental Plan of Michigan
P.O. Box 416
Lansing, MI 48902

Minnesota
Delta Dental Plan of Minnesota
4570 West 77th Street
Minneapolis, MN 55435

Mississippi
Mississippi Dental Services, Inc.
P.O. Box 4205
Jackson, MS 39216

Missouri
Missouri Dental Service
2258 Schuetz Road
St. Louis, MO 63141

Montana
Delta Dental Plan of Montana
See *Delta Plan West.*

Nevada
Delta Dental Plan of Nevada
See *Delta Plan West.*

New Hampshire
New Hampshire Dental Service Corporation
23 School Street
Concord, NH 03301

New Jersey
New Jersey Dental Service Plan
141 South Harrison Street
East Orange, NJ 07018

New Mexico
Delta Dental Plan of New Mexico
7701-A Menaul Boulevard, N.E.
Albuquerque, NM 87110

New York
New York Dental Service Corporation
355 Lexington Avenue
New York, NY 10017

North Carolina
Delta Dental Plan of North Carolina
2310 Myron Drive
Raleigh, NC 27607

Ohio
Delta Dental Plan of Ohio
3620 North High Street
Columbus, OH 43214

Oklahoma
Delta Dental Plan of Oklahoma
2405 N.W. 39th Expressway
Oklahoma City, OK 73112

Oregon
Oregon Dental Service
200 South West Market
Portland, OR 97201

Pennsylvania
Delta Dental of Pennsylvania
23 Old Depot Road
New Cumberland, PA 17070

Rhode Island
Delta Dental Plan of Rhode Island
444 Westminster Mall
Providence, RI 02901

South Carolina
South Carolina Dental Health, Inc.
P.O. Box 8535, Station "A"
Greenville, SC 29604

South Dakota
Delta Dental Plan of South Dakota
P.O. Box 1194
Pierre, SD 57501

Tennessee
Delta Dental Plan of Tennessee
1916 Division Street
Nashville, TN 37203

Utah
Delta Dental Plan of Utah
See *Delta Plan West*.

Vermont
Vermont Dental Service
1109 North Avenue
Burlington, VT 05401

Virginia
Virginia Dental Service Plan, Inc.
1328 Third Street, S.W.
Roanoke, VA 24016

Washington
Washington Dental Service
2208 N.W. Market Street
Seattle, WA 98107

West Virginia
Delta Dental Plan of West Virginia
P.O. Box 728
Charleston, WV 25323

Wisconsin
Wisconsin Dental Service
P.O. Box 26
Stevens Point, WI 54481

Wyoming
Wyoming Dental Service
813 East 16th Street
Cheyenne, WY 82001

Delta Plan West

Includes:
Delta Dental Plan of Montana
Delta Dental Plan of Nevada
Delta Dental Plan of Utah

All correspondence should be
directed to:

Delta Plan West
65 West Louise Avenue
Salt Lake City, UT 84115

or

Dr. Everett L. Lynn
1400 – 8th Avenue
Helena, MT 59601

Inactive Dental Service Corporations

Arkansas
Arkansas Dental Service Corporation
P.O. Box 337
Arkadelphia, AR 71923

District of Columbia
Dental Health Service Corporation
of the District of Columbia
1300 Massachusetts Avenue, N.W.
Washington, D.C. 20005

Nebraska
Nebraska Dental Service Corporation
310 West 6th Street
York, NE 68467

North Dakota
North Dakota Dental Service Corporation
610 Gate City Building
Fargo, ND 58102

Insurance Companies Offering Group Dental Care Coverage

Aetna Life & Casualty
151 Farmington Avenue
Hartford, CT 06115

Bankers Life Company
711 High Street
Des Moines, IA 50307

Beneficial Standard Life Insurance Co.
3700 Wilshire Boulevard
Los Angeles, CA 90010

Benefit Trust Life Insurance Co.
1771 Howard Street
Chicago, IL 60626

Businessmen's Assurance Co.
BMA Tower, P.O. Box 458
Kansas City, MO 64141

California-Western States Life
Insurance Co.
2020 L Street
Sacramento, CA 95814

CNA/ insurance
CNA Plaza
Chicago, IL 60685

Colonial Life Insurance Company
of America
111 Prospect Street
East Orange, NJ 07019

Conger Life Insurance Co.
5050 Biscayne Boulevard
Miami, FL 33147

Connecticut General Life Insurance Co.
Hartford, CT 06115

Continental Assurance Co.
333 South Wabash Avenue
Chicago, IL 60685

Continental Casualty Co.
310 South Michigan Avenue
Chicago, IL 60604

Employers Insurance of Wausau
2000 Westwood Drive
Wausau, WI 54401

The Equitable Life Assurance Society
of the United States
1285 Avenue of the Americas
New York, NY 10019

Federal Life and Casualty Co.
78 West Michigan Avenue
Battle Creek, MI 49016

General American Life Assurance Co.
1501 Locust Street
St. Louis, MO 63103

Great Southern Life Insurance Co.
3121 Buffalo Speedway
Houston, TX 77006

The Guardian Life Insurance
Company of America
201 Park Avenue South
New York, NY 10003

Guardsman Life Insurance Co.
1025 Ashworth Road
Des Moines, IA 50265

Gulf Atlantic Life Insurance Co.
P.O. Box 1054
Dallas, TX 75221

Gulf Life Insurance Co.
1301 Gulf Life Drive
Jacksonville, FL 32207

Hartford Life and Accident Insurance Co.
Hartford Plaza
Hartford, CT 06115

Hartford Life Insurance Co.
Hartford Plaza
Hartford, CT 06115

Home Life Insurance Co.
253 Broadway
New York, NY 10007

Illinois Mutual Life & Casualty Co.
411 Liberty Street
Peoria, IL 61602

Independent Liberty Life Insurance Co.
126 Ottawa Avenue, N.W.
Grand Rapids, MI 49502

John Hancock Mutual Life Insurance Co.
200 Berkeley Street
Boston, MA 02151

Liberty Mutual Insurance Co.
175 Berkeley Street
Boston, MA 02117

Life Insurance Company of Virginia
914 Capitol Street
Richmond, VA 23219

Lincoln National Life Insurance Co.
1301 South Harrison Street
Fort Wayne, IN 46801

Massachusetts Mutual Life Insurance Co.
1295 State Street
Springfield, MA 01111

Metropolitan Life Insurance Co.
One Madison Avenue
New York, NY 10010

The Midland Mutual Life Insurance Co.
250 East Broad Street
Columbus, OH 43215

Monumental Life Insurance Co.
Charles and Chase Streets
Baltimore, MD 21202

Mutual of Omaha Insurance Co.
Dodge at 33rd Street
Omaha, NE 68131

National Casualty Co.
2833 Telegraph Road
Southfield, MI 48076

Nationwide Life Insurance Co.
246 North High Street
Columbus, OH 43216

New York Life Insurance Co.
51 Madison Avenue
New York, NY 10010

Northeastern Life Insurance
  Company of New York
919 Third Avenue
New York, NY 10022

Occidental Life Insurance
  Company of California
Hill & Olive at 12th Street
Los Angeles, CA 90051

Pacific Mutual Life Insurance Co.
523 West Sixth Street
Los Angeles, CA 90014

Paul Revere Life Insurance Co.
Worcester, MA 01608

Pilot Life Insurance Co.
Box 20727
Greensboro, NC 27420

Provident Life and Accident
  Insurance Co.
Fountain Square
Chattanooga, TN 37402

Provident Mutual Life Insurance
  Company of Philadelphia
4601 Market Street
Philadelphia, PA 19139

The Prudential Insurance Company
  of America
Prudential Plaza
Newark, NJ 07101

Republic National Life Insurance Co.
3988 North Central Expressway
Dallas, TX 75204

Sentry Life Insurance Co.
1421 Strongs Avenue
Stevens Point, WI 54481

State Mutual Life Assurance Company
   of America
440 Lincoln Street
Worcester, MA 01605

The Travelers Insurance Co.
One Tower Square
Hartford, CT 06115

The Union Central Life Insurance Co.
Mill and Waycross Roads
Cincinnati, OH 45240

Washington National Insurance Co.
1630 Chicago Avenue
Evanston, IL 60201

Zurich American Life Insurance Co.
111 West Jackson Blvd.
Chicago, IL 60604

Nonprofit Dental Insurance Plan

Group Health Dental Insurance, Inc.
227 West 40th Street
New York, NY 10018

Companies Writing Individual (and Group)
   Dental Insurance

Conger Life Insurance Co.
5050 Biscayne Blvd.
Miami, FL 33147

Illinois Mutual Life & Casualty
411 Liberty Street
Peoria, IL 61602

Mutual of Omaha Insurance Co.
Dodge at 33rd Street
Omaha, NE 68131

Blue Cross/Blue Shield Plans Offering Dental Coverage

Alabama	Kentucky	North Dakota
Arizona	Maine	Ohio
Arkansas	Maryland	Oregon
California	Massachusetts	Pennsylvania
Colorado	Michigan	Puerto Rico
Connecticut	Minnesota	Rhode Island
Delaware	Mississippi	South Carolina
District of Columbia	Missouri	South Dakota
Florida	Montana	Tennessee
Georgia	Nebraska	Texas
Hawaii	Nevada	Utah
Idaho	New Hampshire	Virginia
Illinois	New Jersey	Washington
Indiana	New Mexico	West Virginia
Iowa	New York	Wisconsin
Kansas	North Carolina	Wyoming

To obtain further information about these plans, contact the Blue Cross/Blue Shield office nearest you by referring to Chapter 4, pages 82–86.

REVIEW
QUESTIONS

1. Delta Dental Plans provide _____ dental care coverage on a group basis.

2. Explain the difference between the dentist's fee profile and the physician's fee profile. _____

_____

3. Name the two types of dental coverage.

a. _____

b. _____

4. Explain in your own words how incentive plans work.

_____

_____

_____

_____

5. When is it usually necessary to obtain prior authorization for dental care?

_____

6. Name three reasons why dentists may prefer to submit the treatment form in advance or prior to treatment.

a. _____

b. _____

c. _____

7. Dental fees are based on what two variations?

a. _____

b. _____

8. What does Blue Cross use for coding dental services? _____

_____ How many digits is it? _____

9. If a patient comes in with two group policies from the same insurance carrier, what claim forms need to be submitted? _____

_____

10. What does CDS mean? _____

11. People may receive dental care under the Medicaid program.   T   F

12. Health Maintenance Organizations do not provide dental care.   T   F

13. What is the name of the Medicaid program in California that handles dental care? _____

14. Define these abbreviations.

a. d _____   e. DO _____

b. MOD _____   f. DMF _____

c. m _____   g. ADA _____

d. MO _____   h. DEF _____

15. What do these tooth surfaces mean?

a. lingual _____   e. labial _____

b. distal _____   f. mesial _____

c. occlusal _____

16. California Dental Service is the fiscal intermediary for what state and/or government programs? _____

_____

17. When submitting x-rays with a treatment form, where are they placed on the claim? _____

18. What identification information must x-rays have written on them when submitted with the treatment form? _____

_____

19. When submitting a Denti-Cal claim, what form is used?_____

_____

20. What kind of Medi-Cal identification label is required on a Denti-Cal claim?

_____

Notes:

Notes:

12

Computerized Billing and Insurance*

BEHAVIORAL
OBJECTIVES The Assistant should be able to:

1. State the different ways in which a medical office can utilize a computer system.
2. Explain reasons why a physician would elect to go on a computer system.
3. Learn what to consider before adopting a computer system.
4. Become familiar with the computer coding used for diagnosis and description of services.
5. Identify input and output from the computer.
6. Learn how to complete a Patient Visit Slip.
7. Define Computer terminology and interpret abbreviations.
8. Recognize which output documents are of the most value in a medical practice.
9. Learn how to go over the insurance forms after they have been fed out of the computer to make sure that they are properly completed.
10. Discover what information on computerized patient statements is different from that on manual billing statements.
11. Learn how to follow up on delinquent accounts.

INTRODUCTION

With the advent of automation and the development of larger, multispecialty medical practices has come an increased use of the computer in billing and processing of insurance forms in the medical office. The computer systems available to a medical practice are of three principal types:

1. An *office computer*, which is a machine that can be purchased. This has a limited input capacity, a limited number of users, and a limited lifetime, but it can be utilized independently either by a single physician or by a group practice.

2. The *remote terminal system*, in which information is sent daily from the physician's office by mail or messenger to a bank or data processing center, which then feeds the information into the computer memory. This can accommodate many users because it has a large computer and extensive memory capacity. The user pays a monthly fee for each active account and also may pay a basic charge for each itemized statement or insurance form fed as output from the computer.

*Note: All forms in this chapter are reproduced courtesy of Intellectron International (The Medcobill System), Van Nuys, California.

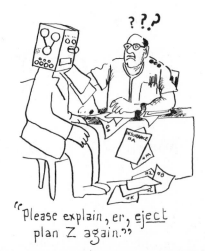

"Please explain, er, eject plan Z again."

3. The *time-share system*, which utilizes a telephone device from the physician's office to feed input into the computer memory. This system can also accommodate many users simultaneously through a large computer and memory. The users share the operating expense. Another major step forward in computer billing is a "talking computer." It gives a patient's up-to-the-minute account balance in reply to doctor/patient I.D. codes sent by Touch-Tone phone, eliminating the need for ledger cards in the office.

There are several reasons why a physician may elect to go onto a computerized billing system. They are:

1. The overhead is lower than under the standard bookkeeping, billing, and collecting procedures.

2. The physician may have better management control and more current information at his disposal.

3. Office efficiency may be increased.

4. The physician may expand his practice more conveniently.

5. Accounts receivable may be monitored more accurately.

6. Collections may be improved.

7. There is better security of records, since many computer firms issue a duplicate set of accounts.

Before a computer system is adopted, the physician should consider the following:

1. Is the company that is going to implement the system experienced in systems analysis? If it is, a member of the firm should perform a system survey on the office. Does the company understand the operation of a medical office?

2. Is the system technically sound? The number one difficulty with the computer system is the introduction of erroneous data. Will the system reject information when the name or number for a particular individual is in error? The system must be able to detect, screen, and eliminate this data. The rejected data must be corrected and resubmitted.

3. Most of the problems attending the use of a computer result from poor planning of the conversion from the former system—manual or bookkeeping machine—to the new computer system. Will a consultant from the computer company call on your office for the first month or two to resolve difficulties with the system and to answer questions? What type of training is provided by the computer company for the medical office personnel?

4. What type of people are administering and marketing the computer system. Are they sales people, computer systems specialists, or management consultants? Do the people servicing the system really understand it?

5. What is the cost of the computer system in comparison to the present system? Find out the specific advantages of the new system.

6. Will personnel changes be needed in the office to make the new system work?

7. Does the system use RVS, CPT, ICDA, or CMIT coding as a basis for recording diagnosis and record transactions?

8. Is the system simple enough that the medical office personnel seldom have to refer to the equipment operating manual?

CODING

Every computer company has its own system of coding information—whether it be by letters or by number—as input to the computer. However, the diagnosis code and the coding used for description of services rendered are fairly standard. For the *diagnosis* code, some computer systems use the *International Classification of Diseases Adapted for Use in the United States*, 8th revision, Volume 2, alphabetical listing. (Volume 1 is the numerical listing used by the medical records department of hospitals.) This is sometimes referred to as ICDA code number and is a four-digit code system. The ICDA is published by the Superintendent of Documents, U.S. Government Printing Office, Washington, D.C. 20402, and can be purchased from the American Hospital Association, 840 North Lake Shore Drive, Chicago, IL 60611. Another code book that is commonly used for the diagnosis code is *Current Medical Information and Terminology* (CMIT), published by the American Medical Association. This also is a four-digit code system. For *description of services rendered*, the *Relative Value Studies* (RVS) or *Current Procedural Terminology* (CPT) five-digit code system is used. See Chapter 2 for detailed information in regard to RVS and CPT coding.

Many times a computer company will have output on the itemized billing statement as well as on the insurance form of both the diagnosis code and the code for description of services. The one problem with the preparation of insurance forms on the computer is that the computer diagnosis is often not detailed enough to satisfy government agencies reviewing such insurance claims.

When a physician adopts a computer system, the computer replaces the manual or pegboard bookkeeping or bookkeeping machine system. To give you an idea of input and output from a computer system, *Medcobill* (a division of Intellectron International, Inc.) has been used as an example of the basic components (Fig. 12–1). Output is shown as weekly, semimonthly, and monthly. The various forms that make up the Medcobill system (numbered in Fig. 12–1) are described in detail in the following section. Abbreviations and terms appearing on the forms are explained in the Glossary (pp. 349, 351, and 352).

FORMS USED IN A TYPICAL COMPUTERIZED BILLING SYSTEM

While the Medical Assistant should be familiar with all of the following forms, not all physicians will want or need all of these forms as output from the computer, since the data included on them overlap considerably.

How the MEDCOBILL system makes the computer work for you

To the Computer (input)

NEW PATIENT INFORMATION

PATIENT VISIT DATA

OTHER INFORMATION

CORRECTION CARD

From the Computer (output)

WEEKLY

AUDIT AND CONTROL

CORRECTION OF ERRORS

FAMILY MASTER FILE

CUMULATIVE TRIAL BALANCE

REQUESTED INSURANCE FORMS

FAMILY MASTER FILE

COMPREHENSIVE INSURANCE LISTING

MONTHLY

PATIENT STATEMENTS

PATIENT LEDGERS

INSURANCE FORMS

DETAILED AGED TRIAL BALANCE

DELINQUENT ACCOUNT REPORT

AGING ANALYSIS

PRACTICE INCOME ANALYSIS

PRACTICE MANAGEMENT REPORT

SEMI-MONTHLY

PATIENT REMINDER NOTICES

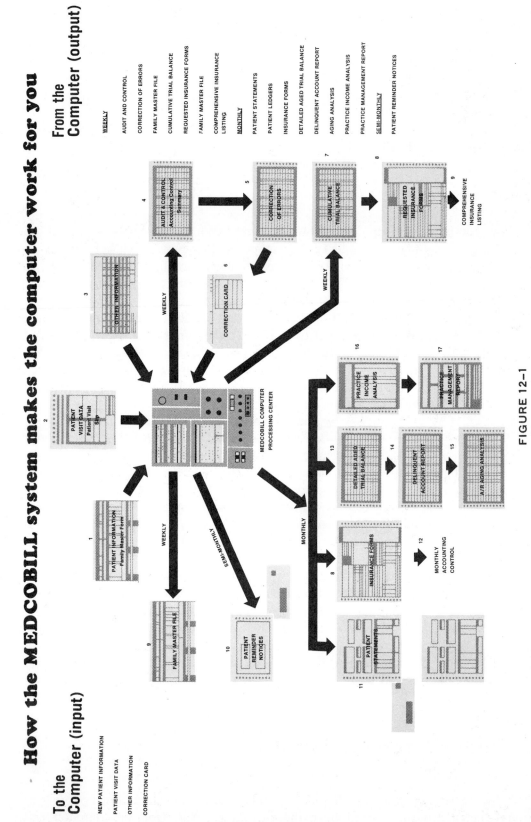

FIGURE 12-1

Comprehensive diagram of the Medcobill computerized billing system, showing the various forms of input and of weekly, semimonthly, and monthly output.

Family Master Form (Fig. 12–2)

This form (similar to the patient history and information sheet) establishes all family insurance and billing information. A Family Master file card is issued weekly on each new patient. (See item number 9 in Fig. 12–1.)

MEDCOBILL	FAMILY MASTER	DIV. INTELLECTRON INTERNATIONAL INC.

GRP. NO.	ACCOUNT NO.	TYPE	LAST	NAME OF RESPONSIBLE PARTY FIRST	M.I.	AREA	HOME PHONE NUMBER
356	078973	B	NAVARRO	MARVIN			241-6048

NUMBER AND STREET	CITY AND STATE
408-B-ALLEN AVE	GLENDALE CA 91201

DATE
01-31-73

PATIENT INFORMATION

FAMILY MEMBER NUMBER	FIRST NAME	M.I.	(LAST, IF DIFFERENT)	SEX	BIRTHDATE MO. DAY YR.	EMP. BY	OCCUPATION	UNION NO.	AUTO	AUTO			P.N.
1	MARVIN	P		M	06 10 32	1	TEACHER		1	1	2		
2	BETTY	J		F	10 01 35		HOMEMAKER		1	1	2		
3	JAMES	B	SMITH	M	02 27 60		STUDENT		1	1	2		

EMPLOYER NO. (1) LA SCHOOL BOARD   EMPLOYER NO.

AGENCY OR INSURANCE INFORMATION

CARRIER 1 BLUE CROSS	CARRIER 2 EQUITABLE	CARRIER
GROUP NO. 1785A	GROUP NO.	GROUP NO.
MEMBER NO. 485-42-3457	MEMBER NO.	MEMBER NO.
SUBSCRIB. NO. (1) 2 3 4 5 6 7 8 9	SUBSCRIB. NO. (1) 2 3 4 5 6 7 8 9	SUBSCRIB. NO. 1 2 3 4 5 6 7 8 9

FIGURE 12–2

Family Master Form for patient information. Similar to a patient history and information sheet.

Patient Visit Slip (Fig. 12–3)

The Patient Visit Slip is personalized to the practice of the physician. It records all information regarding services performed during a patient visit. It is the key to the successful computer billing system and triggers everything automatically, including third party paper work. The assistant fills in the insurance information, account number, name, and date and then places the Patient Visit Slip in the patient's folder before his or her visit. The doctor simply checks the indicated boxes for services, charges, and diagnoses, and hands the slip to the patient. The patient arranges payment at the front desk and the computer does the rest; that is, it gives output in the form of an itemized billing statement and completed insurance form(s), and incorporates some

MEDCOBILL SYSTEM
INTELLECTRON INTERNATIONAL, INCORPORATED

GROUP NO.	DR. NO.	DATE	ACCOUNT NO.	ACCOUNT LAST NAME
999	01	10-11-77	001234	BROWN

FAMILY MEM. NO.	PATIENT FIRST NAME	PATIENT LAST NAME (IF DIFF. FROM ABOVE)
1	JOHN	

IF NOT OFFICE, INDICATE PLACE OF SERVICE: 1 - IN-PATIENT HOSPITAL 2 - OUT-PATIENT HOSPITAL
4 - PATIENT'S HOME 6 - ECF 8 - NURSING HOME 9 - OTHER

SERVICE	RVS		MOD	FEE		SERVICE	RVS		MOD	FEE
NEW						**INJECTION**				
Initial Brief	90000	01		20 —		Penicillin	90705	22		6 —
Init. Limited	90010	02				B12	90705	23		
Init. Intermed.	90015	03								
Init. Comprehen.	90020	04				**IMMUNIZATION**				
ESTABLISHED						Polio	90700	24		
Minimum O.V.	90030	05				Dip Tet	90700	25		
Brief Exam	90040	06								
Limited Exam	90050	07				**SURGERY**				
Intermed. Exam	90060	08				I & D Abscess	10060	26		
Extended Re-Exam	90070	09				Laceration Repair	12000	27		
HOSPITAL										
Initial Brief	90200	10								
Init. Intermed.	90215	11				**PATHOLOGY**				
Init. Comprehen.	90220	12				Blood Type, RH	86100	28		
Brief Exam	90240	13				CBC	85010	29		
Limited Exam	90250	14				Pap Smear	88105	30		
Intermed. Exam	90260	15				Rh Titre	86025	31		
Extended Re-Exam	90270	16				Urinalysis	81000	32		
MEDICINE						Pregnancy Test	83160	33		
EKG	93000	17								
Medication-Suppl	99070	18								
Surgical Tray	99070	19								
Physiotherapy	97000	20				Collect & Handl	99000	34		
Physio-2 Mod.	97050	21				**RADIOLOGY**				
						Chest, 1 View	71010	35		
						Chest, 2 Views	71020	36		
						Foot, Complete	73630	37		
						Pelvis, Limited	72170	38		
						Skull, Complete	70260	39		
						Spine, Complete	70250	40		

4 RECALL	NEXT APPOINTMENT		**TODAY'S TOTAL CHARGES**		
8-02 - 01	DAY:				
4 DIAGNOSIS	DATE:		COURTESY DISC.	00060	5
1. 5/30 6. ___	TIME: ___ AM/PM		CASH PAYMENT	00010	7
	L-1 INS. NOW L-4 INS. MO. END		PERSONAL CHECK	00030	7 26 —
2. ___ 7. ___	MEMO:				
3. ___ 8. ___					

CONDITION CAUSED BY
1 ☐ INJURY
2 ☒ ILLNESS
3 ☐ PREGNANCY

4. ___ 9. ___
5. ___

COMMENCEMENT DATE OF INJURY ☐ ILLNESS ☒ PREGNANCY ☐ | MO. | DAY | YR. |
— — —

☒ NEW ILLNESS   CONDITION DUE TO INJURY ☐ OR SICKNESS ARISING OUT OF PATIENT'S EMPLOYMENT   ☒ NEW PATIENT

IF INJURY, INDICATE HOW SUSTAINED
1 ☐ AUTO ACCIDENT 2 ☐ HOME 3 ☐ OTHER

MEDCOBILL COPY

MEDCOBILL SYSTEM
© COPYRIGHT 1975 INTELLECTRON INTERNATIONAL, INCORPORATED

FIGURE 12-3

Patient Visit Data or Patient Visit Slip.

of the data into month-end printout analyses of various financial aspects of the practice.

Because the Patient Visit Slip has been custom-printed to fit the particular practice, a simple check mark suffices to number-code the charges and procedures for the great majority of patients. For the remainder, the doctor makes the appropriate clinical notation in the open space on the slip. The assistant then completes this by filling in the proper code number, such as the diagnosis code, which she looks up in a master code book sometimes supplied by the computer company. The doctor can revise the Patient Visit Slip whenever the fees or office requirements change. Patient Visit Slips are commonly used with the pegboard bookkeeping system (see Fig. 12–3).

Batch Transmittal Slip (Fig. 12–4)

The Patient Visit Slips are submitted on a daily basis at the end of the day. The Batch Transmittal Slip is placed on top of all of the accumulated Patient Visit Slips. It lists the total amounts of the transaction for the day, including payments and adjustments.

Other Information

Computer companies have different forms to handle the input of additional information obtained after the patient history sheet has already been submitted. Such input might consist of the following:

1. *Change Notice*, used when there is a change in the patient's address or insurance coverage, or for adding another family member (see Fig. 12–5).

2. *Hospital Charges*, used when the physician makes hospital visits (see Fig. 12–6).

3. *Payment Listing*, used to show what monies have been received by mail from patients or from insurance companies (see Fig. 12–7).

4. *Dun Request.* A dun (see Chapter 13) is a phrase or message to promote payment which usually appears on the patient's itemized billing statement when the bill becomes delinquent (see Fig. 12–8).

5. *Insurance Request*, used to generate an insurance form as output for a particular patient (see Fig. 12–14).

6. *Accounts Receivable Adjustments*, used to increase or decrease a balance, to apply or remove a charge, or to apply or remove a payment (see Fig. 12–9).

Accounting Control Summary (Fig. 12–10)

This is a weekly control report that defines each day's charges, payments, and adjustments, and summarizes the week. It is used for balancing. The Assistant pulls her copies of the "batches" and checks each batch total with the batch number listed in the left-hand column of the Accounting Control Summary report. The Assistant makes sure that each batch has reached the computer center by checking the batch numbers listed, and she also checks to see what money is being rejected or held in suspense.

BATCH TRANSMITTAL SLIP

MEDCOBILL SYSTEM
intellectron international, incorporated

TELEPHONE: (213) 988-5670

PREP. BY: _M7_

DATE: _10-9-77_

GROUP _999_

BATCH NO. _068457_

DAILY TRANSACTIONS

CHARGES THIS BATCH 9 _0_

PAYMENTS THIS BATCH 7 _0_

DO NOT WRITE IN THIS SPACE

---

2 **ADJUSTMENTS ONLY**

ADJUSTMENTS 5 _< 22.00 >_

DO NOT COMBINE CHARGES & PAYMENTS WITH ADJUSTMENTS

NUMBER OF DOCUMENTS IN THIS BATCH _____

PATIENT VISIT SLIP NOS.:

BEGIN _____ END _____

VOID SLIP NOS.: _____

INSTRUCTIONS FOR USE OF THIS FORM

A BATCH EACH TYPE OF DOCUMENT SEPARATELY
B USE A SEPARATE FORM FOR EACH BATCH OF TRANSACTIONS OR ADJUSTMENTS.
C ENTER TOTAL CHARGES AND PAYMENTS FROM YOUR ADDING MACHINE TAPES AND ATTACH TAPES TO THIS SLIP.

FILE ORIGINAL FOR YOUR RECORD
MAILING INSTRUCTIONS: ATTACH 2nd & 3rd COPIES TO TICKETS, LISTINGS, ETC., AND MAIL TO MEDCOBILL

LEAVE CARBON INTACT BETWEEN SECOND AND THIRD COPIES

© COPYRIGHT 1975 intellectron international, incorporated

FIGURE 12–4

Batch Transmittal Slip.

GUARANTOR LAST NAME (IN COMPUTER) _DAWSON_   DATE _10-9-77_

medcobill system	FAMILY MASTER	CHANGE NOTICE	© 1975 intellectron international, inc.

GRP. NO.	ACCOUNT NO.	1 TYPE	2 LAST NAME OF RESPONSIBLE PARTY 3 FIRST	4 M.I.	5 AREA	HOME PHONE NUMBER
999	321				013	827-8735

60 CYCLE BILLING	6 NUMBER AND STREET	7	CITY AND STATE
	9715 SAN BRUNO DR		WOODLAND Hills, XY 12345

DATE	9
11-7-77	8

PATIENT INFORMATION

FAMILY MEMBER NUMBER	FIRST NAME	M.I.	(LAST, IF DIFFERENT)	SEX	BIRTHDATE MO.	DAY	YR.	EMP. BY	OCCUPATION	INSURANCE CARRIER AUTO 1	AUTO 2	AUTO 3	1	2	3	P.N.
1																
2																
3																
4																
5																
6																
0																
	12	13	14	15	16			17	18	20	21	22	25	26	27	30
EMPLOYER NO. 1								EMPLOYER NO. 2								

AGENCY OR INSURANCE INFORMATION

31 CARRIER 1		CARRIER 2		CARRIER 3	
32 GROUP NO.		GROUP NO.		GROUP NO.	
33 MEMBER NO.		MEMBER NO.		MEMBER NO.	
34 SUBSCRIB. NO.	1 2 3 4 5 6 7 8 0	SUBSCRIB. NO.	1 2 3 4 5 6 7 8 0	SUBSCRIB. NO.	1 2 3 4 5 6 7 8 0

FIGURE 12-5

Family Master Change Notice.

HOSPITAL CHARGES

MEDCOBILL SYSTEM
Intellectron International, Incorporated
TELEPHONE (213) 988-5670

DATE 10-9-77
GROUP NO. 999
PAGE 1 OF 1

PLACE OF SERVICE CODES (POS CODES)
1 - IN-PATIENT HOSPITAL 2 - OUT-PATIENT HOSPITAL 3 - OFFICE 4 - PATIENT'S HOME 6 - ECF 8 - NURSING HOME 9 - OTHER

DR NO	DATE OF TRANSACTION MO DAY YR	ACCOUNT NUMBER	GUARANTOR LAST NAME	FAM MEM NO	POS CODE	PATIENT FIRST NAME	DIAGNOSTIC CODE	DATE* / HOSPITAL CODE	RVS CODE	TABLE CODE	CHARGES	**INSURANCE NOW MO END
01	10 1 21 77	321	DAWSON	3	1	MIKE	3211		90250		25 00	
03	"	400	Mc Coy	1	1	HAROLD		10-2-77 0021	00480		—	
03	"	"	"	1	1	"			90250		25 00	
03	10 3 77	"	"	1	1	"		10-3-77 0021	"		25 00	
03	"	"	"	1	1	"			00490		—	
02	10 4 77	230	KEARNEY	3	1	JOSEPH	4736		21735		246 00	✓

INSTRUCTIONS

* **HOSPITAL CODE AND DATE:** ENTER HOSPITAL CODE NUMBER AND ADMIT OR DISCHARGE DATE WHEN USING SERVICE CODE 00480 ADMITTED TO HOSPITAL, OR 00490 DISCHARGED FROM HOSPITAL. DO NOT ENTER MONEY PROCEDURES ON THE SAME LINE WITH A HOSPITAL ADMIT OR HOSPITAL DISCHARGE ENTRY.

TRANSACTION DATE: ENTER DATE OF SERVICE.

** CHECK (✓) NOW OR MONTH END IF YOU WISH TO GENERATE A REQUESTED INSURANCE FORM.

© COPYRIGHT 1975 Intellectron International, Incorporated

FIGURE 12–6

Hospital Charges.

MEDCOBILL SYSTEM
intellection international, incorporated
© 1975

PAYMENT LISTING

DATE 10-9-77
GROUP NO. 999
PAGE 1 OF 1

DOCTORS NUMBER	DATE OF PAYMENT	ACCOUNT NUMBER	GUARANTOR LAST NAME	FIRST NAME	INSURANCE CARRIER	INSURANCE ADJUSTMENT SERVICE	INSURANCE ADJUSTMENT AMOUNT (CR)	PAYMENT CODE	CHECK BANK NUMBER	AMOUNT OF PAYMENT
	10-9-77	321	DAWSON	R.				00030	16-332	24 00
	"	400	McCoy	H.	PRUD			00020	16-31	214 50
	"	230	Kearney	E.	MARCH	60071	365	60021	11-121	16 35
	"	141	Long	P.				00010		10 00

TOTAL ADJS. (5) 365

INCLUDE THIS TOTAL ON YOUR BATCH TRANSMITTAL SLIP NEXT TO "CREDIT ADJUSTMENTS"

TOTAL CURRENCY	10 00
TOTAL CHECKS	254 85
TOTAL	264 85

INSTRUCTIONS

1 – MAKE FORM OUT IN DUPLICATE. SEND ORIGINAL TO MEDCOBILL.
2 – ENTER INSURANCE CARRIER NAME ONLY WHEN USING PAYMENT CODE 00020.
3 – USE ADJUSTMENT COLUMN ONLY FOR INSURANCE WRITE OFFS. ALL OTHER ADJUSTMENTS, USE ACCOUNT RECEIVABLE ADJUSTMENT FORM.
4 – ENTER TOTALS IN BOTH PLACES INDICATED ON BOTTOM OF FORM. TEAR ALONG PERFORATION OF SECOND COPY FOR BANK DEPOSIT SLIP. STAMP THE TOP PORTION OF THE SLIP FOR DEPOSIT.

FIGURE 12–7

Payment Listing.

MEDCOBILL SYSTEM / Intellectron International, Inc.

988-5670

DUN REQUEST

DATE 10-31-77

GROUP NO. 999

ACCOUNT NUMBER	GUARANTOR LAST NAME	SERVICE CODE	SERVICE CODES AND MESSAGES PRINTED
321	Dawson	121	112 This account is past due. Please remit.
400	McCoy	612	121 Past Due -- Second Notice.
			134 This account will be placed in outside hands for collection if not paid immediately.
			141 May we have your payment?
			163 Doctor sees you when you are ill. Please return his courtesy by prompt payment.
			192 Have you heard from your insurance company?
			612 May we have your payments regularly each month, please?
			623 Do you have insurance to cover this account? If so, please submit forms.
			632 Future services will be on a cash basis only.
			654 No doubt you have overlooked payment. Your remittance by return mail will be appreciated. Thank you.
			663 Have been very patient. Please remit. -- Second reminder.

AUTOMATIC DUN MESSAGES

The system will enter a message on each account each month, if desired. To request this service fill in the spaces below and sign the form.

Accounts over   30 days: Message Code: ___ 00
Accounts over   60 days: Message Code: ___ 00
Accounts over   90 days: Message Code: ___ 00
Accounts over 120 days: Message Code: ___ 00

Please send all accounts the automatic dun messages indicated above.

Date: _____   Signature: _____

© 1972

FIGURE 12-8

Dun Request.

medcobill system
intellectron international, incorporated

ACCOUNTS RECEIVABLE
ADJUSTMENTS

DATE 10-9-77
GROUP NO. 999
PAGE 1 OF 1

FOR OFFICE USE ONLY

PLACE OF SERVICE CODES

1-IN-PATIENT HOSPITAL   2-OUT-PATIENT HOSPITAL   3-OFFICE   4-PATIENT'S HOME   6-ECF   8-NURSING HOME   9-OTHER

DOCTOR NUMBER	DATE OF TRANSACTION MO. DAY YR.	ACCOUNT NUMBER	GUARANTOR LAST NAME	FAM. MEM. NO.	PLACE OF SERV. CODE	PATIENT FIRST NAME	SERVICE *	APPLY CHARGE ** P	REMOVE CHARGE ** M	APPLY PAYMENT P	REMOVE PAYMENT M	ADJ. TO INCREASE BALANCE P	ADJ. TO DECREASE BALANCE M	REASON FOR ADJUSTMENT
01	10 9 77	321	Dawson	3		Mike	00090						20.00	
03	9 15 77	400	M? Coy	1	3	Harold	90050		20.00					
03	9 15 77	249	M? Coy	1	3	Harold	90050	20.00						
02	10 4 77	230	Kearney	3		Joseph	00060						2.00	
01	10 9 77	127	Mackey	2		Harriet	00030				10.00			
01	10 9 77	357	Mackey	2		Harriet	00030			10.00				

** WHENEVER ENTRIES ARE MADE IN "APPLY CHARGE" OR "REMOVE CHARGE" COLUMNS, ALWAYS INDICATE PLACE OF SERVICE CODE.

* SEE MANUAL FOR USE OF SERVICE CODES

Harold Proctor, M.D.
AUTHORIZED SIGNATURE

NET TOTAL (9): 20.00 / 20.00
NET TOTAL (7): 10.00 / 10.00
NET TOTAL (5): 0 / 22.00

[22.00]

© 1975 intellectron international, incorporated

FIGURE 12-9

Accounts Receivable Adjustments.

meDCOBiLL SYSTEM
intellectron international, incorporated

GROUP 356				PAGE	
REPORT TITLE ACCOUNTING CONTROL SUMMARY				DATE 02/16/73	

BATCH NUMBER	PROCESS DATE	CHARGES	PAYMENTS	ADJUSTMENTS	
12200	02/12/73	135.50	.00	.00	ACCEPTED
		135.50	.00	.00	TOTAL
12210	02/13/73	501.00	.00	.00	ACCEPTED
		25.00	.00	.00	REJECTED
		526.00	.00	.00	TOTAL
12220	02/14/73	.00	1,603.50-	.00	ACCEPTED
		.00	1,603.50-	.00	TOTAL
12230	02/15/73	1,300.00	280.10-	5.00-	ACCEPTED
		.00	10.00-	.00	REJECTED
		1,300.00	290.00-	5.00-	TOTAL
12240	02/16/73	450.00	.00	10.00	ACCEPTED
		450.00	.00	10.00	TOTAL
GROUP 356 TOTALS					
		2,386.50 *	1,883.50- *	5.00 *	ACCEPTED
		25.00 *	10.00- *	.00 *	REJECTED
		2,411.50 **	1,893.50- **	5.00 **	TOTAL
SUSPENSE ITEMS		45.00	10.00-	.00	ACCEPTED
		45.00	10.00-	.00	TOTAL

meDCOBiLL SYSTEM
intellectron international, incorporated

FIGURE 12–10

Accounting Control Summary.

Some examples for rejection might be: no master record sent in on the patient, wrong account number, RVS number missing, and so forth. (For further clarification on rejects, see Fig. 12–11, the Weekly Suspense File Report.) The Accounting Control Summary can also be issued monthly from the computer (see Fig. 12–20).

Weekly Suspense File Report (Fig. 12–11)

Whenever the computer audit discovers an error—such as posting to a wrong account or missing information—the item is placed in "suspense." The Weekly Suspense File Report is a listing of these items. A preprinted card (Fig. 12–12) is also available to make correction easier. Incorrect items will continue to appear on this report until they are corrected.

Cumulative Trial Balance (Fig. 12–13)

This report is issued periodically to bring all of the active accounts up to date. It lists every medical and financial transaction within the month, and notes each patient's current balance (Fig. 12–13A). It also summarizes charges, adjustments, and the number and classification of payments for the week (Fig. 12–13B). It is sometimes referred to as "CUM."

The Cumulative Trial Balance provides a complete listing of all patients in alphabetical sequence, and can be produced daily, weekly, or monthly on some computer systems. It offers the physician total in-office account control and yields an invaluable day-by-day record of the medical practice.

Insurance Request (Fig. 12–14)

Insurance forms are automatically completed and forwarded each week for the doctor's signature if they are requested as output from the computer facility. Some computer firms have a special form to demand or delete an insurance form as output from the computer (see Fig. 12–14). At other times insurance requests are incorporated into a patient visit slip or other form. These can be processed weekly or monthly and thus insurance charges are billed and paid promptly. In some instances the physician may want an insurance form produced that shows only inclusive dates of services.

Some computer companies obtain permission from government authorities or private carriers such as Blue Cross/Blue Shield to use a universal insurance form which is then submitted for all the various insurance companies (see Fig. 12–15). In the Medcobill system, the Patient Visit Slip (Fig. 12–3) shows at the lower left the designations L-1 and L-4, which can be checked to generate an insurance form immediately or monthly. On the form "Hospital Charges" (Fig. 12–6) a form can also be generated immediately or monthly by checking the extreme right column.

Insurance Listing (Fig. 12–16)

This is a weekly comprehensive listing of all insurance forms generated from the computer facility on all patients.

MEDCOBILL SYSTEM
intellection international, incorporated

GROUP 356   THE BROOKS CLINIC   PAGE   01

REPORT TITLE   WEEKLY SUSPENSE FILE REPORT   DATE   02/16/73

DATE	BATCH	ACCT. NO.	CARD OR NO.	FIRST NAME	LAST NAME	FAM. NO.	RVS	MCD	DOCMNT DATE	AMOUNT	TYPE	REMARK
01-15	90	201035	01	INEZ	EL		87000		12-01	5.30	9	NO FAM NO.
01-22	01	218242	01	WILLIAM	RO	1	99647		01-16	14.00	9	NO MASTER RECORD
01-22	01	218242	01	WILLIAM	RO	1	00030		01-16	14.00	-7	NO MASTER RECORD
01-22	02	106098	01	EARL	DU	1	C0010		01-17	5.00	9	INVALID RVS
01-22	99	801457	02	EDDIE	MI	1	S0040		01-14	4.30	-7	INVALID LAST NAME. FILES SHOW RA
02-03	63	018347	03	DOROTHY	HA	2	90705		01-26	8.00	9	INVALID LAST NAME. FILES SHOW VO
02-03	63	018347	03	DOROTHY	HA	2			01-26	4.00	9	INVALID LAST NAME. FILES SHOW VO
02-13	21	105080	01	MARY	RU	1	90500		02-09	12.00	9	NO MASTER RECORD
02-13	21	105080	01	MARY	RO	1	99070		02-09	7.30	9	NO MASTER RECORD
02-13	21	105080	01	MARY	RO	1	88100		02-09	6.00	9	NO MASTER RECORD
02-15	23	107324	01	BOB	SM	1	00030		02-10	10.00	-7	INVALID LAST NAME. FILES SHOW SW

TOTAL CURRENT SUSPENSE GROUP 356   15.00
TOTAL PREVIOUS SUSPENSE GROUP 356   18.00

FIGURE 12–11

Weekly Suspense File Report.

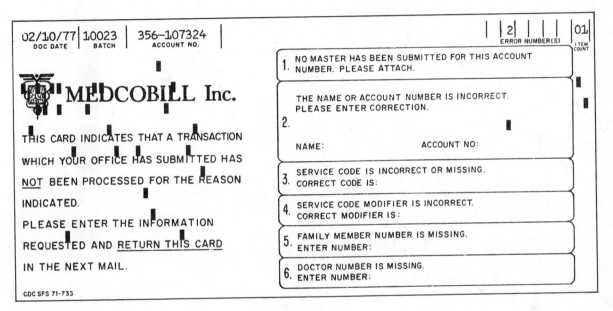

FIGURE 12–12

Correction Card.

CUMULATIVE TRIAL BALANCE

GROUP NO. 356 PERIOD ENDING 08/20/75 CYCLE 3 PAGE 2

ACCOUNT NO.	GUARANTORS NAME	FAMILY MEMBER NAME / NO.	ACCT TYPE	DR. NO.	BTCH	TRANS-DATE	TRANSACTION / DESCRIPTION	CD	DEBIT	CREDIT	BALANCE
078973	NAVARRO MARVIN	2 BETTY	B			0731	PRIOR BALANCE DATB				3900
		2 BETTY		01	43	0804	OFFICE VIS LIMITED EXAM	9	1200		
		2 BETTY			43	0804	SUPP/MATL PENICILLIN	9	1000		
		2 BETTY			44	0804	CHECK *	7		1200	5900
		2 BETTY		01	45	0804	HDR PREG TEST BL-UR IMMUN QUAL	9	1000		*5900
		2 BETTY		01	51	0819	HDR PREG TEST BL-UR IMMUN QUAL	N	1000		
		2 BETTY			91	0819	CHECK *	7		1000	*5900
075724	NEFF ETHELYN	2	B			0731	PRIOR BAL STMNT 08-13 DATB				*5800
075686	NEIDER SUSAN	3 SUSAN				0731	PRIOR BALANCE				2000
		2 SUSAN		02	49	0805	COLL HAND SPEC OFC SIMP	9	400		
		2 SUSAN		01	79	0808	OFFICE VIS LIMITED EXAM	9	1200		
		2 SUSAN		01	49	0815	OFFICE VIS INTERMED EXAM	9	1500		
		2 SUSAN		02	62	0816	COMPR RE-EXAM OR RE-EVAL	9	2250		*7350
065211	NEIL HEDY	4 HEDY	I			0731	PRIOR BALANCE				2650
		2 HEDY	P		82	0818	INS PAYMENT AETNA *	7 N		2650	*00
001354	NORMAN ROBERT	4 MARY	P			0731	PRIOR BALANCE				3600
		2 MARY		02	22	0813	MEDICAL PMT 07-15-75 *	7 N		960	
		2 MARY		02	22	0813	MEDICAL ADJ 07-15-75 *	5 N		240	
		2 MARY		02	24	0819	OFFICE VIS INTERMED EXAM	9 N	1200		
		2 MARY		02	24	0819	XRAY CHEST TWO VIEWS	9 N	1800		
		2 MARY		02	24	0819	INDEX THYROX COL T3-T4 UPTAKE	9 N	1500		
		2 MARY		02	24	0819	BLOOD COUNT COMPLETE	9 N	700		
		2 MARY		02	24	0819	PAP SMEAR SCREEN W/REVIEW	9 N	250		*7850
							CENTRAL DIAGNOSTIC LAB				
							7660 GLORIA AVE				
							VAN NUYS CA 91406				

medcobill system intelligent information, incorporated

© COPYRIGHT 1975 intelligent information, incorporated

A

FIGURE 12–13

Cumulative Trial Balance.

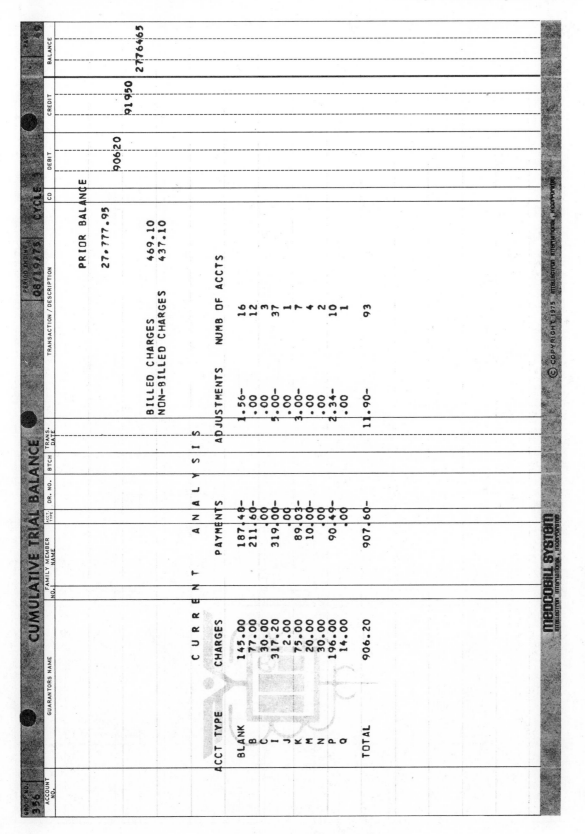

CUMULATIVE TRIAL BALANCE

GROUP NO. 356 | PERIOD ENDING 08/19/75 | CYCLE 3 | PAGE 69

ACCOUNT NO.	GUARANTORS NAME	FAMILY MEMBER NO.	FAMILY MEMBER NAME	ACCT. TYPE	DR. NO.	BTCH	TRANS. DATE	TRANSACTION / DESCRIPTION	CD	DEBIT	CREDIT	BALANCE
								PRIOR BALANCE				
								27,777.95				
										906 20		
											919 50	
												27764 65
								BILLED CHARGES 469.10				
								NON-BILLED CHARGES 437.10				

C U R R E N T   A N A L Y S I S

ACCT TYPE	CHARGES	PAYMENTS	ADJUSTMENTS	NUMB OF ACCTS
BLANK	145.00	187.48-	1.56-	16
B	77.00	211.60-	.00	12
C	30.00	.00	.00	3
I	317.20	319.00-	5.00-	37
J	2.00	.00	.00	1
K	75.00	89.03-	3.00-	7
M	20.00	10.00-	.00	4
N	30.00	.00	.00	2
P	196.00	90.49-	2.34-	10
Q	14.00	.00	.00	1
TOTAL	906.20	907.60-	11.90-	93

MEDCOBILL SYSTEM intellectron international, incorporated

B

FIGURE 12–13 *(Continued)*

MEDCOBILL SYSTEM
INTELLECTRON INTERNATIONAL, INCORPORATED
© 1975

INSURANCE REQUEST

DATE 10-9-77
GROUP NO. 999
PAGE 1 OF 1

ACCOUNT NUMBER	GUARANTOR LAST NAME	FAM MEM NO.	PATIENT FIRST NAME	INS. CARRIER NO.	DIAGNOSIS CODES 1	2	3	4	5	DATES OF SERVICE FROM MO.	DAY	YR.	TO MO.	DAY	YR.
321	Dawson	3	Mike							1	1	77	10	9	77
400	McCoy	1	Harold							9	9	77	10	9	77
230	Kearney	2	Eileen							10	2	77	10	5	77
127	Mackey	2	Harriet							7	8	77	7	8	77

FIGURE 12–14

Insurance Request.

HEALTH INSURANCE
CLAIM FORM

Blue Cross
of Southern California

*READ INSTRUCTIONS BEFORE COMPLETING OR SIGNING THIS FORM

TYPE OR PRINT
☐ MEDICARE ☐ MEDICAID ☐ CHAMPUS ☒ OTHER

Box 60465, Terminal Annex
Los Angeles, California 90060

PATIENT & INSURED (SUBSCRIBER) INFORMATION

1. PATIENT'S NAME (First name, middle initial, last name) BETTY J NAVARRO	2. PATIENT'S DATE OF BIRTH 11 01 40	3. INSURED'S NAME (First name, middle initial, last name) MARVIN NAVARRO
4. PATIENT'S ADDRESS (Street, city, state, ZIP code)	5. PATIENT'S SEX MALE ☐ FEMALE ☒	6. INSURED'S I.D. No. or MEDICARE No. (include any letters) 485 42 3457
	7. PATIENT'S RELATIONSHIP TO INSURED SELF SPOUSE ☒ CHILD OTHER	8. INSURED'S GROUP NO. (Or Group Name) 1785A
9. OTHER HEALTH INSURANCE COVERAGE - Enter Name of Policyholder and Plan Name and Address and Policy or Medical Assistance Number

AETNA | 10. WAS CONDITION RELATED TO: A. PATIENT'S EMPLOYMENT YES ☐ NO ☐ B. AN AUTO ACCIDENT YES ☐ NO ☐ | 11. INSURED'S ADDRESS (Street, city, state, ZIP code) 408 B ALLEN AVE GLENDALE CA 91201 |
| 12. PATIENT'S OR AUTHORIZED PERSON'S SIGNATURE (Read back before signing) I Authorize the Release of any Medical Information Necessary to Process this Claim and Request Payment of MEDICARE/CHAMPUS Benefits Either to Myself or to the Party Who Accepts Assignment Below

SIGNED _____ DATE _____ | | 13. I AUTHORIZE PAYMENT OF MEDICAL BENEFITS TO UNDERSIGNED PHYSICIAN OR SUPPLIER FOR SERVICE DESCRIBED BELOW

SIGNED (Insured or Authorized Person) |

PHYSICIAN OR SUPPLIER INFORMATION

14. DATE OF:	ILLNESS (FIRST SYMPTOM) OR INJURY (ACCIDENT) OR PREGNANCY (LMP)	15. DATE FIRST CONSULTED YOU FOR THIS CONDITION	16. HAS PATIENT EVER HAD SAME OR SIMILAR SYMPTOMS? YES ☐ NO ☐
17 DATE PATIENT ABLE TO RETURN TO WORK	18. DATES OF TOTAL DISABILITY FROM _____ THROUGH _____	DATES OF PARTIAL DISABILITY FROM _____ THROUGH _____
19. NAME OF REFERRING PHYSICIAN		20. FOR SERVICES RELATED TO HOSPITALIZATION GIVE HOSPITALIZATION DATES ADMITTED _____ DISCHARGED _____
21. NAME & ADDRESS OF FACILITY WHERE SERVICES RENDERED (If other than home or office)		22. WAS LABORATORY WORK PERFORMED OUTSIDE YOUR OFFICE? YES ☐ ☒ NO CHARGES:

23. DIAGNOSIS OR NATURE OF ILLNESS OR INJURY, RELATE DIAGNOSIS TO PROCEDURE IN COLUMN D BY REFERENCE TO NUMBERS 1, 2, 3, ETC. OR DX CODE

1.
2. 07-22-75 UPPER RESPIRATORY INFECT
3.
4.

24. A DATE OF SERVICE	B* PLACE OF SERVICE	C FULLY DESCRIBE PROCEDURES, MEDICAL SERVICES OR SUPPLIES FURNISHED FOR EACH DATE GIVEN PROCEDURE CODE (IDENTIFY:) (EXPLAIN UNUSUAL SERVICES OR CIRCUMSTANCES)	D DIAGNOSIS CODE	E CHARGES	F
07/22/75	3	71020 CHEST TWO VIEWS		21 00	
07/22/75	3	81000 URINALYSIS ROUTINE COMPL		3 00	
07/22/75	3	90060 OFFICE VIS INTERMED EXAM		15 00	

| 25. SIGNATURE OF PHYSICIAN OR SUPPLIER (Read back before signing)

SIGNED _____ DATE _____ | 26. ACCEPT ASSIGNMENT (GOVERNMENT CLAIMS ONLY) (SEE BACK) YES ☐ NO ☐ | 27. TOTAL CHARGE 39 00 | 28. AMOUNT PAID | 29. BALANCE DUE |
| | 30. YOUR SOCIAL SECURITY NO. | 31. PHYSICIAN'S OR SUPPLIER'S NAME, ADDRESS, ZIP CODE & TELEPHONE NO. PETER BROOKS, MD 7650 GLORIA AVE VAN NUYS, CA 91406 213-988-5670 I.D. NO. ZZZ123457 | | |
| 32. YOUR PATIENT'S ACCOUNT NO. 356-078973 FORM PREPARED 07/31/75 | 33. YOUR EMPLOYER I.D. NO. 95-633466 | | | |

*PLACE OF SERVICE CODES

1—(IH) — INPATIENT HOSPITAL
2—(OH)—OUTPATIENT HOSPITAL
3—(O) — DOCTOR'S OFFICE

4—(H)—PATIENT'S HOME
5— DAY CARE FACILITY (PSY)
6— NIGHT CARE FACILITY (PSY)

7—(NH) — NURSING HOME
8—(SNF)—SKILLED NURSING FACILITY
9— AMBULANCE

O—(OL)—OTHER LOCATIONS
A—(IL) — INDEPENDENT LABORATORY
B— OTHER MEDICAL/SURGICAL FACILITY

APPROVED BY AMA COUNCIL ON MEDICAL SERVICE 6-74

2331 5/75

FIGURE 12–15

Blue Cross Universal Claim Form as output from the computer.

medcobill system
intellection international, incorporated

		PAGE	01
GROUP 356 THE BROOKS CLINIC			
REPORT TITLE INSURANCE LISTING		DATE	12/21/74

ACCOUNT	LAST NAME	FIRST	DR NO	TYPE	INSURANCE CARRIER	AMOUNT	DATE MAILED	REMARKS
001019-3	BASSETT	LINDA	1	I	MASS MUTUAL LIFE	8.00		
001122-2	STEVESON	PAT	1	I	CONN GENERAL	13.00		
001754-2	TOMMASINO	VIVIAN	1	M	MEDICARE	63.50		
					METROPOLITAN LIFE	63.50		
001850-1	GUNDERSON	KENT	2	P	MEDICAL	25.00		
001925-4	TUCKER	JAMES	2	B	BLUE CROSS	39.00		
003554-1	JOHNSON	WILLIAM	3	I	NEW YORK LIFE	11.00		
012027-1	ROSENBERG	PHIL	2	M	MEDICARE	50.00		
021299-2	FREELEY	JAN	1	I	PHOENIX MUTUAL	175.00		
025787-1	MACGREGOR	WILLIAM	3	B	BLUE CROSS	250.00		
035462-1	THOMAS	ROBERT	4	M	MEDICARE	520.00		
052341-5	SUTTON	PETER	2	I	CONN GENERAL	41.00		
059874-1	PALMER	ARNOLD	1	B	BLUE CROSS	156.00		
					PHOENIX MUTUAL	156.00		
062354-3	ARNETT	MARY	3	I	METROPOLITAN LIFE	75.00		
075329-1	MICHNER	JAMES	1	B	BLUE CROSS	23.50		

FIGURE 12–16

Comprehensive Insurance Listing.

Patient Statements (Fig. 12–17)

An itemized billing statement is released as monthly output from most computerized billing systems. An entire family can be listed on the statement, which shows charges, payments, and the balance due. A computerized statement usually shows a breakdown of the amounts due that are delinquent and how many days delinquent they are (bottom of form in Fig. 12–17). This information is always important from the standpoint of collection of accounts, and is sometimes called "aging analysis."

Notice the phrase or message on the statement to promote payment of a delinquent account. This is sometimes referred to as a "Dun." (See Chapter 13.) If the physician wishes to have monthly itemized statements as output, make sure that the computer company can supply these to the office or mail them out on the mail-out dates for best collection, such as the 8th, 10th, or 12th of the month, or the 20th, 24th, or 27th of the month. Some computer companies will also furnish a year-end tax statement to show only payments made by the patient. This statement is mailed directly to the patient for income tax purposes (see Fig. 12–18).

Patient Ledgers

Some computer companies furnish as an optional feature a duplicate of the patient's statement, which acts as a ledger, or they may print out a ledger if this is desired by the physician's office. This information, plus the details in the weekly cumulative trial balance or the monthly detailed aged trial balance, gives the assistant the equivalent of a monthly ledger card.

Patient Reminder Notices and Requested Recall Listing (Fig. 12–19)

The requested recall listing is a semimonthly report which is optional and depends upon the type of practice involved (Fig. 12–19A). If the physician wishes to have patients reminded that they are due for an appointment, then such a notice can also be generated by the computer (Fig. 12–19B). The notices are sent out by the computer facility or by the assistant. The listing merely shows which message (indicated by a code number) has been sent to which patient.

Monthly Accounting Control (Fig. 12–20)

This is a monthly report given to the auditor or accountant to balance the deposits for the month. It acts as a recap of all of the batches that reach the computer center for processing by the cut-off date (the amount of time before the cut-off date can vary from office to office). At the bottom of the statement is shown the complete month's charges, adjustments, and payments, as well as what cleared this month from last month's suspense file. Note the symbols (+) and (–) on the extreme right hand side of Figure 12–20. These show when to add and subtract figures. The next-to-the-last entries at the bottom of the statement show what is still on suspense for the current month. The totals at the bottom of the page show what figures should match with the Detailed Aged Trial Balance (DATB), described in the next section.

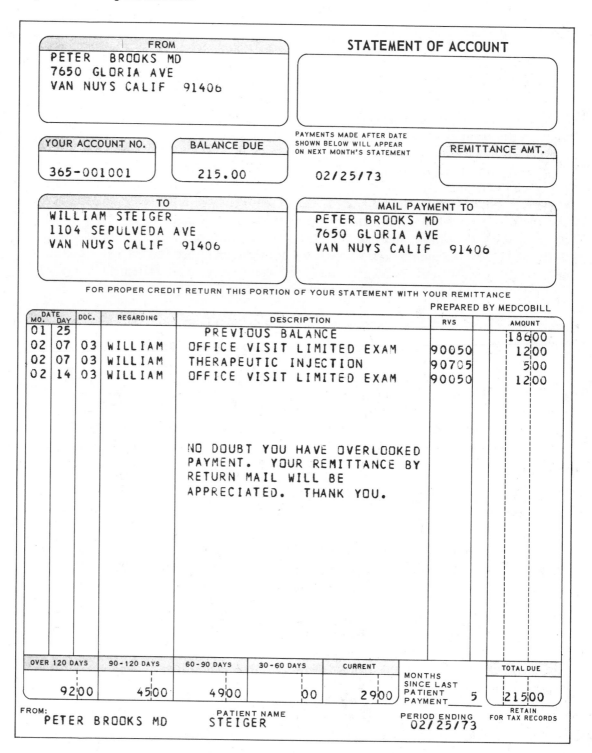

FIGURE 12–17

Patient's Statement of Account—monthly output.

```
                    FRO.                                          LEDGER
  PETER BROOKS        MD              G-10129
  7650 GLORIA AVE
  VAN NUYS CALIF    91406


  YOUR ACCOUNT NO.      BALANCE DUE    PAYMENTS MADE AFTER DATE    REMITTANCE AMT.
                                       SHOWN BELOW WILL APPEAR
                                       ON NEXT MONTH'S STATEMENT
  356-000858


            TO                              MAIL PAYMENT TO
  WILLIAM C CLAUER
  1144 FIRST STREET                  THIS STATEMENT IS FOR
  VAN NUYS CALIF    91406            INFORMATION PURPOSES ONLY
```

FOR PROPER CREDIT RETURN THIS PORTION OF YOUR STATEMENT WITH YOUR REMITTANCE

PREPARED BY MEDCOBILL

DATE MO.	DAY	DOC.	REGARDING	DESCRIPTION	RVS		AMOUNT
				PAYMENTS RECEIVED FROM YOU BY YOUR DOCTOR DURING 1974 ARE LISTED BELOW			
				PAYMENTS RECEIVED FROM INSURANCE CARRIER			65.00
				PAYMENTS RECEIVED FROM PATIENT			45.00

OVER 120 DAYS	90-120 DAYS	60-90 DAYS	30-60 DAYS	CURRENT	MONTHS SINCE LAST PATIENT PAYMENT	TOTAL DUE

FROM: PATIENT NAME   PERIOD ENDING   RETAIN FOR TAX RECORDS

FIGURE 12–18

Patient's Year-to-Date Ledger, showing payments only.

MEDCOBiLL SYSTEM
intellectron international, incorporated

| GROUP | 356 | | | PAGE | 01 |

REPORT TITLE REQUESTED RECALL LISTING   DATE 02/28/73

ACCOUNT	LAST NAME	FIRST NAME	MSG-NO	ELAPSED TIME	VISIT-DATE
100109	DARST	EDITH	01	6 MONTHS	07/29/72
100172	FRICK	LOUISE	01	1 MONTH	01/28/73
100080	FULLERTON	DOREEN	02	6 MONTHS	08/28/72
100335	MEBERG	MARILYN	01	9 MONTHS	05/30/72
100452	ROBERTS	SUE	01	3 MONTHS	10/27/72
100462	ROMERO	LUPE	01	6 MONTHS	08/09/72
100474	SADLER	JUDY	01	12 MONTHS	02/26/72
100820	SMART	CAROL	01	6 MONTHS	08/01/72
101151	PERRY	DONNA	01	2 MONTHS	12/25/72
101196	PETRIE	ELAINE	04	6 MONTHS	07/28/72
101229	SISLER	EVA	01	4 MONTHS	12/05/72
101315	WENZEL	BONNIE	01	6 MONTHS	08/01/72
101365	RIKER	JACK	01	1 MONTH	03/27/72
101484	STRACH	MILLIE	03	6 MONTHS	08/04/72
101604	WILLIAMS	PATRICIA	01	9 MONTHS	07/27/71
101786	DEAN	JAMES	01	6 MONTHS	08/02/72
101851	STEIGER	ROD	01	2 MONTHS	02/27/72
102447	SHANKS	DOROTHY	06	6 MONTHS	08/09/72
102787	FRISS	MARGARET	06	6 MONTHS	07/28/72
102870	PATTERSON	JOYCE	01	6 MONTHS	08/04/72
102915	HARRELSON	SANDRA	01	9 MONTHS	05/28/72
103125	JOHNSON	MARIE	01	12 MONTHS	02/28/72
103143	BERGER	PATTI	01	1 MONTH	01/30/72
103438	FITZ	LOUISE	01	6 MONTHS	07/28/72
103888	HUDDLESTON	MARGARET	01	6 MONTHS	07/28/72

TOTAL NUMBER OF RECALLS MAILED   25

MEDCOBiLL SYSTEM
intellectron international, incorporated

A

FIGURE 12-19

A, Requested Recall Listing shows comprehensive listing of patients to be recalled. B, Patient Reminder Notice.

FROM

PETER BROOKS MD
7650 GLORIA AVENUE
VAN NUYS CALIF 91406

REGARDING MARIE   356-103125

IT IS CUSTOMARY FOR OUR OFFICE
TO REMIND OUR PATIENTS OF THEIR
PERIODIC PROFESSIONAL EXAMINATIONS.
PLEASE CALL THE OFFICE TO
ARRANGE YOUR APPOINTMENT.

362-1234

TO

MARIE   JOHNSON
1152 ADDISON ST
ENCINO, CALIF 91316

MEDCOBILL Inc.

B

FIGURE 12–19 *(Continued)*

medcobill system
intellectron international, incorporated

GROUP 356   PAGE   01

REPORT TITLE   ACCOUNTING CONTROL MONTHLY SUMMARY   DATE   02/28/73

BATCH	DATE	CHARGES	PAYMENTS	ADJUSTMENTS	
12293	02/01/73	205.00	330.00	.00	
12294	02/02/73	142.00	240.00	.00	
12295	02/05/73	187.00	.00	.00	
12296	02/06/73	.00	185.00	28.00	
12297	02/06/73	210.00	.00	.00	
12298	02/07/73	140.00	255.00	.00	
12299	02/08/73	122.50	202.00	.00	
12300	02/09/73	253.50	.00	.00	
12301	02/12/73	135.50	.00	.00	
12302	02/13/73	501.00	.00	.00	
12303	02/14/73	.00	1,603.50	.00	
12304	02/15/73	1,300.00	280.00	5.00-	
12305	02/16/73	450.00	.00	10.00	
12306	02/19/73	288.00	.00	.00	
12307	02/20/73	421.00	322.00	.00	
12308	02/21/73	175.00	144.00	42.00	
12310	02/23/73	224.00	321.00	.00	
12311	02/26/73	177.00	321.00	.00	
12312	02/27/73	147.00	140.00	68.00	
12313	02/28/73	211.00	244.00	.00	
GROUP 356 TOTALS		5,290.50 *	4,587.50 *	143.00 *	
CLEARED FROM PRIOR MONTHS SUSPENSE		254.00	85.00	12.00	(+)
THIS MONTHS SUSPENSE ITEMS		102.00	14.00	.00	(−)
MATCH THESE TOTALS TO THE D. A. T. B.		5,442.50 **	4,658.50 **	155.00 **	

medcobill system
intellectron international, incorporated

FIGURE 12–20

Monthly Accounting Control.

Detailed Aged Trial Balance (Fig. 12–21)

This is the most important document received as output from the computer system. It is sometimes called the "accounts receivable listing" or "cumulative journal." It is the modern-day replacement for the ledger card. Alphabetically listed in detail for each account are the dates, procedures, charges, payments, and adjustments for an entire quarter. The account balance and its age are clearly identified, and the months since the last payment are flagged for follow-up (see Fig. 12–21A).

The physician should review the last page of the monthly report (Fig. 12–21B), which shows the percentages of receivable that are current in comparison with those that are 30, 60, 90, or 120 days overdue. Check the total receivable figure. If this figure exceeds four times the revenue received on an average per month, a check of the person who is responsible for following up on accounts should be made. This form can be used as a collection tool by referring to the patient's name and phone number as listed on the report. Notice that all family members are shown for each account. Notice also that the report shows an aging analysis for each separate family account.

Delinquent Account Record (DAR) Activity Report (Fig. 12–22)

This report is issued every 90 days and automatically identifies the problem accounts (see Fig. 12–22A). The physician selects the period he wishes reported as delinquent: 60, 90, or 120 days. Then any account with that aged balance or over is selectively listed, along with information necessary to follow up the account. There are three categories: new accounts, active prior accounts, and inactive prior accounts. Accounts listed as inactive prior accounts might be turned over to a collection agency. The list of "active prior accounts" gives information to update the "Delinquent Account Record" card, shown in Figure 12–22B.

Aging Analysis (Fig. 12–23)

This is a monthly report showing the age of the physician's accounts receivable as well as the charges and payments. The current balance is analyzed by account type, so that the physician can see how Medicare, Blue Cross, or any other carrier is paying and take appropriate action if the carrier has not paid.

Practice Income Analysis (Fig. 12–24)

This is a monthly report which shows in detail what types of services are being rendered in the physician's practice and where the income is being generated each month and year to date. All procedures, their frequency, and their dollar value are displayed for each physician (and for the entire group), along with any adjustments, courtesy discounts, and payments. This report helps with office management, inventory of supplies, and fee profile studies. For example, if a physician has an x-ray unit in his office but is not generating enough radiologic work to warrant the overhead of extra equipment and personnel, he may decide to send patients out to have x-rays taken.

medcobill system — intellection international, incorporated

DETAIL AGED TRIAL BALANCE

GROUP NO. 356 QTR 3 DATE 08 31 72 PAGE 62

GUARANTOR'S NAME	INS	NO	FAMILY MEMBER NAME	DR. NO.	BATCH	DATE	TRANSACTION/DESCRIPTION	RVS	ED	BALANCE	CURRENT CHARGES	30 DAYS	60 DAYS	90 DAYS	120 DAYS
MARVIN NAVARRO	B	2													950
408 B ALLEN AVE			2BETTY			0630	BALANCE AS OF 6/30/72			2600					
GLENDALE CA 91201			2BETTY	01	23	0703	PERSONAL CHECK	C0030	7 *		-1000				
PHONE-NO. 241-6048			2BETTY	01	75	0712	INSURANCE PAYMENT AETNA	C0020	7 *		-600				
ACCOUNT NO. 078973			2BETTY	01	73	0715	BLUE CROSS PAYMENT	C0230	7 *		-1000				
			2BETTY	01	41	0722	CHEST TWO VIEWS	71020	9		2100				
			2BETTY	01	41	0722	URINALYSIS ROUTINE COMPLETE	81000	9		300				
			2BETTY	01	41	0722	OFFICE VISIT INTERMEDIATE EXAM	90060	9		1500				
			2BETTY	01	43	0730	INS BILLED THRU 7/22 AETNA	C0850	9						
			2BETTY	01	43	0804	OFFICE VISIT LIMITED EXAM	90050	9		1200				
			2BETTY			0804	SUPP/MATL/INJ PENICILLIN	99070	9		1000				
			2BETTY	01	44	0804	PERSONAL CHECK	C0030	7 *		-1200				
			2BETTY	02	44	0804	HCR PREG TEST BL-UR IMMUN QUAL	83160	9		1000				
			2BETTY		51	0819	HCR PREG TEST BL-UR IMMUN QUAL	83160	9		1000				
			2BETTY		91	0819	PERSONAL CHECK	C0030	7 *		-1000				
			1MARVIN	01	82	0822	URINALYSIS ROUTINE COMPLETE	81000	9		300				
			1MARVIN	01	82	0822	OFFICE VISIT COMPR REEXAM	90080	9		2250				
			1MARVIN	01	82	0822	COLL HAND BILL LAB SPEC OFFICE	99000	9		400				
			2BETTY	01	78	0829	HCR PREG TEST BL-UR IMMUN QUAL	83160	9		1000				
			2BETTY		71	0829	BLUE CROSS PAYMENT	C0023	9		-1000				
			2BETTY	01	83	0830	INS BILLED THRU 8/3 BLUE CROSS*	C0850	9						
							0 MONTHS SINCE LAST PAYMENT			*8850	8850				
ETHELYN NEFF	B	2													
9339 E OLIVE ST			2ETHELYN	01	14	0630	BALANCE AS OF 06/30/72			6400		400			
TEMPLE CITY CA 91780			2ETHELYN		88	0728	COLL HAND BILL LAB SPEC OFFICE	99000	9		400				
PHONE-NO. 287-4448			2ETHELYN			0728	PERSONAL CHECK	C0030	7 *	5800	-1000				
ACCOUNT NO. 075724							1 MONTHS SINCE LAST PAYMT			*5800					
SUSAN NEIDER		3												2250	
10978 BLUFFSIDE			2SUSAN	02	49	0630	BALANCE AS OF 06/30/72			2000	2000				
STUDIO CITY CA 91604			2SUSAN	01	79	0805	COLL HAND BILL LAB SPEC OFFICE	90050	9		400				
PHONE-NO. 985-0146			2SUSAN	01	49	0808	OFFICE VISIT LIMITED EXAM	90060	9		1200				
ACCOUNT NO. 075686			2SUSAN	02	62	0815	OFFICE VISIT INTERMEDIATE EXAM	90080	9		1500		2250	2200	2000
						0917	OFFICE VISIT COMPR EXAM	C0110		7350	2250				
						0931	COMMENT								
							3 MONTHS SINCE LAST PAYMT			*7350	5350				
HEDY NEIL	I	4													
7475 MULHOLLAND DR			2HEDY	02	44	0713	OFFICE VISIT CMPR REEXAM	90080	9	2650	2250				
LOS ANGELES CALIF			2HEDY	02	44	0713	COLL HAND BILL LAB SPEC OFFICE	99000	9		400				
PHONE-NO. 876-0700			2HEDY		82	0818	INSURANCE PAYMENT AETNA	C0020	7 *	*00	-2650				
ACCOUNT NO. 065211															

A

FIGURE 12–21

Detailed Aged Trial Balance.

medcobill system
Intellecton International, Incorporated

DETAIL AGED TRIAL BALANCE

GROUP NO.	QTR	DATE	PAGE
356	3	08 / 31 / 72	63

GUARANTORS NAME	RE NO	FAMILY MEMBER NAME	DR. NO.	BATCH	DATE	TRANSACTION/DESCRIPTION	RVS	C D	BALANCE	CURRENT CHARGES	30 DAYS	60 DAYS	90 DAYS	120 DAYS

PRIOR BALANCE   CUR. CHARGES   PAYMENTS   ADJUSTMENTS   BILLED CHARGES   NON-BILLED CHARGES
46,626.42   19,999.42   18,828.72-   260.56-   10,250.40   9,749.02

CURRENT   30 DAYS   60 DAYS   90 DAYS   120 DAYS   BALANCE DUE
12,133.39   15,100.34   5,743.50   3,732.85   10,826.48   47,536.56

                                                                                                 BALANCE
                                                                                                 47,536.56

PERCENTAGES   31.0   12.0   7.0   23.0   100.0
27.0

B

FIGURE 12-21 (Continued)

medcobill system
intellectron international, incorporated

GROUP   356   THE BROOKS CLINIC   PAGE   01

REPORT TITLE   120 DAY DELINQUENCY LISTING   DATE   08/31/74

NAME/ADDRESS	PHONE NO	TYPE	BALANCE	CURRENT	A G I N G				MSLP	LAST PMT	REMARKS
					30	60	90	120			
001234 JAMES C ARNETT 1234 WEST FIRST STREET VAN NUYS CA 91201	988-1234	I	88.00	.00	10.00	.00	.00	78.00	6	10.00 05/15/74	
002354 GERRY FREELEY 3344 EAST GLORIA DRIVE NORTHRIDGE CA 91521	324-3356	I	102.00	.00	.00	30.00	30.00	42.00	5	20.00 07/11/74	
005864 JAMES A MICHNER 9832 VENTURA BLVD ENCINO CA 91009	787-9852	B	140.00	12.00	20.00	40.00	30.00	50.00	2	10.00 07/12/74	
075724 ETHELYN NEFF 9339 E OLIVE ST TEMPLE CITY CA 90124	985-0146	B	58.00	.00	4.00	22.50	22.00	9.50	1	10.00 03/23/74	
017854 WILLIAM STEIGER 3005 CICERO COURT VAN NUYS CA 91405	341-6384		254.00	.00	45.00	54.50	42.00	112.50	7	42.00 01/24/74	
009852 ROBERT L YALE 3598 HOLLYWOOD BLVD SANTA MONICA CA 90123	788-6532	M	85.00	.00	15.00	32.00	12.50	25.50	5	30.00 04/12/74	

DELINQUENT ACCOUNTS   79

TOTAL AMOUNT CURRENT   525.00*
                30 DAYS   1,235.00*
                60 DAYS   2,202.00*
                90 DAYS   1,922.00*
               120 DAYS   8,741.00*

GROUP TOTAL   14,615.00**

medcobill system
intellectron international, incorporated

A

FIGURE 12–22

Delinquent Account Record (DAR) Activity Report.

medcobill system
INTELLECTION INTERNATIONAL, INCORPORATED

GROUP 365
REPORT TITLE DAR ACTIVITY REPORT

PAGE 1
DATE 08/31/75

ACTIVE PRIOR ACCOUNTS

GUARANTOR	ACCOUNT NO	TYPE	CHARGES	PAYMENTS	ADJUSTMENT	BALANCE
ALEXANDER	112591		45.00	45.00		210.00
ANDERSON	217890		25.00			440.00
BENSON	099813			100.00		110.00
CATLETT	224217		30.00	65.00	13.00-	0.00
JOSEPHSON	219640			75.00		50.00
			*100.00	*285.00	*13.00-	
DEAN	225371	B	15.00		50.00-	128.00
EDISON	200106	B	80.00			278.00
YOUNG	212033	B				420.00
			*95.00		*50.00-	
ALLAN	200009	I		50.00		110.00
FRANKLIN	217325	I		15.00		0.00
GAGE	211666	I	25.00	112.50		220.00
HARRISON	191451	I		78.00	6.00-	0.00
SMITH	226525	I		20.00		0.00
			*25.00	*275.50	*6.00-	
ASKEW	219343	M	40.00			310.00
LORING	198972	M		65.00	3.00-	0.00
NORRIS	199001	M		101.00		0.00
RESTIN	202883	M	25.00	40.00		85.00
TASMAN	212676	M			78.50-	0.00
			*65.00	*206.00	*81.50-	
			**285.00	**766.50	**150.50-	

FIGURE 12–22 *(Continued)*

A

medcobill system
intellection international, incorporated

GROUP   365   PAGE   2

REPORT TITLE   DAR ACTIVITY REPORT   DATE   08/31/75

INACTIVE PRIOR ACCOUNTS

GUARANTOR	ACCOUNT NO	TYPE	BALANCE
AAMES	2211C6		72.00
DELONS	218344		122.00
EDWARDS	210971		115.00
EVANS	212242		12.00
IVARS	197360		85.00
KILLIAM	196520		200.00
LESTER	226636		35.00
MARKS	214149		53.50
MORRIS	220086		570.00
ROGERS	227676		65.00
ZALE	199944		100.00
			*1429.50
ARDEN	229191	I	350.00
CARLSON	216666	I	60.00
GORAN	221073	I	100.00
JOHNS	200698	I	75.00
SAFFORD	213533	I	240.00
WATERS	204767	I	80.00
WILLETS	200444	I	100.00
			*1005.00
CHARLES	206540	M	305.00
HUSTON	213267	M	160.00
MORROW	211133	M	12.00
TABOR	222090	M	90.00
ZANE	201313	M	15.00
			*585.00
			**3019.50

medcobill system
intellection international, incorporated

A

FIGURE 12–22 (Continued)

medcobill system
intellectron international, incorporated

GROUP 365

REPORT TITLE   DAR ACTIVITY REPORT

PAGE 3

DATE 08/31/75

NEW ACCOUNTS

GUARANTOR	ACCOUNT NO	TYPE	BALANCE
BLAKE	229414		75.00
BOSCO	196057		40.00
DITMAN	223029		35.00
GRANGER	209103		5.00
HIBBITT	213979		330.00
NADENS	210033		85.00
RIDDELL	221117		15.00
SOUTHARD	222099		100.00
WALLACE	199903		150.00
			*835.00
ANDERS	221273	I	419.00
FOWLER	198081	I	15.00
JESSUP	198666	I	130.00
PAULSON	223479	I	75.00
WYATT	213200		3.00
			*642.00
			**1477.00

© COPYRIGHT 1975 intellectron international, incorporated

FIGURE 12–22 *(Continued)*

A

medcobill system	DELINQUENT ACCOUNT RECORD	DIV. INTELLECTRON INTERNATIONAL, INC.

GRP. NO.	ACCOUNT NO.	TYPE	LAST	NAME OF RESPONSIBLE PARTY	FIRST	M.I.	AREA	HOME PHONE NUMBER
356	197341	I	BALLARD	CHESTER		T	213	360-5217

NUMBER AND STREET	CITY AND STATE
16952 BLANCHE	GRANADA HILLS CA 91344

DATE	
08/31/75	

LAST PAYMENT	EMPLOYER

DATE	AMOUNT	SOURCE	
04/12/75	20.00	PERSONAL	AXTON CORP

ACCOUNT AGEING STATUS

BALANCE	CURRENT	30 DAY	60 DAY	90 DAY	120 DAY	DATE LAST CHARGE	AMT. LAST CHARGE
140.00	.00	20.00	.00	45.00	75.00		

DATE	COMMENT	BALANCE	DATE	COMMENT	BALANCE

B

FIGURE 12-22 *(Continued)*

MEDCOBiLL SYSTEM
Intellectron International, Incorporated

AGING ANALYSIS

GROUP 356 CURRENT MONTH DATE: 06-25-73

MO.	TOTAL / % OF CHANGE	ACCT TYPE	CURRENT	30 DAYS	60 DAYS	90 DAYS	120 DAYS	CHARGES	PAYMENTS
06	265897	I	146302 / 55%	67200 / 25%	32050 / 12%	12400 / 05%	7645 / 03%		
06	297147	P	14008 / 05%	19800 / 06%	66331 / 22%	85200 / 29%	111808 / 38%		
06	654577	M	128690 / 20%	345697 / 53%	105020 / 16%	40150 / 06%	35020 / 05%		
06	152630	B	54800 / 36%	31240 / 20%	12000 / 08%	20000 / 13%	34590 / 23%		
06	43640	C	5000 / 11%	31000 / 71%	3600 / 08%	00 / 00%	4040 / 10%		
06	1049825		649400 / 62%	200575 / 19%	55525 / 05%	40220 / 04%	104105 / 10%		
06	489567	Q	151300 / 31%	132100 / 27%	80327 / 17%	36433 / 07%	89407 / 18%		
06	22992	J	11247 / 49%	5745 / 25%	2300 / 10%	3700 / 16%	00 / 00%		

YEAR TO DATE
CASH FLOW RATIO
100 %

PRIOR BALANCE 31,901.00 YEAR TO DATE

MO.	TOTAL / % OF CHANGE	CURRENT	30 DAYS	60 DAYS	90 DAYS	120 DAYS	CHARGES	PAYMENTS
01	3220086 / 1%	1062388 / 33%	869423 / 27%	418611 / 13%	322250 / 10%	547414 / 17%	1499750	1420500-
02	3220994 / 0%	1064888 / 33%	901878 / 28%	386519 / 12%	320140 / 10%	547569 / 17%	1418650	1389400-
03	3189103 / 1-%	1148106 / 36%	861030 / 27%	382692 / 12%	287019 / 09%	510256 / 16%	1467250	1460100-
04	3096217 / 3-%	1176586 / 38%	805016 / 26%	340583 / 11%	309600 / 10%	464432 / 15%	1504100	1575000-
05	3006037 / 3-%	1137138 / 38%	811630 / 27%	330664 / 11%	305760 / 10%	420645 / 14%	1495650	1500500-
06	2976275 / 1-%	1160747 / 39%	833357 / 28%	357153 / 12%	238103 / 08%	386915 / 13%	1425000	1477200-

FIGURE 12-23

Aging Analysis.

MEDCOBILL SYSTEM — PRACTICE INCOME ANALYSIS

Intellectron International, Incorporated

GROUP 356	S A M P L E	PAGE 1
DOCTOR 01 PETER BROOKS MD		DATE 03/31/72

RVS #	DESCRIPTION	CURRENT MONTH AMOUNT	CURRENT MONTH FREQUENCY	YEAR-TO-DATE AMOUNT	YEAR-TO-DATE FREQUENCY
	M E D I C I N E				
90015	INIT OFFICE VISIT INTERMEDIATE	360.00	12	1,110.00	37
90040	OFFICE VISIT BRIEF	1,608.00	201	4,824.00	603
90060	OFFICE VISIT INTERMEDIATE EXAM	3,107.00	239	9,451.00	717
90080	OFFICE VISIT COMPR REEXAM	540.00	18	1,350.00	45
90250	HOSP LIMITED EXAM	1,781.00	137	5,343.00	411
90360	INTERMEDIATE EXAM ECF	380.00	19	1,140.00	57
90700	IMMUNIZATION	156.00	39	488.00	120
		* 7,932.00	665	23,706.00	1,990
	P A T H O L O G Y				
83440	T-3 OR T-4 UPTAKE RADIOACTIVE	462.50	39	1,386.00	118
84460	TRANSAMINASE SGPT	420.00	43	1,260.00	129
84550	URIC ACID BLOOD CHEMICAL	252.00	44	750.00	130
85010	BLOOD COUNT COMPLETE	348.00	60	1,044.00	176
88100	PAP SMEAR 2 SLIDES	50.00	6	150.00	18
		* 1,532.50	192	4,590.00	571
	S U R G E R Y				
27756	FX TIBIA SHAFT SMP/CMP OPN RED	1,188.00	3	2,576.00	7
45300	PROCTOSIGMOIDOSC DIAG INIT/SUB	45.00	3	200.00	13
63005 80	LAMINEC 1/2 SEGMNTS LUMBAR	2,400.00	2	6,000.00	5
		* 3,633.00	8	8,776.00	25
	TOTAL CHARGES	13,097.50	865	37,072.00	2,586
	A D J U S T M E N T S				
00090	*WRITE OFF	20.60-	3	60.60	8
00070	*ADJUSTMENT	184.00-	10	515.00	27
		* 204.60-	13	575.60	35
	P A Y M E N T S				
00010	*CASH PAYMENT	481.75	45	1,480.00	134
00020	*PRIVATE INSURANCE	2,569.00	140	5,020.00	540
00021	*MEDICAL INSURANCE	1,605.80	50	4,805.00	144
00022	*MEDICARE INSURANCE	729.90	35	2,290.00	105
00023	*BLUE CROSS INSURANCE	1,927.00	121	5,781.00	359
00024	*BLUE SHIELD INSURANCE	2,311.60	135	6,933.00	531
00030	*PERSONAL CHECK	2,532.80	138	7,508.00	538
		* 12,157.85	664	36,817.00	2,351

MEDCOBILL SYSTEM
Intellectron International, Incorporated

FIGURE 12-24

Practice Income Analysis.

Practice Management Report (Fig. 12–25)

This is a monthly report which is a condensed version of both the Aging Analysis and the Practice Income Analysis. It can help with office management because it shows age analysis of accounts receivable along with charges and payments to and from insurance companies. An example of how such a report might benefit a physician is that he can see at a glance where the bulk of his practice rests. If the physician has too many patients on state and government plans and wishes to have a more balanced practice, he can see if any shifting needs to be done with regard to taking on new patients. If there are several doctors in partnership, this report breaks down what charges have been incurred by each doctor in the practice by listing them by code numbers: 01, 02, 03, and so forth.

COMPUTER ABBREVIATIONS AND EXPRESSIONS

ACCT TYPE	Account type
ACCUM	Accumulative (such as accounts receivable monthly listing)
ADJ	Adjust or adjustment
ALPHA ORDER	In order of a, b, c, etc.
APPTS	Appointments
B	Blue Cross (account type)
BTCH	Batch (a number of items taken as a group)
C	Code
C	CPS/Blue Shield (account type)
CD	Action code. Tells computer where to place the transactions (charges, payments, adjustments)
CLU	Compensation, Legal, CHAMPUS
CMIT	Current Medical Information and Terminology
CPT	Current Procedural Terminology
CUM	Cumulative (such as a weekly cumulative trial balance)
CUR CHG	Current charges
CUR CR	Current credits
DAR	Delinquent Activity Record
DELQ	Delinquent
DEP	Dependent
DR NO	Sub number or number of physician in office if more than one doctor is practicing

MEDCOBILL SYSTEM
intellectron international, incorporated

PRACTICE MANAGEMENT REPORT

GROUP 356　　　　NAME THE BROCKS CLINIC　　　　DATE: DEC 74

CHARGES		THIS MONTH	YEAR TO DATE	CHARGES		THIS MONTH	YEAR TO DATE
D O C T O R	01	11,637.50	129,833.00	D O C T O R			
	02	13,404.00	150,727.50				
	03	8,767.50	96,437.00				
	04	10,502.50	103,994.00				
	05	4,316.50	11,622.50				
TOTAL		48,628.00	492,614.00				

CHARGES BY TYPE		THIS MONTH		YEAR TO DATE
1	PRIVATE INSURANCE	1	10,693.00	1	108,375.00
2	MEDI-CAL	2	1,459.00	2	14,773.00
3	MEDICARE	3	3,890.00	3	39,409.00
4	BLUE CROSS	4	8,753.00	4	88,671.00
5	BLUE SHIELD	5	6,322.00	5	64,040.00
6	WORKMENS COMP	6	1,945.00	6	19,705.00
7	NON-INSURANCE	7	15,561.00	7	157,636.00
8		8		8	
9		9		9	
10		10		10	
11		11		11	
TOTAL			48,628.00		492,614.00

PAYMENTS BY TYPE		THIS MONTH		YEAR TO DATE
1	CASH	1	973.00-	1	10,705.00-
2	PERSONAL CHECK	2	13,616.00-	2	134,320.00-
3	PRIVATE INSURANCE	3	9,726.00-	3	99,705.00-
4	MEDI-CAL	4	1,720.00-	4	13,596.00-
5	MEDICARE	5	104.00-	5	36,256.00-
6	BLUE CROSS	6	8,753.00-	6	81,577.00-
7	BLUE SHIELD	7	5,349.00-	7	58,917.00-
8	OTHER	8	1,945.00-	8	18,129.00-
9		9		9	
10		10		10	
11		11		11	
TOTAL			42,186.00-		453,205.00-

YTD CASH FLOW RATIO	92 %		ADJUSTMENTS THIS MONTH	67.00

ACCOUNTS RECEIVABLE	BALANCE	CURRENT	30 DAYS	60 DAYS	90 DAYS	120 DAYS
INSURANCE	41,631.00	23,183.00	11,018.00	6,074.00	1,100.00	256.00
OTHER	21,675.00	10,880.00	5,185.00	2,603.00	2,116.00	891.00
TOTAL	63,306.00	34,063.00	16,203.00	8,677.00	3,216.00	1,147.00

DIV. INTELLECTRON INTERNATIONAL INC.　　　　　　© 1975 intellectron international, incorporated

FIGURE 12–25

Practice Management Report.

DUN	Message or phrase put on delinquent billing statement (see Chapter 13)
ECF	Extended Care Facility
EMP BY	Employed by
EXP	Expense
FM	Family member
GRP	Group
I	Private Carrier (account type)
ICDA	International Classification of Diseases, Adapted
INPUT	What is fed into the computer memory bank
J	Crippled Children Society or Special Category account type
K	CHAMPUS (account type)
M	Member or Medicare (account type)
MEMORY	Storage in computer
MHS	Mail, Hold, Suppress
MI	Middle Initial
MO	Month
MOD	Modifier (pertaining to RVS modifier)
MSG NO	Message Number
MTD	Month-to-date
N	Any or no carrier (account type)
NEW B/FWD	New balance forward
OLD B/FWD	Old balance forward
OUTPUT	Information transferred from internal memory storage to external storage
P	Medi-Cal (account type)
PCT	Percent or percentage
PMT	Payment
PN	Person number (Medi-Cal)
POS CODE	Place of Service code
Q	Medicare/Medi-Cal (account type)
REL CODE	Relation code to family member
RVS	Relative Value Studies
STMT	Statement

SUB NO	Same as DR NO
TR	Treatment
W	Welfare (Medicaid)
YR	Year
YTD	Year-to-date

TO THE STUDENT: Refer to the Appendix, Assignments 30 and 31, pp. 611–621, to complete the insurance forms and work with the Patient Visit Slips pertinent to this chapter.

REVIEW QUESTIONS

1. Name the three different ways in which a medical office can utilize a computer system.

a. _____

b. _____

c. _____

2. State some of the reasons why a physician would elect to go on a computer billing system.

a. _____

b. _____

c. _____

d. _____

e. _____

f. _____

g. _____

3. Name the coding systems that might be used to ascertain the diagnosis code for a computer system.

a. _____

b. _____

4. How many digits is the diagnosis code? _____

5. Name the coding systems that might be used to ascertain the description of services rendered to the patient.

a. _____

b. _____

6. How many digits is the description of service code number? _____

7. What is a Dun Request? _____

_____

8. On a patient's itemized billing statement produced by the computer, what very important item or items appear that are not usually present when a manual bookkeeping system is used? _____

9. What is the most important output for the physician from the computer as far as business dollars and cents are concerned? _____

Why? _____

10. How would the following birthdates appear on a computer insurance form?

June 1, 1960 _____   November 3, 1975 _____

January 9, 1952 _____   March 20, 1902 _____

May 10, 1903 _____   October 25, 1955 _____

11. What about patients such as old Mrs. Broadband? The doctor tells you never to accept Medicare assignments, but you know that he makes an exception for Mrs. Broadband. Can the computer handle exceptions like that? _____

_____

12. You recorded Mrs. Myles' charge after a routine office visit, and the computer's memory bank knew that the patient was insured under Blue Shield, Blue Cross, and Major Medical. The computer printed out insurance forms for all three

policies. Which form(s) would you discard? _____

Which form(s) would apply? _____

13. A patient calls after having been in for an office visit and disputes a charge. How could you straighten things out if all his records were over at the computer

office? _____

_____

14. Mrs. James comes in for an office visit on March 12. She returns again on March 14, 15, and 16. Do you have to complete a form for input for each

visit? _____ What form would you complete? _____

15. You have submitted the address of a patient as input and the following month

the patient moves. What must be done? _____

_____

Notes:

Notes:

13
Credit and Collection

INTRODUCTION

The word "credit" comes from the Latin *credere*, which means "to believe" or "to trust." In the sense in which it is used today, it means a trust in an individual's business integrity and in his financial ability to meet all obligations when they become due.

The assistant's attitude is important in establishing a good patient-physician relationship. She should be courteous at all times but express a firm businesslike approach which will not offend the patient. The patient should be educated regarding the credit and collection procedure of the medical office with his or her first visit to the office or when this first visit is discussed over the telephone. Tell the patient what the fees might be and make a definite arrangement for payment *before* services are performed. Obtain a complete and accurate registration of the patient and secure as much personal history as is necessary for credit responsibility (see Figure 13–1).

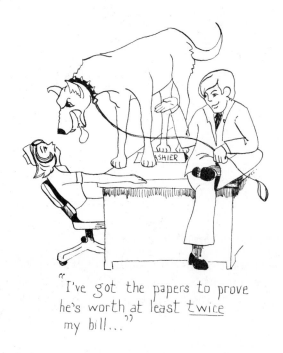

"I've got the papers to prove he's worth at least twice my bill..."

Always leave the patient with a friendly attitude toward the office so he or she will feel free to discuss personal financial problems at any time.

The physician's methods of receiving payment for service and the office policy for the handling of insurance claims should be clearly delineated to all patients. Consistency in this policy, and also in collecting cash, is extremely important. Never badger or intimidate a patient into paying cash. Merely set the policy and educate the patient. Tell the patient the fee and the balance due. Do not say "Would you like to pay now or have a bill sent?"

In some specialty practices the policy is to collect for services as they are rendered while at the same time requiring payment of a small amount towards the performance of future services. An obstetrician-gynecologist, for example, may collect at each prenatal visit a portion of his charge for delivering the baby, so that almost the entire obstetric bill is paid before the child is born. This eliminates having to ask the patient to pay a lump sum after delivery. Some offices are organized to send out statements within 3 days after services are rendered. Many times this can offend patients who did not expect to be billed so soon. Nevertheless, an imbalance in collections can markedly disrupt the overhead ratio. An accurate indication of the degree to which the doctor or assistant is succeeding in educating patients is the collection ratio. *Remember:* the secret to collecting medical fees is simply: "Ask the patient to pay."

COLLECTION TIPS

1. Adopt a specific method of handling accounts so that comprehensive and accurate bookkeeping and accounting records are kept. (See also Chapter 16.)

2. Use a systematic and regular collection follow-up procedure which will make for better collections by your office. Suggestions:

    a. Send an itemized statement within 30 days after treatment. Best results are obtained by presenting the statement at the time of treatment. This is

PATIENT RECORD

Name of Patient_____ Age_____ Birthdate_____ Sex_____
                    Last   First   Middle
Address_____ City_____ Phone_____
                                                    Zip Code
Size of Family_____ House owned_____ Rented_____ Referred by_____

Name of Father or Spouse_____ Name of Mother or Spouse_____

Social Security No._____ Social Security No._____

Father's or Self Employment_____ Mother's or Spouse's Employment_____

_____ _____

Address_____ Address_____

Telephone_____ Telephone_____

Position Held_____ Position Held_____

Salary Per Month_____ Salary Per Month_____

How Long Employed_____ How Long Employed_____

Full Time_____Part Time_____ Full Time_____Part Time_____

Marital Status: Married_____Separated_____Divorced_____

Religion_____Allergic to Any Medication_____

Responsible Person for Medical Payment_____

Name of Insurance Company_____
                                                    Subscriber or Insured
Address_____

Policy Number_____Date of Expiration_____

Previous Physician_____

Address_____

Approximate Date of Last Visit_____

Any Unsettled Balance: Yes_____No_____Amount_____

Driver's License No._____State_____Expiration_____

In Case of Emergency Contact:

Name: _____

Address:_____ Phone:_____

FIGURE 13–1

Patient Registration Record, showing a comprehensive listing of personal and financial information to be obtained from the patient on his or her first visit to the office.

usually called a Patient Visit Slip or Charge Ticket and can be incorporated into manual, pegboard, or computer types of accounting methods. If you send statements by mail, select a mail-out day at the beginning of the month so that the patient will receive the bill near the 15th of the month. You might select the 8th, 10th, or 12th day of the month. If you send statements at the end of the month so that the patient receives the bill on the 1st, you might select the 20th, 24th, or 27th day of the month. *Cycle billing* is a system of billing at spaced intervals on the basis of alphabetical breakdown. It is a time-saving and convenient substitute for once-a-month billing, particularly in larger offices, because it relieves the pressure of having to get all the statements out at one time.

   b. Send a second statement 30 days later.

   c. Send a short, courteous collection letter 15 days after the second statement, if no payment is received. Sometimes a handwritten personal note to the patient will bring results if it is written directly on the billing statement.

   d. Make a courteous telephone call 10 days after the collection letter. If the patient is unable to pay the entire bill, suggest an installment plan.

   e. If the phone call is ignored, a final letter should be sent stating that the account is being placed with a professional collection agency. Many times a letter signed by the physician will bring better results than a letter carrying the secretary's signature.

3. Collections can also be increased by:

   a. Use of colored envelopes or stationery for billing the patient.

   b. Use of commemorative stamps on the envelope.

   c. Enclosing a business reply envelope with every letter requesting payment.

   d. Follow-through on insurance claims.

4. It might also be wise to use a write-it-once bookkeeping system (pegboard system). The patients can be directed to take the Patient Visit Slip or Charge Slip to the appropriate staff member. Some of the advantages of this system are:

   a. Greater accuracy

   b. Time savings

   c. Better collections

5. It is important to know the age of your accounts receivable. This is sometimes referred to as "aging accounts" and is the analysis of the status of the accounts receivable, such as 60, 90, or 120 days delinquent. The information can be shown on each patient's ledger by the use of color tabs, or after sending a warning notice (N) or letter (L), by using codes on the record such as N1, N2 or L1, L2. Many offices also code the patient's charts to match the ledger, perhaps using a green sticker to indicate cash, a red sticker to indicate a Medicaid or Medi-Cal patient, a blue sticker for insurance, and a black sticker to indicate a delinquent account. In this way the physician can tell from the patient's chart the status of the account and determine if there is any need for discussion. Very old accounts continue to cost the physician money, and many accounts over 6 months old prove to be uncollectable. Follow up slow and delinquent accounts by making up an accounts receivable aging record (see Fig. 13-2).

6. Do not spend a lot of time trying to collect "chickenfeed" bills, since this will only cost the physician a great deal of money.

7. A good rule of thumb for accounts receivable is that the ratio should amount to approximately three times the average monthly charge.

ACCOUNTS RECEIVABLE AGE ANALYSIS   Enter credits in parentheses ( ) and subtract when totaling columns & page

Doctor's Name				As of date	Prepared by				Page	of	Pages
Account Name	Phone No.	Present Balance	Over 1 month	2 months	3 months	4 months	6 months	Total	Collection Action		
Amounts Brought Forward											
Amounts Carried Forward											

FIGURE 13–2

Accounts Receivable Age Analysis Record, showing one way in which an office can set up a form to establish an age analysis for accounts.

Directions:

1. List the full name and phone number of each patient.

2. Write in the patient's current total balance in the third column.

3. Break down the total by indicating if a charge is over a month old (put it in the fourth column); over 2 months old (put it in the next column); and so forth.

4. In the second to the last column, put in the total amount owed on the account.

5. Any collection efforts (letters, telephone calls, promises, errors in bills) should be entered in the last column.

6. Give the Accounts Receivable Age Analysis log to the doctor and ask him to indicate in the Collection Action column if he wishes an account turned over to a collection agency or if he wishes any special follow-up procedure. If you wish, you can modify the age analysis columns to read: 30 days; 60 days; 90 days; 120 days.

Insurance Claims Register

In order to reduce collections, it is wise to establish a follow-up procedure on insurance claims. As each form is completed and sent from the physician's office, it can be logged in on an insurance claims register form (see Fig. 13–3). In this way the assistant handling the insurance forms can see at a glance which claims are becoming delinquent and what are the amounts owed to the physician. A Dun Message on an itemized billing statement for those patients who have not brought in an insurance form to complete might look like the one shown in Figure 13–4.

Another method of following up on insurance claims is to keep two copies of each claim for the physician's records, one to be filed by the patient name and the other by carrier name. Or you can simply record the name of the insurance company on each patient's ledger card and keep a file by carrier name only. Then when you are writing to the insurance company all inquiries may be included in a single letter, eliminating writing to the same company three or four times in a two-day period.

Date Claim Filed	Patient Name	Name of Insurance Co.	Where was Claim Sent?	Amount of Claim	Follow-Up Date	Amount Paid	Difference

INSURANCE CLAIMS REGISTER — Page No. _____

FIGURE 13–3

Insurance Claims Register: an example of how a form may be set up to establish an easy way to follow up on insurance claims.

```
                        STATEMENT

                College Hospital and Clinic
                    4567 Broad Avenue
                  Woodland Hills, CA 91364
                       213/486-9002


        ┌                                      ┐
            Mr. Conrad Cashflow
            4508 Penny Street
            Receivable, XY 90002

        └                                      ┘
```

DATE	PROFESSIONAL SERVICE	CHARGE	PAID	BALANCE
2-12-77	OC	15 —		15 —

*WHEN YOU SEND US YOUR INSURANCE FORM, MAY
WE SUGGEST THAT YOU INCLUDE A STAMPED
ENVELOPE ADDRESSED TO YOU OR YOUR INSURANCE
COMPANY. WE ARE REQUESTING THIS DUE TO THE
INCREASED POSTAL RATES AND THE FACT THAT
WE DO NOT CHARGE OUR PATIENTS FOR FILLING
IN THE FIRST INSURANCE FORM. THANK YOU
FOR YOUR COOPERATION.

*Exception Medicare patients.

Pay last amount in this column

CON - CONSULTATION	HCD - HOUSE CALL (DAY)	LAB - LABORATORY
CPX - COMPLETE PHYS EXAM	HCN - HOUSE CALL (NIGHT)	NC - NO CHARGE
E - EMERGENCY	HV - HOSPITAL VISIT	OC - OFFICE CALL
EC - ERROR CORRECTED	INJ - INJECTION	OS - OFFICE SURGERY
ECG - ELECTROCARDIOGRAM	INS - INSURANCE	SE - SPECIAL EXAM

FIGURE 13–4

An example of a Dun Message as it appears on an itemized billing statement, stating the procedure the patient is to follow when submitting an insurance form for completion.

Super Bill

Another method of eliminating paperwork and improving cash flow is by the utilization of "super bill." This term describes a specific method that is usually part of a system for medical office billing and collecting. It is typically a two- or three-part form that shows current fees, description of services, treatment codes, diagnostic information appearing as an ICDA Code number, patient personal data, and insurance requirements. The "super bill" is, in some respects, an Attending Physician's Statement and usually replaces any other form designed for this use. The purpose of the "super bill" is to generate such information at the time of the patient's visit. The physician's signature is *not* required. The completed form is presented or mailed to the patient. Simple instructions tell the patient how to submit his or her own insurance claim. An assignment of benefits is included. One copy of the "super bill" is attached to the insurance claim form, eliminating the need to type insurance information.

There are many varieties of "super bill." It can be a type of Ledger/Statement combination or it may be incorporated into a Transaction Slip. Many systems include a multipart "Super Bill" which has several carbon copies. An example of one of these billing forms is shown in Figure 13–5.

Insurance companies are beginning to recognize the necessity for reducing the administrative detail required on the part of the medical practice in processing insurance claims. Many private companies as well as Blue Cross, Blue Shield, and Medicare now accept one or more versions of the "super bill."

Copy Van

Another method of reducing administrative paperwork and improving cash flow is by the use of Copy Van. This is a system which helps to eliminate peak loads during the billing cycle. It originated as a national franchise called Service Enterprises, and was thought up by Garnett Bowen of Richmond, Virginia. It is now no longer a franchise, and many companies across the nation feature a similar service or system. There is no established fee, nor is there a contract to sign. The control of the accounts receivable remains in the office under the supervision of the medical assistant, and the assistant decides which delinquent notices (Dun Messages) should be sent to each patient. The assistant also decides what day of the month she wants the statements sent out, and then Copy Van does the billing while the assistant continues with her daily duties.

The system works like this: A van comes to the physician's office once each month and parks in the parking lot. It obtains the ledgers for the month, Xeroxes them, returns the originals to the physician's office within 20 minutes or so depending on the volume to be copied, and then stuffs, stamps, and mails the bills to the patients. Some services do microfilming of records for hospitals and for very large practices. The Dun Messages as shown in Figure 13–6 are placed on sticky adhesive labels. These are supplied to the assistant and are coded by number. The assistant may designate which message she wants on a specific ledger. The messages are used over and over again and replaced in their plastic box. In areas that have a large Spanish speaking population, messages such as the following may be used:

Text continued on page 368

STATEMENT

IMPORTANT ➡

One of the attached copies must be included
with any INSURANCE CLAIM – See instructions

CLOSING DATE	ACCOUNT NO.

**CHARGES AND PAYMENTS MADE AFTER THE CLOSING
DATE WILL APPEAR ON YOUR NEXT STATEMENT**

TO INSURE PROPER CREDIT TO YOUR
ACCOUNT RETURN THE UPPER PORTION
OF THIS STATEMENT WITH YOUR PAYMENT

AMOUNT ENCLOSED $ _____

(left margin, vertical text top:) RETURN THIS PORTION WITH YOUR PAYMENT

(left margin, vertical text bottom:) KEEP THIS PORTION FOR TAX & MAJOR MEDICAL PURPOSES

DOCTOR CODE	PATIENT	DATE	DESCRIPTION	DIAGNOSIS ICDA CODE	RVS CODE	AMOUNT

CURRENT	OVER 30 DAYS	OVER 60 DAYS	OVER 90 DAYS	OVER 120 DAYS	TOTAL DUE
UNPAID BALANCES					

PLEASE NOTE: Even though an insurance claim may be pending you will receive a statement each month if your account has an outstanding balance. We cannot accept responsibility for collecting your insurance claim or for negotiating a settlement on a disputed claim. You are responsible for payment of your account within the limits of our credit policy.

(right margin, vertical text:) MEDICOUNT FORM 4045 U (D/M STATEMENT 1-76)

A

FIGURE 13–5

Super Bill is the nickname given a very popular new concept in insurance billing. The statement (*A*), along with two special copies labelled Attending Physicians Statement (*B*), is sent directly to the patient. Simple instructions (*C*) tell the patient how to submit his or her own claim. (An assignment of benefits is included.) The diagnoses appear in ICDA code. The physician's signature is *not* required. The forms have been well received by the insurance carriers as well as by Blue Cross, Blue Shield, and Medicare. Offices using Super Bill have reported improved cash flow.

ATTENDING PHYSICIANS STATEMENT FOR INSURANCE

1

NAME OF PATIENT	AGE	DATE OF BIRTH	SEX	MARITAL STATUS S M W D	RELATION TO SUBSCRIBER:	DOES PATIENT HOLD OTHER COVERAGE ? YES ☐ NO ☐

JOB CONNECTED ILLNESS OR INJURY ? YES ☐ NO ☐	IF ACCIDENT GIVE TIME & PLACE (HOME, WORK, SCHOOL, AUTO, ETC.)	DATE OF ONSET OR ACCIDENT ?	DATE FIRST CONSULTED PHYSICIAN:	PHYSICIAN'S NAME:

CLOSING DATE		ACCOUNT NUMBER	

2

INSURANCE COMPANY

POLICY IDENTIFICATION OR MEDICARE NO.	GROUP

3

I CERTIFY THAT THE SERVICES LISTED BELOW HAVE BEEN RECEIVED & I AUTHORIZE PAYMENT TO BE MADE TO THE OFFICE NAMED HERE ON.

SIGNED   DATE

X

BENEFITS ASSIGNED — VOID IF ALTERED

SEE REVERSE SIDE FOR INSTRUCTIONS

DOCTOR CODE	PATIENT	DATE	DESCRIPTION	DIAGNOSIS ICDA CODE	R V S CODE	AMOUNT

THIS STATEMENT FOR INSURANCE PURPOSES

B

FIGURE 13-5 *(Continued)*

TO PREPARE YOUR OWN INSURANCE CLAIM:

GROUP INSURANCE
1. COMPLETE YOUR PART OF YOUR COMPANY'S FORM.
2. COMPLETE SECTIONS 1. 2. AND 3 ON THE FRONT OF THIS FORM.
3. TAKE OR MAIL THEM TO YOUR INSURANCE CARRIER OR HEALTH PLAN OFFICE.

MEDICARE
1. COMPLETE ITEMS 1 THRU 6 ON YOUR MEDICARE FORM.
2. ATTACH THIS FORM AND MAIL DIRECTLY TO YOUR LOCAL MEDICARE OFFICE.

BLUE SHIELD PATIENTS — COMPLETE SECTIONS 1. 2 AND 3 ON THE FRONT OF THIS FORM AND MAIL TO YOUR INSURANCE CARRIER OR HEALTH PLAN OFFICE.

A SEPARATE CLAIM FORM & STATEMENT ARE USUALLY REQUIRED FOR EACH FAMILY MEMBER RECEIVING SERVICES COVERED BY INSURANCE. IF YOU REQUIRE ANOTHER STATEMENT FOR A THIRD INSURANCE COMPANY OR A THIRD CLAIM PLEASE HAVE A COPY OF THIS STATEMENT MADE AT YOUR LOCAL LIBRARY OR A COMMERCIAL COPYING SERVICE.

TO THE INSURANCE COMPANY

Please expedite payment as your insured will continue to receive monthly statements until the balance is paid.

EXPLANATION OF CODING

ICDA: INTERNATIONAL CLASSIFICATION OF DISEASES ADAPTED, EIGHTH EDITION
Available from the Government Printing Office,
Washington, D.C., in 2 volumes Vol. 1 would be
most useful for insurance companies.

DIAGNOSTIC CODE MODIFIER: P = PRIMARY
S = SECONDARY
R = POSSIBLE/RULE OUT

RVS: CALIFORNIA RELATIVE VALUE STUDIES
A copy of this can be obtained from:
Sutter Publications, Inc.
731 Market Street
San Francisco, CA 94103

C

FIGURE 13–5 *(Continued)*

1. Just a friendly reminder:we have not received a payment on this account in over thirty days.

2. Perhaps you forgot. If so please consider this a friendly reminder that your account has become past due.

3. The previous balance is past due. This has no doubt escaped your attention. A prompt remittance will be appreciated.

4. Please give this account your immediate attention. The previous balance is long past due and settlement must be made without further delay.

5. Please make some effort to pay on account within the next ten days or this account will be turned over to our collection agency.

6. We have received notice from your insurance company that your policy does not cover the above.

7. Since there has been no response from your insurance company, the responsibility for this account rests with you. May we please have a prompt payment?

8. Minimum payment of $_____ will keep your account current.

9. Minimum payment of $_____ will bring your account up to date. Thank you for your cooperation.

10. A small consistent payment will keep this account from Credit Collections, and prove your good faith and respect for services rendered to you. PLEASE CALL.

11. If we are not hearing from you for any reason that we can remedy, please call this office and let us know what it is.

12. After six months postoperative care office visits are no longer included in surgery fee. May we please have your prompt payment?

13. We cannot possibly stock all forms for all types of insurance. Please furnish a form if you wish this billed to your insurance.

14. ANY amount -- LARGE or small, Keep it consistent THAT is all.....

15. Please call our office as we need additional information to complete your patient record.

16. Normal Medicare procedure is to have the patient pay the account. We then will send you a receipt in full along with diagnosis so you can submit it to Medicare.

17. It is the policy of this office not to bill insurance until the account is paid in full, at which time a "Paid in Full" statement will be present.

FIGURE 13-6

Dun messages. These can be placed on sticky labels and kept in a plastic see-through box. They are then ready for use when photocopying ledgers to send out monthly statements. Cash flow is nearly always increased through the use of such notices. (Courtesy of Copy Van of Santa Barbara, California.)

Text continued from page 364

Text continued from page 364

DO YOU HAVE INSURANCE
TO COVER THIS ACCOUNT?
IF SO, PLEASE SUBMIT FORMS.
SI TIENE ASEGURANZA QUE
CUBRA ESTA CUENTA, POR
FAVOR MANDE LAS FORMAS.

NO PAYMENT YET. YOUR
PAYMENT BY RETURN MAIL
WILL BE APPRECIATED. NO
HEMOS RECIBIDO PAGO.
AGRACIERAMOS REMITA
POR CORREO.

THIS ACCOUNT IS PAST DUE.
PLEASE REMIT NOW.
ESTA CUENTA ESTA VENCIDA.
POR FAVOR REMITA HOY.

ACCOUNT WILL BE SENT TO
COLLECTION IF NOT PAID
NOW.
ESTA CUENTA SERA
REMITIDA AL DEPARTMENTO
DE COBROS SI NO SE RECIBE
PAGO HOY.

PAYMENT NEEDED NOW. NO
FURTHER CREDIT WILL BE
EXTENDED.
SE REQUIERE PAGO HOY. NO
SE LE ESTENDERA MAS
CREDITO.

Bonding of Employees

Many times employees who handle cash flow are bonded. Bonding is an insurance contract by which a bonding agency guarantees payment of a certain sum to a physician in case of a financial loss caused by an employee or by some contingency over which the payee has no control. There are two bonding methods that are effective for a practice with three or more office employees:

1. *Position-schedule bond*: This covers a designated job, such as a bookkeeper or nurse, rather than a named individual. If one employee in a category leaves, her replacement is automatically covered.
2. *Blanket-position bond*: This provides coverage for all employees regardless of job title.

Special Fee Services

It is also important to know the policy in your office regarding the following:

1. Phone calls to patients (long distance or local)
2. Broken appointments
3. Completion of insurance forms
4. Narrative reports to other facilities requested by the patient
5. Late charges on fees for professional services
6. Yearly summary of charges for income tax purposes

Charging for any of these special services requires great tact on the part of the assistant, because many times the patient-physician relationship can be destroyed or badly damaged if they are not handled properly.

Professional Courtesy

Professional courtesy is a discount or fee exemption given to certain people at the discretion of the physician. Make sure you know when to bill or not to bill. Sometimes a NO CHARGE (NC) or percentage of the physician's usual and customary fee can be billed. The phrase "By Request" should be typed on the billing statement if the bill has been requested by the doctor's wife. The following are examples of people who may be extended professional courtesy:

1. Physicians and members of their immediate families
2. Parents of physicians
3. Nurses

    4. Medical assistants employed by colleagues
    5. Clergy
    6. Medical assistants' relatives
    7. Pharmacists
    8. Dentists

SERVICE CHARGE

A physician can charge a service charge of 1 per cent or 1½ per cent per month, or 12 per cent or 18 per cent per annum. As long as this policy is noted on the itemized billing statement, it is assumed that the patient knows about it. Usually a verbal discussion of the charge is beneficial for the patient-physician relationship, but this is not necessary if the charge is printed on the itemized billing statement.

TRUTH IN LENDING

When a situation arises in which a patient and his physician together agree upon payment of the bill in more than four installments, then the federal Truth in Lending Act is applicable. At the time a specific agreement is reached between patient and physician, Regulation Z requires that a written disclosure of all pertinent information be made, regardless of the existence of a finance charge. According to the Federal Trade Commission (FTC), the Truth in Lending provision is not applicable and no disclosures are required if a patient decides on his own to pay in installments or whenever convenient. Figure 13–7 shows the disclosure form which is recommended by the Federal Trade Commission. Complete an original and one copy of this form, giving one copy to the patient and retaining one copy for the physician's records. When the assistant is discussing an installment plan she should cover these five major points:

    1. Amount of total debt
    2. Amount of down payment
    3. Estimated date of final payment
    4. Amount of each installment
    5. Date of each payment

TELEPHONE IN DEBT COLLECTING

The telephone has been increasingly used for debt collection in a manner which is in violation of the tariffs of telephone companies and criminal statutes as outlined in Section 22 of the Communication Act. Violations include such practices as calling at odd hours, repeated calls, calls to debtor's friends, relatives, neighbors, employers, or children; calls making threats, calls falsely asserting that credit ratings will be hurt, and calls demanding payment for amounts not owed. The tariff regulations of the telephone company also forbid the use of the telephone for calls which frighten, abuse, torment, or harass another person. A violation of this sort can result in discontinuation of telephone service.

TRUTH IN LENDING FORM FOR PHYSICIANS

Doctor's Name:_____

Doctor's Address:_____

_____

Patient's Name:_____

Patient's Address:_____

_____

Cash price (total fee)   _____

Less cash down payment   _____

Unpaid balance of cash price   _____

Amount financed   _____

FINANCE CHARGE   ___(none)_____

ANNUAL PERCENTAGE RATE   ___(none)_____

Total of payments   _____

Deferred payment price   _____

Patient hereby agrees to pay to_____at
                                                    (physician's name)
his office, the address of which is given above, the total of payments shown

above in _____monthly installments of $_____, first installment being

payable _____, 19_____, and all such installments on the same day

of each consecutive month until paid in full.

_____   _____
        (date)   (signature of patient)

FIGURE 13-7

Truth in Lending Form for Physicians. By filling out this form the physician can provide all information on full disclosure required by the Truth in Lending Act's Regulation Z. The wording shown here must be used, but customary medical terminology may be added in parentheses, as after "Cash price." Note that headings referring to finance charges must be in capital letters and must stand out on the form. The word "none" can be preprinted on the form to show that there are no finance charges. Where there are no such charges, the "Deferred payment price" is the same as the "Cash price." The narrative below the form must be included, but whether the patient later deviates from the periodic payments agreed upon is between him and the physician. Regulation Z imposes no restrictions on the patient. A copy of the form is retained by the doctor and a copy given to the patient.

Collection calls can be effective if you:

1. Call the patient between 8 a.m. and 8 p.m.
2. Ask for the payment with courtesy and firmness.
3. Have the patient write down the payment agreement. (If the patient is to send in half on Friday, ask him or her to write it down, along with the physician's name and address and dates of payment.)
4. Ask the patient to read back to you what he or she has written to make sure there is no misunderstanding.

TRACING A SKIP

If a patient who still owes a balance on his or her account has moved but left no forwarding address, this person is called a "skip." Start tracing as soon as possible. Sometimes an unopened envelope will be returned to your office marked GNO (Gone No Order) or FOE (Forward Order Expired) by the Post Office. This can be avoided by placing the wording "Address Correction Requested" below the doctor's return address on the envelope. The post office will make a search, forward the mail to the new address, and inform you of this new address for a nominal fee when you receive the information (see Fig. 13–8).

The following are some tips for tracing a skip:

1. Call the patient's nearest relative.
2. Call the patient's employer without disclosing to any coworkers the nature of the call.
3. Check with the Department of Motor Vehicles to see if it has been notified of a change of address.
4. Check the City Directory and locate a neighbor or landlord to find out what has happened to the patient.
5. Call the Board of Education to find out the patient's school district and the elementary school closest to his former residence. If the patient has children, call the school to find out the forwarding address or contact the school nurse.
6. If you think the patient may have a criminal record, call the Police Department.
7. Call a self-drive truck rental company near the patient's home. They may have a record of the patient's destination if he moved himself.
8. If the last name is unusual, check the telephone book for the same name and call and ask for the patient.
9. If you know the name of the patient's bank, call and ask if his or her account was transferred or is still open.
10. If the patient might be registered as a student at a local college, call and ask for their help in tracing information.

RETURNED CHECKS

If a patient's check is returned by your bank marked NSF (Not Sufficient Funds) or RTM (Return to Maker), either the patient innocently miscalculated his or her bank balance or the patient is deliberately attempting to stall in making payment. Telephone the patient, but be tactful in discussing the problem. State that you are holding onto

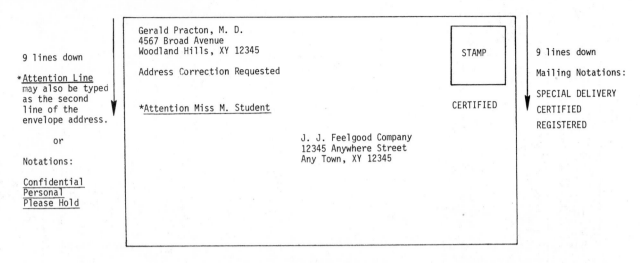

9 lines down

*Attention Line
may also be typed
as the second
line of the
envelope address.

or

Notations:

Confidential
Personal
Please Hold

Gerald Practon, M. D.
4567 Broad Avenue
Woodland Hills, XY 12345

Address Correction Requested

*Attention Miss M. Student

STAMP

CERTIFIED

J. J. Feelgood Company
12345 Anywhere Street
Any Town, XY 12345

9 lines down

Mailing Notations:

SPECIAL DELIVERY
CERTIFIED
REGISTERED

FIGURE 13–8

An example of how to address billing envelope correctly. Note the designation "Address Correction Requested," which tells the Post Office that they are to trace a person who has moved and obtain his new address.

the check and ask when it may be redeposited. If you are unable to reach the patient by phone, write a letter. The following wording is a good model:

Your check dated _____ in the amount of _____ has been returned to our office by the bank marked Insufficient Funds.

Obviously some error led to this problem, but we are sure you would want us to let you know about it. We will hold the check until _____ when we will redeposit it. Please make arrangements so that the check will clear at that time.

If you would prefer to issue another check or to make payment by cash, certified check, or money order, please let us know.

Thank you for your cooperation.

If the patient wishes the check returned to him or her, be sure to photocopy it and keep it in your records, because it serves as an acknowledgment of the debt.

STATUTE OF LIMITATIONS

In regard to collections, the statute of limitations is the maximum time during which a legal collection suit may be rendered against a debtor. To find out the statute of limitation for your state, refer to Table 13–1, Summary of Collection Laws, on pages 374–378. Statutes vary according to three kinds of accounts. These are:

1. *Open book accounts:* accounts which are open to charges made from time to time. Physician's patient accounts are usually open book accounts.

2. *Written contracts:* an agreement by which a patient signs to pay his bill in more than four installments. (See Truth in Lending on page 370.)

3. *Single entry accounts:* accounts having only one entry or charge. Usually these are for a small amount.

Text continued on page 379

TABLE 13–1. SUMMARY OF COLLECTION LAWS.*

Location	Statute of Limitations				Collection Agency Bond and License			General Garnishment Exemption
	Open Accounts Years	Contracts in Writing Years	Domestic Judgments Years	Foreign Judgments Years	Bond	License	Fee	Federal law exempts from garnishment 75% of disposable earnings per work week, or an amount = to 30 × federal minimum hourly wage, whichever is greater. Some state laws still on the books are listed below, but where federal law provides larger exemption, it supersedes the state law.
ALABAMA	2	6	20	20	No	Yes (privilege license)	$150.50 (pop. over 20,000) $38 (pop. under 20,000)	See federal law; except on credit sales, greater of 80% or disposable earnings = to 50 × fed. min. hourly wage, per week.
ALASKA	6	6	10	10	$5,000	Yes	$200 biennially	75% of employee's weekly income, or up to $114 per week of disposable income, whichever is greater.
ARIZONA	3	6	5 Add'l 5 on request	Becomes Ariz. judgment if 20 days' notice and no answer filed.	$3,000	Yes	$ 50 invest. $100 original $100 renewal	See federal law.
ARKANSAS	3	5	10	10	$1,500-$5,000	Yes	Up to $25	$500 head of family; $200 single. Includes personal property except clothing.
CALIFORNIA	2 oral agreement; 4 written book act.	4	10	10	$5,000	Yes	$270 original $160 renewal $ 20 manager $ 10 employee $ 5 emp. ren.	See federal law. Exemptions for non-necessity items.
COLORADO	6	6	20	6	$8,000	Yes	$15	See federal law.
CONNECTICUT	6	3 (Seal) 17	21	Foreign statute applies	$5,000	Yes	$100 $ 50 invest.	75% each week, or greater of $65 or 40 × fed. min. hourly wage.
DELAWARE	3	5	20	20	No	Merc. License	$30	85% of wages.
DISTRICT OF COLUMBIA	3 4 breach of contract seal	3 (seal) 12	6 mun. ct. 12 dist. ct.	Foreign statute applies	No	No	No	See federal law; except 90% of 1st $200 gross wages per month, 80% on excess of $200 & under $500.
FLORIDA	3	5	20	7	$5,000	Yes	$100 $100 renewal $ 50 br. office	See federal law; except 100% head of household.
GEORGIA	4	6	7	5	No	No	No	See federal law.
HAWAII	6	6	6	4	$5,000 ($3,000 each branch)	Yes	$60	95% of 1st $100, 90% of 2nd $100, 80% gross wages in excess of $200 per mo.

*Courtesy of Ray Elliott, Accounts Adjustment Bureau, Oxnard, California. Published in the American Collectors Association, Inc., 1975 Bonded Directory.

TABLE 13–1 (Continued)

Location	Statute of Limitations — Open Accounts Years	Contracts in Writing Years	Domestic Judgments Years	Foreign Judgments Years	Collection Agency Bond and License — Bond	License	Fee	General Garnishment Exemption — Federal law exempts from garnishment 75% of disposable earnings per work week, or an amount = to 30 × federal minimum hourly wage, whichever is greater. Some state laws still on the books are listed below, but where federal law provides larger exemption, it supersedes the state law.
IDAHO	4	5	5 (May renew)	5 (May renew)	Greater of $5,000 or 2 x average monthly net collections previous year plus $2,000 to indemnify state for costs.	Yes	$100 init. exam $100 original $50 renewal	See federal law.
ILLINOIS	5	10	7 (renew up to 10)	Same as domestic after recorded	$25,000	Yes	$50 original $20 renewal	$65 head of family, $50 single, per week, or 85% gross wages, whichever greater, but no more than $200.
INDIANA	6	10 money 20 other	10	10	$5,000	Yes	$50 plus $5 each unlicensed employee $15 br. office	75% of disposable earnings for workweek in excess of 30 × fed. min. hourly wage.
IOWA	5	10	20	20	No	No	No	See federal law.
KANSAS	3	5	5	5	No	No	No	See federal law.
KENTUCKY	5	15	15	15	No	No	No	See federal law.
LOUISIANA	3	5 prom. note 10 other	10	10	No	Yes (Occupational)	$5 for each $5,000	75% disposable earnings per work week, $70 min.
MAINE	6	6	20	20	$3,000	Yes	$100	100%. Money judgment: greater of 75% or amount by which week's earnings exceed 30 × fed. min. hourly wage.
MARYLAND	3	(seal) 12	12	12	No	No	No	Greater of 75% or amount = to $120 × no. of wks. in which wages due were earned; except in Caroline, Worcester, Kent & Queen Anne's Counties, see federal law. Up to $400 in property, $200 of which may be in money.
MASSACHUSETTS	6	20 (seal)	20	20	$10,000	Yes	$100 $50 max. for invest.	1st $100 net wages.
MICHIGAN	6	6	10 (renewable)	10	$5,000 (filed in county)	No	No	See federal law.
MINNESOTA	6	6	10	10	$5,000	Yes	$100	Greater of 75% or amount = to 40 × fed. min. hourly wage.
MISSISSIPPI	3	6	7	7	No	Yes (city only on all businesses)	$15-50	See federal law.
MISSOURI	5	10	3 magistrate court 10 circuit court	10	No	No	No	See federal law; except 90% of week's net pay, head of household.

TABLE 13-1 (Continued)

Location	Statute of Limitations				Collection Agency Bond and License			General Garnishment Exemption
	Open Accounts Years	Contracts in Writing Years	Domestic Judgments Years	Foreign Judgments Years	Bond	License	Fee	Federal law exempts from garnishment 75% of disposable earnings per work week, or an amount = to 30 × federal minimum hourly wage, whichever is greater. Some state laws still on the books are listed below, but where federal law provides larger exemption, it supersedes the state law.
MONTANA	5	8	6 (renewable)	Must obtain domestic judgment	No	No	No	See federal law.
NEBRASKA	4	5	5 (renewable)	5	$2,000	Yes	$100 original $ 50 renewal $ 35 br. office $ 25 br. off. ren.	Greater of 75% disposable earnings (85% if head of household), or 30 × fed. min. hourly wage.
NEVADA	4	6	6	6	$10,000	Yes	$ 25 original $ 15 renewal	See federal law.
NEW HAMPSHIRE	6	6	20	20	No	No	No	50 × fed. min. hourly wage.
NEW JERSEY	6	6 (Seal) 16	20 (May renew for 20 yrs.)	20 (May renew for 6 yrs.)	$5,000 Surety only	No	No	$48 wk. min.; 90% if earnings $7500 a year or less.
NEW MEXICO	4	6	6	6	$3,000 (May be increased by Board)	Yes	$100	Greater of 75% or amount each wk. = to 40 × fed. min. hourly wage.
NEW YORK	Services 6 Merchandise 4	6	20		No ($5,000 in Buffalo)	No Yes	No $50	90% of earnings in last 60 days, except 1st $85 wk. wholly exempt.
NORTH CAROLINA	3	(Seal) 10	7-10	7-10	$5,000	Yes	$50	100% of last 60 days' earnings for family support. Garnishment only by political subdivisions for taxes, ambulance fees, etc.
NORTH DAKOTA	6	6	10 (one renewal)	10	$5,000	Yes	$50	Greater of 75% or amount each wk. = to 40 × fed. min. hourly wage. Personal property, $1500 head of household, $150 single.
OHIO	6	15	5	15	No	No	No	See federal law. Garnishment limited to once a month per employee.
OKLAHOMA	3	5	5	1	No	No	No	See federal law.
OREGON	6	6	10 (renewable)	10	$10,000	Yes	$100 $100 ea. branch	See federal law.
PENNSYLVANIA	6	(Seal) 20	20	20	No	No	No	100%.
RHODE ISLAND	6	6	20	20			No	See federal law.
SOUTH CAROLINA	6	10	6	6	No	Yes (all business)	No	100%.
SOUTH DAKOTA	6	6	20	10	No	No	No	100% of last 60 days' earnings for family support.

TABLE 13-1 (Continued)

Location	Statute of Limitations				Collection Agency Bond and License			General Garnishment Exemption
	Open Accounts Years	Contracts in Writing Years	Domestic Judgments Years	Foreign Judgments Years	Bond	License	Fee	Federal law exempts from garnishment 75% of disposable earnings per work week, or an amount = to 30 × federal minimum hourly wage, whichever is greater. Some state laws still on the books are listed below, but where federal law provides larger exemption, it supersedes the state law.
TENNESSEE	6	6	10	10	$5,000	Yes	$100 $ 50 invest. $ 5 ea. solicitor	Greater of 50% or $20 per wk. head of household, max. $50; greater of 40% or $17.50 per wk. single, max. $40.
TEXAS	2	4	10	10	No	No	No	100% of wages.
UTAH	4	6	8	8 (if reduced to judgment in Utah)	$5,000	Only in Ogden	$5	$80 of disposable earnings for wages paid weekly, $160 if paid bi-weekly, $173.33 if paid semi-monthly, $346.66 if paid monthly.
VERMONT	6	6	8	8	No	No	No	$30 wk. + ½ of earnings in excess of $60 wk.
VIRGINIA	3	5 (seal) 10	10	10	$5,000	Yes	$50	See federal law.
WASHINGTON	3	6	6	6	$5,000	Yes	$100 $100 invest. $ 50 br. office	Greater of 75% or $64 wk. (40 × state min. hourly wage).
WEST VIRGINIA	5	5-10	10	10	$5,000	Yes		80% of wages ($20 per week min.) due or to be due within one year of issuance of execution. Personal property $1,000 for head of household.
WISCONSIN	6	Open-6 (Cognova) 20	6-20	6-10	Yes	Yes	$100 min., orig. investigation $50	Greater of 75% net pay, or 30 × fed. min. wage for each full week of pay period. Special dependent exemption.
WYOMING	8	10	5	10	$2,000	Yes	$20	50% of last 60 days' earnings for family support. See federal law for consumer credit sale, lease or loan.
PUERTO RICO	15		15	15	$5,000	Yes	$100 $100 br. off. $100 ren. $100 invest.	75% of last 30 days' earnings for family support.

TABLE 13-1 (Continued)

Location	Statute of Limitations				Collection Agency Bond and License			Garnishment Exemption	Other
	Open Accounts Years	Contracts in Writing Years	Domestic Judgments Years	Foreign Judgments Years	Bond	License	Fee		
CANADA ALBERTA	6	6	10	10	$5,000-10,000	Yes	$100	Married $200 + $40 each child, single $100.	
BRITISH COLUMBIA	6	6	20	20	10% annual clients' funds handled or $2,500, whichever is greater	Yes	$100	70%, but not less than $200 per mo. head of houshold $100 single	
MANITOBA	6	6	10 (renewable)	6	$5,000	Yes	$100	$75 mo. single; $125 mo. married	
NEW BRUNSWICK	6	20	20		$5,000	Yes	$200	Negotiable bill, draft, note, etc., not overdue. Money due contingently, not absolutely. Money due as officer of crown.	
NEWFOUNDLAND	6	Seal for rent or land—20	20		No	No	No		
NOVA SCOTIA	6	6	20		$5,000	Yes	$50-$250		
ONTARIO	6	6	20	20	$5,000-$25,000 + up to $10,000 for pre-paid colln. service	Yes	$25 main off. $10 br. off. $10 ea. collector $ 5 ren. collector	70% of gross wages. $1,000 on chattels execution.	
PRINCE EDWARD ISLAND	6	6 (Seal) 20	10 (May renew)		$5,000	Yes	$50 orig. $25 ren.	50% single; 50% married, but min. allowance $10 wk.	
QUEBEC	5	5	30	5	$5,000	City only	$150	Federal govt. employee only.	
SASKATCHEWAN	6	6	10	6	$10,000	Yes	$50 $ 5 ea. collector	$200 with 1-3 dep. $225 with 4 or more $100 all others	No exemptions for alimony, separate maintenance, board or lodging, hospital expenses payable to hospital or recoverable by government.

COLLECTION AGENCY

The physician or assistant should seek help in collecting delinquent accounts under the following circumstances:

1. When the patient fails to respond to the physician's letters or telephone calls.
2. When payment terms fail for no valid reason.
3. When repetitious, unfounded complaints occur.
4. When there is a denial of responsibility.
5. When repeated delinquencies occur, with repeated changes of address and/or occupation.
6. When delinquency coexists with serious marital problems.
7. When an obvious financial irresponsibility is exposed.
8. When the patient is a skip (debtor who has moved and neglected to give the office his forwarding address; see p. 372).
9. When any delinquent patient fails to sustain communication.

After a patient's account has been turned over to a collection agency, the patient's financial record should be tagged or removed from the regular file. Frequently after an account has been turned over to a collection agency, the patient will make a payment directly to the physician's office. In this case, call the agency and report the payment. From a malpractice standpoint, it is best to avoid filing suits for collection of fees until counterclaims alleging negligence are barred by the statute of limitations.

CREDIT BUREAUS

Credit bureaus are companies that keep records on individual borrowers. Lending institutions send records of late or unpaid bills and other credit information about borrowers to credit bureaus, where it is placed in the computer files of the individuals involved. These files are then made available to other potential lenders who wish to run credit checks on the individuals. Sometimes an employer may be a member of a credit bureau and in hiring new employees may use the credit bureau to check on an applicant's work history. Many credit bureaus operate a collection department and physicians may turn over their uncollected accounts to them for collection. If a physician belongs to a credit bureau, he or she may obtain the following information by telephone or on a standard computer print-out:

1. Patient's residence and moving habits, as a measure of his permanency
2. Verification of the patient's employment
3. Patient's approximate salary
4. Number of his or her dependents
5. Other merchants' reports on how the patient actually pays bills
6. Any derogatory information such as bankruptcy, use of an alias, and so forth

The Fair Credit Reporting Act of 1971 allows a person to see and to correct his or her credit report. This law states that if a decision is made to refuse a patient credit, based in whole or in part on an adverse credit report from a credit bureau or similar agency, then the name and address of the agency providing the information must be given to the patient. This law does not require the assistant to reveal data or to specify the exact nature of the information obtained from the credit bureau. It only requires that the name and address of the agency be given. Although a patient may not ask for this information, you must volunteer it. Failure to do so can result in legal action.

A form letter should be drawn up that courteously informs the patient that credit has been denied because he or she does not meet credit requirements, leaving blanks for the name and address of the bureau which supplied credit information. By giving one copy to the patient and keeping one for the physician's records, both the patient and the physician—the credit grantor—are protected by the Fair Credit Reporting Act.

The Credit Bureau may also publish bulletins that supply the physician with up-to-date information on people who have moved into the area and bought homes, people who have moved away and their new addresses, deaths, bankruptcy cases, and so forth. In order to find the nearest credit bureau in your area, write to:

American Collectors Association
4040 West 70th Street
Minneapolis, MN 55435
       or
Medical-Dental Hospital Bureaus of America
111 East Wacker Drive
Chicago, IL 60601

FEDERAL BANKRUPTCY LAWS

Bankruptcy laws are federal laws. When a patient files for bankruptcy, he or she becomes a ward of the court and has its protection. When a doctor is notified that a patient has declared bankruptcy, the assistant should no longer send statements or make any individual attempt to collect the account, because a creditor can be fined for contempt of court if he continues to proceed against the debtor. If the account has been turned over to a collection agency and the agency is the one that is notified of the bankruptcy, the situation is the same as if the physician has been notified. If the patient telephones the doctor's office to inform him of the bankruptcy, the verbal communication is valid because notification of bankruptcy does not have to be in writing.

Types of Bankruptcy

There are two types of bankruptcy. They are:

1. *A straight petition in bankruptcy*; sometimes called a Chapter 14. In this situation a person declares those to whom he owes money and is not required to make payment.

2. *A "wage earner's" bankruptcy*; sometimes called a Chapter 13. The debtor pays a fixed amount agreed upon by the court to the trustee in bankruptcy.

If the patient files a straight petition in bankruptcy, the assistant should file a claim on the proper form, which can be obtained from a stationer's store or by writing the referee in bankruptcy. The physician's fee is an unsecured debt. In other words, there is no collateral. Because of this fact it is usually one of the last debts to be paid. If a patient has filed for bankruptcy, there must be a time lapse of six years before he or she can file again. The only exception to this is the Chapter 13 or "wage earner's" bankruptcy.

FEDERAL WAGE GARNISHMENT LAW

The garnishment law attaches a debtor's property, wages, and so forth by the authority of a court so that monies can be used to pay the debt(s). Authority and enforcement are carried out under Title III of the Consumer Credit Protection Act, which became effective on July 1, 1970, and is enforced by Wage and Hour compliance officers located across the United States. This law has two basic provisions: (1) it limits the amount of employee earnings that may be withheld for garnishment in any work week or pay period, and (2) it protects the employee from being fired if his or her pay is garnished for only one debt (regardless of the number of levies that must be made to collect). The law protects everyone receiving all types of personal earnings: wages, salary, commission, bonus, and income from pension or retirement programs. Tips are not considered earnings for purposes of this law. The garnishment law is now a continuous garnishment judgment. In other words, if the debt is not paid off in 90 days it then can be continued for another 90 days.

Restrictions on Garnishment

The amount of total pay subject to garnishment is based on the employee's disposable earnings, which is the amount left after legally required withholdings for federal, state, and local taxes and for Social Security. Deductions such as union dues, health and life insurance, and savings bonds are not considered to be required by law. Garnishment is limited to the lesser of:

1. 25 per cent of disposable earnings in any work week, or
2. Amount by which disposable earnings for that week exceed 30 times the highest current federal minimum wage.

When state garnishment laws conflict with federal laws, the law resulting in the smaller garnishment applies.

Exceptions

The garnishment law does not apply to:

1. Federal government employees
2. Court orders for support of any person
3. Court orders in personal bankruptcy cases
4. State or federal tax levies

For further information contact your local Wage and Hour offices, listed in most telephone directories under U.S. Government, Department of Labor, Employment Standards Administration.

SMALL CLAIMS COURT

A physician may take a claim for an unpaid bill to a small claims court if the amount is under $750. Some offices prefer to handle their delinquent accounts in this manner because it is an inexpensive way to collect. The doctor may send his assistant or bookkeeper to show the records of the account to the judge to verify that it is delinquent. If an account has been turned over to a collection agency, it may not be filed in small claims court but must be filed in a municipal or justice court. The basic data required by the court are:

1. The physician's name, office address, and phone number.
2. The patient's name and address.
3. The amount being claimed.
4. A brief summary of the claim, including the date the physician's bill was due if a series of treatments is involved. Give the date of the last visit or payment and the amount still unpaid.

Filing fees vary by state—even by county within some states—and by the amount of the claim. A small charge to have the summons served on the defendant by a sheriff or other court-appointed officer, plus mileage for the officer who serves it, is also necessary. After a patient has been served, he or she may choose one of four options. They are:

1. Pay the claim to the court clerk, who will forward it on to the physician. The physician will not get back the filing fee or service charges.
2. Ignore the claim, which means that the physician will win by default. In some states you may request a judgment in writing, but in others the assistant must appear on a certain date. When the patient does not show up, the judgment is granted on the spot, and usually your court costs are included.
3. Request a small claims hearing. The court clerk will notify both parties when to appear. If the patient wishes, he or she may file a counterclaim against the physician at this time.
4. Demand a jury trial, which indicates that the case will be taken out of small claims court. The court clerk will notify the physician that he must file a formal complaint in a higher court, which means you will need an attorney to represent you.

The physician or his assistant must appear when instructed or the claim will be dismissed and cannot be refiled. When going to small claims court, each party brings any witnesses, statements, receipts, contracts, notes, dishonored checks, or other evidence. The judge questions both the plaintiff and defendant, reviews the evidence, and then rules. Winning the case gives the physician the legal right to attach a debtor's bank assets, salary, car, personal assets, or real property. The small claims office can show the assistant how to execute a judgment. Judgments are usually effective for many years. There is a small charge if the physician decides to execute against the patient's assets, but the charge is recoverable from the defendant.

ESTATE CLAIMS

Various state time limits and statutes govern the filing of a claim against an estate. See Table 13–2 for information on what the time limits are in your state and on where to file. A billing statement (or in some states a special form) is completed for the collection of a deceased patient's account and is mailed to the estate administrator. If you are unable to obtain the name of the estate administrator, inquire from the probate department of the Superior Court, County Recorder's Office. For ease of reference you might jot this address and telephone number down here. *In my area this is*:

_____
_____
_____
_____

Telephone: _____ / _____

After the name of the estate administrator has been obtained, do the following:

1. Send a duplicate itemized statement of the account to the administrator by certified mail, with return receipt requested.

2. If there is no answer in 10 days, contact the executor or county clerk where the estate is being settled and obtain forms for filing a claim against the estate. Some states do not have special claim forms so an itemized statement is sufficient.

3. The administrator of the estate will accept or reject the claim. If it is accepted, you will receive an acknowledgment of the debt. If it is rejected, the doctor should file a claim against the administrator within a certain amount of time, depending on state laws.

TABLE 13–2. WHEN AND WHERE TO FILE ESTATE CLAIMS.*

When and where to file estate claims

When. The various state laws specify that a doctor must file his claim on an estate within the number of months indicated in the table below, starting:
  (A) From the date a court of probate recognizes an executor or administrator.
  (B) From the date of the first publication of notice to creditors.
  (C) From the date of the second publication.
  (D) From the date of death.
  (E) From a date that has been or will be determined or approved by the court.

The appearance of a range of months indicates that the time limit on filing a claim depends on the amount of the estate, as specified by state law.

Where. A doctor must file his claim with the person or place indicated in the table as follows:
  S As selected by the court.
  P With a court of probate.
  R With the executor or administrator or other representative of the estate, as specified by state law.

State	Time limit (in months)	Where filed	State	Time limit (in months)	Where filed	State	Time limit (in months)	Where filed
Ala.	6 (A)	P	Ky.	9 (D)	R	N.D.	3 (B)	P
Alaska	6 (B)	R	La.	Indefinite	R	Ohio	4 (A)–9 (D)	R
Ariz.	4 (B)	R	Me.	12 (A)	P or R	Okla.	4 (B)	S
Ark.	6 (B)	P or R	Md.	6 (B)	P & R	Ore.	6 (A)	R
Calif.	6 (B)	P or R	Mass.	6 (B)–12 (A)	R	Pa.	12 (D)	R
Colo.	6 (A)	P	Mich.	2–4 (B)	R	R.I.	6 (B)	P
Conn.	6–12 (A)	R	Minn.	4–12 (D)	P	S.C.	5 (B)	P or R
Del.	9 (A)	R	Miss.	6 (B)	P	S.D.	4 (B)	P or R
D.C.	6 (A)	R	Mo.	6 (A)–9 (D)	P & R	Tenn.	1 (A)–9 (B)	P
Fla.	6 (B)	P	Mont.	4 (B)	R	Tex.	12 (A)	R
Ga.	12 (A)	R	Neb.	3–18 (B)	P	Utah	3 (B)	R
Hawaii	4 (B)	R	Nev.	3 (B)	P	Vt.	(E)	S
Idaho	4 (B)	R	N.H.	3–12 (A)	R	Va.	6 (A)	R
Ill.	9 (A)	P	N.J.	6 (A)	R	Wash.	6 (B)	R
Ind.	6 (B)	P	N.M.	6 (B)	P	W. Va.	4–6 (B)	S
Iowa	6 (C)	P	N.Y.	6 (B)–7 (A)	R	Wis.	3–12 (A)	P
Kan.	9 (B)	P	N.C.	6 (B)	R	Wyo.	6 (B)	R

*From Frederick, P.M., and Kinn, M.E.: _The Medical Office Assistant._ Philadelphia, W.B. Saunders Company, 1974, p. 221.

COLLECTION LETTERS

Collection letters should be brief and direct, and should contain the following information:

1. How much is owed.

2. What it is for.
3. What the patient should do about it.
4. When, where, and why the patient should do it.
5. Perhaps how the patient can do it.

Cosmo Graff, M. D.
4567 Broad Avenue
Woodland Hills, CA 91364
213/486-9002

Committee on Physician's Services

Re: Underpayment
Identification No.: *M 18876 782*
Patient: *Peaches Melba*
Type of Service: Plastic & Rec. Surgery
Date of Service: *1-3-77*
Amount Paid: $ *75.00*
My Fees: $ *180.00*

Dear Sirs:

Herewith a request for a committee review of the above named case, since I consider the allowance paid very low having in mind the location, the extent, the type and the necessary surgical procedure performed: *The skin graft, only one inch in diameter, included the lateral third of eyebrow and was full thickness to preserve hair follicles.*

Operative report for the surgery has been sent to you with the claim.

Considering these points I hope that you will authorize additional payment in order to bring the total fee to a more reasonable amount.

Sincerely,

Cosmo Graff

Cosmo Graff, M. D.

mf

FIGURE 13-9

Appeal of Fee Reduction. This letter may be sent to an insurance company after payment has been received which the physician feels should be increased. This simple form requires little time and effort. It has helped physicians to win back many fee cuts made by insurers.

Samples of collection letters that have scored a high record of returns are shown in Figures 13–9 to 13–19. If you have information that will allow you to make the letter more *personal*, then by all means use it.

One final note: If a patient asks the medical assistant to verify what his or her insurance policy will pay on a given surgery or procedure, an Insurance Verification Form (Fig. 13–20) can be sent to the insurance company to find out this information before any procedures are carried out.

Since this is the third statement we have sent you, we feel compelled to call this account to your attention.

Perhaps you have a question concerning your account, or full payment is impossible at this time. Whatever your reason, we request that you get in touch with us in the next two weeks to discuss it with us.

Secretary

We are at a loss to understand why we have not heard from you in the past several months concerning your account.

If payment cannot be made in full, we will be happy to work out some arrangements with you for regular payments to take care of this account promptly and conveniently.

Secretary

For some time we have been expecting word from you concerning your account.

We still feel there must be some reason why you have not responded to our notices. However, since this account is now delinquent, some arrangements must be made at this time to take care of it.

Please let us hear from you at once.

Secretary

We have attempted in every way possible to win your cooperation regarding settlement of your account. Your actions leave us no alternative but to place this account in the hands of a collector.

We still hope to hear from you in the next ten days so this action will not be necessary, however, this is your final notice.

Secretary

FIGURE 13–10

A prime example of the traditional sequence of collection mailings. This series is still favored by some of the leading practice management consultants. Oscar W. Gaarder of Gaarder and Miller, Inc., Madison, Wisconsin, says it's just as productive of payments today as when his firm first started using it 27 years ago, and fully as effective as individually typed letters. (From "The Best Collection Letters We've Ever Seen," by Carole Williams. Medical Economics, December 24, 1973, p. 97.)

LETTER 1

LETTER 2

LETTER 3

THE McGEE-TAYLOR MEDICAL CLINIC
CLARKSDALE, MISSISSIPPI 38614

INTERNAL MEDICINE & CARDIOLOGY
ROBERT RAY McGEE, M.D., F.A.C.P.
WALTER T. TAYLOR, M.D.

December 28, 1972

Dear Mr. Jones:

Our office manager, Mrs. Reisser, informs me that the balance on your account is $86.00 and that there has been no payment made to date after a period of four months.

Please make arrangements to pay your account now.

If you are unable to pay the account in full we will certainly be agreeable to regular monthly payments of whatever amount you are able to handle. Contact Mrs. Reisser by phone or note to arrange this.

If you have problems of which we are unaware in regard to this account please notify Mrs. Reisser.

Sincerely,

Robert Ray McGee

Robert Ray McGee, M.D.

ROB...
WALTER T. TAYLOR, M.D.

January 12, 1973

Dear Mr. Jones:

Over two weeks ago we wrote you requesting that you contact our office manager, Mrs. Reisser, regarding your unpaid balance.

We know that sometimes such things are mislaid or overlooked. This second notice is to request that you contact Mrs. Reisser within one week to discuss this account.

Sincerely,

Robert Ray McGee

Robert Ray McGee, M.D.

...RAY McGEE, M.D., F.A.C.P.
WALTER T. TAYLOR, M.D.

January 22, 1973

Dear Mr. Jones:

As our first letter to you indicated, we are trying to be more than reasonable about your unpaid balance.

Two previous letters have been ignored. If you fail to contact our office manager to arrange a method of paying on this account within ten days it will be necessary to turn it over to a professional collection agency.

Yours truly,

Robert Ray McGee

Robert Ray McGee, M.D.

FIGURE 13-11

This physician got faster collections when he signed the letters himself and wrote more effective collection letters, as shown here in the examples. (From "The Best Collection Letters We've Ever Seen," by Carole Williams. Medical Economics, December 24, 1973, p. 97.)

McCANNE MEDICAL GROUP
J. A. - MONTE O. - LON R. - DON R.
McCANNE, M. D.
1159 NORTH PARK AVENUE
POMONA, CALIFORNIA 91767
TELEPHONE 622-2592

Dear Friend:

As you have failed to respond to repeated statements on your past due account, it is now time when the accountant ordinarily would pick up your account for enforced collection.

However, in your case, Drs. McCanne do not wish to have your account sent to the collectors.

And so, this note is just to let you know that we shall hold your account in this office until you are in a financial position to start making payments again.

Your balance is $_____

I hope all is well with you, and that we shall be able to continue our cordial relationship.

Very sincerely yours,

_____

Secretary

A

STATEMENT
HUGH A. JOHNSON, M. D.
Plastic and Reconstructive Surgery
ROCKFORD MEMORIAL MEDICAL BUILDING
2500 NORTH ROCKTON AVENUE
ROCKFORD, ILLINOIS
61103

4423
Card #11

DATE	DESCRIPTION	CHARGE	PAYMENT	CURRENT BALANCE
	Bal. forward fr. $10.00			21.—
5/31/			—	19.—
6/21/				19.—
			2.—	17.—
8/23/				17.—
9/3/			2.—	15.—
9/6/				15.—
7/			2.—	13.—
	Invoice (2.)		2.—	11.—

COULD YOU SEND IN AT LEAST ONE DOLLAR SOON, IN ORDER TO KEEP THIS ACCOUNT ACTIVE? I WOULD RATHER NOT BRING THIS TO DR. JOHNSON'S ATTENTION.

BOOKKEEPER

PLEASE PAY LAST AMOUNT THIS COLUMN ➡

CODE: NC—No Charge   Consult—Consultation
OV—Office Visit   HV—Hospital Visit
EOR—Hospital Emergency Operating Room

B

FIGURE 13–12

A, This friendly note to delinquents with good past records of paying their medical bills frequently prompts not only partial payments but expressions of gratitude. *B*, In response to this message typed on the overdue bill by the bookkeeper, many patients pay in full immediately to avoid personal embarrassment. (From "The Best Collection Letters We've Ever Seen," by Carole Williams. Medical Economics, December 24, 1973, p. 97.)

Gerald Practon, M. D.
4567 Broad Avenue
Woodland Hills, CA 91364
213/486-9002

April 1, 1977

Mr. Bill Owen
4590 Donation Street
Receivable, CA 90002

Dear Mr. Owen:

Normally, at this time, because your account is long past due, this account would be placed with a collection agency. However, we would prefer to hear from you regarding your preferences in this matter.

Please indicate your choice:

( ) 1. I would prefer to settle this account.
         Please find payment, in full, enclosed.

( ) 2. I would like to make monthly payments of
         $_____, until this account is paid.
         I understand that no interest is being
         charged for this delayed payment schedule.

( ) 3. I would prefer that you assign this account
         to a collection agency for enforcement of
         collection. (Failure to return this letter
         will result in this action).

( ) 4. I would prefer that you cancel the balance
         of my account for the following reason(s):

         Signed_____

Please do not hesitate to call if you have any questions regarding this matter.

Sincerely,

Betty Biller

Betty Biller, Office Manager

FIGURE 13–13

A multipurpose form letter, using the checklist approach.

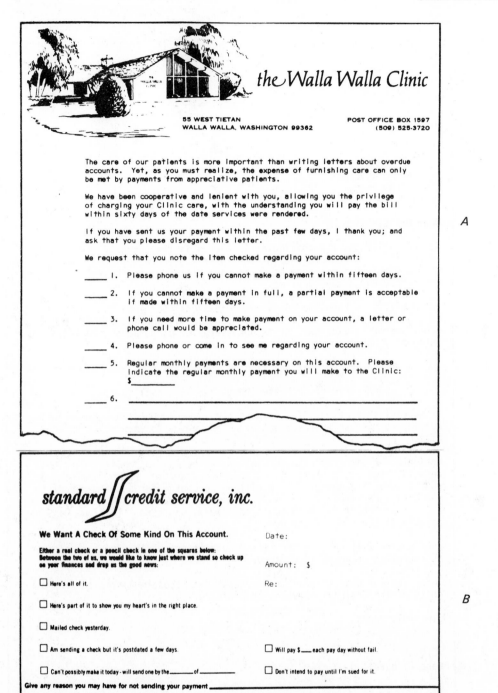

the Walla Walla Clinic

55 WEST TIETAN
WALLA WALLA, WASHINGTON 99362

POST OFFICE BOX 1597
(509) 525-3720

The care of our patients is more important than writing letters about overdue accounts. Yet, as you must realize, the expense of furnishing care can only be met by payments from appreciative patients.

We have been cooperative and lenient with you, allowing you the privilege of charging your Clinic care, with the understanding you will pay the bill within sixty days of the date services were rendered.

If you have sent us your payment within the past few days, I thank you; and ask that you please disregard this letter.

We request that you note the item checked regarding your account:

_____ 1. Please phone us if you cannot make a payment within fifteen days.

_____ 2. If you cannot make a payment in full, a partial payment is acceptable if made within fifteen days.

_____ 3. If you need more time to make payment on your account, a letter or phone call would be appreciated.

_____ 4. Please phone or come in to see me regarding your account.

_____ 5. Regular monthly payments are necessary on this account. Please indicate the regular monthly payment you will make to the Clinic:
$_____

_____ 6. _____

_A_

standard // credit service, inc.

We Want A Check Of Some Kind On This Account.

Date:

Either a real check or a pencil check in one of the squares below:
Between the two of us, we would like to know just where we stand so check up on your finances and drop us the good news:

Amount: $

☐ Here's all of it.

Re:

☐ Here's part of it to show you my heart's in the right place.

☐ Mailed check yesterday.

☐ Am sending a check but it's postdated a few days.

☐ Will pay $_____ each pay day without fail.

☐ Can't possibly make it today - will send one by the _____ of _____

☐ Don't intend to pay until I'm sued for it.

Give any reason you may have for not sending your payment _____

_B_

A business reply envelope is enclosed for your convenience.

R. Reynolds

COLLECTION DEPARTMENT

2501 WEST PETERSON · CHICAGO, ILLINOIS 60659 · PHONE 271-6700

FIGURE 13–14

_A_, Another example of the checklist approach. The Walla Walla Clinic reports "very good success" with this multipurpose form. It covers a wide variety of situations for which the clinic used to send out individually typed letters. _B_, A touch of humor is often effective. Designed to "obtain payment on medical accounts and yet at the same time maintain an amicable relationship," this checklist notice — which might be inappropriate on a doctor's stationery — often leads to "collection on accounts where all other methods have failed," the collection agency reports. (From "The Best Collection Letters We've Ever Seen," by Carole Williams. Medical Economics, December 24, 1973, p. 97.)

Gene Ulibarri, M. D.
4567 Broad Avenue
Woodland Hills, CA 91364
213/486-9002

June 1, 1977

Mr. Conrad Cashflow
4508 Penny Street
Receivable, CA 90002

Dear Mr. Cashflow:

As you well know, the continuing increases in the costs of living are incredible! We too are feeling the spiraling increase, from the price of the simplest items such as cotton and bandaids, to the far more costly laboratory and x-ray supplies.

In an effort to keep the costs of Professional Services to my patients at present levels, in spite of these continually increasing office and other operating expenses, it is necessary for us to adopt the following methods of payment:

    1. Cash or Check at the time of the visit.

    2. BankAmericard or Mastercharge are also available.

If special arrangements for payment are necessary, our Bookkeeper will be glad to discuss this subject with you, prior to your visit to the office.

Patients are directly responsible for the payment of Medical Services. We will, however, prepare any reports necessary for reimbursement from your insurance company. There will be no charge for a claim report to one insurance company. There will, however, be an additional charge of $_____per report for each additional form requested. This fee will be payable at the time of the request.

Full charge will be made for missed appointments unless your appointment is cancelled 24 hours in advance.

Thank you for understanding the necessity of these measures to keep our costs of Professional Services from rising.

Sincerely yours,

Gene Ulibarri, M. D.

mf

FIGURE 13–15

Letter educating the patient on new policies established in an office for credit and collection.

Doctors Business Service
Retail Collection Service

P O Box 23 ● 1315 North Main ● Mitchell, South Dakota 57301 ● Phone 605 996 5531

M. R. KENTON MGR.   J. R. KENTON · PRES.

Medical, dental and hospital bills paid this year are
deductible on your income tax. We suggest for your own
benefit the balance of your account be paid in full on
or before December 31.

Send check or money order in the enclosed self-addressed
envelope to avoid errors and insure proper credit.

If you would like further information in regards to your
benefits from the above procedure, please feel free to
call-phone 605-996-5531.

A

CLARK W. TRUESDALE, M. D.
654 FRANKLIN AVENUE
GLENCOE, MINNESOTA 55336

TELEPHONES
OFFICE 864-3108
RES. 864-3687
IF NO ANS. 864-3121

Our books show that you owe   of which   is
past due by more than 90 days. It is the   90 days
past due that concerns us. We realize that you may be
making payments on this account but the total of such
accounts on our books is such that we find ourselves in the
banking business without the benefit of the interest which
normal banking demands.

Because we are not bankers and because we do not wish to
create an undue burden on you, arrangements have been made
with the First National Bank to loan you the   to bring
your account up to a 90 day basis. Obviously this loan will
carry interest at the current bank rate.

If you can make arrangements to obtain the   from
other sources at less cost it would obviously be to your
advantage to do so. However, one way or another, this
matter must be taken care of by

Complete arrangements can be made at this office.

Sincerely yours,

C. W. Truesdale, M.D.

B

FIGURE 13–16

A, Tax deduction bait. This canny reminder is mailed to reach patients early in November. Those whose medical expenses are large enough to qualify them for an income tax deduction are apt to settle their accounts in full before the year-end deadline. *B*, Bank loan offer. This physician has found that the results are worth the trouble of offering delinquent patients a chance to catch up through a prearranged bank loan — a more discreet approach than if the doctor threatens to charge interest himself. (From "The Best Collection Letters We've Ever Seen," by Carole Williams. Medical Economics, December 24, 1973, p. 97.)

NOTICE OF DELINQUENCY

Date ....

FOR SERVICES RENDERED TO:

....

DUE SINCE ....

Our records indicate you owe $............. which is long past due. Your account cannot be carried any longer without settlement. The account has been reported to The **PROFESSIONAL ACCOUNTS SERVICE, Inc.**

They Are to Wait Ten Days Before Commencing Service. This gives you an opportunity to settle without our resorting to their help.

Your check, or arrangements for settlement, will enable us to advise them that this matter has been satisfactorily closed.

....

Address ....

By ....

DUPLICATE OF THIS NOTICE HAS BEEN SENT TO CREDIT AGENCY

A

Dear _____

On numerous occasions we have notified you of your past due balance and have asked your cooperation. It would appear that you have elected to ignore all of our communications.

We feel that we have afforded you every opportunity to settle your account on an amicable basis. Therefore, your account is being referred to our attorney with instructions to file suit against you for the full principal, plus costs and interest. You shall hear from him shortly.

Very truly yours,

Credit Department

SUMMIT MEDICAL GROUP, P.A.

B

FIGURE 13–17

The showdown stage. *A,* "Pay in 10 days — or else." The collection agency never needs to resort to further action with 30 per cent of the patients who get this notice allowing them exactly 10 days to settle up without any fuss. *B,* No grace period. The usual "Unless we hear from you by _____ we shall. . ." is omitted by design in this no-nonsense letter. The Summit group has found that this approach "prompts the patient to either pay, call, or write immediately." (From "The Best Collection Letters We've Ever Seen," by Carole Williams. *Medical Economics,* December 12, 1973, p. 97.)

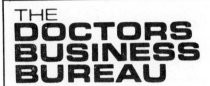

THE
**DOCTORS
BUSINESS
BUREAU**

256 Sutter St. 4th Floor
San Francisco, Ca. 94108
(415) 421-0460

Dear

    *Would it be agreeable with you if we make
arrangements with your employer to have this amount
deducted from your next paycheck?*

    We will wait 72 hours for your reply.

        Very truly yours,

To Agency:

_____ *OK, please make such*

arrangements for me.

Date_____

A

FIGURE 13–18

A, Payroll deduction. It is important to ask the debtor's permission, as this form does; in some states it would be against the law for a creditor to contact or threaten to contact a debtor's employer on his own initiative. Some physicians think this tactic is "too rough." But the collection agency finds it "extremely successful as a follow-up letter, particularly on medium-size accounts." *B*. Notices tailored to size of account. After two monthly statements and a third month "perhaps-you-forgot" reminder have been ignored, doctor-clients of Roger Harrison, practice management consultant of Norman, Oklahoma, use one of these two forms. If the balance due is under $20, the "Final Notice" form is sent. If the account exceeds $20, Harrison has found that the other form works better, with the formidable phrases "auditor of our accounts" and "collection processing." (From "The Best Collection Letters We've Ever Seen," by Carole Williams. Medical Economics, December 12, 1973, p. 97.)

Illustration continued on the following page

B

> ## *Final Notice*
>
> We've been as lenient as we could—more lenient than the credit department of the average business house would have been with an account as old as yours.
>
> However, we cannot continue to let the account run any longer. This is a final notice. The account will be turned for collection unless you make definite arrangements with this office not later than
>
> _____
> DATE
>
> The amount of your account is $_____
>
>
> The auditor of our accounts has classified your account for collection-processing.
>
> The doctor does not want your account handled in this manner. He feels that surely you have encountered circumstances that are most unusual, or that your account would at least show partial-payment each month.
>
> Please talk to us immediately so that we can understand your circumstances, and then seek to help you.
>
> Thanks,
>
>
> R. Harrison
> Business Advisor

FIGURE 13-18 *(Continued)*

CHENANGO BRIDGE MEDICAL GROUP
CHENANGO BRIDGE, N. Y. 13745

CREDIT REMINDER

Your account has been brought to my attention because no payment has been received in the past two regular billings. This may be an oversight. If so, I hope this reminder will bring it to your attention.

I would like to take this opportunity to thank you for your patronage. Should there be any other problems involved, such as insurance, etc., or any dissatisfaction, we would appreciate knowing about it immediately.

If payment in full is not possible or convenient, please call me and arrange a mutually agreeable plan to care for this balance.

Very truly yours,

Ronald E. Brown
Business Manager

A

GREEN ↗

OVERDUE NOTICE

In the two weeks since my reminder letter about your account, we have neither received payment or a communication concerning an arrangement for payment.

I solicit your attention to this matter, because we dislike considering collection action. This costs us money and impairs your credit.

Very truly yours,

Ronald E. Brown
Business Manager

B

YELLOW ↗

FINAL NOTICE

SINCE YOU HAVE NOT RESPONDED TO MY LAST TWO LETTERS, I HAVE NO CHOICE BUT TO START COLLECTION PROCEEDINGS IN TEN DAYS UNLESS THIS BALANCE IS CARED FOR.

RONALD E. BROWN
Business Manager

C

PINK ↗

FIGURE 13-19

Printed on different colors of paper to command extra attention, this medical group's series of letters helped it achieve a 98.3 per cent collection ratio last year (Medicaid accounts excluded). The green "Credit Reminder" (*A*) goes out with the third statement, the yellow "Overdue Notice" (*B*) 15 days later, and the red "Final Notice" (*C*) 30 days after that. (From "The Best Collection Letters We've Ever Seen," by Carole Williams. Medical Economics, December 24, 1973, p. 97.)

```
                          INSURANCE VERIFICATION FORM

                                    Policy:
                                    (  )  Group
Patient:_____   (  )  Individual  #_____

Insurance Company _____

Insurance Co. Address:_____Phone #_____

Employer:_____

Insurance Representative
Releasing Information:_____Date:_____Time:_____
                      (Name)              (Title)

MAJOR MEDICAL:
               Yes      No          % Payable:_____
DEDUCTIBLES:
               Yes      No          Amount: $_____

               time interval:   Year       Month           Other:_____

               per family:   Yes    No    Per Person:  Yes    No
COVERAGE:
          1.  Office visits:    Yes    No    Amount $_____

          2.  Office X-rays & Lab:  Yes    No    Amount $_____

          3.  Hospital surgery:   Yes    No    Limit  $_____ UCR

          4.  Office surgery:    Yes    No    Limit  $_____ UCR

          5.  General anesth.:   Yes    No    Per hr.$_____ Limit $_____
FEE SCHEDULE:

          1.  RVS   Yes    No    1964    1969    1974    conversion factor:_____

          2.  Other:_____

DEPENDENT COVERAGE:

          1.  Wife:     Yes    No    Same?_____

          2.  Children:  Yes    No    Same?_____

IS YOUR FEE SCHEDULE FOR A _____THE SAME AS OTHER MEDICAL SPECIALIST?
                           (Physician's Specialty)
                                                        Yes      No
WHEN CAN I EXPECT PAYMENT AFTER SUBMISSION?_____

REVIEW COPY SENT TO:_____  DATE:_____
                         (Name)

PERSON VERIFYING:_____.  DATE:_____
```

FIGURE 13–20

Insurance Verification Form.

TO THE STUDENT: See the Appendix, Assignments 32, 33, and 34, pp. 622–624, for projects to complete on preparing receipts, composing collection letters, and making up itemized statements.

CREDIT AND COLLECTIONS GLOSSARY

ABA number
Coding system originated by the American Bankers Association for use on checks as a simple way to identify the location of the bank.

Accounts payable
Written contracts or unwritten promises to pay creditors for property such as merchandise, supplies, and equipment purchased on credit or for services rendered.

Accounts receivable
The total amount of money owed to the doctor by patients for professional services rendered.

Aging accounts
Analysis of accounts receivable, showing 60, 90, and 120 days' delinquency.

Bill
Statement sent to the patient for professional services rendered.

Bonding
An insurance contract by which, in return for a stated fee, a bonding agency guarantees payment of a certain sum to an employer in the event of a financial loss to the employer by the act of a specified employee, or by some contingency over which the employer has no control.

Charges
Fees for professional services rendered. (*Note*: "Fees" is the term preferred in current usage.)

Check
An order to pay, and the most common form of money exchange with the exception of actual cash.

Closed accounts
Accounts with a zero balance, or accounts at the end of the year when the final posting is completed.

Collateral
Any possession—such as an automobile, furniture, stocks, or bonds—that secures or guarantees the discharge of an obligation.

Collection ratio
The relationship between the amount of money owed and the amount of money collected in reference to the doctor's accounts receivable.

Credit
From the Latin word *credere*, "to believe" or "to trust." The trust in an individual's business integrity and in his or her financial capacity to meet all obligations when they become due.

Cycle billing	Billing certain portions of the accounts receivable at specified times during the month, usually on the basis of alphabetical breakdown.
Daybook or daysheet	Daily record of each patient seen in the office, hospital, and home, indicating the charges made to each patient and the amounts paid for service, either in cash or by mail. (See also Chapter 16.)
Deposit slip	A form banks provide depositors to use for a detailed listing of items being deposited.
Dun	Message or phrase to remind a delinquent patient about payment (see Figs. 13–4 and 13–6).
Extending	Balance brought forward on the patient's ledger.
Fact sheet	A pamphlet or single information sheet detailing policies of the medical office to the patient on the following subjects: services rendered, appointments, cancelling appointments, telephone, prescriptions and refills, medical fees, insurance, past due accounts, and so forth.
Fee profile	Continuous record of the usual charges submitted for specific services of a physician, compiled over many years.
Fee splitting	Occurs when one doctor gives or receives a commission, rebate, or shares payment with another doctor for a medical service paid by a patient. This is unethical, but not illegal.
Invoice	A bill sent to the doctor for medical supplies, upkeep of machines, and so forth.
Ledger card	Patient's record that shows charges, payments, and balances owed by each patient. This is posted on daily.
Open accounts	Accounts on the books that are open to charges made from time to time.
Payee	Person named on a draft or check as the recipient of the amount shown.
Payments	Cash, checks, or money orders received for professional services rendered.
Petty cash	A small cash fund established for paying small items in the office. (See also Chapter 16.)
Posting	The process of transferring information entered in the journal to the ledger.
Professional courtesy	A discount or exemption from charges given to certain people at the discretion of the physician rendering the service.
Receipt	A record of individual cash payments. Receipts are made out and given to patients when they pay cash, and a carbon copy is retained for the doctor's files.

Reconciliation	A determination of the reason for differences between the balance on the bank statement and the balance on the depositor's books. (See also Chapter 16.)
Restrictive stamp	An endorsement that limits the holder of the check as to the use to be made of the amount collected.
Skip	A debtor who has moved and neglected to give the office his forwarding address.
Stub	Sometimes referred to as voucher. See *voucher*.
Super bill	A method of billing the patient so that the patient may submit the insurance claim himself (see also p. 364 and Fig. 13–5).
Voucher	The left end of the check, which remains in the checkbook after the check has been written and removed. It is used to itemize or to specify the purpose for which the check is drawn. It has no negotiable value.

REVIEW QUESTIONS

1. What are three advantages of the pegboard bookkeeping system?

    a. _____

    b. _____

    c. _____

2. What does cycle billing mean? _____

    _____

3. What are aging accounts? _____

    _____

4. Explain the "super bill" method. _____

    _____

5. What is a dun message? _____

6. Name the two bonding methods.

    a. _____

    b. _____

7. The Truth in Lending provision is applicable when a patient and physician agree upon payment of the bill in more than _____ installments.

8. You send an itemized statement to Mr. Bill Owen. You find out the patient is a skip. What does this mean? _____

_____

9. What is the statute of limitations for collection of accounts in your state?

_____

10. If your physician is a member of a local credit bureau, what information might be of value to know before the physician accepts a patient for extensive treatment? _____

_____

11. Name the two types of bankruptcy.

a. _____

b. _____

12. What does garnishment mean? _____

_____

13. May a physician take a claim for an unpaid bill to small claims court if the amount is $525? _____ Why? _____

_____

14. You have turned over Mr. Bill Lowe's account to a collection agency. If he still does not pay, may his account be filed in small claims court?

_____

15. What is the statute of limitation for filing claims against estates in your state?

_____

16. Mr. Reynolds is now 60 days delinquent on his account. His bill totals $325. What action would you take or what would you send him? _____

_____

17. Mrs. Jeffries owes $250. Her Blue Shield insurance has been billed and the bill is now 90 days delinquent. What action would you take on her bill or what would you send her? _____

_____

18. Miss Bess Baker has a 120 day delinquent bill of $425. You have sent her three notices and telephoned her but without success. The doctor does not want to turn this account over to a collection agency. What other action could be taken? _____

_____

19. Mr. Avery owes the doctor $125 and he comes in for his regular office visit. He tells you he recently had to declare bankruptcy. How would it be best to handle this active account after you have knowledge of this? _____

_____

20. A physician comes in for emergency care for a 4.5 cm. laceration which your doctor sutures. Would you send him a bill? _____ Why? _____

_____

21. Match the expressions in the left column with the definitions in the right column. Write the letters in the blanks.

payee _____

voucher _____

restrictive stamp _____

receipt _____

accounts receivable _____

a. Endorsement on back of check so no one else can cash it

b. Made out when patient pays cash

c. Person named on a check as the recipient of the amount shown

d. Analysis of accounts showing 60, 90, and 120 days delinquency

e. Used to specify purpose for which a check is written

f. The total amount of money owed to the doctor by patients for professional services rendered

Notes:

14
Medical
Ethics and Medical
Professional Liability

BEHAVIORAL

OBJECTIVES *The Assistant should be able to:*

1. Determine the difference between medical ethics, medical etiquette, and medical professional liability.
2. State the two types of medical professional liability insurance.
3. Name the three legal classifications for medical professional liability claims.
4. Discuss common tort liabilities.
5. Understand the Uniform Anatomical Gift Act.
6. Explain three defense actions.
7. Describe informed consent.
8. Learn how to prevent malpractice claims.
9. Understand the Controlled Substances Act of 1970.
10. Formulate procedure for termination of a case.
11. Explain arbitration.
12. State the different kinds of emancipated minors.
13. Learn about subpoena of a witness and subpoena of records.
14. Identify the principles for release and retention of medical records.
15. Define legal terminology.
16. Prepare legally correct medicolegal forms and letters.

INTRODUCTION

This chapter is intended only as a general outline of the various legal matters in which the assistant may be involved. It is not a substitute for legal advice, and the physician and his secretary should always seek the counsel of an attorney about specific questions of law as it relates to medical practice.

Let us first define the difference between medical ethics, medical etiquette, and medical professional liability.

1. *Medical ethics* is concerned with the moral principles and standards in the ideal relationships between the physician and patient and also between the physician and other physicians.

2. *Medical etiquette* has to do with the customs, rules of conduct, courtesy, and manners of the medical profession.

3. *Medical professional liability* is the responsibility that flows from or arises out of medical malpractice, which literally means "bad practice."

The earliest written code of ethical principles and conduct for the medical profession originated in Babylonia about 2500 B.C. and is called the Code of Hammurabi. Then, about the fifth century B.C., Hippocrates, a Greek physician who is known as the Father of Medicine, conceived The Oath of Hippocrates (Fig. 14–1). Our modern code of medical ethics was adopted by the American Medical Association and is known as the Principles of Medical Ethics (Fig. 14–2). Since medical ethics and medical professional liability sometimes overlap, we will discuss both of these in this chapter. There are also principles of ethics for the medical assistant (Fig. 14–3).

The Oath of Hippocrates

I swear by Apollo, the physician, and Aesculapius and health and all-heal and all the Gods and Goddesses that, according to my ability and judgment, I will keep this oath and stipulation:

TO RECKON him who taught me this art equally dear to me as my parents, to share my substance with him and relieve his necessities if required; to regard his offspring as on the same footing with my own brothers, and to teach them this art if they should wish to learn it, without fee or stipulation, and that by precept, lecture and every other mode of instruction, I will impart a knowledge of the art to my own sons and to those of my teachers, and to disciples bound by a stipulation and oath, according to the law of medicine, but to none others.

I WILL FOLLOW that method of treatment which, according to my ability and judgment, I consider for the benefit of my patients, and abstain from whatever is deleterious and mischievous. I will give no deadly medicine to anyone if asked, nor suggest any such counsel; furthermore, I will not give to a woman an instrument to produce abortion.

WITH PURITY AND WITH HOLINESS I will pass my life and practice my art. I will not cut a person who is suffering from a stone, but will leave this to be done by practitioners of this work. Into whatever houses I enter I will go into them for the benefit of the sick and will abstain from every voluntary act of mischief and corruption; and further from the seduction of females or males, bond or free.

WHATEVER, in connection with my professional practice, or not in connection with it, I may see or hear in the lives of men which ought not to be spoken abroad I will not divulge, as reckoning that all such should be kept secret.

WHILE I CONTINUE to keep this oath unviolated may it be granted to me to enjoy life and the practice of the art, respected by all men at all times but should I trespass and violate this oath, may the reverse be my lot.

FIGURE 14–1

The Oath of Hippocrates. (Courtesy of the Judicial Council Opinions and Reports, American Medical Association, 1971.)

PRINCIPLES OF MEDICAL ETHICS

PREAMBLE

These principles are intended to aid physicians individually and collectively in maintaining a high level of ethical conduct. They are not laws but standards by which a physician may determine the propriety of his conduct in his relationship with patients, with colleagues, with members of allied professions, and with the public.

SECTION 1

The principal objective of the medical profession is to render service to humanity with full respect for the dignity of man. Physicians should merit the confidence of patients entrusted to their care, rendering to each a full measure of service and devotion.

SECTION 2

Physicians should strive continually to improve medical knowledge and skill, and should make available to their patients and colleagues the benefits of their professional attainments.

SECTION 3

A physician should practice a method of healing founded on a scientific basis; and he should not voluntarily associate professionally with anyone who violates this principle.

SECTION 4

The medical profession should safeguard the public and itself against physicians deficient in moral character or professional competence. Physicians should observe all laws, uphold the dignity and honor of the profession and accept its self-imposed disciplines. They should expose, without hesitation, illegal or unethical conduct of fellow members of the profession.

SECTION 5

A physician may choose whom he will serve. In an emergency, however, he should render service to the best of his ability. Having undertaken the care of a patient, he may not neglect him; and unless he has been discharged he may discontinue his services only after giving adequate notice. He should not solicit patients.

SECTION 6

A physician should not dispose of his services under terms or conditions which tend to interfere with or impair the free and complete exercise of his medical judgment and skill or tend to cause a deterioration of the quality of medical care.

SECTION 7

In the practice of medicine a physician should limit the source of his professional income to medical services actually rendered by him, or under his supervision, to his patients. His fee should be commensurate with the services rendered and the patient's ability to pay. He should neither pay nor receive a commission for referral of patients. Drugs, remedies or appliances may be dispensed or supplied by the physician provided it is in the best interests of the patient.

SECTION 8

A physician should seek consultation upon request; in doubtful or difficult cases; or whenever it appears that the quality of medical service may be enhanced thereby.

SECTION 9

A physician may not reveal the confidences entrusted to him in the course of medical attendance, or the deficiencies he may observe in the character of patients, unless he is required to do so by law or unless it becomes necessary in order to protect the welfare of the individual or of the community.

SECTION 10

The honored ideals of the medical profession imply that the responsibilities of the physician extend not only to the individual, but also to society where these responsibilities deserve his interest and participation in activities which have the purpose of improving both the health and the well-being of the individual and the community.

FIGURE 14–2

Principles of Medical Ethics. (Courtesy of the Judicial Council Opinions and Reports, American Medical Association, 1971.)

PRINCIPLES OF MEDICAL ETHICS FOR THE MEDICAL ASSISTANT

These principles are intended to aid medical assistants in maintaining a high level of ethical conduct. They are standards by which a medical assistant may determine the propriety of his or her conduct in his or her relationship with patients, with the physician, and with co-workers.

1. Everything you see, hear or read about patients remains confidential and does not leave the office.

2. Never criticize your physician to a patient.

3. Be neat, clean, and dignified, but do not belittle patients.

4. Do not do anything that could be construed as advertising the physician's services, because in many states a physician is not allowed to solicit.

5. If you find out a patient of your physician is under the care of another physician for the same ailment, it is your duty to notify your physician, as it is unethical for two physicians to treat the same patient for the same condition.

6. Maintain a dignified, courteous relationship with all persons in the office—patients, staff, and the physician,—as well as with insurance adjusters, detail men and women, and others that come to the office or telephone the office.

7. Do not collect payment from another physician or members of his family for services unless your employer tells you to do so.

8. Do not discuss a patient's condition within hearing distance of others.

9. Do not discuss a patient with acquaintances—yours or his.

10. Do not leave patients' records exposed on your desk.

11. Do not make critical statements about the treatment given a patient by another physician.

FIGURE 14–3

Principles of Medical Ethics for the Medical Assistant.

Two points about medical etiquette bear mentioning. These are:

1. Never keep another doctor waiting in the reception room. Usher him into the physician's office as soon as the latter is free.

2. Always connect another doctor on the telephone immediately without asking the reason for his call. The only exception to this is if you know the doctor calling is treating one of your patients, and you wish to verify the name to pull the chart for your physician.

MEDICAL PROFESSIONAL LIABILITY INSURANCE

Basically there are two types of medical professional liability insurance. They are:

1. *Claims Made insurance*, which does not protect physicians against suits filed after the policy expires.

2. *Occurrence insurance*, which protects doctors against suits filed after the policy expires.

As mentioned in Chapter 9, an incorporated physician is considered an employee for the purpose of the Workers' Compensation laws. Nevertheless, incorporation does not completely exempt the physician from medical professional liability.

The courts uphold the relationship between a patient and a physician. However, a physician and his staff must be aware of:

1. The physician's obligations to each patient.
2. The physician's liabilities in regard to his service.
3. The patient's obligations to the physician.

The physician-patient relationship begins when the physician performs a service after the patient has requested it. This request can be an implied or direct verbal statement.

Even though a patient carries medical insurance, the contract for treatment is between the physician and patient and the patient is liable for the entire bill. The only exception to this occurs when a person is injured on the job and the matter is referred to Workers' Compensation. Then the contract exists between the physician and the insurance company as far as bills are concerned. If a physician is treating federal or state government patients, he may lose his fee if he fails to follow government guidelines.

A physician is legally responsible for his own conduct and for any actions of his employees performed within the context of their employment. This is referred to as *respondeat superior*, which literally means "let the master answer." If a Registered Nurse gives the wrong injection, the patient can sue the physician, the nurse, or both. On some professional liability policies the nurse is not covered and must have her own insurance coverage. If a physician employs another physician and a nurse, and the nurse, at the direction of the employed physician, gives a treatment and injures the patient, the employer physician and the nurse can be sued but not the employed physician.

If an accident would not ordinarily occur in the absence of negligence, then negligence is either presumed or inferred. This is called *res ipsa loquitur*, or "the thing speaks for itself." Three conditions necessary for res ipsa loquitur are:

1. The accident must be one which normally does not happen unless someone is careless.
2. It must be caused by a situation or instrument within the control of the defendant (physician).
3. It must not have been due to any voluntary action or contribution on the part of the plaintiff (patient). (If the patient is partially responsible for the accident, the situation is known as contributory negligence—see p. 408.)

Expert testimony is sometimes unnecessary in cases tried under res ipsa loquitur and the doctrine of common knowledge.

Most laws governing financial responsibility indicate that a husband is responsible for his wife's debts. A wife is *not always* responsible for her husband's debts. A father is ordinarily responsible for his children's debts if they are minors and are not emancipated (see p. 410). Children may or may not be responsible for the debts of their parents, depending on the circumstances.

It is unwise for a physician to tell a patient or the patient's attorney whether or not he carries professional liability insurance. The mere mention of this fact may plant the seed of a lawsuit in the mind of a dissatisfied patient. Immediately upon being advised of the possibility of a malpractice suit, the physician should notify his insurance carrier. He should not write a letter or make any statement with reference to a professional liability claim or suit, except upon the recommendation of the attorney representing his insurance carrier. A physician should admit error only when his attorney or insurance company tells him to.

Each medical assistant should check with her physician (employer) to see whether or not her name is included in his policy. If it is not, she could well be sued as an individual. It is up to the physician to make certain that all members of his staff are protected.

TYPES OF CLAIMS AND DEFENSES

The three legal classifications for medical professional liability claims are:

1. *Malfeasance claims*, which are based on wrongful treatment of the patient.
2. *Misfeasance claims*, which are based on lawful treatment that has been done in the wrong way.
3. *Nonfeasance claims*, which are based on failure to act when the physician has a duty to do so.

The six common tort liabilities are (for definitions see the glossary on pp. 432–435):

1. Negligence
2. Assault, battery, and false imprisonment or personal restraint of the patient
3. Defamation, libel, and slander
4. Invasion of privacy and breach of confidential communication
5. Liability for the acts of others
6. Fraud or deceit

The three principal defenses in medical professional liability actions are:

1. *Contributory negligence.* This occurs when the patient himself contributes factors which lead to the permanent disability or disfigurement.
2. *Assumption of risk.* When all risks of a particular operation or other medical procedure have been stated to the patient, and he has signed a document giving his informed consent to the procedure, he is presumed to have accepted the risks. The physician may use the signed document in his own defense. For a more comprehensive discussion of informed consent, see the following section.
3. *Statute of limitations.* This is the time limitation upon the institution of a legal action. The time limit varies from state to state. If a suit is filed after the time has expired, the physician has an automatic defense.

SPECIAL CONSIDERATIONS

Informed Consent

After the physician makes a diagnosis and recommends treatment, the patient has a right to decide whether or not to accept that treatment. The physician must tell the patient all the risks of and the alternatives to the procedure he is suggesting. If the

---

Form P-22

CONSENT TO TREATMENT

Date_____ Time_____ A.M.
P.M.

I have been informed by Dr. _____ of the
nature, risks, possible alternative methods of treatment, possible
consequences and possible complications involved in the treat-

ment by means of _____

_____

for the relief of _____.

Nevertheless, I authorize Dr. _____ to administer
such treatment to me.

Signed _____

(Patient or person authorized
to consent for patient)

Witness_____

FIGURE 14–4

Consent to Treatment. This is a general form of consent that is intended for use primarily in connection with the administration of hazardous drugs and treatment normally provided in the physician's office. (From Medicolegal Forms with Legal Analysis, 3rd ed. Office of the General Counsel, 1973, p. 72. Copyright © 1973 American Medical Association. All rights reserved.)

patient decides to accept the risks, and signs a consent form (see Fig. 14–4) to this effect, he is considered to have assumed the risks.

The five elements of informed consent are:

1. The patient's condition must be stated.
2. The proposed treatment must be explained.
3. The risks or consequences of the treatment must be described.
4. Alternative treatment is recommended or given.
5. The chances of possible failure are mentioned.

For proper wording of surgical consent forms, see also Figures 14–14, 14–15, and 14–16.

Emergency Care

A legal patient-physician relationship is not created when emergency care is administered. The "Good Samaritan Law" states that the physician may render first aid and is not liable for any future outcome. Whenever a patient is unconscious or otherwise unable to give valid consent, the physician may do whatever is necessary to preserve life or health. Consent is implied under these circumstances.

If a patient who requires first aid comes into the office when the doctor is not available, the Assistant should do no more than what is absolutely essential. She should get in touch with her physician or with another physician immediately after emergency measures have been taken.

Minors

The age of majority or adulthood varies with the state. Either or both parents having legal custody of a minor may authorize another person to give consent for their child to receive medical treatment and x-rays, but this permission must be set down in writing. The Assistant would be wise to give all parents a consent form to sign so that it will be on file (see Fig. 14–16). List the names of all adults who can give treatment authorization on the patient's chart.

Emancipated Minors

An emancipated minor is a child who falls outside the jurisdiction and custody of his or her parents or guardians. Since the age of majority varies, the term "minor" can designate anyone from an infant to a 20-year-old. A minor is usually considered to be emancipated in the following situations:

1. A minor who is living separate and apart from his parents or guardian, and who is managing his own financial affairs, may personally give consent for medical, surgical, or hospital treatment. Parents are not liable for the cost of care.

2. Any minor who has contracted a lawful marriage can consent to hospital or medical care without approval of parent or guardian. Any subsequent dissolution of the marriage does not deprive the person of this right.

3. A minor who is on active duty in the Armed Forces can give consent for any medical procedure without his parents' knowledge.

4. A minor may personally consent to his or her own medical, surgical, or hospital treatment provided that the treatment is for a communicable disease required by law to be reported by a local health officer, such as infectious hepatitis, measles, mumps, or venereal disease.

5. An unmarried, pregnant minor may give consent for hospitalization and any medical care needed for the pregnancy without consent of the parent(s). If the same minor wishes an abortion, depending on the laws of the state, she may obtain it without parental consent if she meets the criteria set down by the local law.

Termination of a Case

A physician may terminate a contract by:

1. Sending a letter of withdrawal to the patient by registered or certified mail with return of signature card requested.

2. Sending a letter of confirmation of discharge when the patient states he or she no longer wishes care. This should also be sent registered or certified with return receipt requested.

3. Sending a letter stating the patient left the hospital against the advice of the physician. If there is a signed statement in the patient's hospital records to this effect, it will replace sending a letter. If a letter is sent, a copy of the letter and return receipt card from the post office must be filed with the patient's records.

A letter terminating a contract must contain the following information:

1. The physician did not abandon the case.
2. The physician was discharged by the patient, if this is the case.
3. The patient refused to follow the physician's advice.

See Figures 14–5 through 14–8 for the proper wording of letters to patients for termination of a case.

MEDICOLEGAL FORMS AND LETTERS

Figures 14–5 through 14–8 show letters and authorization forms that are commonly used by a physician in his office practice. The Assistant should type a copy of the proper form to be signed by the patient. Use of these forms or letters will avoid many unpleasant situations, will fulfill the physician's legal obligations, and will render better medical services to the patient. After a form has been signed or a letter has been sent, a copy should be filed and retained indefinitely with the patient's records. If a patient should refuse to sign an authorization form, the physician should not proceed with the proposed operation or treatment. Many of these forms were developed by the American Medical Association.

Text continued on page 415

Form A-1

LETTER OF WITHDRAWAL FROM CASE

Dear Mr._____:

I find it necessary to inform you that I am withdrawing from further professional attendance upon you for the reason that you have persisted in refusing to follow my medical advice and treatment. Since your condition requires medical attention, I suggest that you place yourself under the care of another physician without delay. If you so desire, I shall be available to attend you for a reasonable time after you have received this letter, but in no event for more than five days.

This should give you ample time to select a physician of your choice from the many competent practitioners in this city. With your approval, I will make available to this physician your case history and information regarding the diagnosis and treatment which you have received from me.

Very truly yours,

_____, M.D.

FIGURE 14–5

Letter of Withdrawal from Case. (From Medicolegal Forms with Legal Analysis, 3rd ed. Office of the General Counsel, 1973, p. 3. Copyright © 1973 American Medical Association. All rights reserved.)

Form B-1

LETTER TO CONFIRM DISCHARGE BY PATIENT

Dear Mr. _____ :

This will confirm our telephone conversation of today in which you discharged me from attending you as your physician in your present illness. In my opinion your condition requires continued medical treatment by a physician. If you have not already done so, I suggest that you employ another physician without delay. You may be assured that, at your request, I will furnish him with information regarding the diagnosis and treatment which you have received from me.

Very truly yours,

_____ , M.D.

FIGURE 14–6

Letter to Confirm Discharge by Patient. (From Medicolegal Forms with Legal Analysis, 3rd ed. Office of the General Counsel, 1973, p. 5. Copyright © 1973 American Medical Association. All rights reserved.)

Form B-3

STATEMENT OF PATIENT LEAVING HOSPITAL AGAINST ADVICE

This is to certify that I am leaving _____ Hospital at my own insistence and against the advice of the hospital authorities and my attending physician. I have been informed by them of the dangers of my leaving the hospital at this time. I release the hospital, its employees and officers, and my attending physician from all liability for any adverse results caused by my leaving the hospital prematurely.

Signed_____*

I agree to hold harmless the _____ Hospital, its employees and officers, and the attending physician from all liability, with reference to the discharge of the patient named above.

_____
(Husband, wife, parent, etc.)

Date _____

Witness_____

*If the patient refuses to sign such a statement he cannot be forced to do so nor may his release be withheld until he signs. If this occurs, the form should be filled out, witnessed by hospital personnel present and the statement made on the form Signature Refused."

FIGURE 14-7

Statement of Patient Leaving Hospital Against Advice. (From Medicolegal Forms with Legal Analysis, 3rd ed. Office of the General Counsel, 1973, p. 6. Copyright © 1973 American Medical Association. All rights reserved.)

Form B-5

LETTER TO PATIENT WHO
FAILS TO KEEP APPOINTMENT

Dear Mr. _____:

On _____, 19____, you failed to keep your appointment at my office. In my opinion your condition requires continued medical treatment. If you so desire, you may telephone me for another appointment, but if you prefer to have another physician attend you, I suggest that you arrange to do so without delay. You may be assured that, at your request, I am entirely willing to make available my knowledge of your case to the physician of your choice.

I trust that you will understand that my purpose in writing this letter is out of concern for your health and well-being.

Very truly yours,

_____, M.D.

A

Form B-7

LETTER TO PATIENT WHO FAILS TO FOLLOW ADVICE

Dear Mr. _____:

At the time that you brought your son, William, to me for examination this afternoon, I informed you that I was unable to determine without X-ray pictures whether a fracture existed in his injured right arm. I strongly urge you to permit me or some other physician of your choice to make this X-ray examination without further delay.

Your neglect in not permitting a proper X-ray examination to be made of William's arm may result in serious consequences if in fact a fracture does exist.

Very truly yours,

_____, M.D.

B

FIGURE 14-8

A, Letter to Patient Who Fails to Keep Appointment. *B*, Letter to Patient Who Fails to Follow Advice. (From Medicolegal Forms with Legal Analysis, 3rd ed. Office of the General Counsel, 1973, p. 7. Copyright © 1973 American Medical Association. All rights reserved.)

ARBITRATION

Arbitration is an alternative legal method, provided by statute in some states, whereby the patient and physician may agree to resolve any controversy arising between them before an impartial panel, sometimes referred to as a Grievance Committee. The arbitration agreement is a contract between patient and physician prepared by legal counsel for use in the medical office (see Fig. 14–9). A legal agreement covers all present or future claims or disputes of any kind between patient and physician for which the patient might sue the physician, or for which the physician might sue the patient—including collection of the doctor's fees. Arbitration is thus a fairer, faster, and less expensive way of handling disagreements resulting from the patient-physician relationship.

The patient is free to sign the agreement or not. He is not required to sign in order to be seen by the doctor or to receive continuing medical treatment. If he does sign and subsequently changes his mind within 30 days, he can revoke his signature by giving written notice to the doctor stating withdrawal from the arbitration agreement.

Some arbitration contracts, particularly those used in hospitals, include a box which the patient may check to indicate that he is unwilling to accept arbitration but feels he is being forced to sign. This provision may be made when the rules of the hospital specify that the patient must sign an arbitration agreement in order to be admitted. In this instance the patient may disavow the agreement at a later date. A court may set aside the contract on the grounds that at the time the patient was admitted, he was ill and on that basis unable to make a rational judgment.

The tact with which the medical assistant presents the arbitration agreement to the patient and the willingness with which she answers the patient's questions can have considerable bearing on whether or not the court upholds the contract. When the doctor's assistant "speaks for the physician," any representations that she makes can be held against the physician.

An arbitration agreement in no way affects payment by the patient's health insurance. If a claim for professional negligence arises, notify the physician's insurance carrier immediately. Include a copy of any arbitration agreements relating to the patient's care and request that arbitration be invoked. Failure to assert the right to arbitration at the outset can result in a waiver of the arbitration agreement.

SUBPOENA

Subpoena literally means "under penalty." In legal language, it is a writ requiring the appearance of a witness at a trial or other proceeding. Strictly defined, a *subpoena duces tecum* requires the witness both to appear and to bring certain records "in his possession." Frequently, however, the records only may be sent and the physician is not required to go to court. A subpoena is a legal document that has been signed by a judge or by an attorney in the name of a judge. In cases in which a "pretrial of evidence" or deposition is set up, the subpoena may be issued by a notary public, in which event it is called a *notary subpoena*. If an attorney signs it, he must attest it in the name of a judge, the court clerk, or other proper officer.

A subpoena must be personally served or handed to the prospective witness. The acceptance of the paper by someone authorized to accept it is the equivalent of personal service. The subpoena cannot be left on a counter or desk. It must be served

PATIENT-PHYSICIAN ARBITRATION AGREEMENT

1. It is understood that any dispute as to medical malpractice, that is as to whether any medical services rendered under this contract were unnecessary or unauthorized or were improperly, negligently, or incompetently rendered, will be determined by submission to arbitration as provided by California law, and not by a lawsuit or resort to court process except as California law provides for judicial review of arbitration proceedings. Both parties to this contract, by entering into it, are giving up their constitutional right to have any such dispute decided in a court of law before a jury, and instead are accepting the use of arbitration.

2. I voluntarily agree to submit to arbitration any and all claims involving persons bound by this agreement (as set forth in Article 3) whether those claims are brought in tort, contract or otherwise. This includes, but is not limited to, suits for personal injury, actions to collect debts, or **any kind of civil action.**

3. I understand and agree that this Patient-Physician Arbitration Agreement binds me, my heirs, assigns, or personal representative and the undersigned physician, his/her professional corporation or partnership, if any, his/her employees, partners, heirs, assigns, or personal representative, and any consenting substitute physician. I also hereby consent to the intervention or joinder in the arbitration proceeding of all parties relevant to a full and complete settlement of any dispute arbitrated under this agreement, as set forth in the Rules of Arbitration included in this booklet.

4. I agree to accept medical services from the undersigned physician and to pay therefor. I UNDERSTAND THAT I DO **NOT** HAVE TO SIGN THIS AGREEMENT TO RECEIVE THE PHYSICIAN'S SERVICES, AND THAT IF I DO SIGN THE AGREEMENT AND CHANGE MY MIND WITHIN 30 DAYS OF TODAY, THEN I MAY REVOKE THIS AGREEMENT BY GIVING WRITTEN NOTICE TO THE UNDERSIGNED PHYSICIAN WITHIN THAT TIME STATING THAT I WANT TO WITHDRAW FROM THIS ARBITRATION AGREEMENT. After those 30 days, this agreement may be changed or revoked only by a written revocation signed by both parties.

5. I have read and understood the attached explanation of the Patient-Physician Arbitration Agreement and I have read and understood this agreement, and this writing makes up the entire arbitration agreement between me and the undersigned physician.

NOTICE: BY SIGNING THIS CONTRACT YOU ARE AGREEING TO HAVE ANY ISSUE OF MEDICAL MALPRACTICE DECIDED BY NEUTRAL ARBITRATION AND YOU ARE GIVING UP YOUR RIGHT TO A JURY OR COURT TRIAL. SEE ARTICLE 1 OF THIS CONTRACT.

DATED: _____, 19____

_____
(PATIENT)

Physician's Agreement to Arbitrate

In consideration of the above-named patient's promise to be bound by this Patient-Physician Arbitration Agreement, I likewise agree to be similarly bound by its terms, as set forth in this Agreement and in the attached Rules of Arbitration.

DATED: _____, 19____

_____
(PHYSICIAN)

_____
(TITLE—e.g. PARTNER, PRESIDENT, ETC.)

_____
(NAME OF PARTNERSHIP OR PROFESSIONAL CORPORATION)

© California Medical Association, 1975

FIGURE 14–9

Patient-Physician Arbitration Agreement. The Arbitration Agreement is a contract prepared for patient and physician by the legal counsel of the California Medical Association, to be used in the medical office. This contract complies with California law as to content and format.

with the subpoena (witness) fee and mileage fee. In some states provision is made for substitute service by mail or through newspaper advertisements. This is permitted only after all reasonable efforts to effect personal service have failed.

The Assistant should be courteous at all times to the deputy who is serving the subpoena. She should demand the fee when the subpoena is served. Never accept a subpoena without the fee, for in the absence of the fee the subpoena is not legally valid and may be refused.

First find out from the deputy to which doctor the subpoena is addressed. Then ascertain the custodian of records for that doctor if you are not the custodian. If the deputy is uncooperative, tell him that you cannot help unless he lets you see the subpoena so that you know what action to take. If he is antagonistic, ask one of the other doctors what to do.

If a doctor is on vacation, explain that you are not authorized to accept a subpoena on his behalf—if that is indeed the case. Tell the deputy you understand the problem but the doctor is not here and cannot be served. Suggest that he contact the physician's attorney and relay this information to the attorney. Discuss the subpoena problem with one of the other physicians in the office for advice or management.

When the witness fee has been given to the Assistant and the subpoena has been served, the Assistant may then pull the chart, placing the chart and the subpoena on the doctor's desk for review. Willful disregard of a subpoena is punishable as contempt of court. After receiving the subpoena, verify with the court that the case is actually on the calendar.

The medical office should designate one person—preferably the Assistant—as keeper of the medical records. If the subpoena is for medical records only, the Assistant for the specific doctor can then usually accept it, and the physician himself will not be called to court. Another employee cannot accept a subpoena for records, however, since the subpoena is served on the keeper of the records.

The Assistant has a prescribed time in which to produce the records. It is not necessary to show them at the time of service of the subpoena unless the court order so states. Call the attorney who sent the subpoena and ask if the records can be mailed. If he says yes, send them by registered mail with return receipt requested. You will still have to appear in court. If you do not appear, you may be in contempt of court and subject to several days in jail.

Remember never to accept a subpoena or to give records to anyone without the doctor's prior authorization. Before releasing records, make certain that you have a release of records form signed by the patient. Read the record to see that it is complete and that signatures and initials are identifiable.

If you are not mailing the records, remove them to a safe place, preferably under lock and key, so that they cannot be taken away or tampered with before the date appointed for the trial. Make photostatic copies of the records if you are in doubt about their safety. This may be expensive, but it can also prevent a total loss of the records and facilitate discovery of any altering or tampering while they are outside your custody. Number the pages of the records so that you will know if a page is missing when the person copying the records has finished.

On the day of your appearance in court, comply with all instructions given by the court. Do *not* give up possession of the records unless instructed to do so by the judge. Do *not* permit examination of the records by anyone prior to their identification in court. Do *not* leave the chart in the court unless it is in the possession of the judge or jury and a receipt for it has been obtained.

If you have any other questions, call the patient's attorney or the doctor's attorney. Additional information on the Assistant's responsibility for medical records is given in the following section.

MEDICAL RECORDS

Complete and neatly kept patient records can protect a physician in a medical professional liability suit. A letter should be sent to a patient any time there is failure to keep an appointment or to follow the physician's advice (see Figs. 14–7 and 14–8). The patient record as well as any photographs are confidential documents unless a release of information form has been signed by the patient (see Figs. 14–10, 14–11, and 14–12). An exception to the Right of Privacy and Privileged Communication is a physician who is employed by an insurance company, as in Workers' Compensation cases.

Principles for Release of Information

1. Requests from physicians concerned with patient care may be honored with the written consent of the patient.

2. Requests from insurance companies, attorneys, and others concerned from a financial point of view may be honored *only* with the written authorization of the patient.

3. When litigation is involved, information should *not* be released in the absence of a subpoena (see pp. 415 and 417) unless the patient has authorized it.

4. Government and state agencies may have access to records pertaining to government- and state-sponsored programs. See Chapter 7 (p. 168) for an explanation of the Privacy Act of 1974.

5. Information of a psychiatric nature presents special and frequently delicate problems. Usually the psychiatrist or another attending physician concerned with the case should be consulted before records are released.

6. Special care should be exercised in the release of any information to an employer, even with the authorization of the patient.

7. It is preferable not to allow lay persons to examine records so that misunderstandings of technical terms are avoided. However, in some states certain medical records are being made available to patients on an experimental basis to see if this procedure should be allowed in all states.

8. Care must be exercised in the release of any information for publication, since this also constitutes an invasion of the patient's right to privacy and can result in legal action against the physician or health facility releasing such information (see Fig. 14–13).

9. When in doubt about the release of any information, obtain the patient's authorization in writing.

10. When working in a hospital, the Assistant should check with the supervisor at all times to make sure her actions conform with hospital policy. Whether you are working in a hospital or for a doctor, do not hesitate to ask for clarification of matters that are not clear. If you are employed by a health facility which has a policy manual or office procedure manual, familiarize yourself with its rules for the release of information.

Text continued on page 423

Form D-1

AUTHORIZATION FOR DISCLOSURE OF INFORMATION BY PATIENT'S PHYSICIAN

1. I authorize Dr. _____ to disclose complete

information to _____ concerning his medical findings

and treatment of the undersigned from on or about _____

19____ until date of the conclusion of such treatment.

2. Further, I authorize him to testify, without limitation, as to all of his medical findings and the treatment administered to the undersigned, in any legal action, suit, or proceedings to which I am, or may become, a party; and I waive on behalf of myself and any persons who may have an interest in the matter, all provisions of law relating to the disclosure of confidential medical information.

Signed_____

Place_____

Date_____

Witness_____

FIGURE 14–10

Authorization for Disclosure of Information by Patient's Physician. (From Medicolegal Forms with Legal Analysis, 3rd ed. Office of the General Counsel, 1973 p. 9. Copyright © 1973 American Medical Association. All rights reserved.)

Form D-5

AUTHORIZATION FOR EXAMINATION OF PHYSICIAN'S RECORDS

To Dr. _____:

I authorize you to furnish a copy of the medical records of

_____, covering the period from
(state name of patient or "myself")

_____, 19_____ to _____, 19_____ or to allow those

records to be inspected or copied by _____. I release you from all legal responsibility or liability that may arise from this authorization.

Signed_____

Date_____

Witness_____

FIGURE 14-11

Authorization for Examination of Physician's Records. (From Medicolegal Forms with Legal Analysis, 3rd ed. Office of the General Counsel, 1973, p. 11. Copyright © 1973 American Medical Association. All rights reserved.)

Form D-7

AUTHORIZATION TO FURNISH INFORMATION

Date_____Time_____ A.M.
P.M.

I authorize and request the _____ Hospital, and the physicians who attended me while I was a patient in said hos-

pital during the approximate period from _____, 19____ to

_____, 19____, to furnish to _____ all information concerning my case history and the treatment, examinations or hospitalization which I received, including copies of hospital and medical records.

Signed_____

Witness_____

FIGURE 14–12

Authorization to Furnish Information. (From Medicolegal Forms with Legal Analysis, 3rd ed. Office of the General Counsel, 1973, p. 13. Copyright © 1973 American Medical Association. All rights reserved.)

Form E-3

CONSENT TO TAKING AND PUBLICATION OF PHOTOGRAPHS

Patient_____ Place_____ Date_____

In connection with the medical services which I am receiving

from my physician, Dr._____, I consent that photographs may be taken of me or parts of my body, under the following conditions:

1. The photographs may be taken only with the consent of my physician and under such conditions and at such times as may be approved by him.

2. The photographs shall be taken by my physician or by a photographer approved by my physician.

3. The photographs shall be used for medical records and if in the judgment of my physician, medical research, education or science will be benefited by their use, such photographs and information relating to my case may be published and republished, either separately or in connection with each other, in professional journals or medical books, or used for any other purpose which he may deem proper in the interest of medical education, knowledge, or research; provided, however, that it is specifically understood that in any such publication or use I shall not be identified by name.

4. The aforementioned photographs may be modified or retouched in any way that my physician, in his discretion, may consider desirable.

Signed_____
(Patient)

Witness_____

FIGURE 14–13

Consent to Taking and Publication of Photographs. (From Medicolegal Forms with Legal Analysis, 3rd ed. Office of the General Counsel, 1973, p. 31. Copyright © 1973 American Medical Association. All rights reserved.)

Retention of Medical Records

Preservation of medical records is governed by state and local laws. Individual states generally set a minimum of 7 to 10 years, but it is the policy of most physicians to retain medical records on their patients indefinitely. Proof materials such as x-rays, films, laboratory reports, and pathologic specimens should probably be kept indefinitely. In some states a minor may file suit after he or she has attained the legal age for any act performed during childhood which he or she believes to be wrong or harmful. Sometimes a suit may be permitted until 2 to 3 years after the child has reached legal age. Thus it is important to keep records until patients have reached 3 to 4 years beyond the age of majority.

It is true that a person's medical record may be of value not only to the patient in later years but even to his children.

Medical Records and the Assistant

The following are some guidelines for the Assistant in the handling of medical records:

1. Keep the patient records accurate, detailed, and neat.

2. Keep all records until you are positive that they are no longer needed.

3. Remind the doctor to obtain signatures of authorization for operations and other special procedures. Use legal copy pens in your office.

4. When correcting an entry on a patient's record, cross out the wrong entry and write the correct one, then initial it. Never erase or white out any information already recorded on a patient record.

5. Examine insurance reports carefully before sending them out. Be absolutely certain that the insurance form is complete because an insurance firm can sue a physician for incomplete records.

6. Keep a record when a patient fails to return for needed treatment. Post it on the medical record and see that a letter is sent to the patient advising him that further treatment is indicated.

7. Do not release confidential information without the patient's written authorization.

8. Do not attempt to interpret a report or to give any information regarding the outcome of laboratory tests to the patient. Let the doctor do it.

9. If the authorization form containing the signature of the patient is a photocopy, it is necessary to state that the photocopy is approved by the patient. Or write to the patient and obtain an original signed document.

10. If photographs or motion pictures have been taken of the patient, written permission should be in the chart in case the doctor wishes to reuse these materials for scientific purposes.

11. Do not automatically assume that the patient understands instructions for self-treatment at home. Check to make certain by discussing all instructions with the patient. Provide written directions whenever possible, and instruct the patient on what symptoms to report to the physician.

PROFESSIONAL LIABILITY PREVENTION

The Assistant should be aware of her role in claims prevention. She must remember that while acting within the scope of her duties she is the agent of her physician, and the physician is charged with the consequences of her conduct. The Assistant should be polite and courteous to patients regardless of the circumstances. At the reception desk or over the telephone she establishes the doctor-patient relationship even when the patient is calling for information. It is of course impossible for the Assistant to know all of the legal guidelines, and this is not expected of her. However, to aid her in claims prevention, the prevention commandments set forth in 1963 by the American Medical Association Committee on Medicolegal Problems are listed here for her reference. Any special instructions to the Assistant are given in parentheses after the commandment.

Prevention Commandments of American Medical Association Committee on Medicolegal Problems

1. *The physician must care for every patient with scrupulous attention given to the requirements of good medical practice.* In other words, the patient must receive the attention his symptoms demand.

2. *The physician must know and exercise his legal duty to the patient.*

3. *The physician must avoid destructive and unethical criticism of the work of other physicians.* The present physician cannot know the circumstances or condition at the time of prior treatment. (Patients sometimes invite criticism of the methods or results of former physicians. Remember that you are hearing only one side of the story. Do not discuss the other doctor with the patient.)

4. *The physician must keep records which clearly show what was done and when it was done, which clearly indicate that nothing was neglected, and which demonstrate that the care given met fully the standards demanded by the law. If any patient discontinues treatment before he should, or fails to follow instructions, the records should show it; a good method is to preserve a carbon copy of the physician's letter advising the patient against an unwise course.* See Figures 14–5 through 14–8 for proper wording of forms.

5. *The physician must avoid making any statement which constitutes, or might be construed as constituting, an admission of fault on his part. He should instruct employees to make no such statements.* (Remember that the Assistant's position in lawsuits is to say nothing to anyone except as required by the attorney of the physician or by the court of law. If the physician is doing something illegal, the Assistant can be held responsible for being silent.)

6. *The physician must exercise tact as well as professional ability in handling his patients and should insist on a professional consultation if the patient is not doing well, if the patient is unhappy and complaining, or if the family's attitude indicates dissatisfaction.* (The Assistant should tell the doctor immediately if she learns that a new patient is still under treatment by another physician and did not extend this information to the doctor during the initial interview. If a physician feels a specialist is necessary, he is expected to make referral.)

7. *The physician must refrain from overly optimistic prognoses.* (The Assistant should not compare the respective merits of various forms of therapy and should refrain from discussing patients' ailments with them. Patients come to talk to the doctor about their symptoms and you may give them incorrect information. Let the

doctor make the diagnosis. Otherwise, you may seriously embarrass either the physician, yourself, or both.)

8. *The physician must advise his patients of any intended absences from practice and recommend, or make available, a qualified substitute. The patient must not be abandoned.* (See Fig. 14–8.)

9. *The physician must unfailingly secure an "informed" consent (preferably in writing) for medical and surgical procedures and for autopsy.* (The Assistant should not refer to surgical consent forms or other forms as "releases." They are acknowledgment or authorization forms. Help your doctor remember that he needs written consent of parents or legal guardian before he does any surgery on a minor. Sponge counts are mandatory for all surgical procedures. The surgeon should check and double-check to preclude the possibility that a sponge, instrument, or other foreign object still remains in the incision. Even though the object may remain because of the carelessness of another person, the law may impose upon the surgeon the duty to see to the removal of such objects. For examples of authorization for surgery forms, see Figures 14–14, 14–15, and 14–16.

10. *The physician must carefully select and supervise assistants and employees and take great care in delegating duties to them.* (The Assistant should never give an injection to a patient unless the physician is in the office. If, at your doctor's instructions, you give diathermy treatments, remove clothing from the treatment area. Also, towelling at least 1 inch thick should be between the electrode and the patient, since skin moisture will cause a burn. Never apply heat over adhesive tape or a bandage. Patients should be instructed to advise you immediately if they experience more than mild warmth. The Assistant should take every precaution to ensure sterile techniques in any procedure she is performing for the physician.)

11. *The physician must keep abreast of general medical and scientific progress.* (The duty to keep informed applies also to the Assistant in her handling of insurance matters.)

12. *The physician should limit his practice to those fields which are well within his qualifications.* Two legal phrases commonly heard are:

    a. *Standard of reasonable care:* This means that the physician is required to use the same knowledge and skill as other physicians in good standing and of the same general training in the same or similar communities under similar circumstances.

    b. *Standard procedure:* This means any treatment commonly performed by most physicians of similar training.

13. *The physician must frequently check the condition of his equipment and make use of every available safety installation.* (The Assistant should be alert to hazards which may cause injury to the doctor, to the patients, or to herself. Watch for phone and light cords, rugs, or carpets that curl at the edges, wobbly chairs, objects that protrude, and so forth. If you have linoleum floors, do not permit them to be slippery. Do not let equipment get run down.)

14. *The physician should make every effort to reach an understanding with his patient in the matter of fees, preferably in advance of treatment.* (If the Assistant handles the problem of the fee to be charged, she should be sure that the patient understands what services he or she is to receive and what the "extras" may be. In regard to hospital cases, it is advisable to explain that the fee your doctor charges is for his services only, and that operating room, laboratory, anesthesia, and so forth will be charged for in addition to the bed charge.)

15. *The physician must realize that it is dangerous to diagnose or prescribe by telephone.*

16. *The physician should not sterilize a patient solely for the patient's convenience, except after a reasonably complete explanation of the procedure, its risks and possible complications, and after obtaining a signed consent from the patient and the patient's spouse, if the patient is married. Such sterilization is a crime in Connecticut, Kansas, and Utah, and should not be performed in those states. Eugenic sterilization should be performed only in conformity with the law of the state, if any exists. Sterilization for therapeutic purposes may lawfully be performed with the informed consent of the patient and preferably with the informed consent of the patient's spouse, if the patient is married.* Voluntary nontherapeutic surgical sterilization is lawful in the State of California and in many other states, and such operations are permissible for the purpose of family limitation motivated solely by personal or socioeconomic considerations. It is recommended that for every such procedure the physician should obtain from the patient and the spouse, if any, a signed, written recognition of:

  a. The lack of any guarantee of successful sterilization.
  b. The necessity for supplementary contraceptive measures until sterilization can be reasonably assured (particularly after vasectomies).
  c. The risk of tissue breakdown and recanalization with subsequent fertility. See Figure 14–17 for the request for sterilization form.

17. *Except in an actual emergency situation which makes it impossible to avoid doing so, a male physician should not examine a female patient unless an assistant or nurse, or a member of the patient's family, is present.* (The Assistant should make certain that she is present during the examination of a female if the nurse is not available. Assist the patients on and off the examining table. Keep the examining room spotless at all times and be sure the door is closed while the doctor examines a patient. Professional publications should not be available to patients.)

18. *The physician should exhaust all reasonable methods of securing a diagnosis before embarking upon a therapeutic course.* (A legal phrase commonly used is

---

Form P-1

CONSENT TO OPERATION, ANESTHETICS, AND OTHER MEDICAL SERVICES

Date_____Time_____
A.M.
P.M.

1. I authorize the performance upon _____
(*myself or name of patient*)

of the following operation _____
(*state nature and extent of operation*)

to be performed by or under the direction of Dr._____.

FIGURE 14–14

Consent to Operation, Anesthetics, and Other Medical Services. (From Medicolegal Forms with Legal Analysis, 3rd ed. Office of the General Counsel, 1973, pp. 57, 58. Copyright © 1973 American Medical Association. All rights reserved.)

2. I consent to the performance of operations and procedures in addition to or different from those now contemplated, whether or not arising from presently unforeseen conditions, which the above-named doctor or his associates or assistants may consider necessary or advisable in the course of the operation.

3. I consent to the administration of such anesthetics as may be considered necessary or advisable by the physician responsi-

ble for this service, with the exception of _____

(state "none," "spinal anesthesia," etc.)

4. The nature and purpose of the operation, possible alternative methods of treatment, the risks involved, the possible consequences, and the possibility of complications have been ex-

plained to me by Dr._____ and by_____.

5. I acknowledge that no guarantee or assurance has been given by anyone as to the results that may be obtained.

6. I consent to the photographing or televising of the operations or procedures to be performed, including appropriate portions of my body, for medical, scientific or educational purposes, provided my identity is not revealed by the pictures or by descriptive texts accompanying them.

7. For the purpose of advancing medical education, I consent to the admittance of observers to the operating room.

8. I consent to the disposal by hospital authorities of any tissues or body parts which may be removed.

9. I am aware that sterility may result from this operation. I know that a sterile person is incapable of becoming a parent.

10. I acknowledge that all blank spaces on this document have been either completed or crossed off prior to my signing.

(CROSS OUT ANY PARAGRAPHS ABOVE
WHICH DO NOT APPLY)

Signed _____

(Patient or person authorized
to consent for patient)

Witness_____

FIGURE 14–14 (Continued)

negligent diagnosis, which means failure to make necessary tests, take essential x-rays, observe all unusual conditions as the physician's colleagues do under similar circumstances. In dealing with fractures, x-rays should usually be taken before and after reduction, immediately following surgical intervention, and postoperatively during healing to check position and progress. Failure to order sufficient x-rays can create tremendous difficulties in defending a malpractice case. On the other hand, it is also prudent to avoid taking too many x-rays, since some physicians have been sued for exposing the patient to excessive radiation. In the treatment of the patient, there must be no experimentation without the explicit and informed consent of the patient; and then only when there is sufficient reason to believe that such experimentation offers greater potential for benefit to the patient than currently acceptable modes of treatment.)

Form P-2

CONSENT TO OPERATION, ANESTHETICS, AND OTHER MEDICAL SERVICES (ALTERNATE FORM)[10]

Date_____Time_____ A.M. / P.M.

1. I authorize the performance upon _____
   (myself or name of patient)

of the following operation _____
   (state name of operation)

to be performed under the direction of Dr. _____.

2. The following have been explained to me by Dr._____:

   A. The nature of the operation _____
      (describe the operation)

   _____

   _____

   B. The purpose of the operation_____
      (describe the purpose)

   _____

   C. The possible alternative methods of treatment _____

   _____
      (describe the alternative methods)

   D. The possible consequences of the operation _____

   _____
      (describe the possible consequences)

   E. The risks involved _____
      (describe the risks involved)

   _____

   F. The possibility of complications _____

   _____
      (describe the possible complications)

3. I have been advised of the serious nature of the operation and have been advised that if I desire a further and more detailed explanation of any of the foregoing or further information about the possible risks or complications of the above listed operation it will be given to me.

4. I do not request a further and more detailed listing and explanation of any of the items listed in paragraph 2.

Signed _____
   (Patient or person authorized to consent for patient)

Witness_____

---

*This is an alternate form of consent which will provide an opportunity for the physician or hospital to include a detailed disclosure of the operation. The appropriate paragraphs from Form P 1 may be added to this form.

FIGURE 14–15

Consent to Operation, Anesthetics, and Other Medical Services (Alternate Form). (From Medicolegal Forms with Legal Analysis, 3rd ed. Office of the General Counsel, 1973, p. 59. Copyright © 1973 American Medical Association. All rights reserved.)

```
┌──────────────────────────────────────────────────────────────────────────┐
│                    CONSENT FOR SURGERY UPON MINOR                          │
│                                                                            │
│                                                                            │
│ I (We) being the parent, guardian or custodians of_____  │
│ a minor, the age of_____, do hereby authorize, request and direct     │
│ Dr. _____to perform the following operative         │
│ procedure on the person of said minor.                                     │
│                                                                            │
│ ─────────────────────────────────────────────────────────────             │
│                         Operative procedure                                │
│                                                                            │
│ ─────────────────────────────────────────────────────────────             │
│                                                                            │
│ ─────────────────────────────────────────────────────────────             │
│                                                                            │
│ The undersigned to hereby consent to authorize, request and direct the     │
│ surgeons to perform any other operative procedure that, in their judgment,  │
│ is deemed advisable to necessary or required during the operation.         │
│                                                                            │
│ I consent, authorize and request the administration of such anesthetic or  │
│ anesthetics as is deemed suitable by the physician-anesthetist who shall be │
│ chosen by the surgeon.  It is the understanding of the undersigned that the │
│ physician-anesthetist will have full charge of the administration and       │
│ maintenance of the anesthesia, and that this is an independent function     │
│ from the surgery.                                                          │
│                                                                            │
│                                                                            │
│ ───────────────────────────────        ───────────────────────────        │
│   Parent, guardian or custodian                 Dated                      │
│                                                                            │
│                                                                            │
│ ───────────────────────────────        ───────────────────────────        │
│   Parent, guardian or custodian                 Dated                      │
│                                                                            │
│ ───────────────────────────────        ───────────────────────────        │
│            Witness                             Witness                      │
└──────────────────────────────────────────────────────────────────────────┘
```

FIGURE 14–16

Consent for Surgery Upon Minor.

19. *The physician should use conservative and less dangerous methods of diagnosis and treatment whenever possible, in preference to highly toxic agents or dangerous surgical procedures.*

20. *The physician should read the manufacturer's brochure accompanying a toxic agent to be used for diagnostic or therapeutic purposes, and, in addition, should ascertain the customary dosage or usage in this area.*

21. *The physician should be aware of all the known toxic reactions to any drug he uses, together with the proper methods for treating such reactions.* (In preparing medication, the Assistant should check each medication *three* times—when taking it from the shelf, when preparing it for the patient, and when returning the container to the shelf. She should discard outdated medications and be sure to replace them promptly. Do not leave prescription blanks lying on your desk. Lock them up in a safe place. The Assistant should never prescribe, even though she may feel sure that she knows what the doctor would order. Prescribing constitutes the practice of medicine and is unlawful for a nonlicentiate.)

Form P-17

REQUEST FOR STERILIZATION *

A.M.
Date_____ Time_____P.M.

We, the undersigned husband and wife, each being more than twenty-one years of age and of sound mind, request Dr.

_____, and assistants of his choice, to perform upon

_____, the following operation: _____.
   (name of patient)   *(state nature and extent of operation)*

It has been explained to us that this operation is intended to result in sterility although this result has not been guaranteed. We understand that a sterile person is NOT capable of becoming a parent.

We voluntarily request the operation and understand that if it proves successful the results will be permanent and it will thereafter be physically impossible for the patient to inseminate, or to conceive or bear children.

Signed_____
                (Husband)

Signed_____ †
                (Wife)

Witness_____

---

*This form is intended to be used where the primary purpose rather than the incidental result is sterilization.

†The question of the necessity of the consent of the patient's spouse to a voluntary sterilization has never been litigated. It would appear that such consent is not necessary, although it may be desirable. The statutes in Georgia, North Carolina and Virginia which specifically authorize voluntary sterilization require the written consent of the patient's spouse.

FIGURE 14–17

Request for Sterilization. (From Medicolegal Forms with Legal Analysis, 3rd ed. Office of the General Counsel, 1973, p. 69. Copyright © 1973 American Medical Association. All rights reserved.)

UNIFORM ANATOMICAL GIFT ACT

In July 1968 the Uniform Anatomical Gift Act was approved by the National Conference of Commissioners on Uniform State Laws. This act provides that a person 18 years of age or over may give all or any part of his body after death for research, transplant, or placement in a tissue bank. The person wishing to do this merely signs the Uniform Donor Card (Fig. 14–18), which is recognized as a legal document in all 50 states. It is preferable to have one's next of kin co-sign as witnesses, since their permission to carry out the donor's wishes may later be requested. Individuals wishing

UNIFORM DONOR CARD*

OF _____

<small>Print or type name of donor</small>

In the hope that I may help others, I hereby make this anatomical gift, if medically acceptable, to take effect upon my death. The words and marks below indicate my desires.

I give: (a) _____ any needed organs or parts

(b) _____ only the following organs or parts

_____

<small>Specify the organ(s) or part(s)</small>

for the purposes of transplantation, therapy, medical research or education;

(c) _____ my body for anatomical study if needed.

Limitations or special wishes, if any :_____

Signed by the donor and the following two witnesses in the presence of each other:

_____   _____

<small>Signature of Donor   Date of Birth of Donor</small>

_____   _____

<small>Date Signed   City & State</small>

_____   _____

<small>Witness   Witness</small>

This is a legal document under the Uniform Anatomical Gift Act or similar laws.

*The Uniform Donor Card is intended to be carried on the donor's person

FIGURE 14–18

Uniform Donor Card. (From Medicolegal Forms with Legal Analysis, 3rd ed. Office of the General Counsel, 1973, p. 116. Copyright © 1973 American Medical Association. All rights reserved.)

to donate their entire bodies for anatomical study and research should contact their local medical school and make separate arrangements in writing besides signing the Uniform Donor Card. The donation of an organ or tissue essential to the life of another is consistent with most religions and is encouraged. After the card has been signed, it should be placed near the driver's license to facilitate immediate identification. In more than 26 states, the Department of Motor Vehicles issues donor stickers when drivers' licenses are renewed. In the event of a traffic death, the sticker would permit removal of the organ(s). For further information about this subject and to obtain donor cards, write to the National Kidney Foundation, 315 Park Avenue South, New York, NY 10010.

CONTROLLED SUBSTANCES ACT OF 1970

The following is a brief summary of the controlled substance regulations with which the medical assistant should be familiar.

Registration of physicians, hospitals, pharmacies, dentists, veterinarians, and other practitioners is the responsibility of the Drug Enforcement Administration (DEA), which is under the U.S. Department of Justice. The Food and Drug Administration (FDA) continues to have complementary functions in this field. Physicians are required to re-register annually with the Registration Branch, Drug Enforcement Administration, P.O. Box 28083, Central Station, Washington, D.C. 20005, or with their nearest regional office.

If a doctor has offices in more than one region and dispenses and administers drugs listed in any of the five Schedules, he must register at each regional office. If he administers and dispenses drugs at his main office only, then he is required to register at the DEA regional office near his principal office. DEA numbers are issued to qualified registrants by the Drug Enforcement Administration, and the number appears on purchase orders, prescriptions for controlled substances, and other documents of transfer. A physician is required to keep records of drugs he dispenses as listed in the five Schedules for a period of two years. To obtain further information on what drugs are in each Schedule, write for the booklet "Controlled Substance Inventory List," published by the Superintendent of Documents, U.S. Government Printing Office, Washington, D.C. 20402. Copies of the Controlled Substances Act of 1970 can also be obtained from this source.

TO THE STUDENT: Refer to the Appendix, Assignment 35, p. 625, for the project related to this chapter.

GLOSSARY OF MEDICOLEGAL TERMS

arbitration Legal method provided by statute in some states whereby patient and physician may agree to resolve any controversy that may arise between them before an impartial panel (Grievance Committee).

assault Intentional and unlawful attempt to do bodily injury to another person.

assumption of risk If one knowingly pursues a dangerous course, he or she cannot recover damages. If the patient has been informed of the risks and agrees to treatment, he or she cannot sue for damages unless there has been some other factor responsible for the trouble.

battery Unlawful beating or touching of another person. A surgical operation is technically a "battery" regardless of the result, and is excusable only when express or implied consent is given by the patient.

breach of confidential communication	"Breach" means breaking or violation of a law or agreement. In the context of the medical office it means the unauthorized release of information about the patient.
breach of contract	See definition of breach above. If a physician agrees to achieve a particular result for a patient and then fails to do so, he is liable for breach of contract even if he has used the highest degree of skill.
breach of duty	A general term used for violation or omission of a legal or moral duty.
burden of proof	Requires that the patient or the doctor establish the truth as to a particular issue, for instance, the physician's negligence. *Example*: If an instrument is sewn inside a patient's abdomen, it is not the patient but the doctor who has the burden of proof: he must prove that he was not negligent.
civil law	Law that enforces private rights and liabilities, as distinguished from criminal law.
contributory negligence	Want of ordinary care on the part of the person bringing suit, which, in combination with the defendant's (physician's) negligence is part of the cause of injury. *Example*: If a patient does not cooperate with his physician by following all reasonable instructions and this failure contributes to his problem, he cannot collect damages.
defamation	A common tort liability; injury to reputation, i.e., slander or libel.
defendant	The person defending or denying. In a malpractice case this is usually the physician.
deposition	Testimony of a witness made under oath but not in open court and written down to be used when the case comes to trial.
emancipation	Usually used in reference to a minor, and means the child is no longer under parental control.
ethics	Moral principles and standards in the ideal relationships between the physician and patient and also between the physician and other physicians.
etiquette	Customs, rules of conduct, courtesy, and manners of the medical profession.
expert testimony	Testimony given in regard to some scientific, technical, or professional matter by an expert such as a physician.
false imprisonment	A common tort liability; personal restraint.
felony	A major crime for which greater punshment is imposed than for a misdemeanor.

fraud	A common tort liability; deceit. Intentional deception to cause a person to give up property or some lawful right.
Grievance Committee	Impartial panel established by a local medical society to listen to and investigate patients' complaints in regard to medical care or to excessive fees charged by the physician. Also seen in arbitration agreements.
invasion of right of privacy	Unwarranted exploitation of another's personality or personal affairs with which one has no legitimate concern— particularly, intrusion into another's affairs in such a way as to cause mental anguish or humiliation. *Example*: There should be no publication of a patient's medical case record and no showing of a photograph or motion picture from which the identity of the patient is determinable without the knowledge and authorization of the patient.
judgment	The official decision of the court of justice in regard to an action or suit.
libel	Written or graphic statement that damages the reputation or subjects a person to ridicule.
litigation	A lawsuit.
locum tenems	"Holding the place." A deputy, substitute, lieutenant, or representative.
malfeasance	Wrongful treatment of the patient.
misfeasance	Lawful treatment done in the wrong way.
negligence	Omission to do something a reasonable person would do under ordinary circumstances, or the doing of something which a reasonable person would not do under ordinary circumstances. (Negligence can thus work in either of two ways, involving action or omission.)
non compos mentis	Term used when a person is not of sound mind; insane.
nonfeasance	Failure of the physician to do anything in regard to a patient's medical condition, when the physician has a duty to act.
plaintiff	The person who brings suit or action. In a malpractice case this is usually the patient. (Also called *appellant*.)
privileged communication	A confidential communication that may be disclosed only with the patient's permission. Without such permission a doctor and his staff are prohibited from divulging the information contained in such a communication.
proximate cause	Negligence must be shown to be such that the injury would not have occurred if the physician had not acted as he did.

qui facit per alium facit per se	"He who acts through another acts himself."
res gestae	Latin for "things done; deeds." Facts and circumstances attendant to the act in question.
res ipsa loquitur	"The thing speaks for itself." If an accident is inexplicable in terms of ordinary and known experience except by negligence, then negligence is either presumed or inferred.
res judicata	Latin for "thing decided." A matter already decided by judicial authority.
respondeat superior	"Let the master answer." A physician is liable in certain cases for the wrongful acts of his assistant or employees.
slander	A common tort liability. Spoken statement in the presence of others that damages reputation or subjects a person to ridicule.
statute of limitations	Time limit established for filing lawsuits.
subpoena	"Under penalty." A writ that commands a witness to appear at a trial or other proceeding and to give testimony.
subpoena duces tecum	"In his possession." A subpoena that requires the appearance of a witness with his records. Sometimes the judge permits the mailing of records and the physician is not required to appear in court.
suspend	In regard to a lawsuit, this means to interrupt or discontinue the suit temporarily with the intention of resumption at a later date.
tort	Conduct which constitutes a private or civil wrong. The most common liability tort in medicine is tort of negligence.

MEDICOLEGAL REFERENCES

To keep up to date and well informed in the medicolegal field, you might read some journals that frequently have excellent articles and come to the physician's office. They are:

The Journal of Legal Medicine	*MXR – Malpractice X-posure Reports*
M.D.	*Physician's Management*
Medical Economics	*Prism*
Medico-Legal Digest	*Professional Liability Newsletter*
Medical Times	

Some additional reference booklets are:

Professional Liability, published by California Medical Association, Sutter Publications, Inc., 731 Market Street, San Francisco, CA 94103.

Medicolegal Forms with Legal Analysis, published by American Medical Association, 535 North Dearborn Street, Chicago, IL 60610.

Since state laws vary, you should write to the State Board of Medical Examiners and ask for information regarding medicolegal laws or ordinances in your state. For easy reference the following list contains the names as well as the addresses of each state board, since the names of these boards vary from state to state.

DIRECTORY OF STATE BOARDS OF MEDICAL EXAMINERS

Alabama
Alabama State Board of Medical
  Examiners
P.O. Box 946
Montgomery, AL 36102

Alaska
Alaska State Medical Board
Department of Commerce
207 East Northern Lights Blvd.
Anchorage, AK 99503

Arizona
Arizona Board of Medical Examiners
810 West Bethany Home Road
Phoenix, AZ 85013

Arizona Board of Osteopathic Examiners
  in Medicine and Surgery
2020 West Indian School Road
Phoenix, AZ 85015

Arkansas
Arkansas State Medical Board
P.O. Box 102
Harrisburg, AR 72432

California
State of California
Department of Consumer Affairs
Board of Medical Quality Assurance
1020 N Street, Room 434
Sacramento, CA 95814

Colorado
Colorado State Board of Medical
  Examiners
1612 Tremont Place, #715
Denver, CO 80202

Connecticut
Connecticut Medical Examining Board
79 Elm Street
Hartford, CT 06115

Delaware
State of Delaware Board of Examiners
Jesse S. Cooper Building, Room 233
Dover, DE 19901

District of Columbia
Commission of Licensure to Practice the
  Healing Arts in the District of Columbia
Department of Economic Development
Office of Licenses and Permits
Occupational and Professional Licensing
  Division
614 H Street, N.W.
Room 114
Washington, D.C. 20001

Board of Examiners in Medicine and
  Osteopathy
4909 V Street, N.W.
Washington, D.C. 20007

Florida
Florida State Board of Medical Examiners
Los Olas Building, Suite 901
305 South Andrews Avenue
Fort Lauderdale, FL 33301

State of Florida Board of Osteopathic
  Medical Examiners
225 North Causeway
New Smyrna Beach, FL 32069

Georgia
Georgia Composite State Board of
  Medical Examiners
166 Pryor Street, S.W.
Atlanta, GA 30303

Hawaii
Board of Medical Examiners,
  State of Hawaii
P.O. Box 3469
Honolulu, HI 96801

Idaho
Idaho State Board of Medicine
407 West Bannock
Boise, ID 83702

Illinois
State of Illinois
Department of Registration and
  Education
Medical Section
628 East Adams Street
Springfield, IL 62786

Indiana
State of Indiana
Board of Medical Registration
  and Examination
State Board of Health Annex
1375 West 16th Street
Indianapolis, IN 46202

Iowa
Iowa State Board of Medical Examiners
910 Insurance Exchange Building
505 Fifth Street
Des Moines, IA 50309

Kansas
State of Kansas Board of Healing Arts
292 New Brotherhood Building
Kansas City, KS 66101

Kentucky
Kentucky State Board of Medical
  Licensure
3532 Ephraim McDowell Drive
Louisville, KY 40205

Louisiana
Louisiana State Board of Medical
  Examiners
621 Hibernia Bank Building
New Orleans, LA 70112

Maine
State of Maine Board of Registration
  in Medicine
222 Main Street
Waterville, ME 04901

Maryland
Board of Medical Examiners of Maryland
1211 Cathedral Street
Baltimore, MD 21201

Massachusetts
Commonwealth of Massachusetts Board of
  Registration in Medicine
1511 Leverett Saltonstall Building
Government Center
100 Cambridge Street
Boston, MA 02202

Michigan
State of Michigan
Board of Registration in Medicine
Department of Licensing Regulation
1033 South Washington Street
Lansing, MI 48926

State of Michigan
Board of Osteopathic Registration and
  Examination
2424 Burton, S.E.
Grand Rapids, MI 49506

Minnesota
The Minnesota State Board of Medical
  Examiners
Minnesota State Bank Building, Suite 203
200 South Robert Street
St. Paul, MN 55107

Mississippi
Mississippi State Board of Health
P.O. Box 1700
Jackson, MS 39205

Missouri
The State Board of Registration for the
  Healing Arts of Missouri
P.O. Box 4
Jefferson City, MO 65101

Montana
State of Montana
Department of Professional and
　Occupational Licensing
Board of Medical Examiners
LaLonde Building
Helena, MT 59601

Nebraska
Nebraska State Board of Examiners
　in Medicine and Surgery
Lincoln Building, 2nd Floor
1003 "0" Street
Lincoln, NE 68508

Nevada
Nevada State Board of Medical Examiners
3660 Baker Lane
Reno, NV 89502

New Hampshire
The State of New Hampshire Board of
　Registration in Medicine
61 South Spring Street
Concord, NH 03301

New Jersey
The State of New Jersey Board of Medical
　Examiners
Division of Consumer Affairs
28 West State Street
Trenton, NJ 08625

New Mexico
New Mexico Board of Medical Examiners
227 East Palace Avenue
Sante Fe, NM 87501

New Mexico Board of Osteopathic
　Examination and Registration
3800 Wyoming, N.E.
Albuquerque, NM 87111

New York
New York State Board of Medicine
99 Washington Avenue
Albany, NY 12210

North Carolina
Board of Medical Examiners of the
　State of North Carolina
222 North Person Street, Suite 214
Raleigh, NC 27601

North Dakota
North Dakota State Board of Medical
　Examiners
MDU Office Building, Suite 307
400 North 4th Street, Box 1198
Bismarck, ND 58501

Ohio
State of Ohio, State Medical Board
21 West Broad Street
Columbus, OH 43215

Oklahoma
Board of Medical Examiners
State of Oklahoma
730 United Founders Tower
Oklahoma City, OK 73112

Oregon
State of Oregon Board of Medical
　Examiners
Health Division
Department of Human Resources
1002 Loyalty Building
317 S. W. Alder
Portland, OR 97204

Pennsylvania
Commonwealth of Pennsylvania
Department of State
State Board of Medical Education
　and Licensure
279 Boas Street, Box 2649
Harrisburg, PA 17120

Commonwealth of Pennsylvania
Department of State
State Board of Osteopathic Examiners
114 South Main Street
Muncy, PA 17756

Puerto Rico
Commonwealth of Puerto Rico
Board of Medical Examiners
Department of State
P.O. Box 3271
San Juan, PR 00904

Rhode Island
State of Rhode Island and Province
　Plantations
Department of Health
Division of Professional Regulation
104 Health Department Building
75 Davis Street
Providence, RI 02908

South Carolina
State Board of Medical Examiners
of South Carolina
1315 Blanding Street
Columbia, SC 29201

South Dakota
South Dakota State Board of Medical
and Osteopathic Examiners
603 West Avenue North
Sioux Falls, SD 57104

Tennessee
State of Tennessee Board of Medical
Examiners
1826 Clinch Avenue, S.W.
Knoxville, TN 37916

Tennessee State Board for Osteopathic
Physicians
5144 Walnut Grove Road
Memphis, TN 38117

Texas
Texas State Board of Medical Examiners
900 Southwest Tower
211 East 7th Street
Austin, TX 78701

Utah
Utah Department of Registration
Department of Business Regulation
330 East Fourth South
Salt Lake City, UT 84111

Vermont
State of Vermont Board of Medical
Registration
126 State Street
Montpelier, VT 05602

Virginia
Virginia State Board of Medical
Examiners
200 Professional Building
Portsmouth, VA 23704

Washington
The State of Washington
Business and Professions Administration
Division of Professional Licensing
P.O. Box 649
Olympia, WA 98504

West Virginia
The Medical Licensing Board of
West Virginia
State Office Building
1800 Washington Street
Charleston, WV 25305

State of West Virginia Board of
Osteopathy
Route 2, Box 51
Marlington, WV 24954

Wisconsin
State of Wisconsin
Department of Regulation and Licensing
201 East Washington
Madison, WI 53702

Wyoming
Wyoming Board of Medical Examiners
State Office Building
Cheyenne, WY 82002

REVIEW QUESTIONS

1. If an adult gives oral consent for surgery on himself or his child, is this valid in court? _____

2. In medical professional liability cases who is the defendant, generally speaking? _____ Who is the plaintiff? _____

3. If a record is to be given to a new physician, what must the old physician have from the patient? _____

4. If the assistant receives a request from another physician for certain records, what must she do? _____

_____

5. If a statement on an insurance form may be interpreted as placing responsibility on the office for any accident or unfortunate occurrence, what should the assistant do with it? _____

_____

6. If a physician has written on the patient's record, "this patient is a malingerer," what should the assistant do? _____

_____

7. If a physician is requested to give information to an attorney, what must he have from the patient? _____

_____

8. What is the exception to the right to privacy and privileged communication?

_____

_____

9. Who handles the settlement of lawsuits? _____

_____

10. Why should the assistant never write over an entry on a patient's record?

_____

_____

11. Does administering emergency care create the patient-physician relationship?

_____

_____

12. If a physician fails to follow his instructions for government patients, what may happen? _____

_____

13. Can a physician terminate a contract with a patient? _____ If so, how?

_____

_____

14. Define the following terms:

res ipsa loquitur: _____

respondeat superior: _____

subpoena duces tecum: _____

15. Name some of the common tort liabilities _____

_____

_____

16. What is informed consent? _____

_____

_____

17. Can an assistant receive a subpoena for her physician? _____

_____

18. What is the difference between malfeasance, misfeasance, and nonfeasance?

_____

_____

_____

19. A patient comes to Dr. Practon because of pain in the site of an old incision. Dr. Practon immediately sees that the patient has adhesions from previous surgery and that there was improper postsurgical care. He tells the patient that he does not feel he should treat her because of the poor surgical job she received and the lack of care she was given. Was the physician right or wrong? Why?

20. A patient comes into the office just once for treatment. He does not return, because he is dissatisfied with Dr. Practon's treatment. Is it necessary to keep his records when he obviously will not return?_____Why?_____

21. Dr. Practon treated a patient with diathermy, after which she developed a severe rash. Dr. Practon expressed his sympathy, but did not admit that he or his nurse was to blame, saying merely that some people react differently to diathermy. Was the doctor right or wrong? Why?_____

22. According to the facts given in question 21, can the patient sue for malpractice?_____Why?_____

23. A patient in great distress comes in to see Dr. Practon, weeping and saying that she knows she is going to die. You tell her not to worry, that Dr. Practon is a wonderful doctor, and she is going to get well if she just follows what he tells her. Are you right or wrong to tell her this? Why?_____

24. A patient is injured by a short circuit in the laboratory equipment being used on her. Can she sue for malpractice?_____Why?_____

25. Dr. Practon must go to a convention which lasts for 1 week. Is it better for him to go without telling his patients, leaving another doctor on call for them, or to notify each one who has an appointment?_____

26. A patient asks you if Dr. Practon carries malpractice insurance. Do you tell her that he does?_____Why?_____

27.   A patient takes a poorly written prescription of Dr. Practon's to the pharmacy and receives the wrong prescription. Can the patient sue Dr. Practon?

_____

28.   The proper terms for surgical consent forms or other forms sometimes called

"releases" are _____ or _____forms.

29.   The three defenses for medical professional liability actions are:

a. _____

b. _____

c. _____

30.   Most laws governing financial responsibility indicate that a husband is

responsible for his_____ debts. A wife is _____ responsible for her

husband's debts. A father is ordinarily responsible for his _____ debts if they are minors and are not emancipated. Children may or may not be responsible for the

debts of their _____ depending on the circumstances.

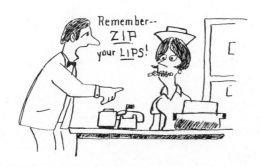

Notes:

15
The Physician's Personal Insurance

BEHAVIORAL

OBJECTIVES *The Assistant should be able to:*

1. State the doctor's personal and business insurance requirements.
2. Prepare pertinent data cards for insurance policies.
3. Explain the two principal types of life insurance policies.
4. Explain some common varieties of life insurance policies.
5. Understand minimum deposit insurance.
6. Describe retirement insurance programs.
7. Learn some pointers on obtaining health insurance.
8. Define disability income insurance.
9. Explain mortgage, fire, and casualty insurance.
10. State the two types of medical professional liability insurance.
11. Evaluate the difference between liability and property insurance.
12. Learn the state laws regarding when a doctor has to obtain workers' compensation insurance.
13. Compare automobile liability insurance and no-fault insurance.
14. Describe different types of insurance protection for business assets.

INTRODUCTION

Doctors spend many years preparing to practice medicine before they see any income. Very few have time to learn how best to manage their earnings once they begin practice, and often they must rely solely on their own limited experience and chance observations to determine their spending and saving decisions. As a result of this casual approach, their personal finances may be poorly planned and utilized. In recent years, however, inflation of office expenses and the spiraling cost of medical professional liability insurance have made physicians increasingly aware of the need for efficient office management and adequate insurance coverage.

The physician should review his or her personal insurance needs thoroughly with a reputable insurance agent who handles property and casualty insurance. An insurance agent should also be consulted before purchasing life insurance or sickness and accident insurance. Insurance policies should be reviewed periodically and revised if necessary. An attorney should examine any lease for office space or any lease that the physician might have with tenants of a building that he or she owns.

The doctor's personal insurance needs usually are:

1. Life Insurance
2. Retirement Insurance Programs
3. Income Protection Insurance
4. Accidental Death and Dismemberment Insurance
5. Health Insurance
6. Disability Income Insurance
7. Mortgage Insurance

A physician can generally obtain group coverage in these categories through his membership in state or county medical societies.

The doctor's business insurance needs are:

1. Fire and Casualty Insurance on home and/or office
2. Medical Professional Liability Insurance
3. Property and Liability Insurance
4. Workers' Compensation Insurance
5. Social Security for the doctor and his employees
6. Unemployment Compensation Insurance
7. Automobile Insurance
8. Office Overhead Expense Insurance

Some physicians, in addition to employee protection required by federal or state laws (e.g., Social Security or Workers' Compensation), also provide other forms of insurance for their employees, such as life insurance, hospital insurance, or Keogh Plans (see pp. 449–450). In some states disability insurance is not mandatory (see Chapter 8), so that some physicians may elect to provide this insurance if sick leave is not given. These fringe benefits can aid a physician in obtaining competent personnel.

MANAGEMENT OF INSURANCE RECORDS

If your physician carries a great deal of insurance coverage, you may find it helpful to set up a form for each policy summarizing the pertinent data. You might also use 5" x 8" cards to record this information, as shown in Figure 15–1. Clip the card containing all of this data to the front of each policy file, or keep it in a bound notebook or card file for easy reference.

Retention of Records

Insurance policies should be kept in a fireproof filing cabinet or in a safety deposit box. They should be retained until the policy lapses if there are no claims pending on the policy. A professional liability policy is kept permanently, however.

Physician's Name _____

Name of Policy _____   Policy # _____

Type of Coverage _____

Insurance Company _____   Insurance Agent _____

Address _____   Phone No. _____

Value of Policy $ _____

Effective Date _____   Expiration Date _____

Annual Premium _____   Renewal Date _____
                                            (quarterly, annual, every 3 yrs.)

Dates of Each Premium Payment _____   Amount $ _____

_____ $ _____

Doctor's age when policy was issued _____
   (if pertinent)

Beneficiary _____

Other Information _____

FIGURE 15–1

Insurance Pertinent Data Card.

LIFE INSURANCE

Life Insurance is a policy through which a doctor contracts with an insurance company to provide payment of a specified amount to his beneficiary or estate if he dies while the policy is in force. Life insurance can be a form of savings and can also be used to supplement a retirement plan. Some professional organizations have established group and franchise plans in which physicians may participate. Many life insurance contracts provide flexibility, so it is wise to analyze the plan periodically and modify it as the physician's family and financial needs change.

Kinds of Policies

1. *Individual Life Insurance* is issued to an individual after he or she has been approved for coverage by the insurance company. The policyholder may be required to have a physical examination. Most individual life insurance is permanent, which means that the majority of people buy it for their lifetime or for a stated number of years. Cash values build up over the years, and the cash value represents the sum the policyholder will receive from the insurance company upon surrendering the policy.

2. *Group Life Insurance* is usually issued without a medical examination and may be obtained through professional medical organizations. Group life insurance is frequently cheaper, but in some instances it can be easily cancelled if the insurance company no longer wants to continue the group. These policies may be renewable only up to a certain age. Read the fine print of the policy for exceptions and exclusions, since these policies vary widely.

Types of Life Insurance

There are many different varieties of programs. The most common types will be described here.

1. *Straight or Ordinary Life Insurance*: This is whole life insurance written under a contract that provides for periodic payment of premiums as long as the policyholder lives. This is the most flexible type of policy and the least expensive kind of permanent protection.

2. *Term Life Insurance*: "Term" insurance usually means temporary coverage for a stated period of time. It is a policy with death benefits but no investment value. As the policyholder ages, either the premium increases or the face value of the policy decreases. This insurance works best during the early years of a physician's practice, when low-cost protection is important. It should be converted at a later time to whole life insurance, which has a cash reserve, because term policies are not renewable after age 65 or 70.

3. *Whole Life Insurance*: "Whole" life is insurance for an individual's entire life. This type of policy has a cash reserve in addition to protection benefits. The policyholder can borrow on the cash reserve at a specified and guaranteed rate. If the insured person dies, the amount of the loan is deducted from the cash value of the policy. The premium remains the same every year.

4. *Limited Payment Life Insurance*: This type of policy gives the physician lifetime protection in return for a limited number of premiums paid over a predetermined time. Since the premiums are paid over a shorter period of time, they will be higher, but the premium remains the same each year. Policies of this type are often used by professional people and others who want their insurance completely paid up before their retirement.

5. *Endowment Insurance*: This policy protects the insured person for a given number of years. At the end of the period, the full amount of the policy is paid to the policyholder, or if the insured person dies before the end of the period, the full amount is paid to the beneficiary. Cash values build up faster in endowment policies because premiums are higher than in other policies. However, the premiums remain the same each year.

A feature that may be added to individual or group policies for an additional premium is *guaranteed renewability*. This means that the insurance company may not refuse to renew the policy if the insured person develops a medical problem that makes him or her a poor insurance risk. If this type of guarantee has not been purchased, most state laws require that a company not wishing to renew a term policy allow conversion of the policy to ordinary life at a premium appropriate to the individual's age.

Minimum Deposit Insurance

This is a form of ordinary life insurance. The doctor buys an ordinary life policy and pays part of the premium with money borrowed from the cash value of the policy. The insurance company gives the policy a cash value immediately which it extracts from the general surplus provided by its other policyholders. The loan comes from the insurance company at a rate that remains constant throughout the life of the policy. In a few years the doctor is borrowing enough to pay all of the premiums due. The loan keeps getting larger. It is possible to postpone interest payments for a few years but then the accrued interest plus the loan will soon exhaust the cash value and the policy may lapse.

If minimum deposit insurance is bought from a mutual company where policyholders are shareholders, then dividends can be used to reduce the premium. Many times the dividends go to purchase term insurance that will provide funds to pay off the loan in case the doctor dies while the term insurance is in force. If the policy comes from a stock company where policyholders are *not* shareholders, then there are no dividends but premiums are lower. In this case the extra term insurance is provided at an increase in the premium. The balance of the loan at the time of death is deducted from the benefits paid. As the loan increases the doctor gets less insurance protection each year.

Minimum deposit insurance is similar to *decreasing term insurance*, which maintains premium rates constant at each renewal but provides fewer benefits as time passes. The advantage of minimum deposit insurance is that the interest payments are tax deductible whereas life insurance premium payments are not. In order to deduct interest on loans made on minimum deposit insurance policies from income taxes, the Internal Revenue Service requires that four of the first seven annual premiums be paid in cash without borrowing. The money paid during the early years of the minimum deposit policy raises its effective cost in comparison with that of term insurance because the cash paid during the early years could be invested at a profit and inflation reduces the value of dollars over time.

RETIREMENT INSURANCE PROGRAMS

Keogh HR-10 Plan

The Keogh Act, which became law on January 1, 1963, states that a doctor may put a certain amount into a retirement fund for himself that is tax-exempt if he also covers all full-time employees who have been with him for three years. The physician may contribute to the fund if an employee has been with him for less than three years if he treats all employees alike. Contributions to the HR-10 Plan are in addition to the employee's salary. The tax law does not exempt these pension funds from taxation but merely postpones taxation until the employee receives the beneficial use of the funds during retirement years.

Types of Plans

Two types of plans under the Keogh Act are:

1. *Fixed Benefit Keogh Plan*: This pays the physician a specific annuity income at retirement. The law's formula allows the physician a life annuity income of $36,000. To achieve this the physician would have to accumulate a fund of approximately $360,000, so that his or her annual contribution would be about $9800. The Fixed Benefit Keogh Plan permits a higher amount tax-free each year than the Defined Contribution Keogh Plan. Under the Fixed Benefit Plan formula entitling the Assistant to $10,000 annuity income at age 65, only $100,000 or so needs to be accumulated over a period of 35 years. A fund of that size can be achieved by an annual contribution of about $900, which is $600 per year less than the physician would pay with a Defined Contribution Plan. The physician has to continue to meet the Fixed-Benefit goal, so that contributions are nonflexible.

2. *Defined Contribution Keogh Plan*: This plan accumulates funds at a specific rate, such as 15 per cent of the physician's gross earnings up to no more than $7500 per year. The ultimate retirement income is an unknown annual amount determined by the size of the fund that has accumulated over the years. The maximum ordinary Keogh contribution for the Assistant could be as high as $1500 a year all of which would come out of the physician's gross income. If an overpayment occurs that is more than 15 per cent of the gross income, a penalty can be enforced. The excess should thus be withdrawn from the plan before annual income tax reports are filed.

In purchasing a Keogh Plan through an insurance agent as opposed to purchasing it through a savings and loan association, it is important to note that some plans do not have a built-in annuity while the plan is in force, and thus the annuity must be purchased at the age of retirement.

POINTERS ON HEALTH INSURANCE

For additional general information on health insurance and definitions of terms, see Chapter 1.

Before purchasing a private health insurance policy, the physician should consider the following:

1. The type and extent of coverage he or she needs.
2. The policy he or she is able to afford.

Deductibles. Be wary of high deductibles. Major medical insurance policies may cover 80 per cent of doctor and hospital costs, but before the coverage is effective you must incur bills in excess of the "deductible" within the calendar year.

Maximum Limits. Almost all policies have a maximum limit on costs. A policy that has a maximum lifetime limit of $10,000 in coverage may sound more than adequate, but if you have even one or two serious illnesses this amount would be quickly exhausted. A limit of $25,000, $50,000, or even $100,000 provides much better protection.

Hospital Expense Benefits. A policy may provide payment up to a specified amount for a hospital room, to a maximum of 30 or 60 days for any illness. Be careful of these narrow limits and about policies written in fixed dollar amounts. An allowance of $125 per day may sound sufficient today, but it will be inadequate in a few years. A good policy will not have fixed dollar coverage but instead will agree to the "reasonable and customary" costs of the hospital room.

Surgical Schedules. Many policies include surgical schedules that give a fixed dollar limit, but these schedules also become outdated with the passage of time.

Pre-existing Conditions. A good policy will not exclude pre-existing conditions, or it will provide coverage for these conditions after a short waiting period. An arrangement may be made in some instances for special inclusions at higher premiums.

Guaranteed Renewability. A policy should include a clause that guarantees your right to renew the policy so that the insurance company cannot cancel it because they consider you a "bad risk." However, guaranteed renewability does not guarantee that the premium will remain the same year after year. Optionally renewable policies may allow an insurance company to refuse to renew coverage at any premium due date.

Waiting Period. There may be a waiting period after the effective date of the insurance policy before any benefits begin for procedures involving tonsils, hemorrhoids, hernia, maternity, or any condition for which the insured received medical attention prior to the effective date. Make sure you check for this limitation.

DISABILITY INCOME INSURANCE

This type of policy helps replace income when a wage earner cannot work because of illness or injury. Sometimes it is called an Income Replacement policy. Two classes of disabilities are recognized: total disability and partial disability. Always check to see for how long benefits are provided. Some policies provide lifetime benefits and some provide only 6 months of benefits, depending on the type of disability.

MORTGAGE INSURANCE

This is one of the basic uses for life insurance. Many family heads purchase life insurance solely for the purpose of paying off any mortgage balance outstanding at their death. Companies may design special policies emphasizing this feature. The insurance is usually made payable to a family beneficiary.

LIABILITY AND PROPERTY INSURANCE

Liability Insurance. If the doctor is the owner or leaser of property, he can be held legally responsible for an injury occurring on the premises where he works or resides. If the doctor leases a suite in a building his responsibility may begin the moment a patient enters the office. But if his office facilities include land and a parking lot for the patients, then the responsibility may extend there also. It is always wise to have insurance coverage for both home and office because the premium cost is modest and accidents do occur.

Property Insurance. In insuring either real or personal property, be sure to distinguish between policies which are based on actual cash value (the original cost of the property less depreciation) and replacement cost value (the cost of the property that must be purchased to replace the lost or damaged property). Remember that as time elapses prices continue to escalate and these policies must be revised from time to time.

FIRE AND CASUALTY INSURANCE ON HOME AND/OR OFFICE

Fire insurance should include coverage not only for the building but also for the value of the furniture and professional equipment. The valuation is usually based on the depreciated or actual sales value at the time of loss, so it is important that an inventory of all items be maintained in a safe place and kept up to date. Since values change, the policy should be reviewed periodically and increased if necessary to cover the current content valuation. If the fire insurance policy for the home does not provide coverage for jewelry and fine art, these items may have to be covered under a special floater or separate policy in case of loss by theft or vandalism.

Many insurance policies include a clause which states that the company does not have to pay full replacement value if a home is not insured for at least 80 per cent of its current replacement value. If it is not insured for 80 per cent or more, depreciation costs can be deducted from your reconstruction bills. Estimated replacement cost covers just the main structure and does not include cost of the lot, driveway, patio, or foundation excavation. The replacement cost for the structure is what it would cost to replace it at today's prices. The contents of the home are usually covered for an amount that is half the policy's face value. Be sure that this is enough to cover the value of your possessions adjusted for depreciation. If it is not enough, get a special endorsement to cover a higher value for the contents.

MEDICAL PROFESSIONAL LIABILITY INSURANCE

Every physician should purchase medical professional liability insurance for protection against financial loss for alleged professional misconduct or for lack of ordinary skill in the performance of a professional act. This coverage is advisable whether the doctor is in solo practice, a partnership, on salary, or in the military. Basically, there are two types of medical professional liability insurance: Claims Made Insurance and Occurrence Insurance. These are explained more fully in Chapter 14. Incorporation does not necessarily limit the physician's liability.

In recent years medical professional liability insurance has become increasingly difficult to obtain. Many companies no longer write it and many group policies have been cancelled. If possible, the physician should have an "umbrella policy" which covers all potential liability risks, such as damages resulting from criminal acts, libel, slander, cosmetic surgery, x-ray, shock therapy, and so forth, depending on his specialty in medicine. The policy should be reviewed by an attorney, but the physician himself should become familiar with its coverage and exclusions, to make sure that it will cover all expenses as well as safeguard his estate in the event of an adverse judgment. The doctor should notify the insurance company immediately whenever a situation arises which might lead to a lawsuit. See Chapter 14 for further discussion of this type of insurance and for sources of additional information.

WORKERS' COMPENSATION INSURANCE

In most states an employer is legally required to assume responsibility for medical payments for injuries or illness sustained on the job by full- or part-time employees. (See Chapter 9 for further information on this subject.) Incorporated physicians are covered under the Workers' Compensation laws. The physician is protecting himself against lawsuits and claims from his employees. A receptionist working in a reception room that is shared by several doctors should be provided adequate insurance coverage by predetermining whose employee she is. In a partnership the individual partners are not subject to Workers' Compensation laws.

Table 15–1 shows the minimum number of employees required by each state before the state Workers' Compensation law comes into effect. There are exemptions in the laws of many states for certain occupations, such as domestic or casual employees, laborers, babysitters, newspaper vendors or distributors, charity workers, and gardeners. Some states also do not require compensation insurance for farm laborers, or they require a larger number of farm employees than the number shown in the table.

TABLE 15–1. MINIMUM NUMBER OF EMPLOYEES FOR STATE WORKERS' COMPENSATION LAW

No. of Employees	1		2	3	4	5
States	Alaska	Minnesota	Oklahoma	Alabama	New Mexico	Arkansas
	Arizona	Montana		Georgia	North Carolina	Mississippi
	California	Nebraska		Michigan	Rhode Island	Missouri
	Colorado	Nevada		Virginia	South Carolina	Tennessee
	Connecticut	New Hampshire				
	Delaware	New Jersey				
	District of Columbia	New York				
	Florida	North Dakota				
	Guam	Ohio				
	Hawaii	Oregon				
	Idaho	Pennsylvania				
	Illinois	Puerto Rico				
	Indiana	South Dakota				
	Iowa	Texas				
	Kansas	Utah				
	Kentucky	Vermont				
	Louisiana	Washington				
	Maine	West Virginia				
	Maryland	Wisconsin				
	Massachusetts	Wyoming				

AUTOMOBILE LIABILITY INSURANCE

This is probably the most easily understood form of liability insurance, since by state law anyone who drives an automobile is required to carry insurance. This type of policy gives protection against losses connected with the use of an automobile and should cover not only damages but also any legal liability resulting from ownership, maintenance, or use of the car. The terms of the contract determine the coverage. Coverage can involve such features as medical payments, collision repairs, public liability, emergency road service, and protection against property damage, theft, fire, or lightning. *Comprehensive coverage* means insurance against any physical loss to an automobile except by collision or upset. This includes loss due to theft, vandalism, hail storm, flood, fire, glass breakage, and other noncollision causes. If the car windshield should become sand-pitted, the repair of the windshield would be covered under comprehensive coverage.

Another type of policy in effect in some states is No-Fault Insurance. Under No-Fault Insurance, each driver's insurance company pays his medical, rehabilitation, and other related expenses as they occur, regardless of who caused the accident. The other driver's insurance company pays his medical and other bills. No one can make a claim against another driver or file suit unless expenses are above amounts specified by the state or injuries sustained are very serious in nature. If an employee is away from work because of automobile injuries, he receives loss of income compensation for a portion of his salary. Some states require No-Fault Insurance coverage, whereas others allow individuals to reject it in writing.

If an employee of the physician uses his or her car in performing a service for the doctor and is involved in an accident, the doctor may be sued as well as the employee. The employee should therefore include the doctor as a co-insured in his or her policy. There are also policies that include coverage for the uninsured motorist should an accident occur with one who does not have insurance.

PROTECTION OF BUSINESS ASSETS

For protection of business assets, several kinds of coverage may be needed. They are:

1. *Physicians' and Surgeons' Floater*: This gives burglary and robbery protection for an office.

2. *Accounts Receivable Insurance*: This covers damage to or loss of accounts receivable records from such risks as fire, vandalism, or theft. Coverage can be obtained under an inland marine floater.

3. *Office Overhead Expense Insurance*: This is written upon the physician who represents the primary source of income for the staff. This insurance can provide some salaries and pay office expenses if the physician is temporarily incapacitated. A good policy might cover the following office expenses: rent or mortgage payments, electricity, telephone, employees' salaries, laundry, depreciation, heat and water, insurance premiums, and other fixed expenses.

STATE INSURANCE COMMISSIONER

If you have complaints about your insurance policy, medical claims, insurance agent, or broker, contact the insurance department of your own state or the state where the company is headquartered. Sometimes this is also referred to as Insurance Commissioner of the state where you reside.

The insurance industry is protected by a special exemption from the Federal Trade Commission Act under the McCarran Act (named for the late Senator Pat McCarran of Nevada). Under this exemption, the FTC cannot attack unfair or deceptive practices if there is any regulation. The regulations vary widely from state to state and by no means are all 50 states equally strict.

Contact the Commissioner in person, by letter, or by telephone. Each complaint should contain:

1. The inquiring person's name, address, and telephone number.
2. The policyholder's name and address if it is different from the person inquiring.
3. The name of the insurance company.
4. The policy period.
5. The policy or claim number.
6. The date of loss.
7. A statement of the complaint, including, if possible, a copy of the policy, medical bills, and any correspondence from the company pertaining to the claim.

If the complaint is against an agent or broker, also include his or her name and address:

1. Name and address of agent or broker.
2. Name and address of the finance company if the premium was financed.

FURTHER INFORMATION

For additional information on insurance write to:

The American Medical Association
535 North Dearborn Street
Chicago, IL 60610

Blue Cross Associations
840 North Lake Shore Drive
Chicago, IL 60611

Group Health Association of American, Inc.
1717 Massachusetts Avenue, N.W.
Washington, D.C. 20005

Health Insurance Institute
277 Park Avenue
New York, NY 10017

TO THE STUDENT: Refer to the Appendix, Assignment 36, pp. 626–627 for the project related to this chapter.

REVIEW QUESTIONS

1. In regard to retention of records, how many years is a professional liability policy kept in a safety deposit box? _____

2. Name the two kinds of life insurance policies.

   a. _____

   b. _____

3. Define "term" in regard to term life insurance. _____

_____

4. Define "whole" in regard to whole life insurance. _____

_____

5. What would you consider to be the main advantage of minimum deposit insurance? _____

6. Name the two types of plans under the Keogh Act. _____

   a. _____

   b. _____

7. What is the other name for Disability Income Insurance? _____

_____

_____

8. Name some types of insurance coverage a physician might need if he or she owns a home.

   a. _____

b. _____

c. _____

d. _____

9. In regard to medical professional liability insurance, explain these two types:

a. Claims Made Insurance _____

_____

b. Occurrence Insurance _____

_____

10. What is the minimum number of employees required in your state before an employer must obtain Workers' Compensation insurance? _____

11. Explain No-Fault Automobile Insurance. _____

_____

_____

_____

12. Name some other kinds of insurance coverage a physician might need for protection of business assets.

a. _____

b. _____

c. _____

Notes:

16
Canadian Medical Office Accounting and Insurance Form Processing*

BY RHODA G. FINNERON

BEHAVIORAL OBJECTIVES   *The Assistant should be able to:*

1. State the important items that should be included on the patient history.
2. Obtain from the patient all information pertinent to insurance billing and summarize it on index cards.
3. State the billing sequence for a typical provincial health insurance plan.
4. Understand the difference between a Provincial Health Insurance Plan and a Supplementary Health and Hospital Care Plan, and know the benefits typically provided by each.
5. Describe the insurance coverage available for Canadians not covered by provincial or supplementary group plans.
6. Describe the coverage available for Landed Immigrants arriving in Canada and Canadian citizens travelling abroad.
7. Bill the patient for in-hospital services provided by his or her private physician.
8. Record disbursements, pay bills, and handle petty cash.
9. Perform a bank reconciliation.
10. Discuss fees with the patient tactfully and completely.
11. Compose a letter to a patient whose account is overdue.

INTRODUCTION

Medical office accounting and the handling of insurance materials are much the same in Canadian doctors' offices as elsewhere. Charges are based on the treatment received by the patient, details of which appear on the patient's chart or history, and are controlled by the scale of charges issued by the Canadian Medical Association,

*I want to thank Dr. B.S. Borden, M.D., my own doctor, who allowed me to use his name; my old friend Mr. P. Creighton, C.A., and a one-time colleague, Mrs. G. Raney, R.N., for all their help. They were all most generous with their time and knowledge. So was my dear old Penny, who always encourages me so much.–R.G.F.

459

which governs the fee guidelines established by provinces. The actual method of payment may vary, however, both within provinces and from one section of the country to another.

Certain things never change. For example: all disbursements are carefully recorded; charges are billed either to the patient or to the patient's insurance carrier; monies owing are collected. All incoming money passes through the bank before being used. Petty cash is accounted for, records are proved and bank reconciliations made. Be sure to read the information on these subjects in Chapters 1, 12, 13, 14, and 15. Information pertinent to Canada will also be found in Chapters 4 (Blue Cross and Blue Shield) and 9 (Workers' Compensation).

The following material on Canadian office practice has been set up for classroom use. It seemed sensible to start with charts/histories, and some exercises on typing them, since they are the basis on which charges to patients are calculated. Following are discussions of disbursements and petty cash, leading up to the processing of insurance forms and the collection of accounts. Medical office procedure exercises are included in the Review Questions at the end of this chapter (pp. 492–495).

THE PATIENT'S CHART, HISTORY, OR RECORD

Upon seeing a patient for the first time, a doctor asks him all sorts of questions, the answers to which go into the patient's history, or chart. This information is used to help the doctor form a correct diagnostic opinion, prescribe a treatment, and decide upon the prognosis, or chances of recovery. Every time the patient sees the doctor, the results of that visit are added to his chart, so that a permanent record of the patient's progress is available to the doctor at all times. The last entry on the patient's history is the date of his discharge and his final condition of health. If the patient dies, this final statement will describe the cause of death, and the history is marked "closed."

The medical history will contain all the details that have been entered on the index card when the Assistant met the patient for the first time (see Fig. 16–1). The doctor

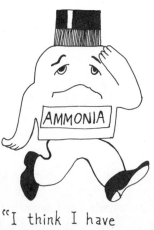

"I think I have walking ammonia."

Penelope (Penny) R.S. Finneron

199 McNicoll Ave., Willowdale, Ont.
M2H 2C2

491-7357 (416)

K.T. Finneron (father)

Patient's Soc. Sec. 82615170

Extended Health:
Confederation Life GH 15900 (Group)
Certificate No. 435408760
Policy Holder Province of Ontario

FIGURE 16-1

Medical insurance index card. In order that medical insurance claims may be processed as quickly and efficiently as possible, take the following information for index cards the first time the patient visits the doctor:
(1) name of patient; (2) mailing address; (3) telephone numbers at home and at business; (4) policyholder's name if the patient is a dependent (e.g., the father of a family, or the single parent cardholder); (5) provincial insurance number; (6) any group number; (7) any group certificate number.

will make a note of the patient's complaint and when it began, and this will be an exact description of the symptoms to the last detail. If the patient has treated himself, the doctor will want to know with what. If the patient thinks he knows what caused the symptoms, the doctor will want to know this too. If the patient has ever seen another doctor for the same complaint, the doctor will want to know about it.

The patient's previous history is called his *anamnesis*, and includes any illnesses or operations he may have had in the past. The treatments he may have had are recorded in his anamnesis, together with a note of any physical handicaps, allergies, and so on. Next the doctor will make a note of his personal history, which will include his smoking, drinking and drug habits, his hobbies, and his work and play habits. The patient's family history will include facts about the health of his parents, brothers and sisters, and other close relatives (see Fig. 16-2).

The doctor will then examine the patient and will record his report on this examination. If any tests or x-rays have been made as part of the examination, they too will be recorded. As a result of the examination, the doctor will try to make a diagnosis. If he is not absolutely sure, this first diagnosis will be tentative and probably subject to further tests, or developments in the patient's condition. What the doctor thinks about the possible outcome of the patient's condition is called his *prognosis*, and is often expressed as simply "good," "poor," or "doubtful."

Any treatment the doctor gives, and any medications ordered, are entered. This may be anything from a medicine for a cough or some kind of pill, to hospitalization. Whatever it is, it is entered under "treatment." All subsequent visits and all changes in medication, treatment, or condition are recorded, and are always dated so that the patient's progress may be observed in a "time sequence." This latter is all-important if the patient returns after a long lapse of time, in the event that similar symptoms appear in other patients, and as statistics of the incidence of a particular disease.

PATIENT RECORD

NAME: FINNERON, Penelope R.S.   REFERRED BY: Doctor B.S. Borden

ADDRESS: 199 McNicoll Avenue, Willowdale, Ontario

AGE: 20

CHIEF COMPLAINT: Upper abdominal pain and heartburn since age of 18 years.

PAST HISTORY: Measles and several attacks of sore throat, appendectomy, hepatitis, tonsillectomy.
After taking "medicine" her heartburn disappeared and at college she took bicarbonate of soda with some lessening of discomfort. About 6 weeks ago she had a severe attack of abdominal pain, followed 3 weeks later by another, both attacks affecting upper abdomen. No relief obtained from usual medication.

HABITS: Alcohol: about three drinks a week. Coffee: about six cups daily. Smoking: large package daily. Appetite: fair.

FAMILY HISTORY: F. 45 a&w, M. 40 a&w. M. very nervous type who has always had "stomach trouble," for which no treatment sought or given. Siblings: 1 m. a&w, 2 f. 1 a. and suffering similar stomach trouble to M.

PHYSICAL EXAMINATION: Tenderness in epigastric region.

X-RAYS: Show irregular erosion of gastric mucosa.

LABORATORY EXAMINATION: Free hydrochloric acid   hemoglobin 11 gm

                            80 degrees   occult blood in stool

            Blood content in gastric   "indicanuria"

            Content:

            gastric juice, 50 cc, obtained in food particles.

            Red blood cells 3,500,000

DIAGNOSIS: Gastric ulcer

TREATMENT: Special bland diet, no alcohol, antacid medication.

PRESCRIBED: Patient to return in two weeks.

FIGURE 16–2

Patient Record format followed when a preprinted form is not utilized for the patient history. Notice the inclusion of complete information on past medical and family background, habits, and current diagnosis and treatment. The paragraph under "Family History" is interpreted as follows: "Father, age 45, alive and well; Mother, age 40, alive and well; mother very nervous type... given. Brothers and sisters: one male, alive and well; two female, one alive and suffering similar stomach trouble to mother."

A hospital's admitting report is done in much the same way, using the hospital's own form (see Fig. 16–3).

THE GOOD INTENT HOSPITAL

Name:	Mr. Arthur Brebner	**Date:**	March 21, 1978
Address:	12 Black Street, Winnipeg, Manitoba.	**Ward or Room:**	357NW
Admitted:	January 24th 1978	**Referring Physician:**	Dr. N.D. Black
Discharged:	February 15th, 1978	**Attending Physician:**	Dr. B.S. Borden

HOSPITAL ADMISSION

CHIEF COMPLAINT: This 39-year-old German-born man, a bus driver, was well until this evening, when, while driving his bus, he developed severe chest pain over the left precordium which radiated up to his throat and down his left arm to the elbow, and was associated with some initial shortness of breath. Pain persisted in these areas for a duration of approximately 2½ hours. There were no palpitations noted.

FAMILY HISTORY: His father died at age 49 from myocardial infarction. No other history of familial diseases. M 60 a&w. Siblings: 1m 1f a&w

PAST HEALTH: Appendectomy in childhood.

PHYSICAL EXAMINATION: The patient was a pleasant male in no acute distress. Examination of the head, neck and chest was clear. Blood pressure 130/88. Pulse 90 per min. regular. Peripheral pulses palpable with no ankle edema. There were no audible murmurs. A pericardial friction rub was heard along the left sternal border.

INVESTIGATION AND COURSE IN HOSPITAL: On admission the patient's Hgb was 13.9 gm, wbc 9700; urinalysis was normal. BUN was 13 mg, and serum electrolytes were normal. Fasting blood sugar was 98 mg. On January 25 SGOT was 32.5 international units and LDH was 27.8 international units. On February 2 the SGOT was 7.4 international units and LDH 27.8 international units. Sed. rate rose only to a level of 32 mm/hr 5 days after admission.

TREATMENT AND PROGRESS: On admission to hospital the patient was treated in the Coronary Intensive Care Unit, but as his condition stabilized and the pericarditis picture became apparent, he was transferred to a semiprivate ward. Blood cultures showed no growth and blood studies were taken but not received at the time of dictation. Patient had an uneventful period in hospital and was allowed to be discharged home on February 15, 1978.

FINAL DIAGNOSIS: Pericarditis — improved. Prognosis — good.

A.B. Burke, M.D.
Assistant Resident in Medicine

FIGURE 16–3

Hospital Admitting Report.

The patient's discharge is noted (a statement of the cause of death is added if he should die), and the file is then marked "closed."

The doctor almost always will take this detailed history; only a very busy doctor with a very experienced Assistant would ask her to undertake this task. If she is asked to do this work, even the most experienced Assistant must take great care that she is absolutely accurate. If a patient complains, for instance, about a pain in his foot, she must say *which* foot. If the pain started two days after his birthday, she must ascertain which birthday. It is important, too, that she not ask personal questions in front of other patients. Further, all extraneous material must be excluded from the medical history. As will be seen, it is no simple task to take an accurate medical history, and any doubts should be taken to the doctor to be sorted out before the final history is made up. It is not "using initiative" to *guess*, and no doctor minds being asked questions in the interest of accuracy and efficiency.

Some doctors prefer to take the history on blank sheets which the Assistant will later type up for them. Others use only a card (see Fig. 16–4). If typed sheets are used, the headings should be prominently displayed, and apart from the text. A simple report type of set-up is most suitable (see Fig. 16–2). The most usual method of recording the history is on preprinted sheets with questions supplied so that the doctor may easily ask them and record the answers. These sheets may be ordered to suit the specialty of the doctor. Examples are shown on pages 462 and 493.

When filling out cards or histories, the doctor may answer the questions either by using "+" (positive) or "o" (negative) signs or by writing in the answers. Medical reports and x-rays are added to the history file, so that the doctor has a complete picture at all times. Sometimes the x-rays have to be kept separately if they are very large.

Reports that might be added to a patient's history are those for blood or urinalysis or for injections or inoculations, and if the patient takes drugs, a record of any that the doctor has dispensed or prescribed will be kept. The narcotics record is kept in a book, and an inventory of all drugs on hand is usually kept with it, along with a note of how they were used.

The Assistant will also file consent forms with the patient's history. These are preprinted for signature by the patient. A typical consent form might be for the use of anaesthesia to set a broken limb, or for an operation. If the service is to be performed on a minor, consent forms will be signed by a parent or guardian. (See Chapter 14, pp. 426–429.)

Medical histories constitute a permanent record of the patient's complaints, treatments, and progress. Although they are generally considered to be the property of the doctor, they can be produced in court, or seen by insurance companies in certain circumstances. (The information given in Chapter 14 generally applies to Canada as well as to the United States.) It is essential that they be kept accurate and up-to-date, and filed properly. They are entirely the responsibility of the secretary once they are given to her care, and carelessness in their handling is a cardinal fault. Without a careful record of all the services provided to each patient and their charges, it is not possible to bill accurately either the provincial health plan or the patient, or to charge any extended health coverage plan to which the patient may belong.

TO THE STUDENT: Turn to pages 490–495 and complete the exercises pertinent to this section of the chapter.

NAME: NEXT OF KIN:

ADDRESS: EMPLOYER:

TELEPHONE: INSURANCE:

FIGURE 16-4

Informal note card used by some physicians for taking the patient history. The Assistant later types up the notes on these cards for the file.

RECORDING DISBURSEMENTS

The Medical Assistant must keep track of every payment made by her doctor on account of his or her practice. This need not be an onerous task if she develops an adequate system.

PAYING THE BILLS

Pay all bills by cheque and, if possible, on fixed days each month. Paying by cheque creates a record so that the expense cannot be overlooked. All transactions relating to the practice should be put through a special current account at the bank. This must be separate from the doctor's personal account. Paying on a specific date makes it easier for the Assistant to schedule her work. Further, if she pays only on certain days, say the 15th and 30th, she will be able to give her doctor a number of cheques to sign at once, rather than having to bother him constantly throughout the month.

The following is a good schedule to keep to for the payment of bills:

1. When a bill is received, check it for errors and file it in the "Unpaid Bills File."

2. On payment days pull the unpaid bills. Prepare the cheques and envelopes.

3. Mark or stamp date paid and cheque number on each bill being paid.

4. Present the cheques with the supporting bills to the doctor for signature.

5. Have the doctor sign the cheques and initial each of the supporting bills to indicate his or her approval.

6. Put the cheques in the envelopes with some form of remittance advice. Typically your supplier will send two copies of his bill, so that you may return one with your payment. If the supplier has not done so, attach a note to the payment indicating what bill(s) the cheque covers.

7. File the paid bills.

8. Record the payments.

FILING THE PAID BILLS

File all paid bills in cheque number order in an arch file or press-type binder. Cheque number order is preferred, because one is typically looking to see what bills were covered by a particular payment. You will find that it is helpful to sort the bills into alphabetical order before writing the cheques. This reduces each month's payments to roughly the same order and so facilitates the search for a specific invoice. You must have a voucher or bill supporting every payment made. A cancelled cheque is proof of payment but it does not show the nature of the payment as does the voucher (bill). If you do not have a bill for some minor disbursement, prepare one yourself and have the doctor approve it.

RECORDING THE PAYMENTS

Each payment is entered in the Disbursements Journal, in cheque number order. The payment is entered twice, once in the "amount paid" column and once in one of the various distribution columns. Use the column appropriate to the disbursement. The purposes of this double entry are to provide an analysis of the disbursements and to permit a proof of the mechanical accuracy of the work.

The procedure for entering in the Disbursements Journal is as follows:

1. Enter each cheque in the manner described above.

2. Examine the doctor's current account bank statement to see if there are any disbursements other than cheques, such as NSF ("Not Sufficient Funds") cheques from patients, bank charges, bank interest, a loan, or the like.

3. Enter such additional disbursements in the same manner as the cheques.

4. At month's end, total all columns and prove the accuracy of your work by cross-adding all the distribution columns to the total of the "Amount Paid" column.

5. At the year's end, summarize the 12 monthly totals and produce grand totals for the year.

PETTY CASH

Inevitably, in the doctor's office, there will be certain disbursements that can be made more conveniently in cash than by cheque. The cheque is to be preferred however, because it creates a record of the payment, which cash does not.

Keeping receipts and vouchers for all cash payments is just as important as keeping accurate records of bills. The Department of National Revenue both can and will disallow, for tax purposes, expenses of the doctor that it feels are not properly supported.

The easiest way for the Medical Assistant to keep track of small cash disbursements is to operate an "imprest" petty cash account. The fund is started by the doctor's issuing a cheque to the Assistant for, say, $50.00. The Assistant cashes it and puts the money in a box. As payments are made, the voucher for each payment is put in the box. At any time, then, the cash on hand and the paid vouchers will total $50.00.

When the cash runs low, prepare a summary of the petty cash disbursements and attach the vouchers. From this point on the summary is treated like any other invoice from a supplier. A cheque is prepared, payable to the Assistant, for the total of the petty cash disbursements as shown on the summary. The cheque is entered in the Disbursements Journal. The Assistant cashes the cheque. Once again the petty cash box has $50.00 in cash in it, while the disbursements are safely recorded in the Disbursements Journal where they should be.

PROVING THE ACCURACY OF YOUR RECORD KEEPING

The effective Medical Assistant will want to prove the accuracy of her record keeping once a month. Both you and the doctor will have confidence in your figures if you have proved them. Furthermore, it is awfully hard to locate errors if you have to search a whole year's records to find them.

The easiest way to prove your work is to compare it with the records the bank maintains. Since banks have been known to make mistakes, the conscientious Assistant will also want to check the accuracy of the bank's work on the doctor's accounts. Seldom will your records and the bank statement agree, at first glance, on how much money is in the doctor's current account. There are four possible causes of differences: (1) deposits recorded by the Assistant but not by the bank until next month; (2) cheques issued and recorded by the Assistant which have not yet cleared back to the bank; (3) errors made by the Assistant; (4) errors made by the bank.

Reconciling the bank's records with the doctor's is accomplished by the following steps:

1. Mark off the deposits shown on the Cash Receipts against the deposits recorded on the Bank Statement.

2. Mark off the cheques returned by the bank against the Disbursements Journal. Make a careful comparison, because it is in this operation that you will find the errors.

3. List the open items (both deposits and cheques) on a reconciliation statement, such as the one shown in Figure 16–5.

SENDING AND COLLECTION OF ACCOUNTS

PROVINCIAL HEALTH INSURANCE PLANS

Most provinces have a Federal Medical Care Program, although not all provinces offer the same coverage. The Canadian Medical Association sets fees for services which apply across Canada, and provincial associations are guided by this indicator. Very often, about 90 per cent of the fees listed by the Provincial Medical Association are paid directly to the physician by the provincial plan. Not all doctors, however, accept the fees provincial programs provide as high enough to cover their services. When this is the case, the fact is always pointed out to patients, who will see a notice to this effect on the doctor's waiting room wall, usually coupled with an invitation to discuss fees with the doctor. If the amount directed to be paid by the Provincial Medical Plan is less than the amount billed, the doctor may prefer to be paid initially by the patient, rather than directly by the provincial authority.

When the doctor prefers to be paid by the patient, the Assistant usually accepts the patient's money and sends the receipted bill to the provincial plan, which in turn reimburses the patient directly for the amount of the covered charges. Some doctors bill the patient, then send a receipted bill which the patient forwards to the provincial plan for reimbursement.

The billing sequence shown in Figure 16–6 is for an Ontario patient, as is the identification card (Fig. 16–7). As shown in the patient's Record of Payment (Fig. 16–6B), the physician billed $20.00. The provincial plan allowed $14.40 (72 per cent) for this service. The doctor billed the patient. Either the doctor or the patient billed the provincial plan by sending the receipted bill in for payment. The provincial plan reimbursed the patient for $14.40, forwarding a check (Fig. 16–6A) and a record for the patient's files. The code for payment (Fig. 16–6C) is shown on the back of the payment record; this record is detached before the check is cashed.

The cost of a provincial plan varies from about $16.00 for an individual to $32.00 for a family each month, up and down the scale.

```
┌─────────────────────────────────────────────────────────────────────┐
│                  BANK RECONCILIATION — CURRENT MONTH                  │
│                                                                       │
│                  Bank Balance per Assistant's Records                 │
│                                                                       │
│  BANK BALANCE — END OF LAST MONTH                      $2,490.75*     │
│                                                                       │
│  ADD CURRENT MONTH'S DEPOSITS FROM                                    │
│    CASH RECEIPTS                                        4,750.30      │
│                                                        ─────────      │
│                                                        $7,241.05      │
│                                                                       │
│  DEDUCT CURRENT MONTH'S PAYMENTS FROM                                 │
│    DISBURSEMENTS JOURNAL                                3,890.03      │
│                                                                       │
│  BANK BALANCE — END OF CURRENT MONTH                                  │
│    PER ASSISTANT                                       $3,351.02      │
│                                                                       │
│                   Bank Balance per Bank's Records                     │
│                                                                       │
│  BANK BALANCE AT CURRENT MONTH'S END                                  │
│    PER BANK STATEMENT                                   $4,870.19     │
│                                                                       │
│  ADD OUTSTANDING DEPOSIT (CREDITED                                    │
│    FIRST DAY OF NEXT MONTH)                             1,850.75      │
│                                                        ─────────      │
│                                                        $6,720.94      │
│                                                                       │
│  DEDUCT OUTSTANDING CHEQUES:                                          │
│                                                                       │
│    NO.  1620   2,000.00                                               │
│         1622     690.07                                               │
│         1623     175.00                                               │
│         1627     504.85                                 3,369.92      │
│                                                                       │
│  BANK BALANCE — END OF CURRENT MONTH                                  │
│    PER BANK                                            $3,351.02      │
│                                                                       │
│  *This figure comes from last month's reconciliation.                │
└─────────────────────────────────────────────────────────────────────┘
```

FIGURE 16–5

Bank reconciliation statement, showing bank balances according to the Assistant's records (*top*) and according to the bank's records (*bottom*).

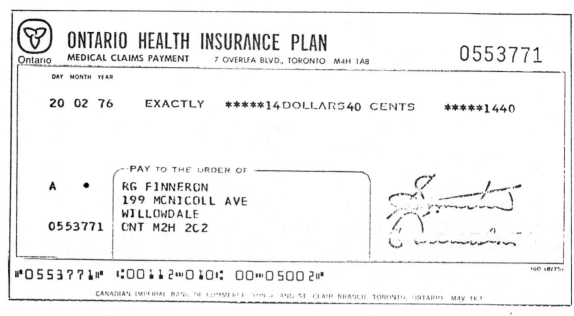

FIGURE 16–6

Forms used by the Ontario Health Insurance Plan (OHIP) to reimburse patients for the portion of service fees covered by the plan. *A*, Cheque. *B*, Record of payment, listing the physician's total charges and the portion of those charges covered by OHIP. *C*, Explanation of the code numbers usually found in the far-right column of the payment record. This explanation is printed on the reverse side of the record.

EXPLANATORY CODES

ELIGIBILITY
J1 SERVICE DATE IS BEFORE THE EFFECTIVE DATE OF OHIP COVERAGE.
J2 SERVICE DATE IS AFTER THE TERMINATION OF COVERAGE DATE.
J7 CLAIM SUBMITTED SIX MONTHS AFTER SERVICE DATE
K4 PATIENT IS OVER THE AGE OF 21 YEARS.
K5 CONTRACT HOLDER IS NOT COVERED UNDER THIS OHIP NUMBER.
K6 SPOUSE NOT COVERED UNDER THIS OHIP NUMBER.
K7 CHILD NOT COVERED UNDER THIS OHIP NUMBER.
K9 DEPENDENT NOT COVERED UNDER THIS SINGLE CONTRACT.
GENERAL
30 THIS SERVICE IS NOT A BENEFIT OF OHIP.
35 OHIP RECORDS SHOW THIS SERVICE RENDERED BY YOU HAS BEEN CLAIMED PREVIOUSLY.
36 OHIP RECORDS SHOW SERVICE HAS BEEN RENDERED BY ANOTHER PRACTITIONER/GROUP.
37 OHIP RECORDS SHOW THIS SERVICE PREVIOUSLY CLAIMED BY YOU.
40 THIS SERVICE ALLOWED ONLY ONCE FOR SAME PATIENT.
50 FEE ALLOWED ACCORDING TO THE CURRENT OMA SCHEDULE OF FEES.
51 SERVICE OUTSIDE OF SPECIALIST'S FIELD ALLOWED AT G.P. RATES.
52 FEE FOR SERVICE ASSESSED BY MEDICAL CONSULTANT.
53 FEE ALLOWED ACCORDING TO APPROPRIATE ITEM IN A PREVIOUS OMA SCHEDULE OF FEES.
54 INTERIM PAYMENT, CLAIM UNDER REVIEW.
55 THIS DEDUCTION IS AN ADJUSTMENT ON AN EARLIER ACCOUNT.
57 THIS PAYMENT IS AN ADJUSTMENT ON AN EARLIER ACCOUNT.
EE ASSESSMENT ALLOWED AT FULL FEE FOR PATIENT PROCEEDING TO HOSPITAL.
CONSULTATIONS
C1 ALLOWED AS REPEAT CONSULTATION.
C2 ALLOWED AT RE-ASSESSMENT FEE.
C3 ALLOWED AT MINOR ASSESSMENT FEE.
DIAGNOSTIC AND THERAPEUTIC PROCEDURES
D1 ALLOWED AS REPEAT PROCEDURE - INITIAL PROCEDURE PREVIOUSLY CLAIMED.
D2 ADDITIONAL PROCEDURES ALLOWED AT 50%.
D3 NOT ALLOWED IN ADDITION TO VISIT FEE.
D4 PROCEDURE ALLOWED AT 50% WITH VISIT.
D5 PROCEDURE ALREADY ALLOWED. VISIT FEE ADJUSTED.
D6 LIMIT OF PAYMENT FOR THIS PROCEDURE REACHED.
D7 NOT ALLOWED IN ADDITION TO OTHER PROCEDURE.
D8 ALLOWED ONLY IN ADDITION TO OTHER PROCEDURE.
FRACTURES
F1 SECOND AND SUBSEQUENT FRACTURES ALLOWED AT 50%.
F2 ALLOWED IN ACCORDANCE WITH TRANSFERRED CARE.
F3 NON-OPERATIVE FRACTURE CASES TERMINATING FATALLY WITHIN 10 DAYS, ALLOWED AT 50%.
F4 FRACT. CASES TREATED OPERATIVELY BUT ARE FATAL WITHIN 10 DAYS AT 75%.
F5 THREE MONTHS AFTER CARE INCLUDED IN FRACTURE FEE.
HOSPITAL VISITS
H1 FEE REDUCED. LEGISLATION REQUIRES ADMIT EXAM WITHIN 72 HRS. OF ADMISSION.
H2 ALLOWED AS SUBSEQUENT VISIT - INITIAL VISIT PREVIOUSLY CLAIMED.
H3 MAXIMUM FEE ALLOWED PER WEEK AFTER 5TH WEEK.
H4 MAXIMUM FEE ALLOWED PER WEEK AFTER 6TH WEEK TO PAEDIATRICIANS.

H5 MAXIMUM FEE ALLOWED PER MONTH AFTER 13TH WEEK.
H6 ALLOWED AS SUPPORTIVE OR CONCURRENT CARE.
H7 ALLOWED AS CHRONIC CARE.
H9 CONCURRENT CARE ALREADY CLAIMED BY ANOTHER DOCTOR.
PAEDIATRIC CARE
P1 MULTIPLE NEWBORN CARE - FOR EACH ADDITIONAL INFANT PAID AT 50%.
P2 MAXIMUM FEE ALLOWED FOR PREMATURE CARE.
P3 MAXIMUM FEE ALLOWED FOR NEWBORN CARE.
P4 FEE FOR NEWBORN CARE DOES NOT APPLY WHEN NEWBORN BABY IS ILL.
P5 OVER AGE FOR PAEDIATRIC RATES OF PAYMENT.
P6 OVER AGE FOR WELL BABY CARE.
OBSTETRICS
O1 FEE FOR OBSTETRIC CARE APPORTIONED.
O2 PREVIOUS PRE-NATAL CARE ALREADY CLAIMED.
O3 PREVIOUS PRE-NATAL CARE ALREADY CLAIMED BY ANOTHER DOCTOR.
O4 OFFICE VISITS RELATING TO PREGNANCY AND CLAIMED PRIOR TO DELIVERY INCLUDED IN OBSTETRIC FEE.
OFFICE AND HOME VISITS
V1 ALLOWED AS REPEAT ASSESSMENT - INITIAL ASSESSMENT PREVIOUSLY CLAIMED.
V2 ALLOWED AS EXTRA PATIENT SEEN IN THE HOME.
V3 NOT ALLOWED IN ADDITION TO PROCEDURAL FEE.
V4 DATE OF SERVICE WAS NOT A SUNDAY OR A STATUTORY HOLIDAY.
V5 ONLY THE OCULO-VISUAL ASSESSMENT ALLOWED WITHIN A 12 MONTH PERIOD.
V6 ALLOWED AS MINOR ASSESSMENT - INITIAL ASSESSMENT ALREADY CLAIMED.
V7 ALLOWED AT SPECIFIC RE-ASSESSMENT FEE.
V8 SERVICE PREV. CLAIMED. THIS SERVICE PAID AT LOWER FEE. O.H.I.P. POLICY.
RADIOLOGY
X1 FEES FOR X-RAY OF ADDITIONAL AREAS IN G.I. TRACT REDUCED BY $5.00.
X2 G.I. TRACT INCLUDES CINE AND VIDEO TAPE.
SURGICAL PROCEDURES
S1 BILATERAL SURGERY, ONE STAGE - ALLOWED AT 50% HIGHER THAN UNILATERAL.
S2 BILATERAL SURGERY, TWO STAGE - ALLOWED AT 75% HIGHER THAN UNILATERAL.
S3 SECOND MAJOR SURGICAL PROCEDURE ALLOWED AT 50%.
S4 THIRD AND ADDITIONAL SURGICAL PROCEDURES ALLOWED AT 25%.
S5 NOT ALLOWED IN ADDITION TO MAJOR SURGICAL FEE.
S6 ALLOWED AS SUBSEQUENT PROCEDURE - INITIAL PROCEDURE PREVIOUSLY CLAIMED.
S7 NORMAL PRE - AND POST-OPERATIVE CARE INCLUDED IN SURGICAL FEE.
HEALTH EXAMINATIONS
R1 ONLY ONE HEALTH EXAM ALLOWED WITHIN A 12 MONTH PERIOD.
R2 10 WELL BABY VISITS ALLOWED UP TO TWO YEARS OF AGE.
R3 2 WELL CHILD EXAMS (AGE 2-5 YEARS) ALLOWED WITHIN A 12 MONTH PERIOD.
R4 ONLY ONE PRIMARY SCHOOL EXAM ALLOWED.
R5 ONLY ONE SECONDARY SCHOOL EXAM ALLOWED.
MAXIMUMS
M1 MAXIMUM FEE ALLOWED FOR THESE SERVICES HAS BEEN REACHED.
M2 MAXIMUM FEE ALLOWANCE FOR RADIOGRAPHIC EXAM HAS BEEN REACHED.

FIGURE 16-6 *(Continued)*

C

Ministry of Health
Ontario

Ontario Health Insurance Plan
Plan d'assurance-santé de l'ontario
Identification Card / *Carte d'identité*

Effective first day of / en vigueur à partir du premier jour de	Surname *Nom*	Init.	Insurance number *Numéro d'assurance*	Supp. Code *Code Supp.*
month *mois* / year *année*				
04 75	FINNERON	RG	82615170	33

When health services required, present this card to the physician, practitioner or hospital. It will be returned. Not valid unless signed on the reverse side.

Quand vous avez besoin de services médicaux, Veuillez présenter cette carte au médecin, au praticien ou à l'hôpital.
Elle vous sera retournée.
Non valide à moins d'être signée au verso.

| GIVE THIS PORTION TO YOUR SPOUSE OR KEEP AS SPARE. | REMETTEZ CETTE PARTIE À VOTRE CONJOINT OU GARDEZ-LA EN RÉSERVE. |

This card is issued to the person named herein, subject to the provisions of the Ontario Health Insurance Plan.

Cette carte est émise au nom de la personne nommément désignée sous réserve dispositions du Plan d'Assurance-Santé de l'Ontario.

Signature of person named herein.   *Signature de la personne nommement désignée.*

Not valid unless signed. Not transferable. There is a penalty for misuse of this identification card.

Non valide à moins d'être signée personnelle. L'emploi abusif de cette carte d'identité est interdit sous peine de sanctions.

FIGURE 16-7

Ontario Health Insurance Plan identification card.

SUPPLEMENTARY PLANS AND GROUP COVERAGE

Many employers or firms offer group coverage under which contributions are deducted at source, both for the provincial plan (for which the employer may pay part of the contribution) and/or for any Extended Health Care Plan (such as Blue Cross) or Supplementary Health and Hospital Plan. The proportion paid by the employer varies widely from the entire amount to some part of it, and the variations occur within each province and from province to province.

Coverage

A Supplementary Health and Hospital Care Plan covers all members of the group. Generally speaking, these plans are drawn up or sponsored by the larger insurance companies, and cover such things as:

1. Ninety per cent of the cost of prescribed drugs or medicines (where Blue Cross might cover 80 per cent).
2. One hundred per cent of semiprivate hospital accommodation to a limit of, say, $20.00 over standard ward care.
3. Outpatient treatment not covered by the provincial plan.
4. Private home nursing.
5. Some services of a chiropractor, osteopath, naturopath, masseur, podiatrist, physiotherapist, or speech therapist, and some of the cost of the services of a psychologist or psychotherapist.
6. Artificial limbs; hospital beds for use in the home, iron lungs, and other kinds of equipment needed for treatment.
7. Ambulance costs over and above the provincial plan allowance.
8. Some dental services or supplies, and eyeglasses and hearing aids.

Where no Supplementary Health and Hospital Plan exists, groups frequently use plans such as Blue Cross to span the difference between what the provincial plan provides and the services offered by the supplementary plans. Blue Cross and other group Extended Health Care Plans are carefully detailed, and very similar. None offers blanket coverage for all medical expenses excluded by a provincial plan. Sometimes drug coverage is 80 per cent as previously mentioned; it may be $50.00 (or some such sum) deductible (that is, the patient pays the first $50.00 and the plan covers the rest); or it may cost so much per prescription—say 25 cents, or 50 cents. Material available from each plan carefully delineates specific benefits (see address list on p. 86). The cost of a supplementary group plan, whether sponsored by Blue Cross or another authority, varies both upwards and downwards from about $2.50 for an individual and $7.10 for a family, generally paid quarterly. There is no precise figure that applies across Canada. This cost is in addition to any provincial plan cost to the individual or family.

INDIVIDUAL (PAY-DIRECT) PLANS

Where no group plan is available to either individual or family, a Pay-Direct Extended Health Care Plan can usually be purchased through one of the carriers offering group coverage. Typically, a single person might pay $16.50 quarterly, and a family $28.50 for the same period, for bridging coverage between the provincial plan and those services covered by a group supplementary plan. It is quite impossible to discuss all the plans offered in Canada in the space of this chapter; therefore one, Blue Cross of Ontario, is shown as a typical example (Fig. 16–8). This plan is semiprivate and pay-direct; the services offered by this individual plan are very similar to those provided by a group plan extended to many people and contributed to at source.

Persons who wish to become members of a provincial plan, and who cannot apply as members of a group, submit applications to the provincial authority where they live in Canada and, if they are eligible, pay the appropriate subscription fee (Fig. 16–9). They are then enrolled in the plan as nongroup participants. Usually, under any provincial plan, the new pay-direct participant is covered on the first day of the third month after enrollment, except when he has become a pay-direct participant as the result of the termination of a group, or his transferral from one. In the latter cases, if he has followed instructions and notified the new plan within 30 days, he remains covered. Similarly, if he is transferring from another province, his new health care insurance coverage will commence on the termination date of the "old" province's plan, provided application for the new medical plan that he wishes to join was made within 30 days of the date entitlement to payment under the original province's plan.

WORKMEN'S COMPENSATION

Much of the information given in Chapter 9 on the American Workers' Compensation laws applies also to Canada. Compensation is paid for working days lost, provided that the worker has sustained a personal injury arising because of and in the course of his employment. If he works Monday to Friday, and is injured on Friday but is able to return to work on Monday, he is not entitled to compensation. If, however, he is injured on Friday and unable to work until the following Wednesday, he is entitled to two days of compensation for Monday and Tuesday. Tax-free compensation is paid at the rate of 75 per cent of the worker's salary. Even if the worker is not eligible for this compensation, necessary medical expenses are paid.

As in the United States, patients requesting treatment under the Workmen's Compensation Act must present a Treatment Memorandum, and the Assistant must file the claim on the appropriate form. For reporting requirements of accidents and waiting periods for income and medical benefits under Workmen's Compensation, see Tables 16–1 and 16–2. Supplies of forms may be obtained from the nearest Workmen's Compensation Office (see address list on pp. 489 and 490). A more complete discussion of Canadian Compensation Laws may be found on pages 704 to 723 of Frederick, P. M., and Kinn, M. E.: *The Medical Office Assistant*, 4th edition (Philadelphia: W. B. Saunders Company, 1974).

PLANS FOR LANDED IMMIGRANTS AND FOREIGN TRAVELLERS

Blue Cross has plans for both landed immigrants and visitors; the plan for visitors is shown in Figure 16–10. Fees for these services may vary, but generally speaking they range from about $10.00 for a single individual entering Canada for a holiday for 21 days, to $68.00 for a family entering for 84 days. Canadians travelling abroad may also obtain temporary additional coverage to bridge the gap between what their provincial plan provides and what is considered necessary extra protection. Although the plan

Text continued on page 479

DETACH HERE

SURNAME		INITIALS

PLEASE PRINT CLEARLY

FOR BLUE CROSS USE ONLY

S | STATUS

EFFECTIVE DATE

ADDRESS (Please Print)

STREET_____ APT. NO._____

CITY_____

POSTAL CODE_____ TELEPHONE NO _____

BILLING FREQUENCY

LAST BILLING DATE

PAID TO DATE

Please complete ONLY ONE of areas (1), (2), (3), or (4) below:

1

I want to enrol in the EHC Pay-Direct Plan. I already have Blue Cross semi-private coverage as follows:

Ident. No._____

Group No._____

Attached is my cheque/money order for
☐ $16.50 single EHC coverage quarterly
☐ $28.50 family EHC coverage quarterly

2

I want to enrol in the EHC Pay-Direct Plan but DO NOT have Blue Cross semi-private coverage. Please enrol me for BOTH EHC Pay-Direct and Blue Cross semi-private coverage. I have attached my cheque/money order for

Total (EHC + Semi-Private)
☐ single $19.50 quarterly ($16.50 + $3.00)
☐ family $34.50 quarterly ($28.50 + $6.00)

3

I want to enrol in the EHC Pay-Direct Plan but DO NOT HAVE Blue Cross semi-private coverage and DO NOT WISH TO ENROL FOR Blue Cross semi-private coverage.

Attached is my cheque/money order for
☐ $16.50 single EHC coverage quarterly
☐ $28.50 family EHC coverage quarterly

4

For semi-private only use this area.

I want to enrol for Blue Cross semi-private hospital accommodation ONLY.

My O.H.I.P. No. is_____
Attached is my cheque/money order for:
☐ $ 6.00 single S.P. Semi-annual
☐ $12.00 family S.P. Semi-annual

Please make your premium cheque or money order payable to: "Ontario Blue Cross".

DO NOT SEND CASH BY MAIL

SIGNATURE_____ DATE_____

DETACH HERE

FIGURE 16–8

Blue Cross of Ontario Extended Health Care and/or Semiprivate "Pay-Direct" Hospital Accommodation for Individual Subscribers. Although payments to this and similar plans are made by individuals on a private basis, the coverage offered closely resembles that provided by group plans paid for by employers.

To obtain this valuable protection for yourself and your family, complete and detach the application card and return to the Blue Cross office of the Province in which you live. An application form for Ontario is shown, together with a list of benefits and limitations. The latter are fairly general throughout all the provinces of Canada. Contact the provincial Blue Cross office for all information, forms, and so forth.

EHC limitations

Extended Health Care pay-direct coverage does NOT pay for:

1. Services normally paid through any provincial hospital plan, any provincial medical plan, Workmen's Compensation Board, other government agencies, or any other source.

2. Doctor's visits in the hospital, home or office, or periodic health check-ups.

3. Treatment for mental illness, tuberculosis or chronic diseases in hospitals other than public general hospitals.

NOTE: A chronic Patient Unit attached to a public general hospital is classified as a separate hospital and Extended Health Care benefits do not apply.

4. Dental care except as provided under "Benefits".

5. Eyeglasses, hearing aids, rest cures, travel for health reasons, insurance examinations, or any treatment for cosmetic purposes.

The benefits listed herein are not available to patients in chronic care hospitals, chronic units of public hospitals, or nursing homes.

EHC benefits

The following benefits are provided when not covered by any government agency:

1. Drugs, serums, injectibles and insulin purchased on the prescription of a medical doctor, except for vitamins and vitamin preparations (unless injected) and patent or proprietary medicines.

2. Private duty nursing by a Registered Nurse who is registered in any province of Canada (not a relative); either in hospital or your home providing it is ordered by the attending physician. Limited to a maximum of 50 eight-hour shifts per subscriber and each eligible dependant during the life of the agreement.

3. Services of a registered or a licensed physiotherapist.

4. Diagnostic services.

5. Difference in cost between semi-private accommodation and a private room (not a suite) in a public general hospital.

6. Dental care when necessitated by a direct accidental blow to the mouth, and not by an object wittingly or unwittingly placed in the mouth when such accident occurs after the effective date of the agreement.

7. Charges up to $10 a day for care in a licensed private hospital, to a maximum of 120 days during the life of the agreement.

8. Purchase or rental of wheelchair, hospital bed, iron lung, oxygen set, artificial limbs or eye, cast, truss, braces or crutches.

9. Radium and radio-isotope treatment and blood transfusions.

10. Ambulance services.

11. Payment to registered clinical psychologists up to $35 for the first visit and $20 per hour for subsequent treatments to a maximum of $200 per person during a benefit year.

12. Payment to registered masseurs up to $7 per treatment for not more than 12 treatments per benefit year per person, but only when we are provided with a certificate by a medical doctor that such treatment is necessary.

13. Payment to qualified speech therapists up to $200 per benefit year per person, but only when we are provided with a certificate by a medical doctor that such treatment is necessary.

14. Payment for medical fees where legal while travelling or residing outside Ontario when such fees are over the Ontario Medical Association Schedule of Fees and are not greater than what would be paid in Ontario if it were legal to provide such benefits in Ontario.

FIGURE 16–8 *(Continued)*

ONTARIO HEALTH INSURANCE COMMISSION
2195 Yonge Street
TORONTO 295, Ontario

NON—GROUP APPLICATION — FORM 105
Not to be used if group facilities are available.

FOR OFFICE USE ONLY

	C. MODE	STATUS	SUPP.
R			
D	EFFECTIVE DATE		
A	PAID TO DATE		

① SURNAME (FAMILY NAME) PLEASE PRINT

Initials of 2 first names

If address is rural route or general delivery, insert name by which you are known—i.e. Tom, Harry, etc.

☐ Mr.
☐ Mrs.
☐ Miss

Postal Address .... (R.R., BOX, OR STREET NUMBER)

NAME OF CITY OR TOWN (PLEASE PRINT)   PROVINCE

HOW TO APPLY AS A NON—GROUP PARTICIPANT

(a) Complete section ① to show surname, initials and address.

(b) Show former Ontario Hospital Insurance number, if any, in section ②.

(c) Check ☒ appropriate box in section ③.

(d) Sign and date application in section ④.

(e) If applicable, complete sections ⑤, ⑥, or ⑦ (over), and note carefully instructions shown in these sections.

(f) If taxable income (amount of income on which you pay taxes after deducting exemptions) is NIL or less than applicable amount shown in section ⑧, enter check mark ☒ in box provided.

② INSERT FORMER ONTARIO HOSPITAL INSURANCE NUMBER (IF ANY)

③ QUARTERLY PREMIUMS (THREE MONTHS)

PERSONS WITH ONE OR MORE ELIGIBLE DEPENDENTS PAY THE FAMILY PREMIUM. NAMES OF DEPENDENTS NOT REQUIRED.

☐ SINGLE PREMIUM: I AM UNMARRIED, SEPARATED, DIVORCED OR WIDOWED, WITHOUT ELIGIBLE DEPENDENT(S).
$33.00 FOR THREE MONTHS.

☐ FAMILY PREMIUM: I HAVE ELIGIBLE DEPENDENT(S).
$66.00 FOR THREE MONTHS.

NOTE: PLEASE MAKE CHEQUE OR MONEY ORDER PAYABLE TO: ONTARIO HEALTH INSURANCE COMMISSION.

NOTE: FUTURE PREMIUMS WILL BE PAYABLE THREE MONTHS PRIOR TO THE BENEFIT PERIOD TO WHICH THEY APPLY.

④ I CERTIFY THAT I AND MY ELIGIBLE DEPENDENTS (IF ANY) ARE RESIDENTS OF ONTARIO AND THAT THE INFORMATION PROVIDED IN THIS APPLICATION IS CORRECT.

I AGREE TO ALLOW THE ONTARIO HEALTH INSURANCE COMMISSION TO VERIFY ALL INFORMATION I HAVE GIVEN IN THIS APPLICATION.

.... (SIGNATURE OF APPLICANT)

DATE ....

IMPORTANT — Please see other side.

BRIEF OUTLINE OF BENEFITS

The following is only a concise description of benefits available under the Plan. More details are available on request.

HOSPITAL CARE

The Plan pays for hospital care which is medically necessary in the treatment of an insured patient in a standard (public) ward of an approved hospital. It also covers a broad range of hospital out-patient services plus medically-prescribed physiotherapy in private non-hospital facilities approved by the Commission.

AMBULANCE SERVICE

Essential and medically-necessary ambulance service is a benefit of the Plan but the insured person is required to pay a small portion of the cost of each trip.

MEDICAL SERVICES

Benefits are provided for medically-necessary physicians' services received at home, in a doctor's office or in hospital. This includes the services of general practitioners and specialists. Payments are made at the rate of 90% of the Ontario Medical Association Schedule of Fees (1971).

OTHER SERVICES

Specified dental surgery performed in hospital is covered up to 90% of the Ontario Dental Association Schedule of Fees (1969) . . . Eye examinations by refraction by an optometrist to determine the need for glasses: $10.00 per person . . . Chiropractic, Osteopathic and Chiropody (Podiatry) services: up to $100.00, plus $25.00 for radiographic examinations,

per person, for each of these three types of services. The dollar maximums quoted above apply to the twelve-month period beginning July 1, each year.

CARE OUTSIDE ONTARIO

Insured physicians' and practitioners' services received outside Ontario are covered to the same extent they would be paid for in Ontario. The amount payable for hospital care is determined by the Commission on the basis of the medical need to obtain the care outside Ontario.

SERVICES NOT COVERED

Any hospital charges for private or semi-private accommodation;

Hospital visits solely for the administration of drugs;

Hospital charges for dental care which is normally provided in the dentist's office; Fees for dental services other than specified;

Eyeglasses, special appliances;

Private duty nursing fees;

Drugs, vaccines, biological serum or extracts or their synthetic substitutes (except when provided in hospital); Drugs taken home from the hospital;

Transportation charges other than approved ambulance service;

Medical examinations required for applications for employment or the continuance of employment, life insurance, schools, camps or recreation;

Payment for any health service other than those provided by approved hospitals or the physicians and practitioners specified in this brochure.

FIGURE 16—9

Blue Cross of Ontario application for nongroup enrollment, Form 105 (1/72). There are changes which may affect coverage, as when the member or the spouse becomes employed where there is an insured group. All information to do with any Provincial Plan is obtainable from that Plan, and anyone writing or telephoning the Plan should quote his or her health insurance number.

TABLE 16-1. EMPLOYERS' AND/OR PHYSICIANS' REPORT OF ACCIDENTS

Jurisdiction	Reporting Requirements	
	Time Limit	Injuries Covered
ALBERTA	24 hours[1]	All injuries
BRITISH COLUMBIA	3 days[1]	All injuries
MANITOBA	3 days[1]	All injuries
NEW BRUNSWICK	3 days[1]	All compensable injuries
NEWFOUNDLAND	3 days	All accidents that disable or require medical aid
NOVA SCOTIA	3 days[1]	All accidents
ONTARIO	3 days[1]	All accidents that disable or require medical aid
PRINCE EDWARD ISLAND	3 days	All accidents that disable or require medical aid
QUEBEC	2 working days	All accidents
SASKATCHEWAN	3 days[1]	All accidents
NORTHWEST TERRITORIES	3 days[1]	All accidents
YUKON TERRITORY	3 days[1]	All accidents in which workman is injured
CANADIAN MERCHANT SEAMEN'S ACT	60 days	All accidents that disable or require medical aid

[1] Insurance carrier and attending physician also required to make report. It should be forthwith by telephone in fatal injury cases, but this is in addition to usual report.

TABLE 16-2. WAITING PERIOD FOR INCOME BENEFITS; MEDICAL BENEFITS

Jurisdiction	Waiting Period
ALBERTA	1 day
BRITISH COLUMBIA	1 day
MANITOBA	1 day
NEW BRUNSWICK	4 days
NEWFOUNDLAND	1 day
NOVA SCOTIA	3 days
ONTARIO	1 day
PRINCE EDWARD ISLAND	1 day
QUEBEC	1 day
SASKATCHEWAN	1 day
NORTHWEST TERRITORIES	1 day
YUKON TERRITORY	1 day
CANADIAN MERCHANT SEAMEN'S ACT	3 days

This is a copy of your Benefits, Limitations and Terms of Agreement. Please retain for your reference.

Benefits: Hospital

1. Hospital Care –

   Option 1 – Hospital care in government approved public general hospitals at regular daily rates up to a maximum of $80.00 (eighty dollars) per day and to a limit of 30 (thirty) days.*

   Option 2 – Hospital care in government approved public general hospitals to 100 per cent of their regular daily rate as set by government for Standard Ward care, to a limit of 30 (thirty) days.*

   NOTE: In larger cities the standard ward rate for hospital care could be in excess of $160.00 (one hundred and sixty dollars) per day.

   Hospitals in Canada charge all-inclusive daily rates.

2. Out-patient and emergency care in hospital to a limit of $500.00 during the life of the agreement.

3. The cost of a local ambulance, at prevailing rates, to the nearest hospital for emergency treatment.

Benefits: Medical-Surgical

1. Medical-Surgical In-patient Hospital Care for a period of 30 (thirty) days with payment up to the current Ontario Medical Association General Practice Schedule of Fees.

2. Medical-Surgical Out-patient and Emergency Hospital Care with payment up to the current Ontario Medical Association General Practice Schedule of Fees, to a maximum of $500.00 during the term of the agreement.

   Visits to the doctor's office or doctor's visits to the home are not covered. This includes visits to doctors' offices located in medical centres and hospitals.

3. Laboratory tests and/or x-rays in a private laboratory or clinic as ordered by a medical doctor, for a specific condition and not for diagnosis only, up to a maximum of $60.00 during the term of agreement.

Limitations:

1. Hospital and Medical-Surgical care will be paid only if rendered in Public General Hospitals for active treatment.

2. Medical-Surgical coverage will be provided only for patients in hospital (except as provided for out-patient and emergency hospital care and in private laboratories or clinics) up to the current Ontario Medical Association General Practice Schedule of Fees.

Exclusions:

1. Hospital and medical care for maternity, any termination of pregnancy, or any condition arising from pregnancy is not covered.

2. Benefits under this agreement are not covered if the patient is entitled to receive same from any government agency or department.

3. Benefits under this agreement are not available for tooth extractions, dental care, cosmetic surgery, plastic surgery, mental or chronic illness, or drugs.

4. **Benefits are not available under this agreement if the patient has come to Canada for the purpose of receiving hospital or Medical-Surgical care or treatment.**

5. No benefits are available beyond the boundaries of Canada or the continental United States of America. (See terms of agreement re limitation on benefits paid in the United States.)

Note: Fill out Option 1 or Option 2 but not both.

* If you are an inpatient in hospital on the expiry date of this agreement, the hospital benefit will continue for the 30 (thirty) days of the hospital benefit.

DETACH HERE

Folds to make envelope   Moisten/Seal

Fold Here

ONTARIO BLUE CROSS
150 FERRAND DRIVE DON MILLS ONTARIO M3C 1H6

Option 2

Application Form

Must be received at an office of Ontario Blue Cross prior to arrival or within 21 days after arrival in Canada. A certificate will be issued.

As a visitor to Canada, I wish to apply for the special Ontario Blue Cross Hospital Medical Plan as checked below to provide for me and/or my family. I have read the literature and understand the conditions relating to this coverage.

Visitor's Place of Residence While in Canada:

(Visitor's) ☐ Mr.

Name: ☐ Mrs. _____ _____

☐ Miss (First Name)   (Family Name)

Address: _____ _____

(Number and Street) (Please Print)   (Apt. Number)

_____ _____

(City or Town) (Please Print)   (Province)

Telephone No. ( ) ☐☐☐ ☐☐☐ ☐☐☐☐

(in Canada) Area Code

Rates and Length of Agreement

Single and Family coverage is available. "Family" means the subscriber, legal spouse, and the unmarried, unemployed children under the age of 21 years.

Coverage is available for periods of 21 days, 42 days, 63 days and 84 days. The agreement may be renewed (requiring additional payment) for one additional period only, provided that benefits have not been used during the preceding period, and if application for renewal is received by Ontario Blue Cross prior to expiry of first period of coverage.

Coverage Option 2

Benefits as listed opposite which include hospital care in government approved public general hospitals to 100 per cent of their regular daily rate as set by government for Standard Ward care, to a limit of 30 (thirty) days.

Coverage Single		Coverage Family	
21 day period	$18.00 ☐	21 day period	$36.00 ☐
42 day period	$27.00 ☐	42 day period	$54.00 ☐
63 day period	$39.00 ☐	63 day period	$78.00 ☐
84 day period	$51.00 ☐	84 day period	$102.00 ☐

Please check coverage desired (above) and attach cheque or money order for

$ _____ Application is not valid unless this portion is completed.

Arrival Date In Canada

Date: _____

Day   Month   Year

Name of Home Country _____

I understand that if this application is received and accepted by Ontario Blue Cross prior to arrival in Canada, benefits commence at 12:01 a.m. on the day of arrival. Otherwise, benefits commence at 12:01 a.m. on the day following receipt of application and payment at Ontario Blue Cross, Don Mills, Ontario or any Ontario Blue Cross district office. **N.B.** No person will be covered under this agreement who is in hospital on the day the agreement becomes effective.

I certify that my visit, or the visit of any member of my family to Canada, is not for the purpose of obtaining hospital or medical care, and further, that as of the date of signing this application I am not aware that I or any member of my family requires hospital or medical care.

Signature of Subscriber or Proxy:

Date: _____

Day   Month   Year

Moisten/Seal

FIGURE 16–10

Ontario Health Plan for visitors to Canada, Form E500 (12/75). Only Option Two is shown — which covers hospital care for the stated period *in full*. Option One offers to cover to the extent of $80.00 per diem only. All questions should be addressed to the provincial Blue Cross office.

shown in Figure 16–11 is for Ontario, other provinces' plans are similar, and information is available on request. Immigrants into Canada pick up the standard application for nongroup enrollment—usually from any bank—fill in the box labelled "New Residents Only," and are covered almost immediately (Fig. 16–12). Anyone entering Ontario on May 10th, for example, would file the application form on arrival and would then be covered from the first day of June: that is, coverage begins the first day of the month succeeding the one in which application was made.

Moisten & Seal

Fold Here

ONTARIO
BLUE CROSS
150 FERRAND DRIVE, DON MILLS, ONTARIO M3C 1H6

APPLICATION FORM

I wish to apply for the special Ontario Blue Cross Hospital Medical Plan as checked below to provide for me and/or my family. I have read and understand the terms and conditions relating to this coverage.

TRAVELLER'S PLACE OF RESIDENCE IN CANADA: (PLEASE PRINT)

(Travellers) MR.
NAME: MRS.
MISS _____ (FIRST NAME) _____ (FAMILY NAME)

CURRENT
MAILING
ADDRESS: (NUMBER AND STREET) _____ (APT. NUMBER)

(CITY OR TOWN) _____ (PROVINCE/STATE)

RATES AND LENGTH OF AGREEMENT

Single and Family coverage is available. "Family" means the subscriber, legal spouse, and the unmarried, unemployed children under the age of 21 years. Coverage is available for periods of 14 days, 21 days, 28 days, 40 days, 60 days, and 120 days or any two periods combined to a maximum of 240 days.

The agreement may be renewed (requiring additional payment) for one additional period **only,** provided that benefits have not been used during the preceding period, and that application for renewal and payment is received by Ontario Blue Cross prior to expiry of the first period of coverage.

COVERAGE SINGLE

14 day period	$ 8.50	☐
21 day period	$ 12.00	☐
28 day period	$ 16.00	☐
40 day period	$ 22.00	☐
60 day period	$ 30.00	☐
120 day period	$ 56.00	☐

COVERAGE FAMILY (including legal wife and all unmarried unemployed children under age 21)

14 day period	$ 17.00	☐
21 day period	$ 24.00	☐
28 day period	$ 32.00	☐
40 day period	$ 44.00	☐
60 day period	$ 60.00	☐
120 day period	$112.00	☐

Please check coverage desired (above) and attach cheque or money order for $_____ (make payable to Ontario Blue Cross). Application is not valid unless this portion is completed.

DEPARTURE DATE: _____
(Day) _____ (Month) _____ (Year)

I understand if this application is received and accepted by Ontario Blue Cross prior to departure date, benefits commence at the time of crossing the border into another country (or if travelling by air, at the time the plane takes off). Otherwise, benefits commence at 12:01 a.m. on the day following receipt of application and payment at Ontario Blue Cross, Don Mills, Ontario or any Ontario Blue Cross district office.

N.B. No person will be covered under this agreement who is in hospital on the day the agreement becomes effective.

I certify that no one covered under the agreement applied for is travelling for the purpose of obtaining hospital or medical treatment, and further, that as of the date of signing this application I am not aware that I or any member of my family requires hospital or medical treatment.

SIGNATURE OF APPLICANT OR PROXY: _____

DATE: _____
Day _____ Month _____ Year

Moisten & Seal

Fold Here

Moisten & Seal – Folds to make envelope

FIGURE 16–11

Ontario Plan for Canadians travelling outside Canada, Form E570 (1/76). Anyone, from any province, planning to travel abroad may take out private short-term health insurance policies. Blue Cross offers one entitled "Health Plan While Outside Canada," and information on it, or on any similar plan, may be obtained from the provincial office of the holder of the plan. The office will be able to outline all benefits and limitations of each plan, and all exclusions.

Terms of the Agreement

a) This health agreement shall be available only to Canadian residents covered by a provincial government health plan and travelling outside the boundaries of Canada. This health agreement shall become effective at the time of crossing the border into another country provided application and payment are received prior to departure date. Otherwise benefits commence at 12:01 A.M. on the day following receipt of application and payment in this office, and shall terminate at the border on the return home or 12 midnight on the expiry date of the agreement, whichever comes first. If travelling by air, the agreement shall become effective at the time the aeroplane takes off in Canada (if application is received prior to departure date) and shall terminate when the aeroplane lands in Canada on the return home, or at 12:00 midnight on the expiry date of the agreement, whichever comes first.

b) The benefits described in this agreement are available to the applicant or if enrolled under a family agreement to the applicant, his legal wife and his unmarried, unemployed children under age 21.

c) All benefits listed herein shall be payable only on the submission of certification by the attending physician that services included in the benefits have been required.

d) It is understood and agreed between the participants in this agreement that no benefits for hospital or medical care shall be paid until after accounts have been appraised by the provincial government health plan and benefits if any have been paid by that plan.

e) Payment will be made by Ontario Blue Cross by cheque, directly to the subscriber, upon receipt and appraisal of the necessary accounts and information concerning the accounts as detailed. Payment will be made in Canadian currency, based on the rate of exchange in effect at the conclusion of the service rendered, as determined by any Canadian Chartered Bank.

ONTARIO BLUE CROSS,
150 FERRAND DRIVE,
DON MILLS, ONTARIO
M3C 1H6   TEL. (416) 429-2661

E-570·1/76·50m

(B) LANDED IMMIGRANT

DATE OF ARRIVAL IN ONTARIO

DAY	MONTH	YEAR

I HAVE BEEN GRANTED THE STATUS OF A LANDED IMMIGRANT BY THE DEPARTMENT OF MANPOWER AND IMMIGRATION.

(REMIT PREMIUMS AS INDICATED IN SECTION ❸.)

FIGURE 16–12

Section of application for nongroup enrollment used by immigrants to Canada who wish to apply for membership in the Ontario Health Insurance Plan (OHIP). In Ontario, Form 105 (1/72) contains the nongroup application form, Part 5 of which, at (B), is for immigrants to Canada. Section 3 of the same card contains the premium scales for married and single people (see Fig. 16–9). All Canadian provinces make plans available to immigrants, and the provincial plan is the place to seek information.

DENTAL COVERAGE

Like most other forms of insurance coverage, dental care protection is not universal throughout the provinces. Some *group* plans cover dental care; others do not. Provincial plans usually cover only those services which must be performed in a hospital, such as the removal of wisdom teeth. The group and individual coverage available to supplement these payments varies with the province and within provinces from none at all to group plans covering any cleaning and scaling necessary, emergency treatment for dental pain, examinations, x-rays, fillings, extractions, inlays, some bridge work, and dentures and repairs to dentures. Between these extremes, plans are found with annual deductibles or with shared-risk (coinsurance—see p. 2) factors. Maximum payment scales are established for diagnostic services, preventative services, treatment services, endodontics, restorative services, and dentures, beyond which the covering agent will not pay. No payment is made for broken appointments, so dentists sometimes claim an examination fee from patients if cancellation was not made in time to call in someone else.

Premium levels for dental insurance vary according to the extent of the coverage selected. The insurance carrier may pay allowable benefits either directly to the dentist or to the subscriber, depending on the dentist's preference. Nothing is paid for what is normally covered by the provincial insurance plan, Workmen's Compensation, or any other government agency. Cosmetic dentistry is also excluded.

For further information on dental insurance, see Chapter 11.

RESPONSIBILITIES OF THE MEDICAL ASSISTANT

Anyone entering the medical secretarial field should obtain all the material she can on the provincial insurance plan of the province where she intends to work. Folders are available containing samples of cards used, together with full instructions regarding eligibility, payment, and billing procedure. Everything covered by a plan is stated in clear terms, so that any patient may be advised by the Assistant and told precisely what to do in case of doubt. All Canadian provincial health authorities may be approached directly at the addresses given on page 489 and are happy to supply pamphlets and answer specific questions about their services. Frequently they will also volunteer guest speakers for class discussion. Blue Cross representatives may be contracted by using the address list on page 86. The wise Assistant (or teacher) will make quite certain that she knows where to go for this help. Mistakes in billing are expensive and may involve lengthy delays in the payment of accounts to the doctor. There is no excuse for them when current and accurate information may be obtained so easily.

The Assistant should also know exactly what benefits are offered as extended health benefits by supplementary carriers such as Blue Cross; all such carriers, in the provinces where they operate, are most cooperative in this regard. All extraprovincial plans extend the coverage offered by the provincial plan and/or the Workmen's Compensation Boards. As has already been indicated, they offer, among other things, semiprivate hospital care for groups or individuals. This is indicated by a code number on the identification card carried by all provincial plan members, and shows up under "Supp.Code/Code Supp." as 33 on the Ontario one shown (see Fig. 16–7).

The Medical Assistant must know what her doctor charges, how to present those charges to the patient, how to handle cash payments, and how to enter them on the patient's charge sheet or ledger sheet from the day book (see p. 467 and Fig. 16–13). Some doctors prefer that the Assistant handle all money matters; most will discuss these with patients personally but are happy to have their assistants do so also. If the Assistant is to handle monetary discussions effectively, she must know exactly what the doctor charges for house calls, office visits, operations, and other services, and she must be familiar with the fee scale laid down by the Provincial Medical Association and/or the Canadian Medical Association. All fixed charges may be quoted by the Assistant to any patient asking about them. If the charge is not fixed, the doctor may prefer to discuss it himself, since anyone asking the price of something is obviously concerned about it, and it is essential that the Assistant be very tactful and helpful about this matter with patients. Any lack of consideration on her part may result in the doctor's loss of the patient. If a charge or fee obviously horrifies a patient, it is necessary to assure him that he will receive every consideration in meeting his bill. Arrangements can and should be made to suit both patient and doctor. If an operation is involved, or any great expense not covered by the insurance carried by the patient (such as cosmetic surgery), the discussion between doctor and patient should be comprehensive, and the patient should be left in no doubt as to the charges involved and exactly what he is getting for his money. Arrangements about payment should be made before—not after—the service or operation is performed, so that there can be no misunderstanding.

However bills are paid, whether by the provincial authority or by the patient, they must be sent out promptly and be accurately stated. Provincial statements are sent in on the proper form. When the doctor does not bill the provincial authority, patients' bills are sent out. Some are coded and itemised; some bear only the words "For professional services rendered" (Fig. 16–14). The Assistant follows the doctor's preference in this, but most patients prefer an itemised account. If a patient dies, the Assistant should send the bill to the estate for collection.

All charges are entered in the day book. When the doctor returns from house calls, those charges and any cash payments the doctor may have received must be entered. Make out charge slips if entries cannot be made immediately (Fig. 16–15A). Never leave this job hanging for several days. Try to do it the first thing each morning. Patients paying at the end of a visit are given a receipt for their money, and those payments are recorded in the day book too. A *day book* is a chronological listing of times at which patients have been seen, into which is entered a record of any payments received in cash, the charge for the service, and any monies received on account (Fig. 16-13A). Always use a receipt book with a carbon, as by the end of the day it will be impossible to remember who paid what.

Charges and monies received are entered on the patients' ledger sheets or cards from the day book (Fig. 16–13B). Everything is recorded, whether it be an office call, house call, or night call: a charge is first recorded in the day book and transferred from there to the ledger sheets, as are all monies coming from patients.

All monies received are paid into the bank daily, weekly, or as the doctor directs (Fig. 16–15B). The amount paid in should tally exactly with the total shown in the day book for that period (Fig. 16–16). The money must never be used without first passing through the bank.

In summary, the doctor's bookkeeping usually consists of the day book, a general ledger, and the patients' ledger sheets or cards. The Medical Assistant should be able to do a bank reconciliation (see Fig. 16–5, p. 469) and read the bank statements. She must know how to deal with petty cash, perform simple bookkeeping up to the trial balance level, and produce a balance sheet and often a statement of income for tax purposes. In

Text continued on page 486

May 12, 1977	Name	Service	Charge	Cash	Received
8:30	J. Brodie	O.C.	5.00		
8:35	M. Matheson	O.C.		10.00	
8:40	R. Finneron	O.C. (daughter)	15.00		
8:45	T. Garnett	O.C. N.P.		5.00	
9:00	A. Courtley	N.C.	6.50		
9:30	J. Forrest	O.C. (prenatal)	25.00		
10:00	T. Shaddock	N.C.	6.50		
10:30	F. Prideaux	CK.			10.00
11:00	J. Hill	CK.			5.00
11:30					
to	HOSPITAL				
4:30					
6:00	F. Allen	N.C.		6.50	
6:15	J. Hay	O.C.	5.00		
6:30	M. Hay	CK.			100.00
			$63.00	$21.50	$115.00

A

FIGURE 16–13

Examples of the bookkeeping duties that the Medical Assistant must be able to handle in order to process insurance claims correctly. *A*, Page from the day book, showing (from left to right) time of service, patient name, service performed, physician's charge for service, and cash and cheques received. Code: O.C., office call; N.C., night call; N.P., new patient; CK., cheque. *B*, Patient ledger card, indicating services, dates performed, and balance due.

| NAME | FINNERON, Rhoda G. | | PHONE | 491-7357 | EMPLOYED BY | | | | |

| ADDRESS | 199 McNicoll Avenue, WILLOWDALE 428 | CHARGE TO Patient |

DATE		DESCRIPTION	FOLIO	DEBIT		CREDIT		BALANCE	
7/2/77		O.C. Pain L. Leg		4	00			4	00
19/3/77		O.C. Insomnia — Menopausal — Inj.		5	00			9	00
3/4/77		CK.				9	00	NIL	
9/10/77		O.C. Daughter Penelope		15	00			15	00

FIGURE 16–13 (Continued)

B

CONSULTATION BY APPOINTMENT

B.S. BORDEN, M.D.   1333 Sheppard Ave. East.
                                     WILLOWDALE, Ont.
                                     494-7442

                              . . . . March 15, ... 19 .77.

Mrs. Rhoda Finneron
199 McNicoll Avenue
Willowdale

FOR PROFESSIONAL SERVICES

Feb. 7
Office call — pain in left leg   4 00

Mar. 7
Office call — insomnia — menopausal   5 00
                                               $ 9 00

PLEASE READ AND COMPLETE THE BACK OF THIS FORM CAREFULLY.

A

FIGURE 16–14

Examples of bills sent to patients when the physician does not bill the provincial authority directly. *A*, Itemized bill, listing type of service in addition to date and charge. *B*, Nonitemized bill, listing date and charge only.

```
            FOR PROFESSIONAL SERVICES      Feb. 7              4  00
                                           Mar. 7              5  00



                                                            $ 9  00



         ·     PLEASE READ AND COMPLETE THE BACK OF THIS FORM CAREFULLY.
```

FIGURE 16-14 *(Continued)*   *B*

the general ledger the cash in the bank will increase each time a deposit is made. The deposit is entered in the day book, on the patients' ledger cards or sheets, and then in the general ledger.

DELINQUENT ACCOUNTS

It is regrettable but true that people who have had treatment from a doctor are often lax in attending to the payment of their bills. If a bill is not paid the second time it is sent, send another when billing time comes around with "overdue" or "please remit" typed or stamped across it. If the doctor prefers not to use this method of reminding, send a letter with the third bill suggesting that a partial payment would be acceptable for the time being and indicating the ways and means of payment that can be worked out. This letter should be signed by the Assistant or the physician. Usually a patient who is having difficulty paying but wishes to do so will reply gladly to such a letter. A patient who has no intention of paying unless forced to do so will not reply. In the latter instance, sending a bill and a second letter to the patient's place of business may be more effective in bringing the patient to settle the account. Married women who do not work can often be reached through their husbands' employers.

Keep reminder letters polite and always sound very reasonable in approaching a patient. When dealing with a patient who has always paid in good time, ask specifically if it is possible to help in any way or if the doctor can help. If the doctor agrees, tardy

CHARGE SLIP

Today's Date

X-ray
Drugs
Injection
Surgery
Consultation   50.00

. . . .
. . . .
. . . .

                                    $50.00

Name of Patient

A

THE CANADIAN DOMINION BANK   ACCOUNT NO. 123456

DATE	LIST CHEQUES				
CURRENT ACCOUNT DEPOSIT CREDIT	15	00	CURRENCY.	50	00
DOCTOR'S NAME	25	00	COIN	5	75
NAME					
SECRETARY'S NAME	75	00	CHEQUES/COUPONS	125	00
DEPOSITED BY			TOTAL	180	75
	10	00	LESS RECEIVED CASH		
TELLER'S	125	00	SIGNATURE . . . . *. . . .	—	—
STAMP	FORWARD TOT.		AMOUNT OF DEPOSIT	180	75

B

FIGURE 16–15

A, Temporary charge slip made out by the Assistant when she is unable to make complete entries in the day book immediately. *B*, Bank deposit slip. If the Assistant had been asked by her doctor to bring back $50.00 for the office petty cash account, the slip would show her signature at the asterisk, $50.00 in the money column to the right of the asterisk, and a total deposit of $130.75.

payers might be called on the telephone. Again, great tact is required in making these calls. The approach should always be that one would like to help however one can; sometimes a patient is genuinely embarrassed by his or her inability to pay a large bill and will jump at the chance to pay over a period of time.

A doctor will rarely take delinquent patients to court, although he may invoke the help of a collection agency. If so, the Assistant stops billing the patient but does report to the agency if the patient pays the outstanding account. The latter is most

DATE		PARTICULARS	CHEQUES		DEPOSITS		BALANCE	
Aug.	15	Balance BF					5765	74
	16	Payroll expenses	410	00			5355	74
	17	Janitor service	50	00			5305	74
	20	Laundry expense	20	41			5285	33
	21	Deposit (see Day Book)			847	17	6132	50
		Telephone	45	00			6087	50
	24	Deposit (see Day Book)			517	00	6604	50

FIGURE 16–16

Cheque book tally sheet, showing correct balance in bank after expenses and deposits.

likely to happen if the patient can pay at all, since it is a great inconvenience for an employer to be approached by a collection agency. Very often this can result in the patient's losing his job.

BILLING FOR IN-HOSPITAL SERVICES

Hospital charges not covered by an insurance plan of some kind are billed before the patient leaves the hospital. All the relative papers will have been sent to the Accounting Department and the bill prepared as soon as it is known when the patient is to be released. The patient goes to the appropriate office on his way out and pays the bill. If he made a deposit against his stay when he entered the hospital, this will be taken into account and he will pay the balance only. The bill is receipted and the patient goes on his way. If the patient is covered by a Federal Provincial Plan, he either pays the entire hospital bill himself and sends the receipted bill in for reimbursement, or, if this is their policy, the hospital will bill the insurance plan directly for covered services.

Sometimes the hospital bill includes all services rendered to the patient during his stay in the hospital; sometimes it covers "bed and board" only. In the latter instance, the patient will receive a bill from the doctor charging him for services performed before, during, and after hospitalization, including anaesthesia, surgery, nonsurgical treatment, drugs, delivery, x-rays, and special therapy. Any service not covered by a Provincial Plan is the patient's financial responsibility.

If the hospital does not bill the Provincial Plan and/or the Extended Health Care Plan directly, the patient is responsible for all charges and costs incurred for both hospital and doctor(s). Any discrepancy between the scale of fees the doctor or hospital charges and what the plan pays is the responsibility of the patient.

The preceding system varies considerably from province to province. Specific guidelines are available in all provinces for the Assistant to follow.

The following are addresses to which to write for information on the health plans for the ten provinces and two territories of Canada.

Alberta
Health Care Insurance Commission
118th Avenue and Groat Road
Box 1360
Edmonton, Alberta T5J 2N3

British Columbia
Medical Services Commission
Department of Health Parliament Buildings
Victoria, British Columbia V8V 1X4

Manitoba
Health Services Commission
Box 925, 599 Empress Street
Winnipeg, Manitoba R3C 2T6

New Brunswick
P.O. Box 6000
Fredericton, New Brunswick E5B 5H1

Newfoundland
Department of Health
Parliament Buildings
St. John's, Newfoundland

Nova Scotia
Health Care Plan
Department of Health
Parliament Buildings
Halifax, Nova Scotia

Ontario
Ontario Health Insurance Plan
Box 1774, Station "R"
Toronto, Ontario M4G 2T3

Prince Edward Island
Health Services Commission
P.O. Box 4500
Charlottetown, Prince Edward Island C1A 7P4

Quebec
Health Insurance Board
P.O. Box 6600
Quebec 2, Quebec

Saskatchewan
Department of Health
Health Building
3211 Albert Street
Regina, Saskatchewan S4S 0A6

Northwest Territories
Health Care Plan
Yellowknife, Northwest Territories X1A 2L9

Yukon
Health Care Plan
Department of Health
Parliament Buildings
Dawson City, Yukon

CANADIAN WORKMEN'S COMPENSATION DIRECTORY

Alberta
Workers' Compensation Board
P. O. Box 2415
Edmonton, Alberta T5J 285

British Columbia
Workers' Compensation Board
5255 Heather Street
Vancouver, British Columbia V5Z 3L8

Manitoba
Worker's Compensation Board
333 Maryland Street
Winnipeg, Manitoba R3G 1M2

New Brunswick
Worker's Compensation Board
Box 160
St. John, New Brunswick

Newfoundland
Workmen's Compensation Board
Philip Place
Elizabeth Avenue East
St. John's, Newfoundland A1A 3B8

Northwest Territories
Worker's Compensation Board
Yellowknife
Northwest Territories XOE 1HO

Nova Scotia
Workmen's Compensation Board
P.O. Box 1150
Halifax, Nova Scotia B3J 2Y2

Quebec
Commission Des Accidents
524 Bourdages Street
Quebec, Quebec G1K 7E2

Ontario
Workmen's Compensation Board
2 Bloor Street East
Toronto, Ontario M4W 3C3

Saskatchewan
Workers' Compensation Board
1840 Lorne Street
Regina, Saskatchewan S4P 2L8

Prince Edward Island
Workmen's Compensation Board
60 Belvedere Avenue
P.O. Box 757
Charlottetown, Prince Edward Island

Yukon
Territorial Secretary-Registrar General
P.O. Box 2703
Whitehorse, Yukon Territory

REVIEW QUESTIONS

1. Why is it important for the Medical Assistant to keep accurate patient histories? _____

_____

_____

2. What items should the Assistant record on the index card when a patient visits the office for the first time?

a. _____   e. _____

b. _____   f. _____

c. _____   g. _____

d. _____

3. What information constitutes the final entry on the patient's history? _____

_____

4. Explain the meaning of the following designation on the patient's chart: F. 60 a&w; M. 55 a. and suffering from angina. Siblings: 3 m. 2 a.; 2 f. a&w.

_____

_____

5. What is an *anamnesis?* _____

6. What is the best way to pay bills sent to the physician's office?

_____

7. Who governs the fees charged by physicians in Canada?

_____

_____

8. What are some of the benefits provided by a Supplementary Health and Hospital Care Plan that may not be provided by a Provincial Health Insurance Plan?

a. _____   d. _____

b. _____   e. _____

c. _____   f. _____

9. What coverage is available in Canada for persons not fully covered by a Provincial Health Insurance Plan or a Supplementary Health and Hospital Care Plan?

_____

_____

_____

10. Are Landed Immigrants to Canada normally covered by Provincial Health

Insurance Plans? _____

_____

11. How soon after enrollment is a pay-direct participant usually covered by a

Provincial Health Insurance Plan? _____

_____

12. Describe the coverage for dental work typically offered by provincial plans

and supplemental group plans. _____

_____

13. What does the Assistant do if the physician decides to employ a collection agency to collect delinquent accounts? _____

_____

14. Why should the Assistant be tactful in discussing money matters with patients? _____

_____

15. What three items make up the doctor's bookkeeping duties?

a. _____

b. _____

c. _____

16. Make up a patient's history from the following details, using the blank patients' record sheet on the facing page.

History notes are for Mrs. Margaret Hay, whose age is 35, and who lives at 1 Wrong Street, Halifax, Nova Scotia. She is off work at present, but her business telephone number is 965-5388 and her home number is 494-8563. She worked for the Halifax General Bank. When she visited Dr. Doe, she was complaining of severe abdominal pain. She said she had had the pain for about 2 hours. She was approximately 35 weeks pregnant. She was having intermittent contractions. She had had no serious illnesses or operations before. Her parents—mother aged 60 and father aged 65—are both alive and well, and she has three brothers and two sisters all in good health. An examination showed no head or neck abnormalities, and the lungs were clear. The heart was regular in rate and rhythm, with no audible murmurs. There was some tenderness over the abdomen, and marked tenderness across the lower portion of the uterus. There was no external bleeding. The uterus was at the level of the xiphoid. On palpation there was a marked tenderness at the lower portion of the uterus, and there were slight irregular contractions. There were no abnormalities of extremities or back. The central nervous system was grossly intact. A provisional diagnosis of abruptio placenta was made. Mrs. Hay was admitted to Halifax General Hospital the day after her visit to Dr. Doe on March 19, 1977. The hospital discharged her on March 28, 1977.

PATIENT RECORD

LAST NAME	FIRST NAME	MIDDLE NAME	BIRTH DATE	SEX	HOME PHONE

ADDRESS   CITY   STATE   ZIP CODE

PATIENT'S OCCUPATION   NAME OF COMPANY

ADDRESS OF EMPLOYER   PHONE

SPOUSE OR PARENT   OCCUPATION

EMPLOYER   ADDRESS   PHONE

INSURANCE

REFERRED BY

PAST ILLNESS AND FAMILY HISTORY

GENERAL PHYSICAL EXAMINATION

HEAD AND NECK

RESPIRATORY SYSTEM

CARDIOVASCULAR SYSTEM

GASTROINTESTINAL SYSTEM

GENITOURINARY SYSTEM

EXTREMITIES AND BACK

NERVOUS SYSTEM

SUMMARY

PROVISIONAL DIAGNOSIS

DATE	PROGRESS

17. Make up an Admission History and combined Operation History for Mr. H.B. Brodie, 1152 Skana Avenue, Vancouver, British Columbia, who was admitted to General Hospital on May 1, 1977. Use the form on the opposite page. Mr. Brodie's room number was 1234; his telephone number is 123-4568, and his age is 67. His private physician, Dr. David Jones, referred him to the ophthalmologist, J.B. Smith, M.D.

On admission, Mr. Brodie's chief complaint was that he had developed bilateral cataracts about 2 years previously. The right cataract was extracted in September, 1975 (18 months earlier), with good results. Since then he had had no major health problems. On physical examination he proved to be a well-developed, well-nourished white male in no acute distress. His heart sounds were normal. His abdomen was negative. His extremities were also negative. Blood pressure was 120/80 and no heart murmurs were apparent. The following diagnosis was made: 1. Cataract left eye. 2. Aphakia right eye.

The operation history showed a preoperative diagnosis of cataract left eye, and the postoperative diagnosis was the same. The operation was an intracapsular cataract extraction—left eye. The description of the operation and operative findings was: under local retrobulbar lidocaine and hyaluronidase, the pre-placed fornix spaced conjunctival flap, using lid sutures, a keratome incision into the anterior chamber was enlarged 180 degrees after two 00000000 corneal scleral sutures were inserted. A superior peripheral iridectomy was performed. Air was inserted into the anterior chamber. Cataract extraction intracapsularily by combined traction and expression with an erysiphake. The wound was closed with a total of 8–0* corneal scleral sutures. Left eye only bandaged. Report signed by J.B. Smith, M.D.

18. Make up a one-paragraph Admission History for a patient who was admitted at 2:00 a.m. on February 11, 1977, with early labour. She went on with rather desultory labour until approximately 10:00 a.m. and then developed stronger labour with dilation to the rim.

The patient made no further progress: the breech did not come down, and in view of the breech presentation with no evidence of further progress, a caesarian section was scheduled. The patient's name is Mrs. John Brown; her address is 1 Cote de Neige, Montreal, P.Q.; age 22; ward 123; telephone number 491-7357; chart no. 1234. Signed by Dr. F.R. Leger.

19. This Operation History is for a Mr. William Bailey. The preoperative diagnosis was chronic ulcer over the medial malleolus, right leg. Postoperative diagnosis was the same. Operation note was: pinch skin graft to ulcer. The right leg was prepared and draped. Some hard-crusted material was removed from the ulcer bed over the medial malleolus of the right leg. The anterolateral aspect of the right thigh was used as the donor site for the pinch skin grafts. These were approximated on the ulcer bed. The donor and recipient sites were then dressed with scarlet red. An Elastoplast dressing was applied to the thigh, and a clean dressing was applied to the right ankle. The patient tolerated the procedure well and was taken back to his room. His operation date was March 22, 1978; room number 801S; surgeon Dr. H. Firth; anaesthetist Dr. M. Matheson; anaesthetic local; operation pinch graft to ulcer. Signed Dr. B.S. Borden.

---

*Both ways of writing this are correct.

THE GENERAL HOSPITAL

NAME: DATE:

ADDRESS: WARD OR ROOM:

ADMITTED: REFERRING PHYSICIAN:

DISCHARGED: ATTENDING PHYSICIAN:

ADMISSION HISTORY

CHIEF COMPLAINT:

GENERAL PHYSICAL EXAMINATION:

ABDOMEN:

EXTREMITIES:

CARDIOVASCULAR SYSTEM:

DIAGNOSIS:

OPERATIVE HISTORY

PREOPERATIVE DIAGNOSIS:

POSTOPERATIVE DIAGNOSIS:

OPERATION:

DESCRIPTION OF OPERATION AND FINDINGS:

Notes:

Appendix

College Hospital and Clinic: A Practice Exercise

BEHAVIORAL OBJECTIVES *The Assistant should be able to:*

1. Abstract from the Patient Record the important information for completing an insurance claim form.
2. Code professional services properly, using RVS or CPT code books.
3. Define abbreviations as they appear on a Patient Record.
4. Learn the proper information to be recorded on the patient's ledger card on submission of the insurance claim.
5. Learn how to complete a Patient Visit Slip for a computerized billing system.
6. Compose effective collection letters.
7. Prepare receipts for patients who pay cash.
8. Prepare an itemized statement for an estate claim and learn what the statutes are for her state.
9. Prepare legally correct medical-legal forms and letters.
10. Prepare pertinent data cards for insurance policies.
11. Complete the most commonly used insurance forms in medical and dental offices.

INSTRUCTIONS

To simulate a more realistic approach, assume that you have been hired as a medical insurance clerk and will be working for an incorporated group of medical doctors, other allied specialists, dentists, and podiatrists. You will be asked to complete various assignments. These doctors will be on the staff of a nearby hospital. On the following pages is the information you will need for reference in order to complete the insurance forms for each job. It would also be wise for you to purchase or obtain the appropriate Relative Value Studies or Current Procedural Terminology code book (see Chapter 2) used in your state so that you will be able to learn the proper codes that must be listed for each professional service rendered when submitting the insurance claim.

Patient Records, ledger cards, and blank insurance forms have been provided. In some instances it has been necessary to omit a lengthy physical examination from the patient record to give you pertinent and concise information. All dollars and cents figures used for doctor's fees on the ledger cards are given only as samples to provide you with experience in totaling up the charges and recording properly the appropriate information on the ledger when the insurance claim is submitted. Many times these fees may appear low. The names and addresses in the appendix are fictitious, and no reference is intended to any person living or dead. No medical advice is to be inferred from the patient records nor any recommendation as to alternative methods of treatment.

In order to learn how to abstract and read doctors' notes, refer to the abbreviation list on pages 501–505 to decode any abbreviations that you do not understand or that appear unfamiliar to you. To reinforce learning these abbreviations, write in their meanings on the Assignment pages. If possible, it is advisable to type all insurance forms, since this is the format in which the insurance carriers wish to receive them for processing. However, if you do not have access to a typewriter, neatly write in the information on the insurance form as you abstract from the Patient Record. Some of the records will be handwritten and some will be typed, to give you a chance at abstracting from both types of medical records. As each Patient Record is used for a particular insurance form, the doctor's signature will appear after the last entry that has been made on the record.

Insurance forms require that the physician's Internal Revenue Service number (IRS number)—sometimes also referred to as a Tax Identification number (Tax I.D. number) or Employer's Identification number (Employer's I.D. number)—be indicated on the claim. Some forms also require a State License number to be given, and in some instances a Provider number issued by an insurance company must also be listed. Refer to the instruction pages for the correct information regarding each doctor on the staff. Notice that some persons on the staff are not M.D.'s but have other degrees (e.g., D.D.S., R.P.T., and so forth). An IRS number or Tax I.D. number (example 95-3664021) is issued when a small business is established. If a group of doctors is practicing together at one location, one number is used by all physicians when reporting. If a private citizen were to establish a Keogh HR-10 Retirement Plan, then he or she would also be issued a Tax I.D. number for reporting purposes. Each doctor has a personal Social Security number and State License number.

If you do not have a background in medical terminology, it might be wise to use as a reference a good medical dictionary, such as *Dorland's Illustrated Medical Dictionary*, 25th edition (Philadelphia, W.B. Saunders Company, 1974). This is also available in a pocket-size edition.

You should begin these assignments after you have completed Chapters 1, 2, and 3. *REMEMBER*: Always read the assignment entirely before attempting to start the project. To complete each type of insurance form properly, refer to the chapter which describes in detail the correct information to be put in each blank or box.

REFERENCE MATERIAL

The dictionaries, texts, magazines, and booklets listed below may be helpful in completing insurance forms. Addresses for obtaining these materials are given in parentheses.

Dictionaries:

Dorland's Illustrated Medical Dictionary, 25th edition. W.B. Saunders Company, 1974. (West Washington Square, Philadelphia, PA 19105.)

Dorland's Pocket Medical Dictionary, 22nd edition. W.B. Saunders Company, 1977.

Texts and Booklets:

Analysis of Workers' Compensation Laws. The Chamber of Commerce of the United States, 1976. (1615 H Street, N.W., Washington, D.C. 20062.)

Current Medical Information and Terminology. American Medical Association, 1971. (535 North Dearborn Street, Chicago, IL 60610.)

Dictionary of Insurance, by Lewis E. Davids. Littlefield, Adams and Company 1974. (81 Adams Drive, Totowa, NJ 07512.)

Evaluation of Industrial Disability, by Packer Thurber, M.D. Oxford University Press, 1960. (1600 Pollitt Drive, Fair Lawn, NJ 07410.)

International Classification of Diseases, Adapted for Use in the United States. U.S. Department of Health, Education and Welfare, Public Health Service, National Center for Health Statistics. Vol. 1: tabular index; Vol. 2: alphabetical index. (Superintendent of Documents, U.S. Government Printing Office, Washington, D.C. 20402.)

Medical Hieroglyphs: Abbreviations and Symbols, by Avice H. Kerr, R.N., B.A. Starling Publications, 1970. (1340 N. Astor Street, Suite 1201, Chicago, IL 60610.)

Physician's Desk Reference (PDR) (for pharmaceutical drug names, descriptions, and so forth). Medical Economics Company, published annually. (P.O. Box 149, Westwood, NJ 07675.)

Simplified Medical Records System, by Burgess L. Gordon. M.D. Publishing Sciences Group, Inc., 1975. (411 Massachusetts Avenue, Acton, MA 01720.)

Source Book of Health Insurance Data 1974-75. Health Insurance Institute, 1975. (277 Park Avenue, New York, NY 10017.)

The Superbill — Guide to a Uniform Billing and/or Claims System, 1974. (Medical Group Management Assn., 4101 East Louisiana Avenue, Second Floor, Denver, CO 80222.)

Your Medicare Handbook. U.S. Department of Health, Education, and Welfare, Social Security Administration, 1976. (Superintendent of Documents, U.S. Government Printing Office, Washington, D.C. 20402.)

Magazines:

Medical Economics. Medical Economics Company. (P.O. Box 149, Westwood, NJ 07675.)

ASSIGNMENTS:

Chapter 3	1, 2, 3
Chapter 4	4, 5, 6, 7, 8
Chapter 5	9, 10
Chapter 6	11, 12, 13, 14, 15, 16
Chapter 7	17, 18, 19
Chapter 8	20, 21, 22, 23, 24
Chapter 9	25, 26, 27
Chapter 10	No assignments
Chapter 11	28, 29
Chapter 12	30, 31
Chapter 13	32, 33, 34
Chapter 14	35
Chapter 15	36
Chapter 16	See Review Questions 16–19 at the end of Chapter 16 (pp. 492–495)

The Patient Records presented in the *Insurance Handbook* include the following doctors' names, specialties, and subspecialties. They will be practicing at:

College Clinic
4567 Broad Avenue
Woodland Hills, XY 12345
tel: 013/486-9002

They are on the staff of:
College Hospital
4500 Broad Avenue
Woodland Hills, XY 12345
tel: 013/487-6789

Clinic IRS number or Tax Identification number: 95-3664021

COLLEGE CLINIC STAFF

Name	Specialty	Soc. Sec. #	State License #
Concha Antrum, M.D.	Otolaryngologist (OTO) or Ear, Nose and Throat Specialist (ENT)	082-19-1707	C 16021
Pedro Atrics, M.D.	Pediatrician (PD)	134-80-7600	D 60123
Bertha Caesar, M.D.	Obstetrician and Gynecologist (OBG)	230-80-6700	A 18174
Perry Cardi, M.D.	Internist (I) *Subspecialty:* Cardiovascular Disease (CD)	557-46-9980	C 21400
Brady Coccidioides, M.D.	Internist (I) *Subspecialty:* Pulmonary Disease (PUD)	670-54-0874	C 48211
Vera Cutis, M.D.	Dermatologist (D)	409-19-8620	C 60021
Clarence Cutler, M.D.	General Surgeon (GS)	410-23-5630	B 76005
Dennis Drill, D.D.S.	Dentist	240-47-8960	7061
Max Gluteus, R.P.T.	Physical Therapist (PT)	507-40-4300	8761

Cosmo Graff, M.D.	Plastic Surgeon (PS)	453-57-9899	C 81046
Malvern Grumose, M.D.	Pathologist (Path)	470-67-2301	A 16025
Gaston Input, M.D.	Internist (I)		
	Subspecialty: Gastroenterologist (GE)	211-09-6734	C 80016
Adam Langerhans, M.D.	Endocrinologist	447-90-6720	C 60511
Cornell Lenser, M.D.	Ophthalmologist (OPH)	322-75-8963	C 60466
Michael Menter, M.D.	Psychiatrist (P)	210-60-5302	C 71402
Arthur O. Dont, D.D.S.	Orthodontist	102-30-4566	8053
Astro Parkinson, M.D.	Neurosurgeon (NS)	210-42-8533	C 26002
Nick Pedro, D.P.M.	Podiatrist	233-08-4300	E 83400
Gerald Practon, M.D.	General Practitioner (GP) or		
	Family Practitioner (FP)	123-45-6789	C 14021
Walter Radon, M.D.	Radiologist (R)	344-09-6540	C 50013
Rex Rumsey, M.D.	Proctologist (Proct)	337-88-9743	C 30421
Sensitiv E. Scott, M.D.	Anesthetist (Anes)	220-45-5655	C 20411
Raymond Skelton, M.D.	Orthopedist (ORS) or (Orthop)	432-11-4589	C 45612
Gene Ulibarri, M.D.	Urologist (U)	990-70-3245	C 64303

ABBREVIATIONS AND SYMBOLS

Abbreviations and symbols may appear on patient records, prescriptions, hospital charts, and patient ledger cards. Abbreviation styles differ, but the current trend is to omit periods in capital letter abbreviations except for doctors' academic degrees. For information on official American Hospital Association policy see Chapter 1, page 10, under the paragraph on Medical and Diagnostic Terminology. The following is a list of the meanings of the abbreviations and symbols seen in this Appendix.

A	allergy	**approx**	approximate
Abdom	abdomen	**apt**	apartment
abt	about	**ASA**	acetylsalicylic acid (aspirin)
ac	before meals		
*Adj	adjustment	**ASCVD**	arteriosclerotic cardiovascular disease
adm	admit, admission, admitted		
		ASHD	arteriosclerotic heart disease
adv	advise		
aet	at the age of	**asst**	assistant
agit	shake or stir	**auto**	automobile
AgNO₃	silver nitrate		
		Ba	barium (enema)
ALL	allergy	***Bal fwd**	balance forward
am	ante meridian (time)	**BI**	biopsy
ant	anterior	**bid**	2 times daily
ante	before	**BMR**	basal metabolic rate
AP	anterior-posterior, anteroposterior	**BP**	blood pressure

*Bookkeeping abbreviations

Brev	sodium brevital	**E**	emergency
		EC	error corrected
C	cervical (vertebrae)	**ECG**	electrocardiogram, electrocardiograph
Ca, CA	cancer, carcinoma		
*c/a	cash on account	**EDC**	estimated date of confinement
cau	caucasian		
CBC	complete blood count	**EENT**	eye, ear, nose, and throat
cc	cubic centimeter	**EKG**	electrocardiogram, electrocardiograph
CC	chief complaint		
chr	chronic	**epith**	epithelial
*ck	check	**ER**	emergency room
cm	centimeter	**ESR**	erythrocyte sedimentation rate
CO	complains of		
comp, compl	complete, comprehensive	**est**	established (patient)
Con, CON, Cons	consultation	**Ex, exam**	examination
		exc	excision
Cont	continue	*Ex MO	express money order
CPX	complete physical examination	**ext**	external
*Cr	credit	**24F, 28F**	French (size of catheter)
C-Section	Cesarean section		
CVA	cardiovascular accident	**FH**	family history
Cysto	cystoscopy	**ft**	foot, feet
		FU	follow-up (examination)
D & C	dilatation and curettage		
dc	discontinue	**Fx**	fracture
DC	discharge		
*def	charge deferred	**gb, GB**	gallbladder
Del	delivery, OB	**GGE**	generalized glandular enlargement
Dg	diagnosis		
dia	diameter	**GI**	gastrointestinal
diag	diagnosis, diagnostic	**GU**	genitourinary
dil	dilate (stretch, expand)		
Disch	discharged	**H**	hospital call
DNA	does not apply	**HBP**	high blood pressure
DNS	did not show	**HC**	hospital call or consultation
DPM	Doctor of Podiatry Medicine		
		HCD	house call (day)
Dr	Doctor	**HCN**	house call (night)
*Dr	debit	**HCVD**	hypertensive cardio-vascular disease
Drs	dressing		
Dx	diagnosis	**Hgb**	hemoglobin
		hist	history

---

*Bookkeeping abbreviations

Hmct	hematocrit
hosp	hospital
H & P	history and physical
hr, hrs	hour, hours
hs	before bedtime
HS	hospital surgery
Ht	height
HV	hospital visit
HX	history
HX PX	history and physical examination
I	injection
IC	initial consultation
I & D	incision and drainage
*I/f	in full
IM	intramuscular (injection)
imp	impression (diagnosis)
inflam	inflammation
init	initial (office visit)
inj, INJ	injection
*ins, INS	insurance
int	internal
intermed	intermediate (office visit)
interpret	interpretation
IV	intravenous (injection)
IVP	intravenous pyelogram
K 35	Kolman (instrument used in urology)
KUB	kidneys, ureters, bladder
L	left; laboratory
Lab, LAB	laboratory
lat	lateral
LMP	last menstrual period
lt	left
ltd	limited (office visit)
L & W	living and well

M	medication; married
med	medicine
mg	milligram(s)
mm	millimeter(s)
mo	month(s)
*MO	money order
N	negative
NA	not applicable
NAD	no appreciable disease
*NC, N/C	no charge
neg	negative
NYD	not yet diagnosed
OB	obstetrical
OC	office call
occ	occasional
ofc	office
OP	outpatient
Op, op	operation
OR	operating room
orig	original
OS	office surgery; left eye
OV	office visit
PA	posterior-anterior, posteroanterior
Para I	woman having borne one child
PC	present complaint
pc	after meals
PD	permanent disability
PE	physical examination
perf	performed
PH	past history
Ph ex	physical examination
phys	physical
PID	pelvic inflammatory disease
pm	post meridian (time)
PND	postnasal drip
PO, P Op	postoperative

---

*Bookkeeping abbreviations

post	posterior	SLR	straight leg raising
postop	postoperative	slt	slight
pre-op	preoperative	Smr	smear
prep	prepared	SOB	shortness of breath
PRN	as necessary (pro re nata)	Sp Gr	specific gravity
Prog	prognosis	SQ	subcutaneous (injection)
P & S	permanent and stationary	STAT	immediately
Pt, pt	patient	surg	surgery
PT	physical therapy		
PTR	patient to return	T	temperature
PX	physical examination	T & A	tonsillectomy and adenoidectomy
		Tb, tb	tuberculosis
Q	every	TD	temporary disability
QD	one time daily, every day	temp	temperature
QH	every hour	tid	three times daily
qid	four times daily	TPR	temperature, pulse, and respiration
QNS	insufficient quantity	Tr, trt	treatment
QOD	every other day	TURB	transurethral resection of bladder
		TURP	transurethral resection of prostate
R	right; residence call; report	TX	treatment
RBC, rbc	red blood cell (count)		
rec	recommend	u	units
re ch	recheck	UA, ua	urinalysis
re-exam	re-examination	UCHD	usual childhood diseases
Reg	regular	UCR	usual, customary, and reasonable (fees)
ret, retn	return	UGI	upper gastrointestinal
rev	review	UPJ	ureteropelvic junction or joint
RHD	rheumatic heart disease	UR	urinalysis
R/O	rule out	URI	upper respiratory infection
*ROA	received on account	Urn	urinalysis
rt	right	UTI	urinary tract infection
RX, Rx, R_X	prescription, any medication or treatment ordered		
		W	work; white
S	surgery	WBC, wbc	white blood cell (count); well baby care
SD	state disability		
SE	special examination		
Sig	directions on prescription		

*Bookkeeping abbreviations

wk	week; work	$\bar{s}$, /s	without
wks	weeks	$\bar{c}c$, $\bar{c}/c$	with correction (eyeglasses)
WNL	within normal limits		
Wr	Wassermann (test for syphilis)	$\bar{s}c$, $\bar{s}/c$	without correction (eyeglasses)
Wt, wt	weight	–	negative
		$\bar{o}$	negative
X	xray, x-ray(s); times (e.g., 3X = 3 times)	Ⓛ	left
		Ⓡ	right
XR	xray, x-ray(s)	♂	male
		♀	female
yr	year	*⊥	charge already made
		*0	no balance due
Symbols		*√	posted
		*($0.00)	credit
$\bar{c}$, /c	with		

---

*Bookkeeping abbreviations

LEDGER CARD

Here is an example of how a ledger card should be completed. You will notice that there are abbreviations at the bottom of the ledger card which pertain to this particular type of practice. However, physicians have this section personalized to their particular practice so that these abbreviations can change from time to time. On pages 501–505 you will find a list of some common codes and symbols used in bookkeeping, as indicated by an asterisk (*).

STATEMENT

College Clinic
4567 Broad Avenue
Woodland Hills, XY 12345
013/486-9002

Mrs. I. M. Hurt
1300 Injury Street
Wound, XY 00345

DATE	PROFESSIONAL SERVICE	CHARGE		PAID		BALANCE	
4-6-77	OC intermed	35	--			35	--
	LAB, UA complete	5	--			40	--
5-10-77	IVP excretory	50	--			90	--
	Diagnostic cysto	45	--			90	--
5-14-77	Init HV, brief	20	--			155	--
5-15-77	Closure of vesicovaginal fistula	150	--			305	--
5-16-77	HV, brief	NC					
5-17-77	HV, brief	NC					
5-18-77	HV, brief	NC					
5-19-77	HV, brief	NC					
5-20-77	HV, brief	NC					
5-21-77	HV, brief	NC					
6-10-77	OC, brief	NC					
6-15-77	Billed Prudential Ins. Co. (4-6 thru 6-10)						
7-17-77	ROA Ins ck			305	--	-0-	

Pay last amount in this column

CON - CONSULTATION
CPX - COMPLETE PHYS EXAM
E - EMERGENCY
EC - ERROR CORRECTED
ECG - ELECTROCARDIOGRAM

HCD - HOUSE CALL (DAY)
HCN - HOUSE CALL (NIGHT)
HV - HOSPITAL VISIT
INJ - INJECTION
INS - INSURANCE

LAB - LABORATORY
NC - NO CHARGE
OC - OFFICE CALL
OS - OFFICE SURGERY
SE - SPECIAL EXAM

Chapter 3:
The Universal Health
Insurance Claim Form

ASSIGNMENT 1

1. Complete the *Universal Health Insurance Claim Form* to Prudential Insurance Company on Mrs. Merry M. Mclean by referring to her Patient Record and ledger card. Date the claim June 15. Dr. Ulibarri accepts assignment.

2. Use your Relative Value Studies or Current Procedural Terminology code book to ascertain the correct five-digit coding for each professional service rendered. Remember to include modifiers if necessary.

3. Record on ledger card when you have billed the insurance company.

Abbreviations pertinent to this record:

Adm _____	mo _____
CC _____	NC _____
Cont _____	OC _____
Cysto _____	Op _____
Disch _____	PC _____
Dx _____	PTR _____
hosp _____	retn _____
HV _____	Sp Gr _____
intermed _____	UA _____
init _____	wk _____
IVP _____	$\bar{c}$ _____

ASSIGNMENT 2

1. Complete the *Universal Health Insurance Claim Form* to Aetna Life and Casualty Company on Mr. Billy S. Rubin by referring to his Patient Record and ledger card. Date the claim August 30. Dr. Ulibarri accepts assignment.

2. Use your Relative Value Studies or Current Procedural Terminology code book to ascertain the correct five-digit coding and modifiers for each professional service rendered.

3. Record when you have billed the insurance company on the ledger card.

Abbreviations pertinent to this record:

Adm _____	mo _____
CA _____	NC _____
CC _____	OC _____
Comp _____	PE _____
Disch _____	phys _____

PATIENT RECORD

Mclean,	Merry	M.	2-2-28	F	013/486-1859
LAST NAME	FIRST NAME	MIDDLE NAME	BIRTH DATE	SEX	HOME PHONE

4919 Dolphin Way,	Woodland Hills,	XY	12345
ADDRESS	CITY	STATE	ZIP CODE

secretary	Porter Company
PATIENT'S OCCUPATION	NAME OF COMPANY

5490 Wilshire Blvd., Merck, XY 12346	013/466-7781
ADDRESS OF EMPLOYER	PHONE

Harry L. Mclean (insured)	computer programmer
SPOUSE OR PARENT	OCCUPATION

IBM Corp. 5616 Wilshire Blvd., Merck, XY 12346	013/664-9023
EMPLOYER	ADDRESS	PHONE

Prudential Ins. Co. 5621 Wilshire Blvd., Merck, XY 12346
NAME OF INSURANCE GROUP

Policy # 8832			6-2-75
BLUE SHIELD OR BLUE CROSS CERT. NO.	GROUP NO.	CURRENT COVERAGE NO.	EFFECTIVE DATE
			459-62-9989
MEDICARE NO.	MEDICAID NO.	EFFECTIVE DATE	SOC. SEC. NO.

REFERRED BY:
Emdee Fine, M. D. 5000 Wilshire Blvd., Merck, XY 12346

DATE	PROGRESS
5-6-77	CC BEGAN ABOUT JUNE 1976. CONSTANT DRIBBLING, WETTING AT NIGHT, USE 15 PADS/DAY. UA SP GR 1.0, FEW BACTERIA, FEW URATES. DX URINARY INCONTINENCE. PTR 4 DAYS FOR DIAGNOSTIC TESTS. G. Uchimi M.D.
5-10-77	IVP 7 CYSTO REVEALED MULTIPLE FISTULA OF BLADDER c̄ 2 OPENINGS INTO URINARY BLADDER AND COPIOUS LEAKAGE INTO VAGINA. CONT TO WORK. G. Uchimi M.D.
5-14-77	ADM TO HOSP. DX: MULTIPLE VESICOVAGINAL FISTULA G. U. M.D.
5-15-77	OP: REPAIR OF VESICOVAGINAL FISTULAE G. U. M.D.
5-16-77	THRU 5-31-77 HV BRIEF DISCH 5-31 TO BE SEEN IN 1 MO G. U. M.D.
6-10-77	RECOVERING RAPIDLY. NO PAIN. NO PC. MAY RETN TO WK 6-20-77 Gene Uchimi M.D.

STATEMENT

College Clinic
4567 Broad Avenue
Woodland Hills, XY 12345
013/486-9002

Mrs. Merry M. Mclean
4919 Dolphin Way
Woodland Hills, XY 12345

DATE	PROFESSIONAL SERVICE	CHARGE		PAID		BALANCE
5-6-77	OC, intermed	35	00			
	LAB, UA complete	5	00			
5-10-77	IVP, excretory	50	00			
	Diagnostic cysto	45	00			
5-14-77	Init Hosp care, brief	20	00			
5-15-77	Closure of vesicovaginal fistulae	150	00			
5-16-77	thru 5-31-77 HV, brief	NC				
6-10-77	OC, brief	NC				

Pay last amount in this column

CON - CONSULTATION	HCD - HOUSE CALL (DAY)	LAB - LABORATORY
CPX - COMPLETE PHYS EXAM	HCN - HOUSE CALL (NIGHT)	NC - NO CHARGE
E - EMERGENCY	HV - HOSPITAL VISIT	OC - OFFICE CALL
EC - ERROR CORRECTED	INJ - INJECTION	OS - OFFICE SURGERY
ECG - ELECTROCARDIOGRAM	INS - INSURANCE	SE - SPECIAL EXAM

HEALTH INSURANCE
CLAIM FORM

READ INSTRUCTIONS BEFORE COMPLETING OR SIGNING THIS FORM

TYPE OR PRINT ☐ MEDICARE ☐ MEDICAID ☐ CHAMPUS ☐ OTHER

PATIENT & INSURED (SUBSCRIBER) INFORMATION

1. PATIENT'S NAME *(First name, middle initial, last name)*	2. PATIENT'S DATE OF BIRTH	3. INSURED'S NAME *(First name, middle initial, last name)*
4. PATIENT'S ADDRESS *(Street, city, state, ZIP code)*	5. PATIENT'S SEX MALE FEMALE	6. INSURED'S I.D. No. or **MEDICARE No.** *(Include any letters)*
	7. PATIENT'S RELATIONSHIP TO INSURED SELF SPOUSE CHILD OTHER	8. INSURED'S GROUP NO. *(Or Group Name)*
9. OTHER HEALTH INSURANCE COVERAGE - Enter Name of Policyholder and Plan Name and Address and Policy or Medical Assistance Number	10. WAS CONDITION RELATED TO: A. PATIENT'S EMPLOYMENT YES NO B. AN AUTO ACCIDENT YES NO	11. INSURED'S ADDRESS *(Street, city, state, ZIP code)*
12. PATIENT'S OR AUTHORIZED PERSON'S SIGNATURE *(Read back before signing)* I Authorize the Release of any Medical Information Necessary to Process this Claim and Request Payment of MEDICARE/CHAMPUS Benefits Either to Myself or to the Party Who Accepts Assignment Below SIGNED _____ DATE _____		13. I AUTHORIZE PAYMENT OF MEDICAL BENEFITS TO UNDERSIGNED PHYSICIAN OR SUPPLIER FOR SERVICE DESCRIBED BELOW SIGNED *(Insured or Authorized Person)*

PHYSICIAN OR SUPPLIER INFORMATION

14. DATE OF: ◄ ILLNESS (FIRST SYMPTOM) OR INJURY (ACCIDENT) OR PREGNANCY (LMP)	15. DATE FIRST CONSULTED YOU FOR THIS CONDITION	16. HAS PATIENT EVER HAD SAME OR SIMILAR SYMPTOMS? YES NO
17. DATE PATIENT ABLE TO RETURN TO WORK	18. DATES OF TOTAL DISABILITY FROM THROUGH	DATES OF PARTIAL DISABILITY FROM THROUGH
19. NAME OF REFERRING PHYSICIAN		20. FOR SERVICES RELATED TO HOSPITALIZATION GIVE HOSPITALIZATION DATES ADMITTED DISCHARGED
21. NAME & ADDRESS OF FACILITY WHERE SERVICES RENDERED *(If other than home or office)*		22. WAS LABORATORY WORK PERFORMED OUTSIDE YOUR OFFICE? YES NO CHARGES

23. DIAGNOSIS OR NATURE OF ILLNESS OR INJURY. RELATE DIAGNOSIS TO PROCEDURE IN COLUMN D BY REFERENCE TO NUMBERS 1, 2, 3, ETC. OR DX CODE

1.
2.
3.
4.

24. A DATE OF SERVICE	B * PLACE OF SERV-ICE	C FULLY DESCRIBE PROCEDURES, MEDICAL SERVICES OR SUPPLIES FURNISHED FOR EACH DATE GIVEN PROCEDURE CODE (IDENTIFY:) *(EXPLAIN UNUSUAL SERVICES OR CIRCUMSTANCES)*	D DIAGNOSIS CODE	E CHARGES	F

SAMPLE

25. SIGNATURE OF PHYSICIAN OR SUPPLIER *(Read back before signing)*	26. ACCEPT ASSIGNMENT (GOVERNMENT CLAIMS ONLY) (SEE BACK) YES NO	27. TOTAL CHARGE	28. AMOUNT PAID 29 BALANCE DUE
SIGNED _____ DATE _____	30. YOUR SOCIAL SECURITY NO.	31. PHYSICIAN'S OR SUPPLIER'S NAME, ADDRESS, ZIP CODE & TELEPHONE NO
32. YOUR PATIENT'S ACCOUNT NO.	33. YOUR EMPLOYER I.D. NO.	I.D. NO.

* PLACE OF SERVICE CODES

1 — (IH) — INPATIENT HOSPITAL	4 — (H) — PATIENT'S HOME	7 — (NH) — NURSING HOME	O — (OL) — OTHER LOCATIONS
2 — (OH) — OUTPATIENT HOSPITAL	5 — DAY CARE FACILITY (PSY)	8 — (SNF) — SKILLED NURSING FACILITY	A — (IL) — INDEPENDENT LABORATORY
3 — (O) — DOCTOR'S OFFICE	6 — NIGHT CARE FACILITY (PSY)	9 — AMBULANCE	B — OTHER MEDICAL/SURGICAL FACILITY

APPROVED BY AMA COUNCIL ON MEDICAL SERVICE 8-74

est _____ Pt _____

exam _____ Retn _____

hist _____ surg _____

hosp _____ TURP _____

HV _____ wk _____

hx _____ wks _____

PATIENT RECORD

Rubin,	Billy	S.	11-9-33	M	013/893-5770
LAST NAME	FIRST NAME	MIDDLE NAME	BIRTH DATE	SEX	HOME PHONE

547 North Oliver Road, Woodland Hills, XY 12345
ADDRESS　　　CITY　　　STATE　　　ZIP CODE

salesman　　　　　　　　Nate's Clothiers
PATIENT'S OCCUPATION　　　NAME OF COMPANY

7786 East Chabner Blvd., Dorland, XY 12347　　　013/349-6605
ADDRESS OF EMPLOYER　　　PHONE

Lydia B. Rubin (wife)　　　homemaker
SPOUSE OR PARENT　　　OCCUPATION

EMPLOYER　　　ADDRESS　　　PHONE

Aetna Life and Casualty Ins. Co. 3055 Wilshire Blvd., Merck, XY 12346
NAME OF INSURANCE GROUP

Subscriber: Billy S. Rubin　　2641　　　　3-5-74
BLUE SHIELD OR BLUE CROSS CERT. NO.　GROUP NO.　CURRENT COVERAGE NO.　EFFECTIVE DATE

505-12-1159

MEDICARE NO.　MEDICAID NO.　EFFECTIVE DATE　SOC. SEC. NO.

REFERRED BY:
U. R. Wright, M. D.　5010 Wrong Road, Torres, XY 12349　　013/907-5440

DATE	PROGRESS
8-7-77	Office exam est pt CC: urinary hesitancy, frequency & post-urinary dribbling since July 15 of this year. Exam revealed hard nodule in testes. Silverman needle biopsy of prostate performed in office. *Gene Ullbani M.D.*
8-10-77	Office exam. Biopsy report positive for Ca of prostate Pt retn in 4 days. *Gene Ullbani M.D.*
8-14-77	OC: explained surgery to pt. Arranged for adm to hosp. *G.U.M.D.*
8-22-77	Adm to hosp. Pt last worked 8-21-77 *Gene Ullbani M.D.*
8-23-77	Surg: TURP, bilateral orchiectomy (scrotal) Est disability 6 wks Pt to be kept under observation for 2 mo & will retn to wk 12-3-77 *Gene Ullbani M.D.*
8-28-77	Disch from hosp. Confined at home for 1 wk. at which time patient will be seen in office. *Gene Ullbani M.D.*

STATEMENT

College Clinic
4567 Broad Avenue
Woodland Hills, XY 12345
013/486-9002

Mr. Billy S. Rubin
547 North Oliver Road
Woodland Hills, XY 12345

DATE	PROFESSIONAL SERVICE	CHARGE		PAID	BALANCE
8-8-77	OC, brief	10	00		
	Biopsy, prostate	15	00		
8-10-77	OC, brief	10	00		
8-14-77	OC, brief	10	00		
8-22-77	Adm hosp, comp hx & PE	25	00		
8-23-77	TURP	200	00		
	Bilateral orchiectomy (scrotal)	100	00		
8-24 thru 8-28-77	HV, brief	NC			

Pay last amount in this column ⬆

CON - CONSULTATION
CPX - COMPLETE PHYS EXAM
E - EMERGENCY
EC - ERROR CORRECTED
ECG - ELECTROCARDIOGRAM

HCD - HOUSE CALL (DAY)
HCN - HOUSE CALL (NIGHT)
HV - HOSPITAL VISIT
INJ - INJECTION
INS - INSURANCE

LAB - LABORATORY
NC - NO CHARGE
OC - OFFICE CALL
OS - OFFICE SURGERY
SE - SPECIAL EXAM

HEALTH INSURANCE
CLAIM FORM

READ INSTRUCTIONS BEFORE COMPLETING OR SIGNING THIS FORM

TYPE OR PRINT ☐ MEDICARE ☐ MEDICAID ☐ CHAMPUS ☐ OTHER

PATIENT & INSURED (SUBSCRIBER) INFORMATION

1. PATIENT'S NAME *(First name, middle initial, last name)*	2. PATIENT'S DATE OF BIRTH	3. INSURED'S NAME *(First name, middle initial, last name)*
4. PATIENT'S ADDRESS *(Street, city, state, ZIP code)*	5. PATIENT'S SEX MALE FEMALE	6. INSURED'S I.D. No. or **MEDICARE No.** *(Include any letters)*
	7. PATIENT'S RELATIONSHIP TO INSURED SELF SPOUSE CHILD OTHER	8. INSURED'S GROUP NO. *(Or Group Name)*
9. OTHER HEALTH INSURANCE COVERAGE - Enter Name of Policyholder and Plan Name and Address and Policy or Medical Assistance Number	10. WAS CONDITION RELATED TO: A. PATIENT'S EMPLOYMENT YES NO B. AN AUTO ACCIDENT YES NO	11. INSURED'S ADDRESS *(Street, city, state, ZIP code)*
12. PATIENT'S OR AUTHORIZED PERSON'S SIGNATURE *(Read back before signing)* *I Authorize the Release of any Medical Information Necessary to Process this Claim and Request Payment of MEDICARE/CHAMPUS Benefits Either to Myself or to the Party Who Accepts Assignment Below* SIGNED DATE		13. *I AUTHORIZE PAYMENT OF MEDICAL BENEFITS TO UNDERSIGNED PHYSICIAN OR SUPPLIER FOR SERVICE DESCRIBED BELOW* SIGNED *(Insured or Authorized Person)*

PHYSICIAN OR SUPPLIER INFORMATION

14. DATE OF: ► ILLNESS (FIRST SYMPTOM) OR INJURY (ACCIDENT) OR PREGNANCY (LMP)	15. DATE FIRST CONSULTED YOU FOR THIS CONDITION	16. HAS PATIENT EVER HAD SAME OR SIMILAR SYMPTOMS? YES NO
17. DATE PATIENT ABLE TO RETURN TO WORK	18. DATES OF TOTAL DISABILITY FROM THROUGH	DATES OF PARTIAL DISABILITY FROM THROUGH
19. NAME OF REFERRING PHYSICIAN		20. FOR SERVICES RELATED TO HOSPITALIZATION GIVE HOSPITALIZATION DATES ADMITTED DISCHARGED
21. NAME & ADDRESS OF FACILITY WHERE SERVICES RENDERED *(If other than home or office)*		22. WAS LABORATORY WORK PERFORMED OUTSIDE YOUR OFFICE? YES NO CHARGES:

23. DIAGNOSIS OR NATURE OF ILLNESS OR INJURY. RELATE DIAGNOSIS TO PROCEDURE IN COLUMN D BY REFERENCE TO NUMBERS 1, 2, 3, ETC. OR DX CODE

1.
2.
3.
4.

24. A DATE OF SERVICE	B * PLACE OF SERV-ICE	C PROCEDURE CODE (IDENTIFY:) FULLY DESCRIBE PROCEDURES, MEDICAL SERVICES OR SUPPLIES FURNISHED FOR EACH DATE GIVEN *(EXPLAIN UNUSUAL SERVICES OR CIRCUMSTANCES)*	D DIAGNOSIS CODE	E CHARGES	F

SAMPLE

25. SIGNATURE OF PHYSICIAN OR SUPPLIER *(Read back before signing)*	26. ACCEPT ASSIGNMENT (GOVERNMENT CLAIMS ONLY) (SEE BACK) YES NO	27. TOTAL CHARGE	28. AMOUNT PAID 29. BALANCE DUE
SIGNED DATE	30. YOUR SOCIAL SECURITY NO.	31. PHYSICIAN'S OR SUPPLIER'S NAME, ADDRESS, ZIP CODE & TELEPHONE NO	
32. YOUR PATIENT'S ACCOUNT NO.	33. YOUR EMPLOYER I.D. NO.		
		I.D. NO.	

* PLACE OF SERVICE CODES

1 — (IH) — INPATIENT HOSPITAL	4 — (H) — PATIENT'S HOME	7 — (NH) — NURSING HOME	O — (OL) — OTHER LOCATIONS
2 — (OH) — OUTPATIENT HOSPITAL	5 — DAY CARE FACILITY (PSY)	8 — (SNF) — SKILLED NURSING FACILITY	A — (IL) — INDEPENDENT LABORATORY
3 — (O) — DOCTOR'S OFFICE	6 — NIGHT CARE FACILITY (PSY)	9 — AMBULANCE	B — OTHER MEDICAL/SURGICAL FACILITY

APPROVED BY AMA COUNCIL ON MEDICAL SERVICE 6-74

ASSIGNMENT 3

1. Complete the *Attending Physician's Statement* to Travelers Insurance Company on Mr. Walter J. Stone by referring to his Patient Record and ledger card. Date the claim June 1. Dr. Input charges $5 for providing information in addition to that required on this form. The doctor is not accepting assignment.

2. Use your Relative Value Studies or Current Procedural Terminology code book to ascertain the correct five-digit coding and modifiers for each professional service rendered. The surgeon, Dr. Cutler, is charging $150 for the cholecystectomy. You are submitting a claim for the assistant surgeon, Dr. Input.

3. Record on ledger card when you have billed the insurance company.

Abbreviations pertinent to this record:

abt _____	hosp _____
adm _____	inflam _____
asst _____	intermed _____
BP _____	OC _____
E _____	ofc _____
ER _____	pt _____
Dx _____	wk _____
Est _____	$\bar{c}$ _____
GB _____	

PATIENT RECORD

Stone,	Walter	J.	3-14-29	M	013/345-0776
LAST NAME	FIRST NAME	MIDDLE NAME	BIRTH DATE	SEX	HOME PHONE

2008 Converse Street,	Woodland Hills,	XY	12345
ADDRESS	CITY	STATE	ZIP CODE

advertising agent	R. V. Black and Associates
PATIENT'S OCCUPATION	NAME OF COMPANY

1267 Broad Street, Woodland Hills, XY 12345	013/345-6012
ADDRESS OF EMPLOYER	PHONE

widow	
SPOUSE OR PARENT	OCCUPATION

EMPLOYER	ADDRESS	PHONE

Travelers Ins. Co. 5460 Olympic Blvd., Woodland Hills, XY 12345

NAME OF INSURANCE GROUP	SUBSCRIBER

Subscriber: Walter J. Bloom Policy # 6754	6-1-75
BLUE SHIELD OR BLUE CROSS CERT. NO. GROUP NO. CURRENT COVERAGE NO.	EFFECTIVE DATE
	456-65-9989

MEDICARE NO.	MEDICAID NO.	EFFECTIVE DATE	SOC. SEC. NO.

REFERRED BY:

brother: John B. Stone   (former patient of Dr. Input)

DATE	PROGRESS
5-3-77	Sun 2AM lst pt had sudden onset of profuse rectal bleeding c̄ nausea & severe abdominal pains; called from home to ER. Consulted c̄ Dr Cutler who recommended pt be admitted for further evaluation & diagnostic treatment. Disabled from wk. BP 130/90 Gaston Input MD
5-4-77	GB series showed prepyloric gastric ulcer, inflam of gb & gallstones present Gaston Input MD
5-5-77	Discharged to home. To be seen in ofc in 1 wk G Input MD
5-18-77	BP 180/100 Return in 2 days G Input MD
5-21-77	BP 180/90 adv to see Dr Cutler for further evaluation & possible surgery Dx: prepyloric gastric ulcer, hypertension, cholecystitis c̄ cholelithiasis. G Input MD
5-26-77	Adm to hosp G Input MD
5-27-77	Cholecystectomy. acted as asst surgeon to Dr Cutler. Pt will resume wk abt 6-22-77 Gaston Input, MD

STATEMENT

College Clinic
4567 Broad Avenue
Woodland Hills, XY 12345
013/486-9002

Mr. Walter J. Stone
2008 Converse Street
Woodland Hills, XY 12345

DATE	PROFESSIONAL SERVICE	CHARGE		PAID		BALANCE	
5-3-77	E service, intermed. exam	50	00				
5-4-77	HV, brief	10	00				
5-5-77	HV, brief	10	00				
5-18-77	OC, intermed exam	15	00				
5-21-77	OC, brief	8	00				
5-27-77	Cholecystectomy	30	00				

Pay last amount in this column

CON - CONSULTATION	HCD - HOUSE CALL (DAY)	LAB - LABORATORY
CPX - COMPLETE PHYS EXAM	HCN - HOUSE CALL (NIGHT)	NC - NO CHARGE
E - EMERGENCY	HV - HOSPITAL VISIT	OC - OFFICE CALL
EC - ERROR CORRECTED	INJ - INJECTION	OS - OFFICE SURGERY
ECG - ELECTROCARDIOGRAM	INS - INSURANCE	SE - SPECIAL EXAM

ATTENDING PHYSICIAN'S STATEMENT

To: _____ Insurance Company

Name of Insured: _____

Address: _____

Name of Patient _____ Relationship to Insured: _____

The following professional services were provided the above named patient as itemized, and on the dates listed below,

for the diagnosis of: _____

Disability related to: ☐ Personal Illness   ☐ Personal Accident   ☐ Occupation   ☐ Pregnancy

Period of Disability: From _____ To _____

DATE	RVS	SERVICE RENDERED	CHARGE
_____	_____	_____	_____
_____	_____	_____	_____
_____	_____	_____	_____
_____	_____	_____	_____
_____	_____	_____	_____
_____	_____	_____	_____
_____	_____	_____	_____
_____	_____	_____	_____
_____	_____	_____	_____
_____	_____	_____	_____
_____	_____	_____	_____
_____	_____	_____	_____
_____	_____	_____	_____

ASSIGNMENT TAKEN _____
MAKE CHECKS PAYABLE TO

> STATE LAW AB 1236 MAKES IT MANDATORY RATHER
> THAN PERMISSIVE THAT INSURANCE COMPANIES
> HONOR ASSIGNMENT OF BENEFITS.

_____ Receipt of $_____ will be required prior to providing additional information
DOCTOR'S SIGNATURE

_____
DOCTOR'S TYPED NAME   LIC. NO.   ADDRESS   TELEPHONE

I HEREBY AUTHORIZE THE DOCTOR(S) WHOSE NAME(S) APPEARS BELOW TO FURNISH THE ABOVE INSURANCE COMPANY ALL INFORMATION WHICH SAID INSURANCE COMPANY MAY REQUEST CONCERNING MY PRESENT ILLNESS OR INJURY. I HEREBY ASSIGN TO THE DOCTOR(S) WHOSE NAME(S) APPEARS BELOW ALL MONEY TO WHICH I AM ENTITLED FOR MEDICAL AND/OR SURGICAL EXPENSE RELATIVE TO THE SERVICE REPORTED BELOW, BUT NOT TO EXCEED MY INDEBTEDNESS TO SAID PHYSICIAN AND SURGEON. IT IS UNDERSTOOD THAT ANY MONEY RECEIVED FROM THE ABOVE NAMED INSURANCE COMPANY, OVER AND ABOVE MY INDEBTEDNESS WILL BE REFUNDED TO ME WHEN MY BILL IS PAID IN FULL. I UNDERSTAND I AM FINANCIALLY RESPONSIBLE TO SAID DOCTOR(S) FOR CHARGES NOT COVERED BY THIS ASSIGNMENT.

NOTE: California law required that Insurance Code Section 556 appear on this claim form.
IT IS UNLAWFUL TO: (a) Present or cause to be presented any false or fraudulent claim for the payment of a loss under a contract of insurance.
(b) Prepare, make, or subscribe any writing, with intent to present or use the same, or allow it to be presented or used in support of any such claim.
Every person who violates any provision of this section is punishable by imprisonment in the State Prison not exceeding three years, or by fine not exceeding one thousand dollars, or by both.

X _____
INSURED OR GUARDIAN SIGNATURE   PATIENT'S SIGNATURE   DATE

Chapter 4:
Blue Cross and Blue Shield

Assignments 4, 5, and 6 have been written for those students in California who will submit claims to Blue Cross. Assignments 7 and 8 have been written for those students in other states who will submit claims to Blue Shield.

ASSIGNMENT 4

1. Complete the *Universal Health Insurance Claim Form** to Blue Cross for Mr. David M. Cash by referring to his Patient Record and ledger card. Date the claim February 27. You have had Mr. Cash sign the release of information portion of the form as well as the assignment of benefits.

2. Use your Relative Value Studies or Current Procedural Terminology code book to ascertain the correct five-digit coding and modifiers for each professional service rendered. Many Blue Cross of Southern California contracts do not pay for the first two office visits but begin payment on the third visit. In such a case, the patient would have to pay for the first two visits. However, on the insurance claim show all visits pertinent to the case.

3. Record on ledger card when you have billed the insurance company.

Abbreviations pertinent to this record:

adv _____	prn _____
dia _____	PT _____
exc _____	retn _____
imp _____	slt _____
N _____	Tr _____
neg _____	wk _____
OC _____	c̄ _____

ASSIGNMENT 5

1. Complete the *Universal Health Insurance Claim Form** to Blue Cross for Mrs. Frances F. Foote by referring to her Patient Record and ledger card. Date the claim October 31. You have had Mrs. Foote sign the release of information portion of the form but no assignment has been taken on this claim.

2. Use your Relative Value Studies or Current Procedural Terminology code book to ascertain the correct five-digit coding and modifiers for each professional service rendered.

3. Record on ledger card when you have billed insurance company.

*See page 331 for help in completing this form.

PATIENT RECORD

Cash,	David	M.	03-15-30	M	013/666-8901
LAST NAME	FIRST NAME	MIDDLE NAME	BIRTH DATE	SEX	HOME PHONE

5729 Redwood Avenue,	Woodland Hills, XY		12345
ADDRESS	CITY	STATE	ZIP CODE

teacher	City Unified School District
PATIENT'S OCCUPATION	NAME OF COMPANY

301 West Third Street,	Dorland, XY 12347	013/667-9018
ADDRESS OF EMPLOYER		PHONE

unmarried	
SPOUSE OR PARENT	OCCUPATION

Century High School, 2031 W. Olympic Blvd., Dorland, XY 12347	013/678-0176
EMPLOYER ADDRESS	PHONE

Blue Cross	Union Local #2	David M. Cash
NAME OF INSURANCE GROUP		SUBSCRIBER

298-34-6754	82099A	2716	1-9-74
BLUE CROSS CERT. NO.	GROUP NO.	CURRENT COVERAGE NO.	EFFECTIVE DATE

			298-34-6754
MEDICARE NO.	MEDICAID NO.	EFFECTIVE DATE	SOC. SEC. NO.

Hugh R. Foot, M. D. 2010 Main Street, Woodland Hills, XY 12345

REFERRED BY:

DATE	PROGRESS
1-4-77	Pt comes in complaining of slt pain in parietal area of skull. Exam N. Some slt redness on parietal area of scalp. Retn in 1 wk for observation. Imp: undetermined. No disability from work. CC
1-11-77	Some slt elevation of skin in parietal area of scalp. Otherwise essentially neg. No warmth over area. Slt pain on pressure. CC
2-3-77	Elevation of skin still persisting. Imp: inflammatory cystic lesion of scalp 1.5 cm. Tr: excision of inflammatory cystic lesion of skin 1.5 cm dia on parietal scalp area. Removed cyst under procaine block; knife dissection; closure of wound c̄ six #000 black silk sutures. Adv to retn in 5 days for removal of sutures. *Clarence Cutler, MD*
2-9-77	Sutures removed & dressed. To retn in 1 wk. *C Cutler, MD*
2-15-77	Parietal area well healed. Retn prn. *C. Cutler, MD.*

STATEMENT

College Clinic
4567 Broad Avenue
Woodland Hills, XY 12345
013/486-9002

Mr. David M. Cash
5729 Redwood Avenue
Woodland Hills, XY 12345

DATE	PROFESSIONAL SERVICE	CHARGE		PAID	BALANCE
1-4-77	OC, ltd	15	00		
1-11-77	OC, brief	10	00		
2-3-77	OC, ltd	15	00		
	Exc inflammatory cystic lesion scalp 1.5 cm dia	20	00		
2-9-77	OC, brief	NC			
2-15-77	OC, brief	NC			

Pay last amount in this column ⬆

CON - CONSULTATION	HCD - HOUSE CALL (DAY)	LAB - LABORATORY
CPX - COMPLETE PHYS EXAM	HCN - HOUSE CALL (NIGHT)	NC - NO CHARGE
E - EMERGENCY	HV - HOSPITAL VISIT	OC - OFFICE CALL
EC - ERROR CORRECTED	INJ - INJECTION	OS - OFFICE SURGERY
ECG - ELECTROCARDIOGRAM	INS - INSURANCE	SE - SPECIAL EXAM

1547

HEALTH INSURANCE
CLAIM FORM

Blue Cross of Southern California

READ INSTRUCTIONS BEFORE COMPLETING OR SIGNING THIS FORM

TYPE OR PRINT ☐ MEDICARE ☐ MEDICAID ☐ CHAMPUS ☐ OTHER

Box 60465, Terminal Annex
Los Angeles, California 90060

PATIENT & INSURED (SUBSCRIBER) INFORMATION

1. PATIENT'S NAME *(First name, middle initial, last name)*	2. PATIENT'S DATE OF BIRTH	3. INSURED'S NAME *(First name, middle initial, last name)*

4. PATIENT'S ADDRESS *(Street, city, state, ZIP code)*

5. PATIENT'S SEX
MALE ☐ FEMALE

6. INSURED'S I.D. No. or **MEDICARE No.** *(include any letters)*

7. PATIENT'S RELATIONSHIP TO INSURED
SELF SPOUSE CHILD OTHER

8. INSURED'S GROUP NO. *(Or Group Name)*

9. OTHER HEALTH INSURANCE COVERAGE - Enter Name of Policyholder and Plan Name and Address and Policy or Medical Assistance Number

10. WAS CONDITION RELATED TO:
A. PATIENT'S EMPLOYMENT
YES ☐ NO
B. AN AUTO ACCIDENT
YES ☐ NO

11. INSURED'S ADDRESS *(Street, city, state, ZIP code)*

12. PATIENT'S OR AUTHORIZED PERSON'S SIGNATURE *(Read back before signing)*
I Authorize the Release of any Medical Information Necessary to Process this Claim and Request Payment of MEDICARE/CHAMPUS Benefits Either to Myself or to the Party Who Accepts Assignment Below

SIGNED   DATE

13. I AUTHORIZE PAYMENT OF MEDICAL BENEFITS TO UNDERSIGNED PHYSICIAN OR SUPPLIER FOR SERVICE DESCRIBED BELOW

SIGNED *(Insured or Authorized Person)*

PHYSICIAN OR SUPPLIER INFORMATION

14. DATE OF: ILLNESS (FIRST SYMPTOM) OR INJURY (ACCIDENT) OR PREGNANCY (LMP)

15. DATE FIRST CONSULTED YOU FOR THIS CONDITION

16. HAS PATIENT EVER HAD SAME OR SIMILAR SYMPTOMS?
YES ☐ NO

17. DATE PATIENT ABLE TO RETURN TO WORK

18. DATES OF TOTAL DISABILITY
FROM   THROUGH

DATES OF PARTIAL DISABILITY
FROM   THROUGH

19. NAME OF REFERRING PHYSICIAN

20. FOR SERVICES RELATED TO HOSPITALIZATION GIVE HOSPITALIZATION DATES
ADMITTED   DISCHARGED

21. NAME & ADDRESS OF FACILITY WHERE SERVICES RENDERED *(If other than home or office)*

22. WAS LABORATORY WORK PERFORMED OUTSIDE YOUR OFFICE?
YES ☐ NO   CHARGES:

23. DIAGNOSIS OR NATURE OF ILLNESS OR INJURY, RELATE DIAGNOSIS TO PROCEDURE IN COLUMN D BY REFERENCE TO NUMBERS 1, 2, 3, ETC. OR DX CODE

1.
2.
3.
4.

24. A DATE OF SERVICE	B* PLACE OF SERV-ICE	C FULLY DESCRIBE PROCEDURES, MEDICAL SERVICES OR SUPPLIES FURNISHED FOR EACH DATE GIVEN PROCEDURE CODE (IDENTIFY:) *(EXPLAIN UNUSUAL SERVICES OR CIRCUMSTANCES)*	D DIAGNOSIS CODE	E CHARGES	F

SAMPLE

25. SIGNATURE OF PHYSICIAN OR SUPPLIER *(Read back before signing)*

SIGNED   DATE

26. ACCEPT ASSIGNMENT *(GOVERNMENT CLAIMS ONLY) (SEE BACK)*
YES ☐ NO

30. YOUR SOCIAL SECURITY NO.

27. TOTAL CHARGE | 28. AMOUNT PAID | 29. BALANCE DUE

31. PHYSICIAN'S OR SUPPLIER'S NAME, ADDRESS, ZIP CODE & TELEPHONE NO.

32. YOUR PATIENT'S ACCOUNT NO.

33. YOUR EMPLOYER I.D. NO.

I.D. NO.

*PLACE OF SERVICE CODES

1-(IH) –INPATIENT HOSPITAL
2-(OH)-OUTPATIENT HOSPITAL
3-(O) –DOCTOR'S OFFICE

4-(H)-PATIENT'S HOME
5- DAY CARE FACILITY (PSY)
6- NIGHT CARE FACILITY (PSY)

7-(NH) –NURSING HOME
8-(SNF) –SKILLED NURSING FACILITY
9- AMBULANCE

O-(OL)-OTHER LOCATIONS
A-(IL) –INDEPENDENT LABORATORY
B– OTHER MEDICAL/SURGICAL FACILITY

2327 1/76

APPROVED BY AMA COUNCIL ON MEDICAL SERVICE 6-74

Abbreviations pertinent to this record:

Adv _____	lt _____
AP _____	neg _____
CC _____	OC _____
compl _____	OP _____
DPM _____	Op _____
dx _____	PO _____
exam _____	re ch _____
interp _____	retn _____
lat _____	wk _____

ASSIGNMENT 6

1. Complete the *Universal Health Insurance Claim Form** to Blue Cross for Charles B. Kamb by referring to his Patient Record and ledger card. Date the claim June 30. You have had Mr. Kamb sign the release of information portion of the form but no assignment has been taken on this claim.

2. Use your Relative Value Studies or Current Procedural Terminology code book to ascertain the correct five-digit coding and modifiers for each professional service rendered.

3. Record on ledger card when you have billed insurance company.

Abbreviations pertinent to this record:

Adv _____	med _____
Ant _____	mg _____
BP _____	mo _____
cc _____	OV _____
D _____	PH _____
Dr _____	post _____
exam _____	Pt _____
HBP _____	retn _____
inj _____	rev _____
intermed _____	W _____
int _____	c̄ _____
ltd _____	♂ _____

---

*See page 331 for help in completing this form.

PATIENT RECORD

Foote,	Frances	F.	08-10-52	F	013/678-0943
LAST NAME	FIRST NAME	MIDDLE NAME	BIRTH DATE	SEX	HOME PHONE

984 North A Street, Woodland Hills,		XY	12345
ADDRESS	CITY	STATE	ZIP CODE

housewife

PATIENT'S OCCUPATION	NAME OF COMPANY

ADDRESS OF EMPLOYER		PHONE

Harry L. Martin	roofer
SPOUSE	OCCUPATION

BDO Construction Co.	340 N. 6th St., Woodland Hills,XY 12345	013/478-9083
EMPLOYER	ADDRESS	PHONE

Blue Cross	Harry L. Martin
NAME OF INSURANCE GROUP	SUBSCRIBER

548-78-8924	16524A	8126	1-1-76
BLUE CROSS CERT. NO.	GROUP NO.	CURRENT COVERAGE NO.	EFFECTIVE DATE

588-90-8701

MEDICARE NO.	MEDICAID NO.	EFFECTIVE DATE	SOC. SEC. NO.

G.U. Curette, M.D., 4780 Main St., Ehrlich, XY 12350

REFERRED BY:

DATE	PROGRESS
10-11-77	CC: discomfort around lt toe. Exam: severe overgrowth of nail into surrounding tissues. X-ray interp: lt foot essentially neg. No gout or arthritis seen. Dx: severe onychocryptosis both margins of lt hallux. Adv to retn as OP to hosp for surgery on lt hallux. No disability from work. *Nick Pedra, DPM*
10-13-77	Op: wedge resection for repair of ingrown nails, Retn 1 wk for PO re ch. Pt may continue to work. No disability. *N Pedra DPM*
10-20-77	Lt hallux healing well. No retn necessary. *Nick Pedra, DPM*

STATEMENT

College Clinic
4567 Broad Avenue
Woodland Hills, XY 12345
013/486-9002

Mrs. Frances F. Foote
984 North A Street
Woodland Hills, XY 12345

DATE	PROFESSIONAL SERVICE	CHARGE		PAID		BALANCE
10-11-77	OC brief	9	00			
	AP & Lat x-rays lt foot	15	00			
10-13-77	Exc nail & nail matrix, compl	150	00			
10-20-77	OC, brief	NC				

Pay last amount in this column

CON - CONSULTATION	HCD - HOUSE CALL (DAY)	LAB - LABORATORY
CPX - COMPLETE PHYS EXAM	HCN - HOUSE CALL (NIGHT)	NC - NO CHARGE
E - EMERGENCY	HV - HOSPITAL VISIT	OC - OFFICE CALL
EC - ERROR CORRECTED	INJ - INJECTION	OS - OFFICE SURGERY
ECG - ELECTROCARDIOGRAM	INS - INSURANCE	SE - SPECIAL EXAM

1547

HEALTH INSURANCE
CLAIM FORM

Blue Cross of Southern California

READ INSTRUCTIONS BEFORE COMPLETING OR SIGNING THIS FORM

TYPE OR PRINT ☐ MEDICARE ☐ MEDICAID ☐ CHAMPUS ☐ OTHER

Box 60465, Terminal Annex
Los Angeles, California 90060

PATIENT & INSURED (SUBSCRIBER) INFORMATION

1. PATIENT'S NAME (First name, middle initial, last name)	2. PATIENT'S DATE OF BIRTH	3. INSURED'S NAME (First name, middle initial, last name)

4. PATIENT'S ADDRESS (Street, city, state, ZIP code)	5. PATIENT'S SEX MALE ☐ FEMALE	6. INSURED'S I.D. No. or **MEDICARE No.** (include any letters)

7. PATIENT'S RELATIONSHIP TO INSURED   SELF   SPOUSE   CHILD   OTHER

8. INSURED'S GROUP NO. (Or Group Name)

9. OTHER HEALTH INSURANCE COVERAGE - Enter Name of Policyholder and Plan Name and Address and Policy or Medical Assistance Number	10. WAS CONDITION RELATED TO: A. PATIENT'S EMPLOYMENT YES ☐ NO B. AN AUTO ACCIDENT YES ☐ NO	11. INSURED'S ADDRESS (Street, city, state, ZIP code)

12. PATIENT'S OR AUTHORIZED PERSON'S SIGNATURE (Read back before signing)
I Authorize the Release of any Medical Information Necessary to Process this Claim and Request Payment of MEDICARE/CHAMPUS Benefits Either to Myself or to the Party Who Accepts Assignment Below

SIGNED _____ DATE

13. I AUTHORIZE PAYMENT OF MEDICAL BENEFITS TO UNDERSIGNED PHYSICIAN OR SUPPLIER FOR SERVICE DESCRIBED BELOW

SIGNED (Insured or Authorized Person)

PHYSICIAN OR SUPPLIER INFORMATION

14. DATE OF:	ILLNESS (FIRST SYMPTOM) OR INJURY (ACCIDENT) OR PREGNANCY (LMP)	15. DATE FIRST CONSULTED YOU FOR THIS CONDITION	16. HAS PATIENT EVER HAD SAME OR SIMILAR SYMPTOMS? YES ☐ NO

17. DATE PATIENT ABLE TO RETURN TO WORK	18. DATES OF TOTAL DISABILITY FROM THROUGH	DATES OF PARTIAL DISABILITY FROM THROUGH

19. NAME OF REFERRING PHYSICIAN	20. FOR SERVICES RELATED TO HOSPITALIZATION GIVE HOSPITALIZATION DATES ADMITTED DISCHARGED

21. NAME & ADDRESS OF FACILITY WHERE SERVICES RENDERED (If other than home or office)	22. WAS LABORATORY WORK PERFORMED OUTSIDE YOUR OFFICE? YES ☐ NO CHARGES:

23. DIAGNOSIS OR NATURE OF ILLNESS OR INJURY, RELATE DIAGNOSIS TO PROCEDURE IN COLUMN D BY REFERENCE TO NUMBERS 1, 2, 3, ETC. OR DX CODE

1.
2.
3.
4.

24. A DATE OF SERVICE	B* PLACE OF SERV- ICE	C FULLY DESCRIBE PROCEDURES, MEDICAL SERVICES OR SUPPLIES FURNISHED FOR EACH DATE GIVEN PROCEDURE CODE (IDENTIFY:) (EXPLAIN UNUSUAL SERVICES OR CIRCUMSTANCES)	D DIAGNOSIS CODE	E CHARGES	F

SAMPLE

25. SIGNATURE OF PHYSICIAN OR SUPPLIER (Read back before signing) SIGNED _____ DATE	26. ACCEPT ASSIGNMENT (GOVERNMENT CLAIMS ONLY) (SEE BACK) YES ☐ NO 30. YOUR SOCIAL SECURITY NO.	27. TOTAL CHARGE	28. AMOUNT PAID	29. BALANCE DUE

31. PHYSICIAN'S OR SUPPLIER'S NAME, ADDRESS, ZIP CODE & TELEPHONE NO.

32. YOUR PATIENT'S ACCOUNT NO.	33. YOUR EMPLOYER I.D. NO.

I.D. NO.

*PLACE OF SERVICE CODES

1–(IH) –INPATIENT HOSPITAL	4–(H)–PATIENT'S HOME	7–(NH) –NURSING HOME	O–(OL)–OTHER LOCATIONS
2–(OH)–OUTPATIENT HOSPITAL	5– DAY CARE FACILITY (PSY)	8–(SNF) –SKILLED NURSING FACILITY	A–(IL) –INDEPENDENT LABORATORY
3–(O) –DOCTOR'S OFFICE	6– NIGHT CARE FACILITY (PSY)	9– AMBULANCE	B– OTHER MEDICAL/SURGICAL FACILITY

2327 1/76

APPROVED BY AMA COUNCIL ON MEDICAL SERVICE 6-74

PATIENT RECORD

Kamb,	Charles	B.	01-26-27	M	013/467-2601
LAST NAME	FIRST NAME	MIDDLE NAME	BIRTH DATE	SEX	HOME PHONE

2600 West Nautilus Street,	Woodland Hills,	XY	12345
ADDRESS	CITY	STATE	ZIP CODE

TV actor	Amer. Federation of TV & Radio Artists (AFTRA)
PATIENT'S OCCUPATION	NAME OF COMPANY

30077 Ventura Blvd., Woodland Hills, XY 12345	013/466-3331
ADDRESS OF EMPLOYER	PHONE

Jane C. Kamb	housewife
SPOUSE	OCCUPATION

EMPLOYER	ADDRESS	PHONE

Blue Cross	Charles B. Kamb	
NAME OF INSURANCE GROUP	SUBSCRIBER	

246-31-2201	26071	Union Local TV-303 4133	1-30-76
BLUE CROSS CERT. NO.	GROUP NO.	CURRENT COVERAGE NO.	EFFECTIVE DATE

			246-31-2201
MEDICARE NO.	MEDICAID NO.	EFFECTIVE DATE	SOC. SEC. NO.

Mr. O.S. Tomy (friend)
REFERRED BY:

DATE	PROGRESS
6-1-77	New pt ♂ comes in complaining of nasal bleeding for 2½ mo c̄ headaches & nasal congestion. PH pt has had HBP for 1yr Taking med Serpasil prescribed by dr in Ohio. Lab work done in office – normal. Exam revealed nasal hemorrhage BP 200/120. Gave inj IM adrenosem salicylate 5 mg/1cc, used cautery, ant & post nasal packs. Adv retn tomorrow. Ordered previous med records from dr in Ohio. Di recurrent epistaxis due to hypertension. No disability from work. S Practon MD
6-2-77	Removed nasal packs. Inj IM 5mg/cc adrenosem salicylat post nasal pack BP 180/100 adv retn in 3 days S Practon MD
6-5-77	Removed post pack & replaced. BP 200/100 Adv retn in 4 days for recheck S Practon MD
6-9-77	Removed post pack BP 180/120 Adv retn 3 days SPMD
6-12-77	Rev previous med records Pt referred to Dr Perry, Cardi (int) for future care re HBP No dis from work Gerald Practon MD

STATEMENT

College Clinic
4567 Broad Avenue
Woodland Hills, XY 12345
013/486-9002

Mr. Charles B. Kamb
2600 West Nautilus Street
Woodland Hills, XY 12345

DATE	PROFESSIONAL SERVICE	CHARGE		PAID		BALANCE	
6-1-77	Lee & White Clotting Time (coagulation)	5	00				
	Platelet Count (Rees-Ecker)	3	00				
	Inj 5 mg/1cc Adrenosem	5	00				
	Salicylate Sterile Tray (nasal packs,	2	00				
	syringe, med. etc.)						
	Post nasal packs c̄ cauteri-						
	zation & ant packs (init OC						
	intermed incl)	25	00				
6-2-77	Sterile Tray	2	00				
	Subsequent post packing	5	00				
	Inj 5 mg/1cc Adrenosem Salicyl	5	00				
6-5-77	Sterile Tray	2	00				
	Subsequent post packing	5	00				
6-9-77	OC, ltd removal post packs	7	00				
6-12-77	OC intermed, rev of records, referred to int.	10	00				

Pay last amount in this column

CON - CONSULTATION	HCD - HOUSE CALL (DAY)	LAB - LABORATORY
CPX - COMPLETE PHYS EXAM	HCN - HOUSE CALL (NIGHT)	NC - NO CHARGE
E - EMERGENCY	HV - HOSPITAL VISIT	OC - OFFICE CALL
EC - ERROR CORRECTED	INJ - INJECTION	OS - OFFICE SURGERY
ECG - ELECTROCARDIOGRAM	INS - INSURANCE	SE - SPECIAL EXAM

1547

HEALTH INSURANCE
CLAIM FORM

READ INSTRUCTIONS BEFORE COMPLETING OR SIGNING THIS FORM

Blue Cross
of Southern California

TYPE OR PRINT ☐ MEDICARE ☐ MEDICAID ☐ CHAMPUS ☐ OTHER

Box 60465, Terminal Annex
Los Angeles, California 90060

PATIENT & INSURED (SUBSCRIBER) INFORMATION

1. PATIENT'S NAME *(First name, middle initial, last name)*	2. PATIENT'S DATE OF BIRTH	3. INSURED'S NAME *(First name, middle initial, last name)*

4. PATIENT'S ADDRESS *(Street, city, state, ZIP code)*

5. PATIENT'S SEX
MALE ☐ FEMALE

6. INSURED'S I.D. No. or **MEDICARE No.** *(include any letters)*

7. PATIENT'S RELATIONSHIP TO INSURED
SELF SPOUSE CHILD OTHER

8. INSURED'S GROUP NO. *(Or Group Name)*

9. OTHER HEALTH INSURANCE COVERAGE - Enter Name of Policyholder and Plan Name and Address and Policy or Medical Assistance Number

10. WAS CONDITION RELATED TO:

A. PATIENT'S EMPLOYMENT
YES ☐ NO

B. AN AUTO ACCIDENT
YES ☐ NO

11. INSURED'S ADDRESS *(Street, city, state, ZIP code)*

12. PATIENT'S OR AUTHORIZED PERSON'S SIGNATURE *(Read back before signing)*
I Authorize the Release of any Medical Information Necessary to Process this Claim and Request Payment of MEDICARE/CHAMPUS Benefits Either to Myself or to the Party Who Accepts Assignment Below

SIGNED _____ DATE _____

13. I AUTHORIZE PAYMENT OF MEDICAL BENEFITS TO UNDERSIGNED PHYSICIAN OR SUPPLIER FOR SERVICE DESCRIBED BELOW

SIGNED *(Insured or Authorized Person)*

PHYSICIAN OR SUPPLIER INFORMATION

14. DATE OF:
ILLNESS (FIRST SYMPTOM) OR INJURY (ACCIDENT) OR PREGNANCY (LMP)

15. DATE FIRST CONSULTED YOU FOR THIS CONDITION

16. HAS PATIENT EVER HAD SAME OR SIMILAR SYMPTOMS?
YES ☐ NO

17. DATE PATIENT ABLE TO RETURN TO WORK

18. DATES OF TOTAL DISABILITY
FROM _____ THROUGH _____

DATES OF PARTIAL DISABILITY
FROM _____ THROUGH _____

19. NAME OF REFERRING PHYSICIAN

20. FOR SERVICES RELATED TO HOSPITALIZATION GIVE HOSPITALIZATION DATES
ADMITTED _____ DISCHARGED _____

21. NAME & ADDRESS OF FACILITY WHERE SERVICES RENDERED *(If other than home or office)*

22. WAS LABORATORY WORK PERFORMED OUTSIDE YOUR OFFICE?
YES ☐ NO CHARGES:

23. DIAGNOSIS OR NATURE OF ILLNESS OR INJURY, RELATE DIAGNOSIS TO PROCEDURE IN COLUMN D BY REFERENCE TO NUMBERS 1, 2, 3, ETC. OR DX CODE

1.
2.
3.
4.

24. A DATE OF SERVICE	B* PLACE OF SERVICE	C FULLY DESCRIBE PROCEDURES, MEDICAL SERVICES OR SUPPLIES FURNISHED FOR EACH DATE GIVEN — PROCEDURE CODE (IDENTIFY:) (EXPLAIN UNUSUAL SERVICES OR CIRCUMSTANCES)	D DIAGNOSIS CODE	E CHARGES	F

SAMPLE

25. SIGNATURE OF PHYSICIAN OR SUPPLIER *(Read back before signing)*

SIGNED _____ DATE _____

26. ACCEPT ASSIGNMENT *(GOVERNMENT CLAIMS ONLY) (SEE BACK)*
YES ☐ NO

30. YOUR SOCIAL SECURITY NO.

27. TOTAL CHARGE

28. AMOUNT PAID

29. BALANCE DUE

31. PHYSICIAN'S OR SUPPLIER'S NAME, ADDRESS, ZIP CODE & TELEPHONE NO.

32. YOUR PATIENT'S ACCOUNT NO.

33. YOUR EMPLOYER I.D. NO.

I.D. NO.

*PLACE OF SERVICE CODES

1–(IH) –INPATIENT HOSPITAL
2–(OH) –OUTPATIENT HOSPITAL
3–(O) –DOCTOR'S OFFICE
4–(H)–PATIENT'S HOME
5– DAY CARE FACILITY (PSY)
6– NIGHT CARE FACILITY (PSY)
7–(NH) –NURSING HOME
8–(SNF) –SKILLED NURSING FACILITY
9– AMBULANCE
O–(OL)–OTHER LOCATIONS
A –(IL) –INDEPENDENT LABORATORY
B– OTHER MEDICAL/SURGICAL FACILITY

2327 1/76

APPROVED BY AMA COUNCIL ON MEDICAL SERVICE 6-74

ASSIGNMENT 7

1. Complete the *Blue Shield Form* for Mrs. Hortense N. Hope by referring to her Patient Record and ledger card.* Date the claim July 31.

2. Use your Relative Value Studies or Current Procedural Terminology code book to ascertain the correct five-digit coding and modifiers for each professional service rendered.

3. Record on ledger card when insurance company has been billed.

Abbreviations pertinent to this record:

adv _____	PRN _____
Drs _____	Pt _____
exam _____	PTR _____
lt _____	retn _____
NC _____	♀ _____
OC _____	

Note: For those completing this claim in California, assume Dr. Practon is a member physician of Blue Shield.

ASSIGNMENT 8

1. Complete the *Blue Shield Form* for Mrs. Louise K. Herman by referring to her Patient Record and ledger card.* Date the claim May 31. You have had Mrs. Herman sign an Assignment of Benefits Form for Dr. Rumsey and you will be attaching this to the claim. Complete the *Assignment of Benefits Form* on page 535.

2. Use your Relative Value Studies or Current Procedural Terminology code book to ascertain the correct five-digit coding and modifiers for each professional service rendered.

3. Record on ledger card when the insurance company has been billed.

Abbreviations pertinent to this record:

adv _____	int _____
cc _____	OC _____
diag _____	ofc _____
DNS _____	perf _____
dx _____	pre-op _____
exam _____	prn _____
exc _____	pt _____
ext _____	retn _____
init _____	wk _____

Note: For those completing this claim in California, assume Dr. Rumsey is a member physician of Blue Shield.

PATIENT RECORD

Hope,	Hortense	N.	4-12-46	F	013/666-7821
LAST NAME	FIRST NAME	MIDDLE NAME	BIRTH DATE	SEX	HOME PHONE

247 Lantern Pike, Woodland Hills, XY 12345

ADDRESS	CITY	STATE	ZIP CODE

clerk typist   R and S Manufacturing Company

PATIENT'S OCCUPATION		NAME OF COMPANY

2271 West 74 Street, Torres, XY 12349   013/466-5890

ADDRESS OF EMPLOYER	PHONE

Harry J. Hope   carpenter

SPOUSE	OCCUPATION

Jesse Construction Co. 3861 S. Orange St., Torres, XY 12349   013/765-2318

EMPLOYER	ADDRESS	PHONE

Blue Shield   Hortense N. Hope

NAME OF INSURANCE GROUP	SUBSCRIBER

585537AT   T8471811A

BLUE SHIELD	CERT. NO.	GROUP NO.	CURRENT COVERAGE NO.	EFFECTIVE DATE
				321-45-8809
MEDICARE NO.	MEDICAID NO.	EFFECTIVE DATE	SOC. SEC. NO.	

husband

REFERRED BY:

DATE	PROGRESS
7-1-77	New ♀ pt comes in complaining of lt great toe. Exam reveals slight infection of lt great toe. Drained and cleaned nail lt great toe. Adv to retn in 2 days. *Gerald Procton, MD*
7-3-77	Excised entire lt great toenail under total toe procaine block. Drs applied. PTR in 5 days for checkup. *G. Procton, MD*
7-7-77	Nail bed healing well. Retn PRN. *Gerald Procton, MD*

STATEMENT

College Clinic
4567 Broad Avenue
Woodland Hills, XY 12345
013/486-9002

Mrs. Hortense N. Hope
247 Lantern Pike
Woodland Hills, XY 12345

DATE	PROFESSIONAL SERVICE	CHARGE		PAID	BALANCE
7-1-77	Brief exam & drainage lt great toenail	15	00		
7-3-77	Excision entire lt great toenail under total toe procaine block	20	00		
	Sterile Tray (itemized)	5	00		
7-7-77	OC, brief	NC			

Pay last amount in this column

CON - CONSULTATION	HCD - HOUSE CALL (DAY)	LAB - LABORATORY
CPX - COMPLETE PHYS EXAM	HCN - HOUSE CALL (NIGHT)	NC - NO CHARGE
E - EMERGENCY	HV - HOSPITAL VISIT	OC - OFFICE CALL
EC - ERROR CORRECTED	INJ - INJECTION	OS - OFFICE SURGERY
ECG - ELECTROCARDIOGRAM	INS - INSURANCE	SE - SPECIAL EXAM

NOTE: Please do not detach this stub. Detach the last copy and one carbon. 25683

Send Blue Shield of California the balance of the form with carbon insert intact. See Reverse side for billing instructions.

TAB SET

FOR BLUE SHIELD USE ONLY

SERVICE REPORT
MC 163 (REV. 10/75)

PATIENT'S NAME			
LAST		FIRST	MIDDLE INITIAL

COMPLETE FOR MEDI-CAL PROGRAM

CALIFORNIA MEDICAL ASSISTANCE PROGRAM
PATIENT'S IDENTIFICATION NUMBER.

COMPLETE FOR BLUE SHIELD SUBSCRIBERS

GROUP NO.   SECTION NO.

PATIENT'S ADDRESS
STREET

CO.	AID	CASE NO.	FBU	PERS. NO.

SUBSCRIBER NO.

CITY   STATE   ZIP CODE

SUBSCRIBER'S NAME (IF PATIENT IS A DEPENDENT)   LAST   FIRST   MIDDLE INITIAL

PATIENT'S RELATIONSHIP TO SUBSCRIBER

☐ SELF   ☐ SPOUSE   ☐ CHILD

SUBSCRIBER'S EMPLOYER

PATIENT'S BIRTHDATE
MONTH   DAY   YR.   AGE

PATIENT'S SEX

☐ MALE   ☐ FEMALE

FOR PROVIDER'S USE ONLY

CONDITION CAUSED BY: ☐ INJURY   ☐ ILLNESS   ☐ PREGNANCY

IF INJURY: INDICATE DATE, HOW AND WHERE SUSTAINED

☐ AUTO ACCIDENT
☐ HOME
☐ OTHER

DATE OF INJURY
MO.   DAY   YR.

IF PREGNANCY, DATE OF COMMENCEMENT

IS THIS A NEW ILLNESS?   ☐ NO   ☐ YES

IS CONDITION DUE TO INJURY OR SICKNESS ARISING OUT OF PATIENT'S EMPLOYMENT?   IS THIS A NEW PATIENT?

☐ NO   ☐ YES   ☐ NO   ☐ YES

IF PATIENT WAS REFERRED INDICATE: ☐ FROM
☐ TO   DOCTOR

IF TREATED IN HOSPITAL OR NURSING HOME
I.P. OR O.P. INDICATE NAME AND LOCATION

ADMISSION DATE
MO.   DAY   YR.

DISCHARGE DATE
MO.   DAY   YR.

OTHER GROUP HOSPITAL, MEDICAL COVERAGE INCLUDING MEDICARE.   ☐ NO   ☐ YES

NAME OF COMPANY OR PLAN   HEALTH INSURANCE CLAIM NO.   LETTER

DIAGNOSIS AND CONCURRENT CONDITIONS

NAME AND ADDRESS OF PROVIDER OF SERVICE   PROVIDER NO.

DATE THIS FORM WAS PREPARED ▶

WAS LABORATORY WORK PERFORMED IN YOUR OFFICE?

☐ NO (IF NO, ENTER NAME AND ADDRESS OF LABORATORY BELOW)   ☐ YES

AMOUNT CHARGED TO PHYSICIAN BY LABORATORY

$

THIS IS TO CERTIFY THAT THE FOREGOING INFORMATION IS TRUE, ACCURATE AND COMPLETE. I UNDERSTAND THAT PAYMENT AND SATISFACTION OF THIS CLAIM WILL BE FROM FEDERAL AND STATE FUNDS, AND THAT ANY FALSE CLAIMS, STATEMENTS, OR DOCUMENTS OR CONCEALMENT OF A MATERIAL FACT, MAY BE PROSECUTED UNDER APPLICABLE FEDERAL OR STATE LAWS.

SIGNATURE OF PROVIDER OF SERVICE (REQUIRED FOR MEDI-CAL PROGRAM) ▶

PLACE OF SERVICE CODES

FAMILY PLANNING SERVICES? (MEDI-CAL)   ☐ NO   ☐ YES

1=IN-PATIENT HOSPITAL   2=OUT-PATIENT HOSPITAL   3=OFFICE   4=PATIENTS' HOME
8=NURSING HOME   9=OTHER

BLUE SHIELD USE ONLY	DATE OF SERVICE			PROCEDURE NUMBER		DESCRIBE EACH SERVICE OR APPLIANCE SEPARATELY	FOR BLUE SHIELD USE ONLY	YOUR FEE	PLACE OF SERV CODE	FOR BLUE SHIELD USE ONLY
LINE NO.	LAST DAY	MO.	DAY	YR.	← SMA NUMBER → UNIT MODIFIER RVS NUMBER					

SAMPLE

TOTAL

SPECIAL PAYEE NAME		CN		CD		CLM MSG	DIAG	TYPE OF SERVICE	UNITS	LOC	MSG	TOTAL
SPECIAL PAYEE NO. AND STREET		SPECIAL PAYEE CITY, STATE					ZIP CODE					

CLAIM TYPE	PAY CODE	CPC	MDE	FEE	PROF	HOSP	MISC	QUAL	REL	PERS	ORIG EFF DATE	EXPL	DATE OF CHG OR CX	D/S
1	2	3	4	5	6	7	8	9	10					

1

PATIENT RECORD

Herman,	Louise	K.	11-04-36	F	013/266-9085
LAST NAME	FIRST NAME	MIDDLE NAME	BIRTH DATE	SEX	HOME PHONE

13453 Burbank Boulevard, Woodland Hills,		XY	12345
ADDRESS	CITY	STATE	ZIP CODE

budget analyst	City Unified School District
PATIENT'S OCCUPATION	NAME OF COMPANY

900 North 9th Street, Saunders, XY 12348	913/666-0985
ADDRESS OF EMPLOYER	PHONE

Harold D. Herman	salesman
SPOUSE	OCCUPATION

V. X. Paint Supply Co. 335 Burbank Blvd., Woodland Hills, XY 12345		013/457-8009
EMPLOYER	ADDRESS	PHONE

Blue Shield	Louise K. Herman
NAME OF INSURANCE GROUP	SUBSCRIBER

623711CT		T2097700C		1-1-76
BLUE SHIELD	CERT. NO.	GROUP NO.	CURRENT COVERAGE NO.	EFFECTIVE DATE

			519-36-0018
MEDICARE NO.	MEDICAID NO.	EFFECTIVE DATE	SOC. SEC. NO.

Raymond Skelton, M. D.

REFERRED BY:

DATE	PROGRESS
5-6-77	Pt referred by Dr Skelton c̄c̄ bleeding hemorrhoids anoscopy exam revealed dr int & ext. hemorrhoids & 2 infected rectal polyps. Adv. retn 2 days for removal of hemorrhoids & Polyps. _RR M.D._
5-8-77	In ofc. perf int & ext hemorrhoidectomy; proctosigmoidoscopy then perf for removal of Polyps. Adv sitz baths daily. Pt adv to retn 1 wk will be off W.K from 5-8 thru 5-14 _Rex Rumsey M.D._
5-15-77	D.N.S.
5-17-77	Progressing well. no pain, no discomfort. Retn prn. _Rex Rumsey M.D._

STATEMENT

College Clinic
4567 Broad Avenue
Woodland Hills, XY 12345
013/486-9002

Mrs. Louise K. Herman
13453 Burbank Boulevard
Woodland Hills, XY 12345

DATE	PROFESSIONAL SERVICE	CHARGE		PAID	BALANCE	
5-6-77	Init comprehensive pre-op exam	50	00			
	Anoscopy, diag	25	00			
5-8-77	Int & ext hemorrhoidectomy	75	00			
	Proctosigmoidoscopy exc rectal polyps, complicated	60	00			
	Sterile Tray (itemized)	10	00			
5-17-77	OC, brief	NC				

Pay last amount in this column

CON - CONSULTATION	HCD - HOUSE CALL (DAY)	LAB - LABORATORY
CPX - COMPLETE PHYS EXAM	HCN - HOUSE CALL (NIGHT)	NC - NO CHARGE
E - EMERGENCY	HV - HOSPITAL VISIT	OC - OFFICE CALL
EC - ERROR CORRECTED	INJ - INJECTION	OS - OFFICE SURGERY
ECG - ELECTROCARDIOGRAM	INS - INSURANCE	SE - SPECIAL EXAM

ASSIGNMENT OF BENEFITS AND INFORMATION RELEASE

PATIENT'S NAME_____

PHYSICIAN'S NAME AND ADDRESS:

I HEREBY AUTHORIZE THE _____TO PAY
DIRECTLY TO THE DOCTORS SURGICAL AND MEDICAL EXPENSE INSURANCE
BENEFITS TO WHICH I MAY BE ENTITLED UNDER THE DOCTOR'S INSURANCE
PROVISION OF:

GROUP POLICY #_____SUBSCRIBER #_____

THIS WILL APPROVE THE RELEASE OF NECESSARY INFORMATION TO MY
INSURANCE COMPANY FOR PURPOSES OF SUBMITTING A CLAIM AGAINST MY
MEDICAL INSURANCE POLICY.

SIGNATURE OF PATIENT_____

SIGNATURE OF INSURED_____DATE_____

ASSIGNMENT OF BENEFITS AND INFORMATION RELEASE

PATIENT'S NAME_____

PHYSICIAN'S NAME AND ADDRESS:

I HEREBY AUTHORIZE THE _____TO PAY
DIRECTLY TO THE DOCTORS SURGICAL AND MEDICAL EXPENSE INSURANCE
BENEFITS TO WHICH I MAY BE ENTITLED UNDER THE DOCTOR'S INSURANCE
PROVISION OF:

GROUP POLICY #_____SUBSCRIBER #_____

THIS WILL APPROVE THE RELEASE OF NECESSARY INFORMATION TO MY
INSURANCE COMPANY FOR PURPOSES OF SUBMITTING A CLAIM AGAINST MY
MEDICAL INSURANCE POLICY.

SIGNATURE OF PATIENT_____

SIGNATURE OF INSURED_____DATE_____

NOTE: Please do not detach this stub. Detach the last copy and one carbon. 25683
Send Blue Shield of California the balance of the form with carbon insert intact. See Reverse side for billing instructions.

TAB SET

FOR BLUE SHIELD USE ONLY

SERVICE REPORT
MC 163 (REV. 10/75)

PATIENT'S NAME			
LAST	FIRST	MIDDLE INITIAL	

PATIENT'S ADDRESS
STREET

CITY	STATE	ZIP CODE

SUBSCRIBER'S NAME (IF PATIENT IS A DEPENDENT)
LAST   FIRST   MIDDLE INITIAL

SUBSCRIBER'S EMPLOYER

COMPLETE FOR MEDI-CAL PROGRAM
CALIFORNIA MEDICAL ASSISTANCE PROGRAM
PATIENT'S IDENTIFICATION NUMBER.

CO.	AID	CASE NO.	FBU	PERS. NO.

COMPLETE FOR BLUE SHIELD SUBSCRIBERS
GROUP NO.   SECTION NO.

SUBSCRIBER NO.

PATIENT'S RELATIONSHIP TO SUBSCRIBER
☐ SELF ☐ SPOUSE ☐ CHILD

PATIENT'S BIRTHDATE
MONTH   DAY   YR.   AGE

PATIENT'S SEX
☐ MALE ☐ FEMALE

FOR PROVIDER'S USE ONLY

CONDITION CAUSED BY: ☐ INJURY ☐ ILLNESS ☐ PREGNANCY

IF INJURY: INDICATE DATE, HOW AND WHERE SUSTAINED

☐ AUTO ACCIDENT
☐ HOME
☐ OTHER

DATE OF INJURY
MO. DAY YR.

IF PREGNANCY, DATE OF COMMENCEMENT

IS THIS A NEW ILLNESS? ☐ NO ☐ YES

IS CONDITION DUE TO INJURY OR SICKNESS ARISING OUT OF PATIENT'S EMPLOYMENT?
☐ NO ☐ YES   IS THIS A NEW PATIENT? ☐ NO ☐ YES

IF PATIENT WAS REFERRED INDICATE: ☐ FROM ☐ TO DOCTOR

NAME AND ADDRESS OF PROVIDER OF SERVICE   PROVIDER NO.

DATE THIS FORM WAS PREPARED ▶

IF TREATED IN HOSPITAL OR NURSING HOME
I.P. OR O.P. INDICATE NAME AND LOCATION

ADMISSION DATE
MO. DAY YR.

DISCHARGE DATE
MO. DAY YR.

OTHER GROUP HOSPITAL, MEDICAL COVERAGE INCLUDING MEDICARE. ☐ NO ☐ YES

NAME OF COMPANY OR PLAN   HEALTH INSURANCE CLAIM NO.   LETTER

DIAGNOSIS AND CONCURRENT CONDITIONS

WAS LABORATORY WORK PERFORMED IN YOUR OFFICE?

☐ NO (IF NO. ENTER NAME AND ADDRESS OF LABORATORY BELOW)   ☐ YES

AMOUNT CHARGED TO PHYSICIAN BY LABORATORY
$

THIS IS TO CERTIFY THAT THE FOREGOING INFORMATION IS TRUE, ACCURATE AND COMPLETE. I UNDERSTAND THAT PAYMENT AND SATISFACTION OF THIS CLAIM WILL BE FROM FEDERAL AND STATE FUNDS, AND THAT ANY FALSE CLAIMS, STATEMENTS, OR DOCUMENTS OR CONCEALMENT OF A MATERIAL FACT, MAY BE PROSECUTED UNDER APPLICABLE FEDERAL OR STATE LAWS.

SIGNATURE OF PROVIDER OF SERVICE (REQUIRED FOR MEDI-CAL PROGRAM) ▶

PLACE OF SERVICE CODES
1=IN-PATIENT HOSPITAL   2=OUT-PATIENT HOSPITAL   3=OFFICE   4=PATIENTS' HOME
8=NURSING HOME   9=OTHER

FAMILY PLANNING SERVICES? (MEDI-CAL) ☐ NO ☐ YES

BLUE SHIELD USE ONLY LINE NO.	DATE OF SERVICE			PROCEDURE NUMBER RVS NUMBER / SMA NUMBER — UNIT MODIFIER	DESCRIBE EACH SERVICE OR APPLIANCE SEPARATELY	FOR BLUE SHIELD USE ONLY	YOUR FEE	PLACE OF SERV CODE	FOR BLUE SHIELD USE ONLY
	LAST DAY	MO.	DAY	YR.						

SAMPLE

SPECIAL PAYEE NAME   CN   CD   CLM MSG   DIAG

SPECIAL PAYEE NO. AND STREET   SPECIAL PAYEE CITY, STATE   ZIP CODE

TYPE OF SERVICE	UNITS	LOC	MSG	TOTAL
D/S				

CLAIM TYPE	PAY CODE	CPC	MDE	FEE	PROF	HOSP.	MISC	QUAL	REL	PERS	ORIG EFF DATE	EXPL	DATE OF CHG OR CX
1	2	3	4	5	6	7	8	9	10				

1

Chapter 5:
Medicaid and Medi-Cal

ASSIGNMENT 9

1. Complete a *Medi-Cal Treatment Authorization Request* for Stephen M. Drake's hospital admission. Date the form May 6.

2. Complete the *Medi-Cal (Blue Shield) Form* for Stephen M. Drake by referring to his Patient Record and ledger card. Date the claim May 26. Place an adhesive label at the proper location on the form, identify whether it is MEDI or POE, and show month and year on label to indicate current eligibility.

3. Use your Relative Value Studies or Current Procedural Terminology code book to ascertain the correct five-digit coding and modifiers for each professional service rendered.

4. Record on ledger card when Medi-Cal has been billed.

Abbreviations pertinent to this record:

adm _____	imp _____
adv _____	inflam _____
cc _____	NC _____
comp _____	phys _____
exam _____	Pt _____
hosp _____	Temp _____
HV _____	wk _____
IM _____	

ASSIGNMENT 10

1. Complete the *Medi-Cal (Blue Shield) Form* for Barry L. Brook by referring to his Patient Record and ledger card. Date the claim May 31. Place an adhesive label at the proper location on the form, identify whether it is MEDI or POE, and show month and year on label to indicate current eligibility.

2. Use your Relative Value Studies or Current Procedural Terminology code book to ascertain the correct five-digit coding and modifiers for each professional service rendered.

3. Record on ledger card when you have billed Medi-Cal.

Abbreviations pertinent to this record:

cc _____	L _____
ER _____	lt _____
Fx _____	N _____
hosp _____	pt _____
Imp _____	Tx _____
hist _____	wks _____

PATIENT RECORD

Drake,	Stephen	M.	04-03-63	M	013/277-5831
LAST NAME	FIRST NAME	MIDDLE NAME	BIRTH DATE	SEX	HOME PHONE

2317 Charnwood Avenue, Woodland Hills,		XY	12345
ADDRESS	CITY	STATE	ZIP CODE

student	
PATIENT'S OCCUPATION	NAME OF COMPANY

ADDRESS OF EMPLOYER		PHONE

Mrs. Virginia B. Drake (mother)	None- family on welfare	
SPOUSE OR PARENT	OCCUPATION	

EMPLOYER	ADDRESS	PHONE

NAME OF INSURANCE GROUP	SUBSCRIBER

BLUE SHIELD OR BLUE CROSS CERT. NO.	GROUP NO.	CURRENT COVERAGE NO.	EFFECTIVE DATE
	19-37-1524033-1-62		566-09-0081
MEDICARE NO.	MEDICAID NO.	EFFECTIVE DATE	SOC. SEC. NO.

James B. Jeffers, M.D., 100 S. Broadway, Woodland Hills, XY 12345
REFERRED BY:

DATE	PROGRESS
5-1-77	Pt comes in complaining of severe sore throat since April 4. Exam shows much enlargement & inflam of tonsils. Temp 101.2 Did complete phys exam. Gave penicillin 5 cc IM. Imp: Acute tonsillitis. *G Practon, MD*
5-6-77	Pt comes in again with severe sore throat. Mother states Stephen has had bouts of tonsillitis since age 6. Adv. tonsillectomy. Phoned for TAR authorization: 3 p.m., Log # 102, authorized by Mrs. Jane Michaels. Pt admitted to hosp for 2 days stay during which time surgery will be performed. *G Practon, M D*
5-7-77	Tonsillectomy and hospital visit. Pt doing well. *G Practon MD*
5-8-77	Brief hospital visit made and pt discharged. To be seen in office in 10 days. *Gerald Practon, MD*
5-18-77	No complaints. Temp 98.1. Return if necessary. *Gerald Practon, MD*

STATEMENT

College Clinic
4567 Broad Avenue
Woodland Hills, XY 12345
013/486-9002

Mrs. Virginia B. Drake
2317 Charnwood Avenue
Woodland Hills, XY 12345

Re: Professional services - Stephen M. Drake

DATE	PROFESSIONAL SERVICE	CHARGE		PAID	BALANCE
5-1-77	OC, comp.	30	00		
	Penicillin inj	5	00		
5-6-77	OC, brief				
	Adm to hosp, intermed hist & phys exam, initial hospital card	25	00		
5-7-77	Tonsillectomy	100	00		
5-8-77	HV, brief	NC			
5-18-77	OC, brief	NC			

Pay last amount in this column

CON - CONSULTATION	HCD - HOUSE CALL (DAY)	LAB - LABORATORY
CPX - COMPLETE PHYS EXAM	HCN - HOUSE CALL (NIGHT)	NC - NO CHARGE
E - EMERGENCY	HV - HOSPITAL VISIT	OC - OFFICE CALL
EC - ERROR CORRECTED	INJ - INJECTION	OS - OFFICE SURGERY
ECG - ELECTROCARDIOGRAM	INS - INSURANCE	SE - SPECIAL EXAM

E-Z-OUT ®

INSTRUCTIONS

UARCO BUSINESS FORMS
OAKLAND. CALIF.

DOCTOR:—USE TYPEWRITER OR BALL POINT PEN. AFTER EXAMINATION MAIL WHITE, YELLOW AND BLUE FORMS WITH CARBONS BETWEEN TO
COUNTY WELFARE DEPARTMENT NAMED ON PATIENT'S IDENTIFICATION CARD. RETAIN PINK COPY FOR YOUR FILES.

NO.**389472**

STATE OF CALIFORNIA

MEDICAL ASSISTANCE PROGRAM

MEDICAL
TREATMENT AUTHORIZATION REQUEST

FOR DOCTOR'S USE	FOR COUNTY USE

FOR DOCTOR'S USE

NAME AND ADDRESS OF PATIENT

AGE | SEX | PATIENTS IDENTIFICATION | PERS. NO.

CO. | AID | CASE NO. | FBU

NAME OF COUNTY

DOCTOR PLEASE PRINT YOUR NAME AND ADDRESS HERE

THE ABOVE NAMED PATIENT IS IN NEED OF ADDITIONAL TREATMENT WHICH WILL EX-CEED THE AMOUNT AUTHORIZED WITHOUT PRIOR APPROVAL. INITIAL DIAGNOSTIC IM-PRESSIONS:

AUTHORIZATION IS REQUESTED TO CLAIM PAYMENT FOR THE FOLLOWING
RECOMMENDED TREATMENT:

FOR COUNTY USE

DOCTOR:

☐ YOU ARE AUTHORIZED TO CLAIM PAY-MENT FOR TREATMENT AS RECOMMENDED BY YOU. AUTHORIZATION EXPIRES IN_____ DAYS.

☐ REQUEST DENIED.
COMMENTS:

SAMPLE

☐ YOU ARE AUTHORIZED TO CLAIM PAY-MENT FOR TREATMENT CHECKED "YES".

AUTHORIZATION EXPIRES IN_____ DAYS.

DESCRIPTION (BE SPECIFIC)	PROCEDURE NO.	CHARGES	AUTHORIZED		EXPLANATION
			YES	NO	

SIGNATURE | DEGREE | DATE

NOTE: COUNTY AUTHORIZATION DOES NOT GUARANTEE PAYMENT. PAYMENT IS SUBJECT TO PATIENTS ELIGIBILITY. BE SURE THE IDENTIFICATION CARD IS CURRENT BEFORE RENDERING SERVICE.

COUNTY WELFARE DEPARTMENT

BY_____

DATE_____

MC - 161 (REV. 8-69)

263328

NOTE: Please do not detach this stub. Detach the last copy and one carbon.   25683

Send Blue Shield of California the balance of the form with carbon insert intact. See Reverse side for billing instructions.

TAB SET

FOR BLUE SHIELD USE ONLY

SERVICE REPORT
MC 163 (REV. 10/75)

PATIENT'S NAME		
LAST	FIRST	MIDDLE INITIAL

COMPLETE FOR MEDI-CAL PROGRAM	COMPLETE FOR BLUE SHIELD SUBSCRIBERS

CALIFORNIA MEDICAL ASSISTANCE PROGRAM
PATIENT'S IDENTIFICATION NUMBER.

GROUP NO.	SECTION NO.

PATIENT'S ADDRESS
STREET

CO.	AID	CASE NO.	FBU	PERS. NO.

CITY   STATE   ZIP CODE

SUBSCRIBER NO.

SUBSCRIBER'S NAME (IF PATIENT IS A DEPENDENT)
LAST   FIRST   MIDDLE INITIAL

PATIENT'S RELATIONSHIP TO SUBSCRIBER
☐ SELF   ☐ SPOUSE   ☐ CHILD

SUBSCRIBER'S EMPLOYER

PATIENT'S BIRTHDATE
MONTH   DAY   YR.   AGE

PATIENT'S SEX
☐ MALE   ☐ FEMALE

CONDITION CAUSED BY: ☐ INJURY ☐ ILLNESS ☐ PREGNANCY

NAME AND ADDRESS OF PROVIDER OF SERVICE   PROVIDER NO.

IF INJURY: INDICATE DATE, HOW AND WHERE SUSTAINED

FOR PROVIDER'S USE ONLY

☐ AUTO ACCIDENT
☐ HOME
☐ OTHER

DATE OF INJURY
MO.   DAY   YR.

IF PREGNANCY, DATE OF COMMENCEMENT

IS THIS A NEW ILLNESS?   ☐ NO   ☐ YES

IS CONDITION DUE TO INJURY OR SICKNESS ARISING OUT OF PATIENT'S EMPLOYMENT?
☐ NO   ☐ YES

IS THIS A NEW PATIENT?
☐ NO   ☐ YES

IF PATIENT WAS REFERRED INDICATE: ☐ FROM   ☐ TO   DOCTOR

DATE THIS FORM WAS PREPARED ▶

IF TREATED IN HOSPITAL OR NURSING HOME
I.P. OR O.P. INDICATE NAME AND LOCATION

ADMISSION DATE
MO.   DAY   YR.

DISCHARGE DATE
MO.   DAY   YR.

WAS LABORATORY WORK PERFORMED IN YOUR OFFICE?

☐ NO (IF NO, ENTER NAME AND ADDRESS OF LABORATORY BELOW)   ☐ YES

AMOUNT CHARGED TO PHYSICIAN BY LABORATORY
$

OTHER GROUP HOSPITAL, MEDICAL COVERAGE INCLUDING MEDICARE. ☐ NO ☐ YES

NAME OF COMPANY OR PLAN   HEALTH INSURANCE CLAIM NO.   LETTER

THIS IS TO CERTIFY THAT THE FOREGOING INFORMATION IS TRUE, ACCURATE AND COMPLETE. I UNDERSTAND THAT PAYMENT AND SATISFACTION OF THIS CLAIM WILL BE FROM FEDERAL AND STATE FUNDS, AND THAT ANY FALSE CLAIMS, STATEMENTS, OR DOCUMENTS OR CONCEALMENT OF A MATERIAL FACT, MAY BE PROSECUTED UNDER APPLICABLE FEDERAL OR STATE LAWS.

DIAGNOSIS AND CONCURRENT CONDITIONS

SIGNATURE OF PROVIDER OF SERVICE (REQUIRED FOR MEDI-CAL PROGRAM) ▶

PLACE OF SERVICE CODES
1=IN-PATIENT HOSPITAL   2=OUT-PATIENT HOSPITAL   3=OFFICE   4=PATIENTS' HOME
8=NURSING HOME   9=OTHER

FAMILY PLANNING SERVICES? (MEDI-CAL)   ☐ NO   ☐ YES

BLUE SHIELD USE ONLY LINE NO.	DATE OF SERVICE LAST DAY	MO.	DAY	YR.	PROCEDURE NUMBER RVS NUMBER SMA NUMBER / UNIT MODIFIER	DESCRIBE EACH SERVICE OR APPLIANCE SEPARATELY	FOR BLUE SHIELD USE ONLY	YOUR FEE	PLACE OF SERV CODE	FOR BLUE SHIELD USE ONLY
									TOTAL	

SAMPLE

SPECIAL PAYEE NAME		CN	CO	CLM MSG	DIAG				TOTAL

SPECIAL PAYEE NO. AND STREET		SPECIAL PAYEE CITY, STATE		ZIP CODE	T Y P E O F S E R V I C E	U N I T S	L O C	M S G	

CLAIM TYPE	PAY CODE	CPC	MOE	FEE	PROF	HOSP	MISC	QUAL	REL	PERS	ORIG. EFF. DATE	EXPL	DATE OF CHG. OR CX	D/S
1	2	3	4	5	6	7	8	9	10					

PATIENT RECORD

Brook	Barry	L.	02-03-70	M	013-487-9770
LAST NAME	FIRST NAME	MIDDLE NAME	BIRTH DATE	SEX	HOME PHONE

3821 Ocean Drive,	Woodland Hills,	XY	12345
ADDRESS	CITY	STATE	ZIP CODE

child
PATIENT'S OCCUPATION   NAME OF COMPANY

ADDRESS OF EMPLOYER   PHONE

Robert D. Brook (father)   None - family on welfare (father totally disabled)
SPOUSE OR PARENT   OCCUPATION

EMPLOYER   ADDRESS   PHONE

NAME OF INSURANCE GROUP   SUBSCRIBER

BLUE SHIELD OR BLUE CROSS CERT. NO.	GROUP NO.	CURRENT COVERAGE NO.	EFFECTIVE DATE
	54-32-7681533-1-03		776-09-1931
MEDICARE NO.	MEDICAID NO.	EFFECTIVE DATE	SOC. SEC. NO.

Virginia B. Drake (friend)
REFERRED BY:

DATE	PROGRESS
5-28-77	11:30 PM Sunday New pt seen in ER at hosp. Pt twisted Ⓛ knee while playing baseball at Grove Playground. X-rays were ordered N for Fx. Imp: effusion + ligament strain lt knee. Tx: aspirated lt knee & removed 5 cc bloody fluid. Applied long leg cylinder cast. Pt to be seen in office in 2 wks. Raymond Skelton MD

STATEMENT

College Clinic
4567 Broad Avenue
Woodland Hills, XY 12345
013/486-9002

Mr. Robert D. Brook
3821 Ocean Drive
Woodland Hills, XY 12345

Re: Professional Services - Barry L. Brook

DATE	PROFESSIONAL SERVICE	CHARGE		PAID		BALANCE	
5-28-77	Init. intermed exam & hist	35	00				
	Aspiration lt knee	10	00				
	Application long leg cylinder cast lt leg	25	00				

Pay last amount in this column

CON - CONSULTATION	HCD - HOUSE CALL (DAY)	LAB - LABORATORY
CPX - COMPLETE PHYS EXAM	HCN - HOUSE CALL (NIGHT)	NC - NO CHARGE
E - EMERGENCY	HV - HOSPITAL VISIT	OC - OFFICE CALL
EC - ERROR CORRECTED	INJ - INJECTION	OS - OFFICE SURGERY
ECG - ELECTROCARDIOGRAM	INS - INSURANCE	SE - SPECIAL EXAM

NOTE: Please do not detach this stub. Detach the last copy and one carbon.
25683
Send Blue Shield of California the balance of the form with carbon insert intact. See Reverse side for billing instructions.

TAB SET

FOR BLUE SHIELD USE ONLY

SERVICE REPORT
MC 163 (REV. 10/75)

PATIENT'S NAME LAST ... FIRST ... MIDDLE INITIAL	**COMPLETE FOR MEDI-CAL PROGRAM**
PATIENT'S ADDRESS STREET	**CALIFORNIA MEDICAL ASSISTANCE PROGRAM PATIENT'S IDENTIFICATION NUMBER.**
CITY ... STATE ... ZIP CODE	CO. AID CASE NO. FBU PERS. NO.

COMPLETE FOR BLUE SHIELD SUBSCRIBERS
GROUP NO.   SECTION NO.

SUBSCRIBER NO.

SUBSCRIBER'S NAME (IF PATIENT IS A DEPENDENT)   LAST   FIRST   MIDDLE INITIAL

PATIENT'S RELATIONSHIP TO SUBSCRIBER
☐ SELF ☐ SPOUSE ☐ CHILD

SUBSCRIBER'S EMPLOYER

PATIENT'S BIRTHDATE MONTH DAY YR.   AGE

PATIENT'S SEX ☐ MALE ☐ FEMALE

FOR PROVIDER'S USE ONLY

CONDITION CAUSED BY: ☐ INJURY ☐ ILLNESS ☐ PREGNANCY

IF INJURY: INDICATE DATE, HOW AND WHERE SUSTAINED
☐ AUTO ACCIDENT
☐ HOME
☐ OTHER

DATE OF INJURY MO. DAY YR.

IF PREGNANCY, DATE OF COMMENCEMENT

IS THIS A NEW ILLNESS? ☐ NO ☐ YES

IS CONDITION DUE TO INJURY OR SICKNESS ARISING OUT OF PATIENT'S EMPLOYMENT? ☐ NO ☐ YES

IS THIS A NEW PATIENT? ☐ NO ☐ YES

IF PATIENT WAS REFERRED INDICATE ☐ FROM ☐ TO DOCTOR

NAME AND ADDRESS OF PROVIDER OF SERVICE   **PROVIDER NO.**

DATE THIS FORM WAS PREPARED ▶

IF TREATED IN HOSPITAL OR NURSING HOME I.P. OR O.P. INDICATE NAME AND LOCATION

ADMISSION DATE MO. DAY YR.

DISCHARGE DATE MO. DAY YR.

WAS LABORATORY WORK PERFORMED IN YOUR OFFICE?
☐ NO (IF NO, ENTER NAME AND ADDRESS OF LABORATORY BELOW)   ☐ YES

AMOUNT CHARGED TO PHYSICIAN BY LABORATORY $

OTHER GROUP HOSPITAL, MEDICAL COVERAGE INCLUDING MEDICARE. ☐ NO ☐ YES

NAME OF COMPANY OR PLAN   HEALTH INSURANCE CLAIM NO.   LETTER

DIAGNOSIS AND CONCURRENT CONDITIONS

THIS IS TO CERTIFY THAT THE FOREGOING INFORMATION IS TRUE, ACCURATE AND COMPLETE. I UNDERSTAND THAT PAYMENT AND SATISFACTION OF THIS CLAIM WILL BE FROM FEDERAL AND STATE FUNDS, AND THAT ANY FALSE CLAIMS, STATEMENTS, OR DOCUMENTS OR CONCEALMENT OF A MATERIAL FACT, MAY BE PROSECUTED UNDER APPLICABLE FEDERAL OR STATE LAWS.

SIGNATURE OF PROVIDER OF SERVICE (REQUIRED FOR MEDI-CAL PROGRAM) ▶

PLACE OF SERVICE CODES

FAMILY PLANNING SERVICES? (MEDICAL) ☐ NO ☐ YES

1=IN-PATIENT HOSPITAL   2=OUT PATIENT HOSPITAL   3=OFFICE   4=PATIENTS' HOME
8=NURSING HOME   9=OTHER

BLUE SHIELD USE ONLY	DATE OF SERVICE	PROCEDURE NUMBER	DESCRIBE EACH SERVICE OR APPLIANCE SEPARATELY	FOR BLUE SHIELD USE ONLY	YOUR FEE	PLACE OF SERV CODE	FOR BLUE SHIELD USE ONLY
LINE NO. / LAST DAY	MO. DAY YR.	RVS NUMBER — SMA NUMBER — UNIT MODIFIER					

SAMPLE

SPECIAL PAYEE NAME	CN	CO	CLM MSG	DIAG	T Y P E O F S E R V I C E	U N I T S	L O C	M S G	TOTAL
SPECIAL PAYEE NO AND STREET	SPECIAL PAYEE CITY, STATE		ZIP CODE		D/S				

CLAIM TYPE	PAY CODE	CPC	MDE	FEE	PROF	HOSP	MISC	QUAL	REL	PERS	ORIG EFF DATE	EXPL	DATE OF CHG OR CX
1	2	3	4	5	6	7	8			10			

1

Assignments 11, 12, 13, and 14 have been written for Medicare claims and assignments 15 and 16 have been written for Medicare/Medicaid (Medi-Cal) claims.

Chapter 6:
Medicare and Medi-Medi

ASSIGNMENT 11

1. Complete the *Request for Medicare Payment*, directing it to your local fiscal intermediary. Refer to Elsa M. Mooney's Patient Record and ledger card for information. Date the claim December 21. Dr. Cardi is accepting assignment in this particular case. Mrs. Mooney has already met her deductible for the year, owing to previous medical expenses from another physician.

2. Use your Relative Value Studies or Current Procedural Terminology code book to ascertain the correct five-digit coding and modifiers for each professional service rendered.

3. Record on ledger card when you have billed Medicare.

Abbreviations pertinent to this record:

ASCVD	N
EKG	OC
exam	Pt
intermed	ret
interpret	Rx
init	c̄
mo	

ASSIGNMENT 12

1. Complete the *Request for Medicare Payment*, directing it to your local fiscal intermediary. Refer to Peter F. Donlon's Patient Record and ledger card for information. Date the claim May 14. Dr. Antrum is not accepting assignment in this case. Mr. Donlon has met his deductible for the year, owing to previous care by Dr. Antrum in February. (This part of the case has been omitted from the Patient Record for the sake of brevity.)

2. Use your Relative Value Studies or Current Procedural Terminology code book to ascertain the correct five-digit coding and modifiers for each professional service rendered.

3. Record on the ledger card when you have billed Medicare.

Abbreviations pertinent to this record:

adm	intermed
a.m.	NC
auto	OC

PATIENT RECORD

Mooney,	Elsa	M.	02-06-10	F	013/452-4968
LAST NAME	FIRST NAME	MIDDLE NAME	BIRTH DATE	SEX	HOME PHONE

5750 Canyon Road,	Woodland Hills,	XY	12345
ADDRESS	CITY	STATE	ZIP CODE

retired secretary
| PATIENT'S OCCUPATION | | NAME OF COMPANY |

ADDRESS OF EMPLOYER	PHONE

husband deceased
| SPOUSE OR PARENT | OCCUPATION |

EMPLOYER	ADDRESS	PHONE

Medicare
| NAME OF INSURANCE GROUP | SUBSCRIBER |

BLUE SHIELD OR BLUE CROSS CERT. NO.	GROUP NO.	CURRENT COVERAGE NO.	EFFECTIVE DATE

321-10-2653B			321-10-2653
MEDICARE NO.	MEDICAID NO.	EFFECTIVE DATE	SOC. SEC. NO.

George Gentle, M. D. 1000 N. Main Street, Woodland Hills, XY 12345
REFERRED BY:

DATE	PROGRESS
12-15-77	New pt comes in complaining of chest pain & shortness of breath.
	Exam essentially N
	EKG done to rule out myocardial infarction
	Imp: ASCVD — angina pectoris
	Given Rx & advised to ret. in 1 mo.
	Perry Cardi, M.D.

STATEMENT

College Clinic
4567 Broad Avenue
Woodland Hills, XY 12345
013/486-9002

Mrs. Elsa M. Mooney
5750 Canyon Road
Woodland Hills, XY 12345

DATE	PROFESSIONAL SERVICE	CHARGE		PAID	BALANCE
12-15-77	Init. OC, intermed	15	00		
	EKG c̄ interpret & report	25	00		

Pay last amount in this column

CON - CONSULTATION	HCD - HOUSE CALL (DAY)	LAB - LABORATORY
CPX - COMPLETE PHYS EXAM	HCN - HOUSE CALL (NIGHT)	NC - NO CHARGE
E - EMERGENCY	HV - HOSPITAL VISIT	OC - OFFICE CALL
EC - ERROR CORRECTED	INJ - INJECTION	OS - OFFICE SURGERY
ECG - ELECTROCARDIOGRAM	INS - INSURANCE	SE - SPECIAL EXAM

REQUEST FOR MEDICARE PAYMENT

MEDICAL INSURANCE BENEFITS—SOCIAL SECURITY ACT (See Instructions on Back—**Type or Print Information**)

Form Approved
OMB No.
72-RO730

NOTICE—Anyone who misrepresents or falsifies essential information requested by this form may upon conviction be subject to fine and imprisonment under Federal Law.

PART I—PATIENT TO FILL IN ITEMS 1 THROUGH 6 ONLY

When completed, send this form to:

Copy from YOUR OWN HEALTH INSURANCE CARD *(See example on back)*

1 Name of patient (First name, Middle initial, Last name)

2 Health insurance claim number *(Include all letters)*

☐ Male ☐ Female

3 Patient's mailing address   City, State, ZIP code

Telephone Number

4 Describe the illness or injury for which you received treatment *(Always fill in this item if your doctor does not complete Part II below)*

Was your illness or injury connected with your employment?
☐ Yes   ☐ No

5 If any of your medical expenses will be or could be paid by another insurance organization or government agency (including FEHB), show below.

Name and address of organization or agency

Policy or Identification Number

Note: If you **Do Not** want information about this Medicare claim released to the above upon its request, check (X) the following block ☐

6 I authorize any holder of medical or other information about me to release to the Social Security Administration or its intermediaries or carriers any information needed for this or a related Medicare claim. I permit a copy of this authorization to be used in place of the original, and request payment of medical insurance benefits either to myself or to the party who accepts assignment below.

Signature of patient *(See instructions on reverse where patient is unable to sign)*

SIGN HERE ▶

Date signed

PART II—PHYSICIAN OR SUPPLIER TO FILL IN 7 THROUGH 14

7 A. Date of each service	B. Place of service (*See Codes below)	C. Fully describe surgical or medical procedures and other services or supplies furnished for each date given	Procedure Code	D. Nature of illness or injury requiring services or supplies *(diagnosis)*	E. Charges *(If related to unusual circumstances explain in 7C)*	Leave Blank
					$	

SAMPLE

8 Name and address of physician or supplier *(Number and street, city, State, ZIP code)*

Telephone No.

Physician or supplier code

9 Total charges $

10 Amount paid $

11 Any unpaid balance due $

12 Assignment of patient's bill
▶ ☐ I accept assignment *(See reverse)* ☐ I do not accept assignment.

13 Show name and address of person or facility which furnished service *(if other than your own office or patient's home)*

14 Signature of physician or supplier *(A physician's signature certifies that a physician's services were personally rendered by the physician or under the physician's personal direction).*
▶

Date signed

*O—Doctor's Office
IL—Independent Laboratory

H—Patient's Home *(If portable X-ray services, identify the supplier)*
IH—Inpatient Hospital

SNF—Skilled Nursing Facility
OH—Outpatient Hospital

OL—Other Locations
NH—Nursing Home

FORM SSA 1490 (2) (CA) (11-75)

Department of Health, Education, and Welfare
Social Security Administration

ER _____   PO _____

est _____   postop _____

hosp _____   Pt _____

hrs _____   surg _____

Imp _____   c̄ _____

PATIENT RECORD

Donlon,	Peter	F.	08-09-04	M	013/762-3580
LAST NAME	FIRST NAME	MIDDLE NAME	BIRTH DATE	SEX	HOME PHONE

1840 East Chevy Chase Drive,	Woodland Hills,	XY	12345
ADDRESS	CITY	STATE	ZIP CODE

retired chef
PATIENT'S OCCUPATION   NAME OF COMPANY

ADDRESS OF EMPLOYER   PHONE

wife deceased
SPOUSE OR PARENT   OCCUPATION

EMPLOYER   ADDRESS   PHONE

Medicare
NAME OF INSURANCE GROUP   SUBSCRIBER

BLUE SHIELD OR BLUE CROSS CERT. NO.   GROUP NO.   CURRENT COVERAGE NO.   EFFECTIVE DATE

987-65-4321A			987-65-4321
MEDICARE NO.	MEDICAID NO.	EFFECTIVE DATE	SOC. SEC. NO.

Martha Frederick, M. D. 1000 N. Main Street, Woodland Hills, XY 12345
REFERRED BY:

DATE	PROGRESS
5-1-77	Est. pt injured in auto accident. Dr. called to ER (Sunday) from outside hosp at 3 a.m. Pt complains of acute headache & 2.0 cm laceration of nose. Request ER consult c̄ neurologist, Dr. Parkinson, who recommended pt be admitted to hosp. Sutured 2.0 cm laceration of nose. Imp: Acute cephalgia, nasal laceration, deviated septum. *Concha Antrum, MD.*
5-4-77	Discharged from hosp. See hosp records for daily notes. *CA, MD*
5-7-77	Sutures removed. Recommended to have surg. *Ca MD*
5-9-77	Adm to hosp. *Concha Antrum, MD*
5-10-77	Septoplasty. Pt doing well after surg. *C Antrum, MD*
5-11-77	Hosp visit. Pt seems to be improving. No hemorrhaging. *C Antrum MD*
5-12-77	Severe postop nasal hemorrhage. Dr detained 2 hrs c̄ pt. *Concha Antrum MD*

STATEMENT

College Clinic
4567 Broad Avenue
Woodland Hills, XY 12345
013/486-9002

Mr. Peter F. Donlon
1840 East Chevy Chase Drive
Woodland Hills, XY 12345

DATE	PROFESSIONAL SERVICE	CHARGE		PAID		BALANCE	
5-1-77	ER Service, intermed	50	00				
	Suture 2.0 cm laceration of nose	25	00				
5-2-77	HV, brief	15	00				
5-3-77	HV, brief	NC					
5-4-77	HV, brief	NC					
5-7-77	OC, intermed	20	00				
5-10-77	Septoplasty	100	00				
5-11-77	HV, brief	NC					
5-12-77	PO nasal hemorrhage	35	00				

Pay last amount in this column

CON - CONSULTATION	HCD - HOUSE CALL (DAY)	LAB - LABORATORY
CPX - COMPLETE PHYS EXAM	HCN - HOUSE CALL (NIGHT)	NC - NO CHARGE
E - EMERGENCY	HV - HOSPITAL VISIT	OC - OFFICE CALL
EC - ERROR CORRECTED	INJ - INJECTION	OS - OFFICE SURGERY
ECG - ELECTROCARDIOGRAM	INS - INSURANCE	SE - SPECIAL EXAM

☆ U.S.GPO:1976-0-210-833/40

REQUEST FOR MEDICARE PAYMENT

MEDICAL INSURANCE BENEFITS—SOCIAL SECURITY ACT (See Instructions on Back—**Type or Print Information**)

Form Approved
OMB No.
72–RO730

NOTICE—Anyone who misrepresents or falsifies essential information requested by this form may upon conviction be subject to fine and imprisonment under Federal Law.

PART I—PATIENT TO FILL IN ITEMS 1 THROUGH 6 ONLY

When completed, send this form to:

Copy from YOUR OWN HEALTH INSURANCE CARD (See example on back) ➡

1 Name of patient (First name, Middle initial, Last name)

2 Health insurance claim number (Include all letters)

☐ Male   ☐ Female

3 Patient's mailing address — City, State, ZIP code — Telephone Number

4 Describe the illness or injury for which you received treatment (Always fill in this item if your doctor does not complete Part II below)

Was your illness or injury connected with your employment?
☐ Yes   ☐ No

5 If any of your medical expenses will be or could be paid by another insurance organization or government agency (including FEHB), show below.

Name and address of organization or agency

Policy or Identification Number

Note: If you **Do Not** want information about this Medicare claim released to the above upon its request, check (X) the following block ☐

6 I authorize any holder of medical or other information about me to release to the Social Security Administration or its intermediaries or carriers any information needed for this or a related Medicare claim. I permit a copy of this authorization to be used in place of the original, and request payment of medical insurance benefits either to myself or to the party who accepts assignment below.

Signature of patient (See instructions on reverse where patient is unable to sign)

Date signed

SIGN HERE ➡

PART II—PHYSICIAN OR SUPPLIER TO FILL IN 7 THROUGH 14

7 A. Date of each service	B. Place of service (*See Codes below)	C. Fully describe surgical or medical procedures and other services or supplies furnished for each date given / Procedure Code	D. Nature of illness or injury requiring services or supplies (diagnosis)	E. Charges (If related to unusual circumstances explain in 7C)	Leave Blank
				$	

SAMPLE

8 Name and address of physician or supplier (Number and street, city, State, ZIP code)

Telephone No.

Physician or supplier code

9 Total charges $

10 Amount paid $

11 Any unpaid balance due $

12 Assignment of patient's bill
➡ ☐ I accept assignment (See reverse) ☐ I do not accept assignment.

13 Show name and address of person or facility which furnished service (if other than your own office or patient's home)

14 Signature of physician or supplier (A physician's signature certifies that a physician's services were personally rendered by the physician or under the physician's personal direction).

Date signed

➡

*O—Doctor's Office
IL—Independent Laboratory

H—Patient's Home (If portable X-ray services, identify the supplier)
IH—Inpatient Hospital

SNF—Skilled Nursing Facility
OH—Outpatient Hospital

OL—Other Locations
NH—Nursing Home

FORM SSA 1490 (2) (CA) (11-75)

Department of Health, Education, and Welfare
Social Security Administration

ASSIGNMENT 13

1. Complete the *Request for Medicare Payment*, directing it to your local fiscal intermediary. Refer to Jeremiah W. Diffenderffer's Patient Record and ledger card for information. Date the claim June 13. Dr. Coccidioides is not accepting assignment in this case. Mr. Diffenderffer has met his deductible for the year, owing to previous care by Dr. Coccidioides in March. (This part of the case has been omitted from the Patient Record for the sake of brevity.)

2. Use your Relative Value Studies or Current Procedural Terminology code book to ascertain the correct five-digit coding and modifiers for each professional service rendered. In this case, the doctor is being billed by the outside labs for the x-rays and bronchogram.

3. Record on the ledger card the proper information when you have billed Medicare.

Abbreviations pertinent to this record:

Adv _____ PA _____

AP _____ phys _____

CPX _____ pt _____

est _____ re-exam _____

exam _____ tid _____

HCN _____ wk _____

Imp _____

ASSIGNMENT 14

1. Complete the *Request for Medicare Payment*, directing it to your local fiscal intermediary. Refer to Raymond D. Fay's Patient Record and ledger card for information. Date the claim December 31. Dr. Antrum is accepting assignment in this case. Mr. Fay has met his deductible for the year, owing to previous care by another physician.

2. Use your Relative Value Studies or Current Procedural Terminology code book to ascertain the correct five-digit coding and modifiers for each professional service rendered.

3. Record on the ledger card the proper information when you have billed Medicare.

Abbreviations pertinent to this record:

exam _____ OC _____

Imp _____ OV _____

inj _____ Pt _____

ltd _____ retn _____

N _____ X _____

PATIENT RECORD

Diffenderffer,	Jeremiah	W.	08-24-01	M	013/471-9930
LAST NAME	FIRST NAME	MIDDLE NAME	BIRTH DATE	SEX	HOME PHONE

120 Elm Street,	Woodland Hills,	XY	12345
ADDRESS	CITY	STATE	ZIP CODE

retired painter
PATIENT'S OCCUPATION   NAME OF COMPANY

ADDRESS OF EMPLOYER   PHONE

deceased
SPOUSE   OCCUPATION

EMPLOYER   ADDRESS   PHONE

Medicare
NAME OF INSURANCE GROUP   SUBSCRIBER

BLUE SHIELD OR BLUE CROSS CERT. NO.   GROUP NO.   CURRENT COVERAGE NO.   EFFECTIVE DATE

731-32-7401T   731-32-7401
MEDICARE NO.   MEDICAID NO.   EFFECTIVE DATE   SOC. SEC. NO.

John M. Diffenderffer (brother)
REFERRED BY:

DATE	PROGRESS
6-1-77	Est pt phoned. Dr. ordered chest x-rays to be taken at Clay Radiologists 614 Elm St., Woodland Hills, XY 12345 & bilateral bronchogram at Wilcox Med. Arts Lab 6299 Winnetka Ave., Woodland Hills, XY 12345. *B. Coccidioides, MD.*
6-2-77	PA & AP chest x-rays showed pulmonary emphysema. Bilateral bronchogram showed pulmonary emphysema. *B. Coccidioides, MD.*
6-5-77	Pt given comprehensive physical re-exam. Imp: recurrent pneumonitis Adv bed rest. *B Coccidioides, MD*
6-12-77	HCN 8 P.M., limited exam, administered medication (Athemol 25 tabs tid) Imp: recurrent pneumonitis, exertional dyspnea. Adv bed rest. To be seen in 1 wk. *B. Coccidioides, M.D*

STATEMENT

College Clinic
4567 Broad Avenue
Woodland Hills, XY 12345
013/486-9002

Mr. Jeremiah W. Diffenderffer
120 Elm Street
Woodland Hills, XY 12345

DATE	PROFESSIONAL SERVICE	CHARGE		PAID		BALANCE	
	Balance fwd					Ꝋ	
6-2-77	Chest x-rays	40	00				
	Bilateral bronchogram	25	00				
6-5-77	CPX	35	00				
6-12-77	HCN & medication	18	00				

Pay last amount in this column

CON - CONSULTATION	HCD - HOUSE CALL (DAY)	LAB - LABORATORY
CPX - COMPLETE PHYS EXAM	HCN - HOUSE CALL (NIGHT)	NC - NO CHARGE
E - EMERGENCY	HV - HOSPITAL VISIT	OC - OFFICE CALL
EC - ERROR CORRECTED	INJ - INJECTION	OS - OFFICE SURGERY
ECG - ELECTROCARDIOGRAM	INS - INSURANCE	SE - SPECIAL EXAM

☆ U.S. GPO:1976-0-210-833/40

REQUEST FOR MEDICARE PAYMENT

MEDICAL INSURANCE BENEFITS—SOCIAL SECURITY ACT (See Instructions on Back—**Type or Print Information**)

Form Approved
OMB No.
72-RO730

NOTICE—Anyone who misrepresents or falsifies essential information requested by this form may upon conviction be subject to fine and imprisonment under Federal Law.

PART I—PATIENT TO FILL IN ITEMS 1 THROUGH 6 ONLY

When completed, send this form to:

Copy from **YOUR OWN HEALTH INSURANCE CARD** (See example on back)

1 Name of patient (First name, Middle initial, Last name)

2 Health insurance claim number (Include all letters)

☐ Male   ☐ Female

3 Patient's mailing address   City, State, ZIP code   Telephone Number

4 Describe the illness or injury for which you received treatment (Always fill in this item if your doctor does not complete Part II below)

Was your illness or injury connected with your employment?
☐ Yes   ☐ No

5 If any of your medical expenses will be or could be paid by another insurance organization or government agency (including FEHB), show below.

Name and address of organization or agency   Policy or Identification Number

Note: If you **Do Not** want information about this Medicare claim released to the above upon its request, check (X) the following block ☐

6 I authorize any holder of medical or other information about me to release to the Social Security Administration or its intermediaries or carriers any information needed for this or a related Medicare claim. I permit a copy of this authorization to be used in place of the original, and request payment of medical insurance benefits either to myself or to the party who accepts assignment below.

Signature of patient (See instructions on reverse where patient is unable to sign)   Date signed

SIGN HERE ▶

PART II—PHYSICIAN OR SUPPLIER TO FILL IN 7 THROUGH 14

7 A. Date of each service	B. Place of service (*See Codes below)	C. Fully describe surgical or medical procedures and other services or supplies furnished for each date given		D. Nature of illness or injury requiring services or supplies (diagnosis)	E. Charges (If related to unusual circumstances explain in 7C)	Leave Blank
			Procedure Code			
					$	

SAMPLE

8 Name and address of physician or supplier (Number and street, city, State, ZIP code)

Telephone No.

9 Total charges $

Physician or supplier code

10 Amount paid $

11 Any unpaid balance due $

12 Assignment of patient's bill
▶ ☐ I accept assignment (See reverse) ☐ I do not accept assignment.

13 Show name and address of person or facility which furnished service (if other than your own office or patient's home)

14 Signature of physician or supplier (A physician's signature certifies that a physician's services were personally rendered by the physician or under the physician's personal direction).
▶

Date signed

*O—Doctor's Office   H—Patient's Home (If portable X-ray services, identify the supplier)   SNF—Skilled Nursing Facility   OL—Other Locations
IL—Independent Laboratory   IH—Inpatient Hospital   OH—Outpatient Hospital   NH—Nursing Home

FORM SSA 1490 (2) (CA) (11-75)

Department of Health, Education, and Welfare
Social Security Administration

PATIENT RECORD

Fay,	Raymond		02-03-02	M	013/788-9090
LAST NAME	FIRST NAME	MIDDLE NAME	BIRTH DATE	SEX	HOME PHONE

333 North Pencil Avenue,	Woodland Hills,	XY	12345
ADDRESS	CITY	STATE	ZIP CODE

retired railroad engineer	Santa Fe Railroad
PATIENT'S OCCUPATION	NAME OF COMPANY

ADDRESS OF EMPLOYER		PHONE

Marilyn B. Fay	housewife	
SPOUSE OR PARENT	OCCUPATION	

EMPLOYER	ADDRESS	PHONE

Medicare		
NAME OF INSURANCE GROUP	SUBSCRIBER	

BLUE SHIELD OR BLUE CROSS CERT. NO.	GROUP NO.	CURRENT COVERAGE NO.	EFFECTIVE DATE
WA 887-66-1235			887-66-1235
MEDICARE NO.	MEDICAID NO.	EFFECTIVE DATE	SOC. SEC. NO.

George Gentle, M. D. 1000 N. Main Street, Woodland Hills, XY 12345
REFERRED BY:

DATE	PROGRESS
10-31-77	New pt complains of dizziness for 3 days. Exam essentially N.
	Imp: food & inhalant allergy. Retn in 4 days for tests. _C Antrum_
11-4-77	Audiometric hearing tests (air, bone, and speech) - N.
	Vestibular function test - normal
	10 intradermal allergy tests _C Antrum MD_
11-10-77	Bilateral mastoid X
	OV ltd. Pt to retn daily for desensitization inj _C Antrum MD_
11-11-77	OC minimal desensitization inj
thru	" " " "
12-11-77	Improved & discharged ③⓪ _C Antrum MD_

STATEMENT

College Clinic
4567 Broad Avenue
Woodland Hills, XY 12345
013/486-9002

Mr. Raymond D. Fay
333 North Pencil Avenue
Woodland Hills, XY 12345

DATE	PROFESSIONAL SERVICE	CHARGE		PAID		BALANCE	
10-31-77	OC intermed	20	00				
11-4-77	Audiometric hearing test (air, bone, and speech)	15	00				
	Vestibular function test	15	00				
	10 intradermal allergy tests	50	00				
11-10-77	Bilateral mastoid x-rays	35	00				
	OC, ltd	15	00				
11-11-77	thru 12-11-77 Desensitization inj (30) @ $5 ea						

Pay last amount in this column

CON - CONSULTATION	HCD - HOUSE CALL (DAY)	LAB - LABORATORY
CPX - COMPLETE PHYS EXAM	HCN - HOUSE CALL (NIGHT)	NC - NO CHARGE
E - EMERGENCY	HV - HOSPITAL VISIT	OC - OFFICE CALL
EC - ERROR CORRECTED	INJ - INJECTION	OS - OFFICE SURGERY
ECG - ELECTROCARDIOGRAM	INS - INSURANCE	SE - SPECIAL EXAM

☆ U. S. GPO:1976-0-210-833/40

REQUEST FOR MEDICARE PAYMENT

MEDICAL INSURANCE BENEFITS—SOCIAL SECURITY ACT (See Instructions on Back—**Type or Print Information**)

Form Approved
OMB No.
72–RO730

NOTICE—Anyone who misrepresents or falsifies essential information requested by this form may upon conviction be subject to fine and imprisonment under Federal Law.

PART I—PATIENT TO FILL IN ITEMS 1 THROUGH 6 ONLY

When completed, send this form to:

Copy from
YOUR OWN
HEALTH
INSURANCE
CARD
(See example
on back)

1 Name of patient (First name, Middle initial, Last name)

2 Health insurance claim number
(Include all letters)

☐ Male   ☐ Female

3 Patient's mailing address   City, State, ZIP code   Telephone Number

4 Describe the illness or injury for which you received treatment (Always fill in this item if your doctor does not complete Part II below)

Was your illness or injury connected with your employment?
☐ Yes   ☐ No

5 If any of your medical expenses will be or could be paid by another insurance organization or government agency (including FEHB), show below.

Name and address of organization or agency   Policy or Identification Number

Note: If you Do Not want information about this Medicare claim released to the above upon its request, check (X) the following block ☐

6 I authorize any holder of medical or other information about me to release to the Social Security Administration or its intermediaries or carriers any information needed for this or a related Medicare claim. I permit a copy of this authorization to be used in place of the original, and request payment of medical insurance benefits either to myself or to the party who accepts assignment below.

Signature of patient (See instructions on reverse where patient is unable to sign)   Date signed

SIGN
HERE ▶

PART II—PHYSICIAN OR SUPPLIER TO FILL IN 7 THROUGH 14

7 A. Date of each service	B. Place of service (*See Codes below)	C. Fully describe surgical or medical procedures and other services or supplies furnished for each date given	Procedure Code	D. Nature of illness or injury requiring services or supplies (diagnosis)	E. Charges (If related to unusual circumstances explain in 7C)	Leave Blank
					$	

SAMPLE

8 Name and address of physician or supplier (Number and street, city, State, ZIP code)

Telephone No.

Physician or supplier code

9 Total charges $

10 Amount paid $

11 Any unpaid balance due $

12 Assignment of patient's bill
▶ ☐ I accept assignment (See reverse) ☐ I do not accept assignment.

13 Show name and address of person or facility which furnished service (if other than your own office or patient's home)

14 Signature of physician or supplier (A physician's signature certifies that a physician's services were personally rendered by the physician or under the physician's personal direction).
▶

Date signed

*O—Doctor's Office   H—Patient's Home (If portable X-ray services, identify the supplier)   SNF—Skilled Nursing Facility   OL—Other Locations
IL—Independent Laboratory   IH—Inpatient Hospital   OH—Outpatient Hospital   NH—Nursing Home

FORM SSA 1490 (2) (CA) (11-75)

Department of Health, Education, and Welfare
Social Security Administration

ASSIGNMENT 15

1. Complete the *Request for Medicare Payment,* directing it to your local Medicaid (Medi-Cal) fiscal intermediary. Refer to Mrs. Helen P. Nolan's Patient Record and ledger card for information. Date the claim May 31. Dr. Rumsey is accepting assignment in this Medi-Medi case. For Medi-Cal, place an adhesive label at the proper location on the form, identify whether it is MEDI or POE, and show month and year on label to indicate current eligibility.

2. Use your Relative Value Studies or Current Procedural Terminology code book to ascertain the correct five-digit coding and modifiers for each professional service rendered.

3. Record on the ledger card the proper information when you have billed Medicare/Medicaid (Medi-Cal). On July 1 you will receive a check from Medicare for $120 and on July 15 you will receive a check from Medicaid (Medi-Cal) for $40. Record these payments on the ledger and show the adjustment (write-off).

Abbreviations pertinent to this record:

Adm	OC
Adv	phys
BP	prep
Dx	prn
exam	Pt
ext	Rx
hosp	slt
int	wk
NC	c̄

ASSIGNMENT 16

1. Complete the *Request for Medicare Payment*, directing it to your local Medicaid (Medi-Cal) fiscal intermediary. Refer to Mr. Harris Fremont's Patient Record and ledger card for information. Date the claim October 31. The podiatrist accepts assignment in this Medi-Medi case. For Medi-Cal processing, place an adhesive label at the proper location on the form, identify whether it is MEDI or POE, and show month and year on label to indicate current eligibility.

2. Use your Relative Value Studies or Current Procedural Terminology code book to ascertain the correct five-digit coding and modifiers for each professional service rendered.

3. Record on the ledger card the proper information when you have billed Medicare/Medicaid (Medi-Cal).

PATIENT RECORD

Nolan,	Helen	P.	05-10-07	F	013/660-9878
LAST NAME	FIRST NAME	MIDDLE NAME	BIRTH DATE	SEX	HOME PHONE

2588 Cedar Street,	Woodland Hills,	XY	12345
ADDRESS	CITY	STATE	ZIP CODE

housewife	
PATIENT'S OCCUPATION	NAME OF COMPANY

ADDRESS OF EMPLOYER	PHONE

James J. Nolan	retired journalist
SPOUSE	OCCUPATION

EMPLOYER	ADDRESS	PHONE

Medicare/Medi-Cal	
NAME OF INSURANCE GROUP	SUBSCRIBER

BLUE SHIELD OR BLUE CROSS CERT. NO.	GROUP NO.	CURRENT COVERAGE NO.	EFFECTIVE DATE
732-32-1573A	19-60-2358490-1-01		732-32-1573
MEDICARE NO.	MEDICAID NO.	EFFECTIVE DATE	SOC. SEC. NO.

James B. Jeffers, M.D., 100 S. Broadway, Woodland Hills, XY 12345
REFERRED BY:

DATE	PROGRESS
5-1-77	This new pt comes in complaining of constipation & some rectal bleeding & pain. Exam reveals int & ext hemorrhoids. BP 120/80
	Dx: hemorrhoids; int & ext bleeding; anal fistula
	Rx: Adv hospitalization for removal of hemorrhoids *R Rumsey, MD*
5-7-77	Adm to hosp - phys exam & prep hosp records *R Rumsey, MD*
5-8-77	Hemorrhoidectomy c̄ fistulectomy *R Rumsey MD*
5-9-77	Hosp visit, brief. Pt comfortable, slt pain *Rex Rumsey MD*
5-10-77	Hosp visit, no pain *R Rumsey MD*
5-11-77	Hosp visit. Discharged. To be seen in office in 1 wk *R Rumsey, MD*
5-17-77	Well healed, no pain, return prn. *Rex Rumsey, MD*

STATEMENT

College Clinic
4567 Broad Avenue
Woodland Hills, XY 12345
013/486-9002

Mrs. Helen P. Nolan
2588 Cedar Street
Woodland Hills, XY 12345

DATE	PROFESSIONAL SERVICE	CHARGE		PAID		BALANCE
5-1-77	OC, intermed	15	00			
5-7-77	Initial HV, ltd	15	00			
5-8-77	Hemorrhoidectomy c̄ fistul-ectomy	150	00			
5-9-77	HV, brief	NC				
5-10-77	HV, brief	NC				
5-11-77	HV, brief	NC				
5-17-77	OC, brief	NC				

Pay last amount in this column

CON - CONSULTATION	HCD - HOUSE CALL (DAY)	LAB - LABORATORY
CPX - COMPLETE PHYS EXAM	HCN - HOUSE CALL (NIGHT)	NC - NO CHARGE
E - EMERGENCY	HV - HOSPITAL VISIT	OC - OFFICE CALL
EC - ERROR CORRECTED	INJ - INJECTION	OS - OFFICE SURGERY
ECG - ELECTROCARDIOGRAM	INS - INSURANCE	SE - SPECIAL EXAM

☆ U.S.GPO:1976-0-210-833/40

REQUEST FOR MEDICARE PAYMENT

MEDICAL INSURANCE BENEFITS—SOCIAL SECURITY ACT (See Instructions on Back—**Type or Print Information**)

Form Approved
OMB No.
72-R0730

NOTICE—Anyone who misrepresents or falsifies essential information requested by this form may upon conviction be subject to fine and imprisonment under Federal Law.

PART I—PATIENT TO FILL IN ITEMS 1 THROUGH 6 ONLY

When completed, send this form to:

Copy from YOUR OWN HEALTH INSURANCE CARD (See example on back) ▶

1 Name of patient (First name, Middle initial, Last name)

2 Health insurance claim number (Include all letters)

☐ Male ☐ Female

3 Patient's mailing address   City, State, ZIP code   Telephone Number

4 Describe the illness or injury for which you received treatment (Always fill in this item if your doctor does not complete Part II below)

Was your illness or injury connected with your employment?
☐ Yes ☐ No

5 If any of your medical expenses will be or could be paid by another insurance organization or government agency (including FEHB), show below.

Name and address of organization or agency   Policy or Identification Number

Note: If you **Do Not** want information about this Medicare claim released to the above upon its request, check (X) the following block ☐

6 I authorize any holder of medical or other information about me to release to the Social Security Administration or its intermediaries or carriers any information needed for this or a related Medicare claim. I permit a copy of this authorization to be used in place of the original, and request payment of medical insurance benefits either to myself or to the party who accepts assignment below.

Signature of patient (See instructions on reverse where patient is unable to sign)   Date signed

SIGN HERE ▶

PART II—PHYSICIAN· OR SUPPLIER TO FILL IN 7 THROUGH 14

7

A. Date of each service	B. Place of service (*See Codes below)	C. Fully describe surgical or medical procedures and other services or supplies furnished for each date given / Procedure Code	D. Nature of illness or injury requirng services or supplies (diagnosis)	E. Charges (If related to unusual circumstances explain in 7C)	Leave Blank
				$	

SAMPLE

8 Name and address of physician or supplier (Number and street, city, State, ZIP code)

Telephone No.

Physician or supplier code

9 Total charges $

10 Amount paid $

11 Any unpaid balance due $

12 Assignment of patient's bill
▶ ☐ I accept assignment (See reverse) ☐ I do not accept assignment.

13 Show name and address of person or facility which furnished service (if other than your own office or patient's home)

14 Signature of physician or supplier (A physician's signature certifies that a physician's services were personally rendered by the physician or under the physician's personal direction).   Date signed

▶

*O—Doctor's Office   H—Patient's Home (If portable X-ray services, identify the supplier)   SNF—Skilled Nursing Facility   OL—Other Locations
IL—Independent Laboratory   IH—Inpatient Hospital   OH—Outpatient Hospital   NH—Nursing Home

FORM **SSA 1490** (2) (CA) (11-75)

Department of Health, Education, and Welfare
Social Security Administration

Abbreviations pertinent to this record:

Adv _____	mo _____
AP _____	N _____
DPM _____	OC _____
exam _____	Pt _____
ft _____	retn _____
Imp _____	rt _____
lat _____	Rx _____
lt _____	

PATIENT RECORD

Fremont,	Harris	-	07-10-03	M	013/899-0109
LAST NAME	FIRST NAME	MIDDLE NAME	BIRTH DATE	SEX	HOME PHONE

735 North Center Street,	Woodland Hills,	XY	12345
ADDRESS	CITY	STATE	ZIP CODE

retired baseball coach
PATIENT'S OCCUPATION   NAME OF COMPANY

ADDRESS OF EMPLOYER   PHONE

Emily B. Fremont	housewife	
SPOUSE	OCCUPATION	

EMPLOYER   ADDRESS   PHONE

Medicare/Medi-Cal
NAME OF INSURANCE GROUP   SUBSCRIBER

BLUE SHIELD OR BLUE CROSS CERT. NO.	GROUP NO.	CURRENT COVERAGE NO.	EFFECTIVE DATE
454-01-9569A	5610-0020205-000		454-01-9569
MEDICARE NO.	MEDICAID NO.	EFFECTIVE DATE	SOC. SEC. NO.

Raymond Skelton, M.D. 4567 Broad Avenue, Woodland Hills, XY 12345
REFERRED BY:

DATE	PROGRESS
10-2-77	Pt referred by Dr. Skelton. Pt has gout. He comes in complaining of discomfort around toes of both feet. Exam shows overgrowth & hooking & curving of nails. X-rays of rt & lt feet essentially N Gout seen. Rx trimmed away overgrowth & adv to retn for further care in 3 days. Imp: onychauxis & onychocryptosis *Nick Pedro DPM*
10-5-77	Treated rt & lt feet, more thorough trimming of overgrowth & callus formation. To retn in 1 mo. *Nick Pedro DPM*

STATEMENT

College Clinic
4567 Broad Avenue
Woodland Hills, XY 12345
013/486-9002

Mr. Harris Fremont
735 North Center Street
Woodland Hills, XY 12345

DATE	PROFESSIONAL SERVICE	CHARGE		PAID	BALANCE
10-2-77	OC, ltd	10	00		
	AP & Lat x-rays lt ft	15	00		
	AP & Lat x-rays rt ft	15	00		
10-5-77	OC, brief	9	00		

Pay last amount in this column

CON - CONSULTATION	HCD - HOUSE CALL (DAY)	LAB - LABORATORY
CPX - COMPLETE PHYS EXAM	HCN - HOUSE CALL (NIGHT)	NC - NO CHARGE
E - EMERGENCY	HV - HOSPITAL VISIT	OC - OFFICE CALL
EC - ERROR CORRECTED	INJ - INJECTION	OS - OFFICE SURGERY
ECG - ELECTROCARDIOGRAM	INS - INSURANCE	SE - SPECIAL EXAM

☆ U.S.GPO:1976-0-210-833/40

REQUEST FOR MEDICARE PAYMENT

MEDICAL INSURANCE BENEFITS—SOCIAL SECURITY ACT (See Instructions on Back—**Type or Print Information**)

Form Approved
OMB No.
72-RO730

NOTICE—Anyone who misrepresents or falsifies essential information requested by this form may upon conviction be subject to fine and imprisonment under Federal Law.

PART I—PATIENT TO FILL IN ITEMS 1 THROUGH 6 ONLY

When completed, send this form to:

Copy from YOUR OWN HEALTH INSURANCE CARD (See example on back)

1 Name of patient (First name, Middle initial, Last name)

2 Health insurance claim number (Include all letters) ☐ Male ☐ Female

3 Patient's mailing address   City, State, ZIP code   Telephone Number

4 Describe the illness or injury for which you received treatment (Always fill in this item if your doctor does not complete Part II below)

Was your illness or injury connected with your employment? ☐ Yes ☐ No

5 If any of your medical expenses will be or could be paid by another insurance organization or government agency (including FEHB), show below.

Name and address of organization or agency   Policy or Identification Number

Note: If you **Do Not** want information about this Medicare claim released to the above upon its request, check (X) the following block ☐

6 I authorize any holder of medical or other information about me to release to the Social Security Administration or its intermediaries or carriers any information needed for this or a related Medicare claim. I permit a copy of this authorization to be used in place of the original, and request payment of medical insurance benefits either to myself or to the party who accepts assignment below.

Signature of patient (See instructions on reverse where patient is unable to sign)   Date signed

SIGN HERE ▶

PART II—PHYSICIAN OR SUPPLIER TO FILL IN 7 THROUGH 14

7 A. Date of each service	B. Place of service (*See Codes below)	C. Fully describe surgical or medical procedures and other services or supplies furnished for each date given — Procedure Code	D. Nature of illness or injury requirng services or supplies (diagnosis)	E. Charges (If related to unusual circumstances explain in 7C)	Leave Blank
				$	

8 Name and address of physician or supplier (Number and street, city, State, ZIP code)

Telephone No.

9 Total charges $

Physician or supplier code

10 Amount paid $

11 Any unpaid balance due $

12 Assignment of patient's bill
▶ ☐ I accept assignment (See reverse) ☐ I do not accept assignment.

13 Show name and address of person or facility which furnished service (if other than your own office or patient's home)

14 Signature of physician or supplier (A physician's signature certifies that a physician's services were personally rendered by the physician or under the physician's personal direction).

Date signed

▶

*O—Doctor's Office
IL—Independent Laboratory
H—Patient's Home (If portable X-ray services, identify the supplier)
IH—Inpatient Hospital
SNF—Skilled Nursing Facility
OH—Outpatient Hospital
OL—Other Locations
NH—Nursing Home

FORM SSA 1490 (2) (CA) (11-75)

Department of Health, Education, and Welfare
Social Security Administration

Chapter 7:
CHAMPUS, CHAMPVA,
and VA Outpatient Clinic

ASSIGNMENT 17

1. Complete the *CHAMPUS* claim for, directing it to your local CHAMPUS fiscal intermediary. Refer to Miss Rosa M. Sandoval's Patient Record and ledger card for information. Date the claim May 31. Let us assume the patient's mother brings in a completed Non-Availability Statement DD Form 1251 which shows approval of the physician to treat the patient. Dr. Atrics is not accepting assignment but is completing the claim for the patient's convenience. The family of this patient has not previously met its deductible.

2. Use your Relative Value Studies or Current Procedural Terminology code book to ascertain the correct five-digit coding and modifiers for each professional service rendered.

3. On May 11 Mrs. Sandoval makes a partial payment by check of $60. Record the proper information on the ledger card for the payment as well as noting when you have billed CHAMPUS (May 31).

Abbreviations pertinent to this record:

Adv _____	prn _____
a.m. _____	pt _____
ER _____	retn _____
exam _____	Rt _____
FU _____	Surg _____
HV _____	T _____
Imp _____	Temp _____
OC _____	wk _____
ofc _____	c̄ _____

ASSIGNMENT 18

1. Complete the *CHAMPUS* claim form, directing it to your local CHAMPUS fiscal intermediary. Refer to Mrs. Darlene B. Drew's Patient Record and ledger card for information. Date the claim February 3. Let us assume the patient brings in a completed Non-Availability Statement DD Form 1251 which shows approval of the physician to treat the patient. Dr. Ulibarri is accepting assignment. This patient met her deductible last November when seen by a previous physician.

2. Use your Relative Value Studies or Current Procedural Terminology code book to ascertain the correct five-digit coding and modifiers for each professional service rendered.

3. Record the proper information on the ledger card when you have billed CHAMPUS.

PATIENT RECORD

Sandoval,	Rosa	M.	11-01-73	F	013/456-3322
LAST NAME	FIRST NAME	MIDDLE NAME	BIRTH DATE	SEX	HOME PHONE

209 West Maple Street,	Woodland Hills,	XY	12345
ADDRESS	CITY	STATE	ZIP CODE

child
PATIENT'S OCCUPATION   NAME OF COMPANY

ADDRESS OF EMPLOYER   PHONE

Maria B. Sandoval (mother) housewife
SPOUSE OR PARENT   OCCUPATION

Hernan J. Sandoval (father) Army Staff Sargeant,Active Status
EMPLOYER   ADDRESS   PHONE

Service # 886-91-0999   Soc.Sec.# 886-91-0999, HHC, 3rd Batt., 25th Infantry
NAME OF INSURANCE GROUP   SUBSCRIBER

Grade 9, A.P.O., New York, New York 10030

BLUE SHIELD OR BLUE CROSS CERT. NO.	GROUP NO.	CURRENT COVERAGE NO.	EFFECTIVE DATE
CHAMPUS I.D. card # 73485		01-01-77	994-02-1164
MEDICARE NO.	MEDICAID NO.	EFFECTIVE DATE Pt's	SOC. SEC. NO.
		Exp.Date 1-1-82	

Hilda M. Mendez (friend)
REFERRED BY:

DATE	PROGRESS
5-1-77	Sunday 3 a.m. pt seen in ER hosp complaining of pain rt ear
	for 3 days. Exam revealed fluid & pus rt ear. Temp 101°
	Adv mother a myringotomy was necessary. Imp: Rt otitis media
	Pt admitted to hosp same day. Surg: rt myringotomy c̄
	aspiration. *Pedro Atrics, MD*
5-2-77	Discharged. To be seen in ofc for FU. *P Atrics MD*
5-3-77	No pain rt ear. Pt progressing to retn in 1 wk T 98 *P Atrics MD*
5-10-77	T 98, no fluid or pus in rt ear. No pain. Retn prn
	Pedro Atrics, MD

STATEMENT

College Clinic
4567 Broad Avenue
Woodland Hills, XY 12345
013/486-9002

Mr. Hernan J. Sandoval
209 West Maple Street
Woodland Hills, XY 12345

Re: Prof. Serv. for Rosa M. Sandoval

DATE	PROFESSIONAL SERVICE	CHARGE		PAID	BALANCE	
5-1-77	ER	40	00			
	Rt myringotomy c̄ aspiration	50	00			
5-2-77	HV brief	10	00			
5-3-77	OC, limited	10	00			
5-10-77	OC, limited	10	00			

Pay last amount in this column

CON - CONSULTATION	HCD - HOUSE CALL (DAY)	LAB - LABORATORY
CPX - COMPLETE PHYS EXAM	HCN - HOUSE CALL (NIGHT)	NC - NO CHARGE
E - EMERGENCY	HV - HOSPITAL VISIT	OC - OFFICE CALL
EC - ERROR CORRECTED	INJ - INJECTION	OS - OFFICE SURGERY
ECG - ELECTROCARDIOGRAM	INS - INSURANCE	SE - SPECIAL EXAM

☆ U. S. GOVERNMENT PRINTING OFFICE: 1970 - 390 - 777

| SERVICES AND/OR SUPPLIES PROVIDED BY CIVILIAN SOURCES (EXCEPT HOSPITALS) CIVILIAN HEALTH AND MEDICAL PROGRAM OF THE UNIFORMED SERVICES (CHAMPUS) | SEE INSTRUCTIONS ON REVERSE |

SECTION I *(To be completed by patient or other responsible family member. Please print or type)*

| PATIENT DATA | SERVICE MEMBER DATA |

1. NAME *(last, first, middle initial)*
2. DATE OF BIRTH
7. NAME OF SPONSOR *(last, first, middle initial)*

3. ADDRESS *(Include Zip Code)*
8 a. SERVICE NUMBER | b. SOCIAL SECURITY ACCOUNT NUMBER | 9. GRADE

10. ORGANIZATION AND DUTY STATION *(Home Port for Ships)* *(Address for Retired)*

4. PATIENT IS A *(Check one)*
☐ (1) SPOUSE ☐ (2) DAUGHTER ☐ (3) SON ☐ (4) RETIREE

5. IDENTIFICATION CARD *(DD Form 1173, DD Form 2 or PHS Form 1866—3)*
CARD NO.
| MONTH | DAY | YEAR |
EFFECTIVE DATE
EXPIRATION DATE

11. SPONSOR'S OR RETIREE'S BRANCH OF SERVICE
☐ (1) USA ☐ (2) USAF ☐ (3) USMC ☐ (4) USN
☐ (5) USCG ☐ (6) USPHS ☐ (7) ESSA

6. BASIS FOR CARE - ACTIVE DUTY DEPENDENTS ONLY *(Check one)*
☐ (1) RESIDING APART FROM SPONSOR ☐ (2) RESIDING WITH SPONSOR DD FORM 1251 ATTACHED ☐ (3) OUTPATIENT
☐ (4) OTHER *(Specify)*

12. STATUS
☐ (1) ACTIVE DUTY ☐ (2) RETIRED ☐ (3) DECEASED

13. CERTIFICATION

I certify to the best of my knowledge and belief the above information in Section I is correct. To the extent that I have authority to do so I hereby authorize the release of medical records in this case to both the contractor and the Government.
If a RETIRED MEMBER or dependent of a retired or deceased member, I certify that to the best of my knowledge and belief, that *(Check appropriate box)* *(Delete portion in parenthesis not applicable)*

☐ (I am not) (the patient is not) enrolled (neither is sponsor) in any other insurance, medical service, or health plan provided by law or through employment.

☐ (I am) (the patient is) enrolled (so is sponsor) in another insurance, medical service, or health plan provided by law or through employment; however the particular benefits claimed on this form are not payable under the other plan.

Name (print or type) | (Relationship to Patient) | Date | Signature

SECTION II *(To be completed by Source of Care)*

14. NAME AND ADDRESS OF SOURCE OF CARE *(Include Zip Code)*
a. SOURCE OF CARE LOCATION CODE | b. PROVIDER OF SERVICES
☐ (1) ATTENDING PHYSICIAN
☐ (2) OTHER *(Specify)*
c. PATIENT STATUS
☐ (1) INPATIENT
☐ (2) OUTPATIENT

15. NAME AND TITLE OF INDIVIDUAL ORDERING CARE
16. INCLUSIVE DATES OF CARE
| | MONTH | DAY | YEAR | | MONTH | DAY | YEAR |
FROM | | | | TO | | |

17. DIAGNOSIS *(Use standard nomenclature)*
a. INTL STAT CODE

(Check when applicable) ☐ services were necessary for treatment of a bonafide medical emergency
b. 12 - BREAK CODE

18. RELATED HOSPITALIZATION *(If applicable)*
FROM | TO

19. ENTER ESTIMATED OR ACTUAL DATE OF DELIVERY IN MATERNITY CASES. LIST BY DATE SURGICAL OPERATIONS AND/OR CARE FURNISHED INCLUDING VISITS FOR WHICH SEPARATE CHARGES ARE CLAIMED *(Type or print)* *(Attach additional sheets if required)*

DATE(S) OF SERVICE	a. ITEM OR DESCRIPTION OF SERVICE	b. CHARGES	c. PROCEDURE CODE
		$	
d. TOTAL CHARGES THIS STATEMENT FOR CARE AUTHORIZED		$	
e. (PAID BY) OR (DUE FROM) PATIENT *(Cross out one)*		$	
f. DUE FROM GOVERNMENT TO SOURCE OF CARE		$	
g. DUE PATIENT OR SPONSOR, REIMBURSEMENT		$	

20. CERTIFICATION BY SOURCE OF CARE

I certify that the services and / or supplies listed hereon were performed or authorized by the attending physician, dentist or other professional personnel in charge, that payment due from the Government has not been received, and that, except for the amount payable by the patient in accordance with the terms of the Civilian Health and Medical Program of the Uniformed Services, the amount paid by the Government will be accepted as payment in full for the authorized services and / or supplies listed hereon.
I further certify that I am not an intern, resident or otherwise in training status for which I am receiving compensation for services listed on this claim.

Name (print or type) | Title | Date | Signature

The persons signing this form are advised that the willful making of a false or fraudulent statement herein renders them liable to prosecution under applicable Federal Laws.

DA FORM 1 JUN 67 1863 - 2 (Civilian Sources) | REPLACES DA FORM 1863 - 2, 1 SEP 61, WHICH IS OBSOLETE. | Form Approved Comptroller General, U. S., 22 Sep 67

1

Abbreviations pertinent to this record:

Adm _____	PE _____
BP _____	Pt _____
CC _____	RBC _____
cc _____	Rec _____
DC _____	Retn _____
Dx _____	Rx _____
Ex _____	tid _____
FU _____	UA _____
Hosp _____	WBC _____
I & D _____	c̄ _____

PATIENT RECORD

Drew,	Darlene	B.	12-22-37	F	013/466-1002
LAST NAME	FIRST NAME	MIDDLE NAME	BIRTH DATE	SEX	HOME PHONE

720 Ganley Street,	Woodland Hills,	XY	12345
ADDRESS	CITY	STATE	ZIP CODE

seamstress	J. B. Talon Company
PATIENT'S OCCUPATION	NAME OF COMPANY

2111 Ventura Road, Merck, XY 12346	013/733-0156
ADDRESS OF EMPLOYER	PHONE

Harry M. Drew	U.S. Navy Lieutenant Commander (L/C)	Active Status
SPOUSE OR PARENT	OCCUPATION	

Service # 221-96-0711	Soc.Sec.# 221-96-0711	Grade 12
EMPLOYER	ADDRESS	PHONE

P.O. Box 2927, APO New York, NY 09194	
NAME OF INSURANCE GROUP	SUBSCRIBER

BLUE SHIELD OR BLUE CROSS CERT. NO.	GROUP NO.	CURRENT COVERAGE NO. 1-1-76	EFFECTIVE DATE 450-10-3762

MEDICARE NO. CHAMPUS ID Card # 67531	MEDICAID NO.	EFFECTIVE DATE Exp. date 1-1-80	Pt's SOC. SEC. NO.

James B. Jeffers, M.D., 100 S. Broadway, Woodland Hills, XY 12345
REFERRED BY:

DATE	PROGRESS
1-13-77	CC New pt comes in complaining of very large, tender mass in periurethral orifice, milked out 10 cc greenish pus. U.A.–WBC & RBC's loaded. Pt feels much better. R̂ Terramycin 20 caps T.I.D Retn 5 days ⊕ suburethral cyst. Took culture
1-18-77	Cyst is filled up again. Rec. hospitalization culture shows pseudomonas organism.
1-28-77	Adm To College Hosp. Pt scheduled for cystoscopy and retrograde pyelogram.
1-29-77	Surg: I&D of large suburethral cyst c̄ evacuation of pus, marsupialization of urethral diverticulum + packing c̄ Iodoform
1-30-77	Hosp visit Pt. improved
1/31-77 +	Hosp visit no fever BP 120/80
2/1-77	Hosp visit Improved
2-2-76	DC from hosp To be seen in office next week for F/U Ex Gene Ulibarri M.D.

STATEMENT

College Clinic
4567 Broad Avenue
Woodland Hills, XY 12345
013/486-9002

Mrs. Harry M. Drew
720 Ganley Street
Woodland Hills, XY 12345

DATE	PROFESSIONAL SERVICE	CHARGE	PAID	BALANCE
1-13-77	OC intermediate	15 00		
	UA, routine	4 00		
	Drainage of deep periurethral abscess	20 00		
1-18-77	OC brief	8 00		
1-28-77	Init hosp care, intermed	35 00		
1-29-77	Marsupialization of urethral diverticulum	45 00		

Pay last amount in this column

CON - CONSULTATION	HCD - HOUSE CALL (DAY)	LAB - LABORATORY
CPX - COMPLETE PHYS EXAM	HCN - HOUSE CALL (NIGHT)	NC - NO CHARGE
E - EMERGENCY	HV - HOSPITAL VISIT	OC - OFFICE CALL
EC - ERROR CORRECTED	INJ - INJECTION	OS - OFFICE SURGERY
ECG - ELECTROCARDIOGRAM	INS - INSURANCE	SE - SPECIAL EXAM

☆ U. S. GOVERNMENT PRINTING OFFICE: 1970 - 390 - 777

SERVICES AND/OR SUPPLIES PROVIDED BY CIVILIAN SOURCES (EXCEPT HOSPITALS) CIVILIAN HEALTH AND MEDICAL PROGRAM OF THE UNIFORMED SERVICES (CHAMPUS)	SEE INSTRUCTIONS ON REVERSE

SECTION I *(To be completed by patient or other responsible family member. Please print or type)*

PATIENT DATA	SERVICE MEMBER DATA

1. NAME *(last, first, middle initial)*   2. DATE OF BIRTH   7. NAME OF SPONSOR *(last, first, middle initial)*

3. ADDRESS *(Include Zip Code)*   8 a. SERVICE NUMBER   b. SOCIAL SECURITY ACCOUNT NUMBER   9. GRADE

10. ORGANIZATION AND DUTY STATION *(Home Port for Ships)* *(Address for Retired)*

4. PATIENT IS A *(Check one)*
☐ (1) SPOUSE ☐ (2) DAUGHTER ☐ (3) SON ☐ (4) RETIREE

5. IDENTIFICATION CARD *(DD Form 1173, DD Form 2 or PHS Form 1866–3)*
CARD NO.   MONTH DAY YEAR
EFFECTIVE DATE
EXPIRATION DATE

11. SPONSOR'S OR RETIREE'S BRANCH OF SERVICE
☐ (1) USA ☐ (2) USAF ☐ (3) USMC ☐ (4) USN
☐ (5) USCG ☐ (6) USPHS ☐ (7) ESSA

6. BASIS FOR CARE - ACTIVE DUTY DEPENDENTS ONLY   *(Check one)*
☐ (1) RESIDING APART FROM SPONSOR ☐ (2) RESIDING WITH SPONSOR DD FORM 1251 ATTACHED ☐ (3) OUTPATIENT
☐ (4) OTHER *(Specify)*

12. STATUS
☐ (1) ACTIVE DUTY ☐ (2) RETIRED ☐ (3) DECEASED

13. CERTIFICATION
    I certify to the best of my knowledge and belief the above information in Section I is correct. To the extent that I have authority to do so I hereby authorize the release of medical records in this case to both the contractor and the Government.
    If a RETIRED MEMBER or dependent of a retired or deceased member, I certify that to the best of my knowledge and belief, that *(Check appropriate box)* *(Delete portion in parenthesis not applicable)*

☐ (I am not) (the patient is not) enrolled (neither is sponsor) in any other insurance, medical service, or health plan provided by law or through employment.

☐ (I am) (the patient is) enrolled (so is sponsor) in another insurance, medical service, or health plan provided by law or through employment; however the particular benefits claimed on this form are not payable under the other plan.

Name (print or type)   (Relationship to Patient)   Date   Signature

SECTION II *(To be completed by Source of Care)*

14. NAME AND ADDRESS OF SOURCE OF CARE *(Include Zip Code)*

a. SOURCE OF CARE LOCATION CODE   b. PROVIDER OF SERVICES
☐ (1) ATTENDING PHYSICIAN
☐ (2) OTHER *(Specify)*
c. PATIENT STATUS
☐ (1) INPATIENT
☐ (2) OUTPATIENT

15. NAME AND TITLE OF INDIVIDUAL ORDERING CARE

16. INCLUSIVE DATES OF CARE
FROM   MONTH DAY YEAR   TO   MONTH DAY YEAR

17. DIAGNOSIS *(Use standard nomenclature)*
(Check when applicable) ☐ services were necessary for treatment of a bonafide medical emergency

a. INTL STAT CODE
b. 12 - BREAK CODE

18. RELATED HOSPITALIZATION *(If applicable)*
FROM   TO

19. ENTER ESTIMATED OR ACTUAL DATE OF DELIVERY IN MATERNITY CASES. LIST BY DATE SURGICAL OPERATIONS AND/OR CARE FURNISHED INCLUDING VISITS FOR WHICH SEPARATE CHARGES ARE CLAIMED   *(Type or print)*   *(Attach additional sheets if required)*

DATE(S) OF SERVICE	a. ITEM OR DESCRIPTION OF SERVICE	b. CHARGES	c. PROCEDURE CODE
		$	

d. TOTAL CHARGES THIS STATEMENT FOR CARE AUTHORIZED		$	
e. (PAID BY) OR (DUE FROM) PATIENT *(Cross out one)*		$	
f. DUE FROM GOVERNMENT TO SOURCE OF CARE		$	
g. DUE PATIENT OR SPONSOR, REIMBURSEMENT		$	

20. CERTIFICATION BY SOURCE OF CARE
    I certify that the services and / or supplies listed hereon were performed or authorized by the attending physician, dentist or other professional personnel in charge, that payment due from the Government has not been received, and that, except for the amount payable by the patient in accordance with the terms of the Civilian Health and Medical Program of the Uniformed Services, the amount paid by the Government will be accepted as payment in full for the authorized services and / or supplies listed hereon.
    I further certify that I am not an intern, resident or otherwise in training status for which I am receiving compensation for services listed on this claim.

Name (print or type)   Title   Date   Signature

The persons signing this form are advised that the willful making of a false or fraudulent statement herein renders them liable to prosecution under applicable Federal Laws.

DA FORM 1 JUN 67   1863 - 2   (Civilian Sources)   REPLACES DA FORM 1863 - 2, 1 SEP 61, WHICH IS OBSOLETE.   Form Approved Comptroller General, U. S., 22 Sep 67

1

ASSIGNMENT 19

1. Complete the *CHAMPUS* claim form, directing it to your local CHAMPUS fiscal intermediary. Refer to Mrs. Mae I. Abbreviate's Patient Record and ledger card for information. Date the claim January 31. Assume that the patient brings in a completed Non-Availability Statement DD Form 1251 which shows approval of the physician to treat the patient. Dr. Coccidioides is not accepting assignment but is completing the claim for the patient's convenience. This patient has not previously met her deductible.

2. Use your Relative Value Studies or Current Procedural Terminology code book to ascertain the correct five-digit coding and modifiers for each professional service rendered. X-rays in this case were taken at Speedy Radiology Service at 4300 Broad Avenue, Woodland Hills, XY 12345, and laboratory work was sent to Laboratory Associates, 4100 Broad Avenue, Woodland Hills, XY 12345. The doctor is submitting the bill for x-rays and outside laboratory work.

3. Record the proper information on the ledger card when you have billed CHAMPUS. Since billing space is limited on the claim form, it might be wise to type in "See attached itemized statement" and include a copy of the statement indicating RVS or CPT code numbers.

Abbreviations pertinent to this record:

abdom _____	PH _____
aet _____	PND _____
BP _____	Prog _____
Ca _____	pt _____
CC _____	PTR _____
D & C _____	PX _____
Dx _____	RBC _____
EENT _____	Rx _____
FH _____	Surg _____
GB _____	T & A _____
GGE _____	TPR _____
GI _____	u _____
Ht _____	UCHD _____
I _____	URI _____
LMP _____	W _____
L & W _____	WBC _____
NYD _____	wk _____
OS _____	wt _____
Para I _____	yr _____
PE _____	$\bar{c}$ _____

ō——————————————————— ♀ ———————————————————

X ———————————————————

PATIENT RECORD

Abbreviate,	Mae	I.	01-02-32	F	013/985-7667
LAST NAME	FIRST NAME	MIDDLE NAME	BIRTH DATE	SEX	HOME PHONE

4667 Symbol Road,	Woodland Hills,	XY	12345
ADDRESS	CITY	STATE	ZIP CODE

typist	U. R. Wright Company
PATIENT'S OCCUPATION	NAME OF COMPANY

6789 Abridge Road, Woodland Hills, XY 12345	013/988-7540
ADDRESS OF EMPLOYER	PHONE

Shorty S. Abbreviate	Army Staff Sargeant, Active Status
SPOUSE	OCCUPATION

Service # 023-19-7866	Soc. Sec. # 023-19-7866, HHC, 2nd Batt., 27th Infantry
EMPLOYER	ADDRESS	PHONE

Grade 12, A.P.O., New York, New York 10030	
NAME OF INSURANCE GROUP	SUBSCRIBER

BLUE SHIELD OR BLUE CROSS CERT. NO.	GROUP NO.	CURRENT COVERAGE NO.	EFFECTIVE DATE
CHAMPUS ID Card # 97600		01-01-77	865-04-2311
MEDICAID NO.		EFFECTIVE DATE	Pt's SOC. SEC. NO.
		Exp.Date 1-1-82	

Jane B. Accurate (friend)

REFERRED BY:

DATE	PROGRESS
1-14-77	Pt 45 W ♀ in for complete PE; CC recent URI of 2 wk duration; PND, chest pain & cough; Sweat, chills & sputum c̄ pus X 5 days.
	PH removal of T & A aet 6, UCHD; Para I, D & C aet 41; Surg on OS after accident last yr.
	FH: Father expired c̄ Ca of kidney aet 63; Mother L & W after GB surg.
	PX: Ht 5' 7", Wt 150#, EENT ō except OS opaque; LMP 12-18-77; Chest: Dyspnea & rales, BP 120/80; TPR normal, Abdomen ō. GGE;
	WBC 7,800; RBC 4.2 Prog: NYD. Chest x-rays reveal a cavity c̄ a fluid level. Sputum specimen sent for culture & sensitivity tests.
	Dx: lung abscess. Rx Penicillin G 10 million u/day IV for 4 days. *Brady Coccidioides MD*
1-15-77	Penicillin G 10 million units IV Pt doing well *B C. MD*
1-16-77	Penicillin G 10 million units IV ordered bilateral bronchography *BCMD*
1-17-77	Penicillin G 10 million units IV *B. Coccidioides MD*
1-18-77	Penicillin G 10 million units IV Pt doing well. Few residual shadows on repeat of chest x-ray. PTR in 1 wk. *Brady Coccidioides, MD*

STATEMENT

College Clinic
4567 Broad Avenue
Woodland Hills, XY 12345
013/486-9002

Mrs. Shorty S. Abbreviate
4667 Symbol Road
Woodland Hills, XY 12345

PROCEDURE CODE	DATE	PROFESSIONAL SERVICE	CHARGE		PAID		BALANCE	
	1-14-77	OC, comprehensive	50	00				
		PA, AP & Lat chest x-rays	50	00				
		Sputum culture for single organism (outside lab)	25	00				
		Sensitivity study up to 10 discs	20	00				
		Collection of sputum specimen	3	00				
		Penicillin inj 10 million u	7	00				
	1-15-77	OC, ltd	10	00				
		Penicillin inj 10 million u	7	00				
	1-16-77	OC, ltd	10	00				
		Penicillin inj 10 million u	7	00				
		Bilateral bronchography	50	00				
	1-17-77	OC, ltd	10	00				
		Penicillin inj 10 million u	7	00				
	1-18-77	OC, ltd	10	00				
		Penicillin inj 10 million u	7	00				
		AP & PA chest x-rays	30	00				

Pay last amount in this column

CON - CONSULTATION	HCD - HOUSE CALL (DAY)	LAB - LABORATORY
CPX - COMPLETE PHYS EXAM	HCN - HOUSE CALL (NIGHT)	NC - NO CHARGE
E - EMERGENCY	HV - HOSPITAL VISIT	OC - OFFICE CALL
EC - ERROR CORRECTED	INJ - INJECTION	OS - OFFICE SURGERY
ECG - ELECTROCARDIOGRAM	INS - INSURANCE	SE - SPECIAL EXAM

☆ U. S. GOVERNMENT PRINTING OFFICE: 1970 - 390 - 777

SERVICES AND/OR SUPPLIES PROVIDED BY CIVILIAN SOURCES (EXCEPT HOSPITALS)
CIVILIAN HEALTH AND MEDICAL PROGRAM OF THE UNIFORMED SERVICES (CHAMPUS)

SEE INSTRUCTIONS ON REVERSE

SECTION I *(To be completed by patient or other responsible family member. Please print or type)*

PATIENT DATA	SERVICE MEMBER DATA

1. NAME *(last, first, middle initial)* 2. DATE OF BIRTH

7. NAME OF SPONSOR *(last, first, middle initial)*

3. ADDRESS *(Include Zip Code)*

8 a. SERVICE NUMBER b. SOCIAL SECURITY ACCOUNT NUMBER 9. GRADE

10. ORGANIZATION AND DUTY STATION *(Home Port for Ships) (Address for Retired)*

4. PATIENT IS A *(Check one)*
☐ (1) SPOUSE ☐ (2) DAUGHTER ☐ (3) SON ☐ (4) RETIREE

5. IDENTIFICATION CARD *(DD Form 1173, DD Form 2 or PHS Form 1866—3)*
CARD NO.
EFFECTIVE DATE MONTH DAY YEAR
EXPIRATION DATE

11. SPONSOR'S OR RETIREE'S BRANCH OF SERVICE
☐ (1) USA ☐ (2) USAF ☐ (3) USMC ☐ (4) USN
☐ (5) USCG ☐ (6) USPHS ☐ (7) ESSA

6. BASIS FOR CARE - ACTIVE DUTY DEPENDENTS ONLY *(Check one)*
☐ (1) RESIDING APART FROM SPONSOR ☐ (2) RESIDING WITH SPONSOR DD FORM 1251 ATTACHED ☐ (3) OUTPATIENT
☐ (4) OTHER *(Specify)*

12. STATUS
☐ (1) ACTIVE DUTY ☐ (2) RETIRED ☐ (3) DECEASED

13. CERTIFICATION
I certify to the best of my knowledge and belief the above information in Section I is correct. To the extent that I have authority to do so I hereby authorize the release of medical records in this case to both the contractor and the Government.
If a RETIRED MEMBER or dependent of a retired or deceased member, I certify that to the best of my knowledge and belief, that *(Check appropriate box)* *(Delete portion in parenthesis not applicable)*

☐ (I am not) (the patient is not) enrolled (neither is sponsor) in any other insurance, medical service, or health plan provided by law or through employment.

☐ (I am) (the patient is) enrolled (so is sponsor) in another insurance, medical service, or health plan provided by law or through employment; however the particular benefits claimed on this form are not payable under the other plan.

Name (print or type) (Relationship to Patient) Date Signature

SECTION II *(To be completed by Source of Care)*

14. NAME AND ADDRESS OF SOURCE OF CARE *(Include Zip Code)*

a. SOURCE OF CARE LOCATION CODE

b. PROVIDER OF SERVICES
☐ (1) ATTENDING PHYSICIAN
☐ (2) OTHER *(Specify)*

c. PATIENT STATUS
☐ (1) INPATIENT
☐ (2) OUTPATIENT

15. NAME AND TITLE OF INDIVIDUAL ORDERING CARE

16. INCLUSIVE DATES OF CARE
FROM MONTH DAY YEAR TO MONTH DAY YEAR

17. DIAGNOSIS *(Use standard nomenclature)*

a. INTL STAT CODE

(Check when applicable) ☐ services were necessary for treatment of a bonafide medical emergency

b. 12 - BREAK CODE

18. RELATED HOSPITALIZATION *(If applicable)*
FROM TO

19. ENTER ESTIMATED OR ACTUAL DATE OF DELIVERY IN MATERNITY CASES. LIST BY DATE SURGICAL OPERATIONS AND/OR CARE FURNISHED INCLUDING VISITS FOR WHICH SEPARATE CHARGES ARE CLAIMED *(Type or print)* *(Attach additional sheets if required)*

DATE(S) OF SERVICE	a. ITEM OR DESCRIPTION OF SERVICE	b. CHARGES	c. PROCEDURE CODE
		$	

d. TOTAL CHARGES THIS STATEMENT FOR CARE AUTHORIZED		$	
e. (PAID BY) OR (DUE FROM) PATIENT *(Cross out one)*		$	
f. DUE FROM GOVERNMENT TO SOURCE OF CARE		$	
g. DUE PATIENT OR SPONSOR, REIMBURSEMENT		$	

20. CERTIFICATION BY SOURCE OF CARE
I certify that the services and / or supplies listed hereon were performed or authorized by the attending physician, dentist or other professional personnel in charge, that payment due from the Government has not been received, and that, except for the amount payable by the patient in accordance with the terms of the Civilian Health and Medical Program of the Uniformed Services, the amount paid by the Government will be accepted as payment in full for the authorized services and / or supplies listed hereon.
I further certify that I am not an intern, resident or otherwise in training status for which I am receiving compensation for services listed on this claim.

Name (print or type) Title Date Signature

The persons signing this form are advised that the willful making of a false or fraudulent statement herein renders them liable to prosecution under applicable Federal Laws.

DA FORM 1 JUN 67 1863 - 2 (Civilian Sources) REPLACES DA FORM 1863 - 2, 1 SEP 61, WHICH IS OBSOLETE. Form Approved Comptroller General, U. S., 22 Sep 67

1

Chapter 8:
Unemployment Compensation Disability

ASSIGNMENT 20

1. To familiarize you with what information the employee must furnish, this assignment will encompass completing both the *Claim Statement of Employee* and the *Doctor's Certificate*. Mr. Broussard is applying for state disability benefits and he does not receive sick leave pay from his employer. Date the Claim Statement of Employee November 5 and date the Doctor's Certificate November 10. Remember that this is not a claim for payment to the physician, so no ledger card has been furnished for this patient.

Abbreviations pertinent to this record:

exam _____ retn _____

hosp _____ rt _____

imp _____ SLR _____

lt _____ wk _____

pt _____ WNL _____

ASSIGNMENT 21

1. Let us assume that the Claim Statement of Employee has been completed satisfactorily by Mr. Fred E. Thorndike. Complete the *Doctor's Certificate* portion of the First Claim Form and date it December 2. In completing this portion of the assignment look at only the first entry made by Dr. Practon on November 25.

2. Mr. Thorndike returns to see Dr. Practon on December 7, at which time his disability needs to be extended. Complete the *Physician's Supplementary Certificate* by referring to the entry made during the second visit and date the Certificate December 7. Remember that this is not a claim for payment to the physician, so no ledger card has been furnished for this patient.

Abbreviations pertinent to this record:

Dx _____ SD _____

PE _____ slt _____

Pt _____ wk _____

reg _____ wks _____

PATIENT RECORD

Broussard,	Jeff	L.	03-09-32	M	013/466-2490
LAST NAME	FIRST NAME	MIDDLE NAME	BIRTH DATE	SEX	HOME PHONE

3577 Plain Street,	Woodland Hills,	XY	12345
ADDRESS	CITY	STATE	ZIP CODE

carpenter Payroll # 2156	Ace Construction Company
PATIENT'S OCCUPATION	NAME OF COMPANY

4556 West Eighth Street,	Dorland, XY 12347	013/477-8900
ADDRESS OF EMPLOYER		PHONE

Harriet M. Broussard	secretary
SPOUSE	OCCUPATION

Merit Accounting Co.	6743 Main St., Woodland Hills, XY 12345	013/478-0980
EMPLOYER	ADDRESS	PHONE

Blue Cross	Jeff L. Broussard
NAME OF INSURANCE GROUP	SUBSCRIBER

466-23-9979	82098-A	6131	1-1-75
BLUE SHIELD OR BLUE CROSS CERT. NO.	GROUP NO.	CURRENT COVERAGE NO.	EFFECTIVE DATE
			566-12-0090
MEDICARE NO.	MEDICAID NO.	EFFECTIVE DATE	SOC. SEC. NO.

Harold B. Hartburn (friend)
REFERRED BY:

DATE	PROGRESS
10-21-77	On 8-15-77 after swinging a golf club, pt had sudden onset of severe pain in low back with radiation to lt side. Pt unable to work on 8-16 but resumed wk on 8-17 and has been working full time but doing no lifting while working. Exam showed SLR strongly positive on lt, on rt causes pain into lt side. Neurological exam WNL. *Raymond Skelton, MD*
10-29-77	10 a.m. Pt admitted to College Hosp. Myelogram ordered. *RS MD*
10-30-77	Myelogram showed huge defect L4-5 on lt. Imp: acute herniated disc L4-5 on lt. *Raymond Skelton, MD*
11-1-77	Operation: Lumbar laminectomy & disc excision L4-5. Pt seen daily in hosp. *Raymond Skelton, MD*
11-10-77	3 p.m. Discharged to home. Will retn to wk 12-15-77. *Raymond Skelton, MD*

CLAIM STATEMENT OF EMPLOYEE

COMPLETE *ALL* ITEMS. IF INCOMPLETE, THIS FORM WILL BE RETURNED, CAUSING A DELAY IN BENEFIT PAYMENTS.

1. Print your full name:

Mr.	FIRST	INITIAL	LAST
Mrs.			
Miss			
Ms.			

Your mailing address:
STREET ADDRESS, P.O. OR R.F.D.   APT. NO.   CITY OR TOWN   STATE & ZIP CODE

Your home address: (if different from mailing address)
STREET ADDRESS, P.O. OR R.F.D.   APT. NO.   CITY OR TOWN   STATE & ZIP CODE

Male ☐   Female ☐   Year of birth _____

2. IMPORTANT: Enter Your Social Security Account Number

3. What was the first *full* day you were too sick to work even if it was a Saturday, Sunday, holiday, or normal day off?   MONTH   DATE   YEAR

4. What was the last day you worked BEFORE THIS DISABILITY?   MONTH   DATE   YEAR

5. Employer's Business Name:

Employer's Business Address: NUMBER AND STREET   CITY   STATE & ZIP CODE

6. Your occupation with this employer: Your Badge or Payroll number:

Were you an employer or self-employed individual?   Yes ☐   No ☐

Did you work more than 14 days during your last period of employment which ended on the date shown in item (4) above?   Yes ☐   No ☐

Did you stop work because of sickness or injury? If "NO," please give reason: Yes ☐   No ☐

Has your employer continued or will he continue your pay, by means of sick leave, vacation, pension, gift or other means?   Yes ☐   No ☐

7. Was this disability caused by your work? If "YES," describe HOW: Yes ☐   No ☐

Are you claiming or receiving Workers' Compensation Benefits for *any* on-the-job injuries or illnesses during the period covered by this claim?   Yes ☐   No ☐

8. Have you recovered from your disability?   MONTH   DATE   YEAR   Yes ☐   No ☐
If "YES," enter date of recovery:

9. Have you returned to work for any day, part time or full time after the date shown in item (3) above?   Yes ☐   No ☐
If "YES," please enter such dates:

FOR DEPARTMENT USE ONLY

Office: 2

Comp:

2503 B

2501 H

5006

By

10. I hereby claim benefits and certify that for the period covered by this claim I was unemployed and disabled, that the foregoing statements including any accompanying statements are to the best of my knowledge and belief true, correct and complete. I hereby further authorize my attending physician, practitioner or hospital to furnish and disclose all facts concerning my physical condition that are within his knowledge.

Claim signed on: MONTH   DATE   YEAR   Claimant's signature: (DO NOT PRINT)   TELEPHONE NUMBER

Under Section 2101 of the California Unemployment Insurance Code, it is a misdemeanor wilfully to make a false statement or knowingly to conceal a material fact in order to obtain the payment of any benefits, such misdemeanor being punishable by imprisonment not exceeding six months or by a fine not exceeding $500 or both.

If your signature is made by mark (X) it must be attested by two witnesses with their addresses
SIGNATURE – WITNESS   SIGNATURE – WITNESS
ADDRESS   ADDRESS

If an authorized agent is filing for benefits in the claimant's behalf, a DE 2522 "Appointment of Representative for INCAPACITATED Claimant," must accompany this claim form. When a Form DE 2522 is used, the representative must complete item 10, above, by signing the claimant's name followed by the representative's signature. (Form DE 2522 is available at any department office.)

FOLD ON THIS LINE   FOLD ON THIS LINE

MOISTEN GLUE AND FOLD UP ON THIS LINE
PLEASE DO NOT STAPLE

DOCTOR'S CERTIFICATE

Certification may be made by a licensed physician and surgeon, osteopath, chiropractor, dentist, podiatrist, optometrist, or an authorized medical officer of a United States Government facility. All items on this sheet must be completed.

SAMPLE

11. I attended the patient for his present medical problem from: MONTH   DAY   YEAR   To   MONTH   DAY   YEAR   At intervals of: _____

12. History: _____

(State the nature, severity and the bodily extent of the incapacitating disease or injury.)

Findings: _____

Diagnosis: _____

13. Diagnosis confirmed by X-ray or other tests?   YES ☐   NO ☐   Findings: _____

14. Is this patient now pregnant or has she been pregnant since the date of treatment as reported above?   YES ☐   NO ☐   If "Yes," date pregnancy terminated or future EDC:

Is the maternity care routine?   YES ☐   NO ☐   If "No," state nature and severity of *maternal* pathology:

15. Operation: Performed [_____] (ENTER DATE)   Type of operation:

To be performed [_____]

16. Has the patient at any time during your attendance for this medical problem, been incapable of performing his regular work?   YES ☐   NO ☐   If "Yes," his disability commenced on:

17. APPROXIMATE date, in your opinion, disability (if any) should end or has ended sufficiently to permit patient to resume his regular or customary work. Even if considerable question exists, make SOME "estimate". This is a requirement of the Code, and the claim will be delayed if such date is not entered. Such answers as "Indefinite" or "don't know" will not suffice.   (ENTER DATE) [_____]

18. In your opinion, is this disability the result of "occupation" either as an "industrial accident" or as an "occupational disease"?   YES ☐   NO ☐   (This should include aggravation of pre-existing conditions by occupation)

19. Have you reported this OR A CONCURRENT DISABILITY to any insurance carrier as a Workers' Compensation Claim?   YES ☐   NO ☐   If "Yes," to whom? (Name of carrier or firm)

20. Further comments (if indicated): _____

21. In what HOSPITAL was or is patient confined as a registered bed patient?   Hospital name and address: _____ Zip code

22. **Date** and **hour** entered as a registered bed patient and discharged from such Hospital pursuant to your orders:

ENTERED	STILL CONFINED	DISCHARGED
on , 19 , at A.M. P.M.	on , 19	on , 19 , at A.M. P.M.

23. I hereby certify that the above statements in my opinion truly describe the patient's disability (if any) and the estimated duration thereof, and that I am a _____ (TYPE OF DOCTOR) licensed to practice by the State of _____

_____ PRINT OR TYPE DOCTOR'S NAME   _____ SIGNATURE OF ATTENDING DOCTOR

_____ NO. AND STREET   CITY   ZIP CODE   _____ STATE LICENSE NUMBER   TELEPHONE NO.   DATE OF SIGNING THIS FORM

PATIENT RECORD

Thorndike,	Fred	E.	02-17-34	M	013/465-7820
LAST NAME	FIRST NAME	MIDDLE NAME	BIRTH DATE	SEX	HOME PHONE

5784 Helen Street,	Woodland Hills,	XY	12345
ADDRESS	CITY	STATE	ZIP CODE

salesman	Payroll No. 6852	Easy On Paint Company
PATIENT'S OCCUPATION		NAME OF COMPANY

4586 West 20th Street, Woodland Hills, XY 12345	013/467-8898
ADDRESS OF EMPLOYER	PHONE

Jennifer B. Thorndike	housewife
SPOUSE OR PARENT	OCCUPATION

EMPLOYER	ADDRESS	PHONE

Pacific Mutual Insurance Co.	Fred E. Thorndike
NAME OF INSURANCE GROUP	SUBSCRIBER

120 So. Main Street, Merck, XY 12346	Group # 6709		1-9-75
BLUE SHIELD OR BLUE CROSS CERT. NO.	GROUP NO.	CURRENT COVERAGE NO.	EFFECTIVE DATE

			549-23-8721
MEDICARE NO.	MEDICAID NO.	EFFECTIVE DATE	SOC. SEC. NO.

John Diehl (friend)
REFERRED BY:

DATE	PROGRESS
11-25-77	On or about 11-3-77 pt began to have chest pain & much coughing. On 11-24-77 pt too ill to work & decided to file for SD benefits. Pt states illness is not work connected & he does not receive sick leave pay PE: Pt examined & complained of productive cough of 3 wks duration & chest pain. Chest xrays confirmed dx - bronchitis. Pt will be capable of returning to wk 12/8/77 Gerald Practon MD
12-7-77	Pt complains of recurring chest pain & slt cough. Will extend disability to 12/15/77 at which time pt can resume reg work. No complications anticipated. Gerald Practon, MD

DOCTOR'S CERTIFICATE

Certification may be made by a licensed physician and surgeon, osteopath, chiropractor, dentist, podiatrist, optometrist, or an authorized medical officer of a United States Government facility. All items on this sheet must be completed.

SAMPLE

11. I attended the patient for his present medical problem from: _MONTH DAY YEAR_ To _MONTH DAY YEAR_ At intervals of: _____

12. History: _____

(State the nature, severity and the bodily extent of the incapacitating disease or injury.)

Findings: _____

Diagnosis: _____

13. Diagnosis confirmed by X-ray or other tests? YES ☐ NO ☐ Findings: _____

14. Is this patient now pregnant or has she been pregnant since the date of treatment as reported above? YES ☐ NO ☐ If "Yes," date pregnancy terminated or future EDC:

Is the maternity care routine? YES ☐ NO ☐ If "No," state nature and severity of *maternal* pathology:

15. Operation: Performed [_____ (ENTER DATE)] Type of operation:
To be performed [_____]

16. Has the patient at any time during your attendance for this medical problem, been incapable of performing his regular work? YES ☐ NO ☐ If "Yes," his disability commenced on:

17. APPROXIMATE date, in your opinion, disability (if any) should end or has ended sufficiently to permit patient to resume his regular or customary work. Even if considerable question exists, make SOME "estimate". This is a requirement of the Code, and the claim will be delayed if such date is not entered. Such answers as "Indefinite" or "don't know" will not suffice. (ENTER DATE) [_____]

18. In your opinion, is this disability the result of "occupation" either as an "industrial accident" or as an "occupational disease"? YES ☐ NO ☐ (This should include aggravation of pre-existing conditions by occupation)

19. Have you reported this OR A CONCURRENT DISABILITY to any insurance carrier as a Workers' Compensation Claim? YES ☐ NO ☐ If "Yes," to whom? (Name of carrier or firm)

20. Further comments (if indicated): _____

21. In what HOSPITAL was or is patient confined as a registered bed patient? Hospital name and address: _____

Zip code _____

22. **Date** and **hour** entered as a registered bed patient and discharged from such Hospital pursuant to your orders:

ENTERED	STILL CONFINED	DISCHARGED
on _____ , 19 ___ , at ___ A.M. P.M.	on _____ , 19 ___	on _____ , 19 ___ , at ___ A.M. P.M.

23. I hereby certify that the above statements in my opinion truly describe the patient's disability (if any) and the estimated duration thereof, and that I am a _____ (TYPE OF DOCTOR) licensed to practice by the State of _____

_____
PRINT OR TYPE DOCTOR'S NAME

_____
SIGNATURE OF ATTENDING DOCTOR

_____
NO. AND STREET   CITY   ZIP CODE

_____
STATE LICENSE NUMBER   TELEPHONE NO.   DATE OF SIGNING THIS FORM

PHYSICIAN'S SUPPLEMENTARY CERTIFICATE

File _____ 8721 _____ Patient _Fred E. Thorndike_____ Date Issued _12-6-77_____

1. **To be completed by your present physician ONLY if he finds that you will be unable to work on and beyond the date entered here**___ _December 8,_ _____19 _77_ .

2. Are you still treating patient?_____   Date of last treatment_____19_____.

3. What **complications,** if any, or what **present condition** would tend to make the patient disabled **longer than normally expected** for this type of illness or injury?_____

_____ VOID _____

_____

4. Date patient recovered, or will recover sufficiently (even if under treatment) to be able to perform his regular and customary work
_____19_____.

I hereby certify that the above statements in my opinion truly describe the claimant's condition and the estimated duration thereof.

_____19_____   _____
            Date   Doctor's Signature

DE 2525X Rev. 11 (3-74)

ASSIGNMENT 22

1. Assume that the Claim Statement of Employee has been completed satisfactorily by Mr. James T. Fujita. Complete the *Doctor's Certificate* portion of the First Claim Form and date it December 15. Remember that this is not a claim for payment to the physician, so no ledger card has been furnished for this patient.

Abbreviations pertinent to this record:

exam _____   SD _____

Imp _____   WBC _____

neg _____   wk _____

pt _____

PATIENT RECORD

Fujita,	James	T.	03-27-34	M	013/677-2881
LAST NAME	FIRST NAME	MIDDLE NAME	BIRTH DATE	SEX	HOME PHONE

3538 South A Street, Woodland Hills, XY 12345		
ADDRESS	CITY	STATE ZIP CODE

electrician	Payroll No. 8834	Macy Electric Company
PATIENT'S OCCUPATION		NAME OF COMPANY

2671 North C Street, Woodland Hills, XY 12345	013/677-2346
ADDRESS OF EMPLOYER	PHONE

Mary J. Fujita	housewife
SPOUSE OR PARENT	OCCUPATION

EMPLOYER	ADDRESS	PHONE
Atlantic Mutual Ins. Co.	111 S. Main St.,	James T. Fujita
NAME OF INSURANCE GROUP		SUBSCRIBER

Woodland Hills, XY 12345	Policy # F20015		1-3-76
BLUE SHIELD OR BLUE CROSS CERT. NO.	GROUP NO.	CURRENT COVERAGE NO.	EFFECTIVE DATE

			567-43-8898
MEDICARE NO.	MEDICAID NO.	EFFECTIVE DATE	SOC. SEC. NO.

Cherry Hotta (aunt)
REFERRED BY:

DATE	PROGRESS
12-7-77	Today pt could not go to work & came for exam complaining of pain in abdomen, nausea, no vomiting. Will file for SD benefits. Pt states illness is not work connected & he receives sick leave pay of $50/wk. Exam neg except abdomen showed tenderness all over with voluntary guarding. WBC 10,000. Imp: mesenteric adenitis. Advised strict bed rest at home & bland diet. To return in 1 wk. _Gaston Input MD_
12-15-77	Exam showed normal abdomen. WBC 7,500. Pt will be capable of returning to work 12-22-77. _Gaston Input MD_

DOCTOR'S CERTIFICATE

Certification may be made by a licensed physician and surgeon, osteopath, chiropractor, dentist, podiatrist, optometrist, or an authorized medical officer of a United States Government facility. All items on this sheet must be completed.

11. I attended the patient for his present medical problem from: MONTH   DAY   YEAR   To   MONTH   DAY   YEAR   At intervals of:

12. History: _____

(State the nature, severity and the bodily extent of the incapacitating disease or injury.)

Findings: _____

Diagnosis: _____

13. Diagnosis confirmed by X-ray or other tests?   YES ☐   NO ☐   Findings:

14. Is this patient now pregnant or has she been pregnant since the date of treatment as reported above?   YES ☐   NO ☐   If "Yes," date pregnancy terminated or future EDC:

   Is the maternity care routine?   YES ☐   NO ☐   If "No," state nature and severity of *maternal* pathology:

15. Operation: Performed ☐ (ENTER DATE)   Type of operation:
   To be performed ☐

16. Has the patient at any time during your attendance for this medical problem, been incapable of performing his regular work?   YES ☐   NO ☐   If "Yes," his disability commenced on:

17. APPROXIMATE date, in your opinion, disability (if any) should end or has ended sufficiently to permit patient to resume his regular or customary work. Even if considerable question exists, make SOME "estimate". This is a requirement of the Code, and the claim will be delayed if such date is not entered. Such answers as "Indefinite" or "don't know" will not suffice.   (ENTER DATE)

18. In your opinion, is this disability the result of "occupation" either as an "industrial accident" or as an "occupational disease"?
   YES ☐   NO ☐   (This should include aggravation of pre-existing conditions by occupation)

19. Have you reported this OR A CONCURRENT DISABILITY to any insurance carrier as a Workers' Compensation Claim?
   YES ☐   NO ☐   If "Yes," to whom? (Name of carrier or firm)

20. Further comments (if indicated): _____

21. In what HOSPITAL was or is patient confined as a registered bed patient?   Hospital name and address:

   Zip code

22. **Date** and **hour** entered as a registered bed patient and discharged from such Hospital pursuant to your orders:

ENTERED		STILL CONFINED	DISCHARGED	
on , 19 , at	A.M. P.M.	on , 19	on , 19 , at	A.M. P.M.

23. I hereby certify that the above statements in my opinion truly describe the patient's disability (if any) and the estimated duration thereof, and that I am a_____ licensed to practice by the State of _____
   (TYPE OF DOCTOR)

_____   _____
PRINT OR TYPE DOCTOR'S NAME   SIGNATURE OF ATTENDING DOCTOR

_____   _____
NO. AND STREET   CITY   ZIP CODE   STATE LICENSE NUMBER   TELEPHONE NO.   DATE OF SIGNING THIS FORM

ASSIGNMENT 23

1. Mr. Jake J. Burrows has previously applied for state disability benefits. After two months he is referred to another doctor for further care. Complete the form and date it July 25. You will notice that this form is almost identical to the Doctor's Certificate and is mailed to the claimant to secure the certification of a new physician or to clarify a specific claimed period of disability. In completing this part of the assignment look at only the first three entries on the Patient Record.

2. Complete the *Request for Additional Medical Information Form* by looking at the last entry made on Mr. Burrows' record and date the report August 15. Remember that this is not a claim for payment to the physician, so no ledger card has been furnished for this patient.

Abbreviations pertinent to this record:

approx _____ Imp _____

C 5/6 _____ Pt _____

exam _____ retn _____

hosp _____ c̄ _____

ASSIGNMENT 24

1. Mr. Vincent P. Michael is applying for state disability benefits. Complete the *Doctor's Certificate* portion of the form and date it September 21. Assume that the Claim Statement of Employee has been completed satisfactorily by Mr. Michael. Remember that this is not a claim for payment to the physician, so no ledger card has been furnished for this patient.

Abbreviations pertinent to this record:

approx _____ Imp _____

CVA _____ mm _____

ESR _____ pt _____

L _____ retn _____

hr _____ wk _____

PATIENT RECORD

Burrows,	Jake	J.	04-26-30	M	013/478-9009
LAST NAME	FIRST NAME	MIDDLE NAME	BIRTH DATE	SEX	HOME PHONE

319 Barry Street,	Woodland Hills,	XY	12345
ADDRESS	CITY	STATE	ZIP CODE

assembler	Convac Electronics Company
PATIENT'S OCCUPATION	NAME OF COMPANY

3440 West 7th Street, Woodland Hills, XY 12345	013/467-9008
ADDRESS OF EMPLOYER	PHONE

Jane B. Burrows	housewife
SPOUSE OR PARENT	OCCUPATION

EMPLOYER	ADDRESS	PHONE

Blue Shield	Jake J. Burrows
NAME OF INSURANCE GROUP	SUBSCRIBER

T8471811A	585537AT		1-1-76
BLUE SHIELD OR BLUE CROSS CERT. NO.	GROUP NO.	CURRENT COVERAGE NO.	EFFECTIVE DATE

			457-99-0801
MEDICARE NO.	MEDICAID NO.	EFFECTIVE DATE	SOC. SEC. NO.

Clarence Butler, M. D. 300 Sixth Avenue, Woodland Hills, XY 12345
REFERRED BY:

DATE	PROGRESS
6-2-77	Pt referred by Dr. Butler. Pt states on 4-19-77 was wrestling $\bar{c}$ son and jerked his neck the wrong way. 2 days later had much pain & muscle spasm cervical region. X-rays show degenerated disc C5/6. Exam - limited range of neck motion & limited abduction both shoulders. Imp: Degenerated cervical disc C5/6. Pt to be hospitalized. Myelogram ordered. *R Skelton MD*
7-24-77 9:00 a.m.	Pt hospitalized at College Hosp. Myelogram positive at C5/6 Scheduled for surgery. *Raymond Skelton MD*
7-25-77	Disc excision & anterior cervical fusion at C5/6. Pt will remain in hosp. indefinitely. Approx date of retn to work 11-1-77. *RS MD*
8-15-77	Pt is being seen monthly. Has some restriction of cervical motion. No muscle spasm. Very little cervical pain. To retn to work 11-1-77. *Raymond Skelton MD*

MOISTEN GLUE AND FOLD UP ON THIS LINE
PLEASE DO NOT STAPLE

SAMPLE

In order that any disability insurance to which you may be entitled may be paid without undue delay, please have the physician who treats or treated you during the period indicated below complete this form and return it to us at his earliest convenience.

Henry B. Garcia
Claims Examiner

6-2 thru 7-25-77   0801
Period Dates   File No.

1. I attended the patient for his present medical problem from:

Month   Day   Year   Month   Day   Year   At intervals of:
To

2. History:

(State the nature, severity and the bodily extent of the incapacitating disease or injury)

Findings:

Diagnosis:

3. Diagnosis confirmed by X-ray or other tests?   Yes ☐   No ☐   Findings:

4. Is this patient now pregnant or has she been pregnant since the date of treatment as reported above?   Yes ☐   No ☐   If "Yes", date pregnancy Terminated or future EDC:

Is the maternity care routine?   Yes ☐   No ☐   If "No", state nature and severity of maternal pathology:

5. Operation: Performed [   ]   Type of Operation:
                 (Enter Date)
To be performed [   ]

6. Has the patient at any time during your attendance for this medical problem, been incapable of performing his regular work?   Yes ☐   No ☐   If "Yes", his disability commenced on:

7. APPROXIMATE date, in your opinion, disability (if any) should end or has ended sufficiently to permit patient to resume his regular or customary work. Even if considerable question exists, make SOME "estimate". This is a requirement of the Code, and the claim will be delayed if such date is not entered. Such answers as "Indefinite" or "Don't know" will not suffice.   (Enter Date)

8. In your opinion, is this disability the result of "occupation" either as an "Industrial accident" or as an "occupational disease"? (This should include aggravation of pre-existing conditions by occupation)   Yes ☐   No ☐

9. Have you reported this OR A CONCURRENT DISABILITY to any insurance carrier as a Workmen's Compensation Claim?   Yes ☐   No ☐   If "Yes", to whom? (Name of carrier or firm)

10. Further comments (if indicated):

11. In what HOSPITAL was or is patient confined as a registered bed patient?   Hospital name and address:

Zip Code

12. Date and hour entered as a registered bed patient and discharged from such Hospital pursuant to your orders:

ENTERED		STILL CONFINED	DISCHARGED	
on , 19 , at	A.M. P.M.	on , 19	on , 19 , at	A.M. P.M.

13. I hereby certify that the above statements in my opinion truly describe the patient's disability (if any) and the estimated duration thereof, and that I am a _____ licensed to practice by the State of _____
(TYPE OF DOCTOR)

_____   _____
PRINT OR TYPE DOCTOR'S NAME   SIGNATURE OF ATTENDING DOCTOR

NO. AND STREET   CITY   ZIP CODE   STATE LICENSE NO.   TELEPHONE NO.   DATE OF SIGNING THIS FORM

Certification may be made by a licensed physician and surgeon, osteopath, chiropractor, dentist, podiatrist, optometrist, or an authorized medical officer of a United States Government facility. All items on this sheet must be completed.

STATE OF CALIFORNIA
EMPLOYMENT DEVELOPMENT DEPARTMENT

.

REFER TO
↓

0801   – Our File No.
Jake J. Burrows   – Your Patient
                        – Regular Work

SAMPLE

REQUEST FOR ADDITIONAL
MEDICAL INFORMATION

.

Raymond Skelton, M. D.
4567 Broad Avenue
Woodland Hills, XY 12345

.

The original basic information and estimate of duration of your patient's disability
have been carefully evaluated. At the present time, the following additional information based upon the progress and present condition of this patient is requested.
This will assist the Department in determining eligibility for further disability
insurance benefits. Return of the completed form as soon as possible will be appreciated.

D. ALLEN TREAT, M.D., MEDICAL DIRECTOR

CLAIMS EXAMINER   **DOCTOR: PLEASE COMPLETE EITHER PART A OR B. DATE AND SIGN**

PART A   IF YOUR PATIENT HAS RECOVERED SUFFICIENTLY TO BE ABLE TO RETURN TO HIS REGULAR OR
          CUSTOMARY WORK LISTED ABOVE, PLEASE GIVE THE DATE_____19____.

PART B   THIS PART REFERS TO PATIENT WHO IS STILL DISABLED.

          Are you still treating the patient   YES ☐   NO ☐   _____19____.
                                                                  Date of last treatment.

          What are the medical circumstances which continue to make your patient disabled?

          _____

          _____

          _____

          _____

          _____

          What is your present estimate of the date your patient will be able to perform his
          regular or customary work listed above?   Date_____19___

          Further Comments:_____

          _____

          _____

          _____

          Date_____19___   _____
                                                      Doctor's Signature

          ENCLOSED IS A STAMPED PREADDRESSED ENVELOPE FOR YOUR CONVENIENCE
          SE

DE 2547 REV. 13 (12-73)   △ OSP

PATIENT RECORD

Michael,	Vincent	P.	05-17-15	M	013/567-9001
LAST NAME	FIRST NAME	MIDDLE NAME	BIRTH DATE	SEX	HOME PHONE

1529½ Thompson Boulevard,	Woodland Hills,	XY	12345
ADDRESS	CITY	STATE	ZIP CODE

assembler "A"	Burroughs Corporation
PATIENT'S OCCUPATION	NAME OF COMPANY

5411 North Lindero Canyon Road, Woodland Hills, XY 12345	013/560-9008
ADDRESS OF EMPLOYER	PHONE

Helen J. Michael	housewife
SPOUSE OR PARENT	OCCUPATION

EMPLOYER	ADDRESS	PHONE

Blue Shield	Vincent P. Michael
NAME OF INSURANCE GROUP	SUBSCRIBER

T8411981A	677899 AT		1-1-75
BLUE SHIELD OR BLUE CROSS CERT. NO.	GROUP NO.	CURRENT COVERAGE NO.	EFFECTIVE DATE

			562-90-8888
MEDICARE NO.	MEDICAID NO.	EFFECTIVE DATE	SOC. SEC. NO.

Robert T. Smith (friend)
REFERRED BY:

DATE	PROGRESS
9-20-77	Pt complains of having had the flu, headache and of being tired. Pt unable to go to work today. Exam shows weakness of L hand. Hyperreflexia on L. X-ray shows cardiomegaly and slight pulmonary congestion. ESR 46 mm/hr. Imp: Post flu syndrome, transient ischemia attack; possible CVA. Pt to retn in 1 wk. Approx. date to retn to work 10-16-77. *Brady Coccidioides, MD*

DOCTOR'S CERTIFICATE

Certification may be made by a licensed physician and surgeon, osteopath, chiropractor, dentist, podiatrist, optometrist, or an authorized medical officer of a United States Government facility. All items on this sheet must be completed.

11. I attended the patient for his present medical problem from: MONTH   DAY   YEAR   To   MONTH   DAY   YEAR   At intervals of:

12. History:

(State the nature, severity and the bodily extent of the incapacitating disease or injury.)

Findings:

Diagnosis:

13. Diagnosis confirmed by X-ray or other tests?   YES ☐   NO ☐   Findings:

14. Is this patient now pregnant or has she been pregnant since the date of treatment as reported above?   YES ☐   NO ☐   If "Yes," date pregnancy terminated or future EDC:

Is the maternity care routine?   YES ☐   NO ☐   If "No," state nature and severity of *maternal* pathology:

15. Operation: Performed ☐ (ENTER DATE)   Type of operation:
To be performed ☐

16. Has the patient at any time during your attendance for this medical problem, been incapable of performing his regular work?   YES ☐   NO ☐   If "Yes," his disability commenced on:

17. APPROXIMATE date, in your opinion, disability (if any) should end or has ended sufficiently to permit patient to resume his regular or customary work. Even if considerable question exists, make SOME "estimate". This is a requirement of the Code, and the claim will be delayed if such date is not entered. Such answers as "Indefinite" or "don't know" will not suffice.   (ENTER DATE) ☐

18. In your opinion, is this disability the result of "occupation" either as an "industrial accident" or as an "occupational disease"?
YES ☐   NO ☐   (This should include aggravation of pre-existing conditions by occupation)

19. Have you reported this OR A CONCURRENT DISABILITY to any insurance carrier as a Workers' Compensation Claim?
YES ☐   NO ☐   If "Yes," to whom? (Name of carrier or firm)

20. Further comments (if indicated):

21. In what HOSPITAL was or is patient confined as a registered bed patient?   Hospital name and address:

Zip code

22. **Date** and **hour** entered as a registered bed patient and discharged from such Hospital pursuant to your orders:

ENTERED		STILL CONFINED	DISCHARGED	
on , 19 , at	A.M. P.M.	on , 19	on , 19 , at	A.M. P.M.

23. I hereby certify that the above statements in my opinion truly describe the patient's disability (if any) and the estimated duration thereof, and that I am a_____ licensed to practice by the State of _____
(TYPE OF DOCTOR)

_____
PRINT OR TYPE DOCTOR'S NAME

_____
SIGNATURE OF ATTENDING DOCTOR

_____
NO. AND STREET   CITY   ZIP CODE

_____
STATE LICENSE NUMBER   TELEPHONE NO.   DATE OF SIGNING THIS FORM

Chapter 9 :
Workers' Compensation

ASSIGNMENT 25

    1. Complete the *Doctor's First Report of Occupational Injury or Illness* for this nondisability type of claim. Date the form May 24. The ledger card could be photocopied after inserting RVS or CPT code numbers and sent along with the report as a billing statement to the insurance carrier. X-rays would be billed by the hospital as inpatient diagnostic workup.

Abbreviations pertinent to this record:

AP _____	neg _____
apt _____	PD _____
DC _____	Pt _____
Dr _____	reg _____
Ex _____	R/O _____
hosp _____	Tr _____
lat _____	Tx _____
lt _____	♂ _____

ASSIGNMENT 26

    1. Complete the *Doctor's First Report of Occupational Injury or Illness* for this temporary disability type of claim. Date the form November 12. Remember to complete the report using only the information pertinent up to and including November 12, which means referring to only the first two entries on the Patient Record.

    2. Send in a *Surgeon's Report* on December 29 and submit a complete billing in triplicate to the insurance company. Use the patient's Social Security number as the case number. Be sure to include RVS or CPT code numbers for each professional service rendered. Dr. Parkinson is a graduate of Columbia University Medical School, June, 1950.

Abbreviations pertinent to this record:

Cons _____	PT _____
DC _____	qd _____
Dg _____	reg _____
HV _____	R _____
intermed _____	TD _____
OC _____	trt _____
P & S _____	W _____
p.m. _____	

PATIENT RECORD

Hiranuma,	Glen	M.	12-24-25	M	013/467-3383
LAST NAME	FIRST NAME	MIDDLE NAME	BIRTH DATE	SEX	HOME PHONE

4372 Hanley Avenue,	Woodland Hills,	XY	12345
ADDRESS	CITY	STATE	ZIP CODE

house painter		Pittsburgh Paint Co.(commercial paint-
PATIENT'S OCCUPATION		NAME OF COMPANY ing company)

3725 Bonfeld Avenue, Woodland Hills, XY 12345	013/486-9070
ADDRESS OF EMPLOYER	PHONE

Esme M. Hiranuma	housewife
SPOUSE OR PARENT	OCCUPATION

EMPLOYER	ADDRESS	PHONE

State Compensation Ins.Fund 14156 Magnolia Blvd.,Torres,XY 12349

NAME OF INSURANCE GROUP		SUBSCRIBER

Policy # 016-2432-211

BLUE SHIELD OR BLUE CROSS CERT. NO.	GROUP NO.	CURRENT COVERAGE NO.	EFFECTIVE DATE
			558-40-9960

MEDICARE NO.	MEDICAID NO.	EFFECTIVE DATE	SOC. SEC. NO.

Pittsburgh Paint Co.

REFERRED BY:

DATE	PROGRESS
5-22-77	At 9:30 a.m. this ♂ pt was painting an apt ceiling. Pt slipped & fell from ladder & hit lt side of body. Apt located at 3540 W. 87 St., Woodland Hills, XY 12345. Pt notified employer immediately. Taken to College Hosp where x-rays of lt hip, lt femur, & cervical spine were taken (2 views ea AP & Lat)--all neg. (Dr. was called to hosp at request of employer & saw pt at 5 p.m.) Ex & Tr for abrasions, multiple contusions & sprain of lt shoulder. Pt to be kept in hosp to R/O head trauma & will be DC 5-27-77. No PD expected. No further Tx after DC from hosp. Pt will resume reg work 6-1-77. *Gerald Procton, M.D.*

STATEMENT

College Clinic
4567 Broad Avenue
Woodland Hills, XY 12345
013/486-9002

State Compensation Ins. Fund
14156 Magnolia Boulevard
Torres, XY 12349

DATE	PROFESSIONAL SERVICE	CHARGE	PAID	BALANCE
	Re: Inj: Glen M. Hiranuma			
	Date of Inj: 5-22-77			
	Emp: Pittsburgh Paint Co.			
5-22-77	Hosp exam & initial treatment	50 00		

Pay last amount in this column

CON - CONSULTATION	HCD - HOUSE CALL (DAY)	LAB - LABORATORY
CPX - COMPLETE PHYS EXAM	HCN - HOUSE CALL (NIGHT)	NC - NO CHARGE
E - EMERGENCY	HV - HOSPITAL VISIT	OC - OFFICE CALL
EC - ERROR CORRECTED	INJ - INJECTION	OS - OFFICE SURGERY
ECG - ELECTROCARDIOGRAM	INS - INSURANCE	SE - SPECIAL EXAM

DOCTOR'S FIRST REPORT
OF
OCCUPATIONAL INJURY OR ILLNESS

STATE OF CALIFORNIA
AGRICULTURE AND SERVICES AGENCY
DEPARTMENT OF INDUSTRIAL RELATIONS
DIVISION OF LABOR STATISTICS AND RESEARCH
P. O. Box 965, San Francisco, Calif. 94101

Immediately after first examination mail one copy **directly** to the Division of Labor Statistics and Research. Failure to file a report with the Division is a misdemeanor. (Labor Code Section 6413.5) Answer all questions fully.

☞ **A. INSURANCE CARRIER**

Do not write in this space

1. **EMPLOYER**
2. Address (No., St. & City)
3. Business (Manufacturing shoes, building construction, retailing men's clothes, etc.)

4. **EMPLOYEE** (First name, middle initial, last name) .... Soc. Sec. No.
5. Address (No., St. & City)
6. Occupation .... Age .... Sex
7. Date injured .... Hour .... M. Date last worked
8. Injured at (No., St. & City) .... County
9. Date of your first examination .... Hour .... M. Who engaged your services?
10. Name other doctors who treated employee for this injury

11. **ACCIDENT OR EXPOSURE:** Did employee notify employer of this injury? .... Employee's statement of cause of injury or illness:

12. **NATURE AND EXTENT OF INJURY OR DISEASE** (Include all objective findings, subjective complaints, and diagnoses. If occupational disease state date of onset, occupational history, and exposures.)

13. X-rays: By whom taken? (State if none)
    Findings:

14. Treatment:

15. Kind of case (Office, home or hospital) .... If hospitalized, date .... Estimated stay
    Name and address of hospital
16. Further treatment (Estimated frequency and duration)
17. Estimated period of disability for: Regular work .... Modified work
18. Describe any permanent disability or disfigurement expected (State if none)

19. If death ensued, give date
20. **REMARKS** (Note any pre-existing injuries or diseases, need for special examination or laboratory tests, other pertinent information.)

SAMPLE

Name .... Degree .... [PERSONAL SIGNATURE OF DOCTOR]
(Type or print)

Date of report .... Address (No., St. & City)

FORM 5021 (REV. 1) .... *Use reverse side if more space required* .... D OSP

PATIENT RECORD

Giovanni,	Carlos	A.	10-24-45	M	013/677-3485
LAST NAME	FIRST NAME	MIDDLE NAME	BIRTH DATE	SEX	HOME PHONE

89 Beaumont Court,	Woodland Hills,	XY	12345
ADDRESS	CITY	STATE	ZIP CODE

TV repairman	Giant Television Co. (tv repair co)
PATIENT'S OCCUPATION	NAME OF COMPANY

8764 Ocean Avenue, Woodland Hills, XY 12345	013/627-8851
ADDRESS OF EMPLOYER	PHONE

Maria B. Giovanni	housewife
SPOUSE OR PARENT	OCCUPATION

EMPLOYER	ADDRESS	PHONE
State Compensation Ins.Fund 600 S. Lafayette Park Pl., Ehrlich, XY 12350		
NAME OF INSURANCE GROUP	SUBSCRIBER	

Policy # 57780

BLUE SHIELD OR BLUE CROSS CERT. NO.	GROUP NO.	CURRENT COVERAGE NO.	EFFECTIVE DATE
			556-48-9699

MEDICARE NO.	MEDICAID NO.	EFFECTIVE DATE	SOC. SEC. NO.

Giant Television Co.
REFERRED BY:

DATE	PROGRESS
11-11-77	Today at 2 PM Pt was thrown from roof of private home (2231 Duarte St. Woodland Hills XY 12345, in Woodland Hills County) states "when I was attaching the base of an antenna, the weight of the antenna shifted & threw me off the roof". Saw Pt at College Hosp at 5 PM as inpatient. Pt was referred by employer Dg: x-rays - fractured skull. Pt also suffered cerebral concussion + R subdural hematoma A Parkinson MD
11-12-77	Performed R frontal parietal craniotomy & removed subdural hematoma Pt will be seen qd. TD: pt will be disabled until 1-1-78. Possible cranial defect & head disfigurement resulting. Pt to be hospitalized for approx 2 wks for further tr. Astro Parkinson MD
11-14-77	PT seen in cons by Dr. Cosmo Graff who stated unable to correct cranial defect. APMD
11-30-77	DC from hosp. Permanent cranial defect resulting from surgery. APMD
12-29-77	No further trt necessary. PT able to resume reg W on 1-15-78 Case P & S. Astro Parkinson MD

STATEMENT

College Clinic
4567 Broad Avenue
Woodland Hills, XY 12345
013/486-9002

State Compensation Insurance Fund
600 South Lafayette Park Place
Ehrlich, XY 12350

DATE	PROFESSIONAL SERVICE	CHARGE		PAID		BALANCE	
	Re: Inj: Carlos A. Giovanni						
	Date of Inj: 11-11-77						
	Emp: Giant Television Co.						
11-11-77	HV, intermed	30	00				
11-12-77	Craniotomy remove subdural						
	hematoma	600	00				
11-13 thru 11-30-77	HV brief	NC					
12-29-77	OC, intermed	NC					

Pay last amount in this column

CON - CONSULTATION	HCD - HOUSE CALL (DAY)	LAB - LABORATORY
CPX - COMPLETE PHYS EXAM	HCN - HOUSE CALL (NIGHT)	NC - NO CHARGE
E - EMERGENCY	HV - HOSPITAL VISIT	OC - OFFICE CALL
EC - ERROR CORRECTED	INJ - INJECTION	OS - OFFICE SURGERY
ECG - ELECTROCARDIOGRAM	INS - INSURANCE	SE - SPECIAL EXAM

DOCTOR'S FIRST REPORT
OF
OCCUPATIONAL INJURY OR ILLNESS

STATE OF CALIFORNIA
AGRICULTURE AND SERVICES AGENCY
DEPARTMENT OF INDUSTRIAL RELATIONS
DIVISION OF LABOR STATISTICS AND RESEARCH
P. O. Box 965, San Francisco, Calif. 94101

Immediately after first examination mail one copy **directly** to the Division of Labor Statistics and Research. Failure to file a report with the Division is a misdemeanor. (Labor Code Section 6413.5) Answer all questions fully.

A. INSURANCE CARRIER

Do not write in this space

1. **EMPLOYER**
2. Address (No., St. & City)
3. Business (Manufacturing shoes, building construction, retailing men's clothes, etc.)

4. **EMPLOYEE** (First name, middle initial, last name) Soc. Sec. No.
5. Address (No., St. & City)
6. Occupation Age Sex
7. Date injured Hour M. Date last worked
8. Injured at (No., St. & City) County
9. Date of your first examination Hour M. Who engaged your services?
10. Name other doctors who treated employee for this injury

11. **ACCIDENT OR EXPOSURE:** Did employee notify employer of this injury? Employee's statement of cause of injury or illness:

12. **NATURE AND EXTENT OF INJURY OR DISEASE** (Include all objective findings, subjective complaints, and diagnoses. If occupational disease state date of onset, occupational history, and exposures.)

13. X-rays: By whom taken? (State if none)
Findings:

14. Treatment:

15. Kind of case (Office, home or hospital) If hospitalized, date Estimated stay
Name and address of hospital
16. Further treatment (Estimated frequency and duration)
17. Estimated period of disability for: Regular work Modified work
18. Describe any permanent disability or disfigurement expected (State if none)

19. If death ensued, give date

20. **REMARKS** (Note any pre-existing injuries or diseases, need for special examination or laboratory tests, other pertinent information.)

SAMPLE

Name Degree [PERSONAL SIGNATURE OF DOCTOR]
(Type or print)
Date of report Address (No., St. & City)

FORM 5021 (REV. 1) *Use reverse side if more space required* D OSP

STANDARD FORM FOR

SURGEON'S REPORT

INDUSTRIAL ACCIDENT BOARD

SAMPLE

State's	File:
Number	Carrier:
For:	Employer:

Carrier's File No. _____

(The spaces above not to be filled in by Employer)

THE PATIENT

1. Name of Injured Person _____ Age _____ Sex _____
2. Address: No. and St. _____ City or Town _____ State _____
3. Name and Address of Employer _____

THE ACCIDENT

4. Date of accident _____ Hour _____ M. Date disability began _____
5. State in patient's own words where and how accident occurred _____

THE INJURY

6. Give accurate description of nature and extent of injury and state your objective findings _____

7. Will the injury result in (a) Permanent defect? _____ If so, what? _____
   (b) Facial or head disfigurement? _____
   (Permanent disability such as loss of whole or part of fingers, facial or head disfigurement, etc., must be accurately marked on chart on reverse side of this report.)

8. Is accident above referred to the only cause of patient's condition? _____ If not, state contributing causes _____

9. Is patient suffering from any disease of the heart, lungs, brain, kidneys, blood, vascular system or any other disabling condition not due to this accident? _____ Give particulars _____

10. Has patient any physical impairment due to previous accident or disease? _____ Give particulars _____

11. Has normal recovery been delayed for any reason? _____ Give particulars _____

TREATMENT

12. Date of your first treatment _____ Who engaged your services? _____
13. Describe treatment given by you _____
14. Were X-rays taken? _____ By whom? _____ When? _____
    (NAME AND ADDRESS)
15. X-ray diagnosis _____
16. Was patient treated by anyone else? _____ By whom? _____ When? _____
    (NAME AND ADDRESS)
17. Was patient hospitalized? _____ Name and address of hospital _____
18. Date of admission to hospital _____ Date of discharge _____
19. Is further treatment needed? _____ For how long? _____

DIS-ABILITY

20. Patient was/will be able to resume regular work on _____
21. Patient was/will be able to resume light work on _____
22. If death ensued, give date _____

REMARKS: (Give any information of value not included above) _____

I am a duly licensed physician in the State of _____
I was graduated from _____ Medical School in _____ Year _____
Date of this report _____ (Signed) _____ Telephone _____
This report must be signed personally by physician. Address _____

FORM U-101   PHYSICIANS' RECORD CO., BERWYN, ILLINOIS · PRINTED IN U.S.A.   **SURGEON'S REPORT**

ASSIGNMENT 27

1. Complete the *Doctor's Final (Or Monthly) Report and Bill*. Date it October 17. The case number will be the patient's Social Security number. Remember to complete the report using only the information pertinent up to and including October 16, which means referring to the first four entries on the Patient Record. Be sure to include RVS or CPT code numbers for each professional service rendered.

2. Mr. Weston returns to see Dr. Input on January 3. Complete a *Doctor's Supplemental Report* and date it January 4, 1978. The January 3, 1978, office visit was limited and the doctor's fee was $15.00. Record the proper information on the ledger card for all the above transactions.

Abbreviations pertinent to this record:

adv _____	PD _____
CO _____	Pt _____
DC _____	retn _____
exam _____	Rev _____
Hx _____	Rt _____
Imp _____	slt _____
inj _____	trt _____
med _____	wks _____
orig _____	

PATIENT RECORD

Weston,	Keith	P.	01-03-38	M	013/567-8898
LAST NAME	FIRST NAME	MIDDLE NAME	BIRTH DATE	SEX	HOME PHONE

4201 Huntington Drive, Woodland Hills,		XY	12345
ADDRESS	CITY	STATE	ZIP CODE

delivery man	Hathaway Service Co. (parcel delivery co)
PATIENT'S OCCUPATION	NAME OF COMPANY

200 Holloway Drive, Woodland Hills, XY 12345	013/466-7887
ADDRESS OF EMPLOYER	PHONE

Jane F. Weston	housewife
SPOUSE OR PARENT	OCCUPATION

EMPLOYER	ADDRESS	PHONE

State Compensation Ins.Fund 14156 Magnolia Blvd., Torres, XY 12349

NAME OF INSURANCE GROUP	SUBSCRIBER

Policy # 578099

BLUE SHIELD OR BLUE CROSS CERT. NO.	GROUP NO.	CURRENT COVERAGE NO.	EFFECTIVE DATE
			174-98-0080
MEDICARE NO.	MEDICAID NO.	EFFECTIVE DATE	SOC. SEC. NO.

Hathaway Service Company

REFERRED BY:

DATE	PROGRESS
10-1-77	CO recurrent pain lower rt abdomen. Records forwarded from prior exams for evaluation. Orig inj 8-18-76 at 2 p.m. Hx & exam showed right inguinal hernia. Reviewed prior med records & assessed data & evaluations. Imp: rt recurrent inguinal hernia. Recommended trt: herniorrhaphy *G. Ingut MD*
10-10-77	Pt admitted to College Hosp. *D Ingut MD*
10-11-77	Surg: R recurrent inguinal herniorrhaphy. Pt to be seen daily in hosp. *Gaston Ingut MD*
10-16-77	Pt cond satisfactory. DC & adv to rest at home for 5 wks. Pt to be seen monthly. Pt able to retn to work 12-30-77. No PD anticipated. *G Ingut MD*
1-3-78	Pt continues to have slt pain. Unable to work on 12-30-77 Some pain on forward bending & lt lateral bending. To retn in 1 mo for re-exam. Pt should be able to resume work on 1-30-78 Full recovery undetermined at this time. *Gaston Ingut MD.*

STATEMENT

College Clinic
4567 Broad Avenue
Woodland Hills, XY 12345
013/486-9002

State Compensation Insurance Fund
14156 Magnolia Boulevard
Torres, XY 12349

DATE	PROFESSIONAL SERVICE	CHARGE		PAID	BALANCE
	Re: Case No. 174-98-0080				
	Inj: Keith P. Weston				
	Date of Inj: 8-18-76				
	Emp: Hathaway Service Co.				
10-1-77	Extensive rev of prior medical records and assessment of data, evaluation & written report	50	00		
10-10-77	Hospital exam limited, follow-up	25	00		
10-11-77	Rt recurrent inguinal herniorrhaphy	300	00		
10-11-77	HV brief	NC			
10-12-77	HV brief	NC			
10-13-77	HV brief	NC			
10-14-77	HV brief	NC			
10-15-77	HV brief	NC			
10-16-77	HV brief	NC			

Pay last amount in this column

CON - CONSULTATION	HCD - HOUSE CALL (DAY)	LAB - LABORATORY
CPX - COMPLETE PHYS EXAM	HCN - HOUSE CALL (NIGHT)	NC - NO CHARGE
E - EMERGENCY	HV - HOSPITAL VISIT	OC - OFFICE CALL
EC - ERROR CORRECTED	INJ - INJECTION	OS - OFFICE SURGERY
ECG - ELECTROCARDIOGRAM	INS - INSURANCE	SE - SPECIAL EXAM

● SAMPLE ●

STATE COMPENSATION INSURANCE FUND

14156 MAGNOLIA BOULEVARD, TORRES, XY 12349

DOCTOR'S FINAL (OR MONTHLY) REPORT AND BILL

Monthly itemized bills required on all cases under continuing treatment.
Services beginning late in month and extending into succeeding month may be itemized on one statement.

CASE No._____

EMPLOYER_____

EMPLOYEE_____

DATE OF INJURY_____ SERVICES FOR MONTH OF_____ 19____

Patient refused treatment_____19____ Patient able to return to work_____19____

Patient stopped treatment Patient discharged as cured_____19____
    without orders_____19____ Condition at time of last visit_____

Patient entered hospital_____19____

Further treatment anticipated? _____ _____ _____
                       (Yes)   (No)

Any other charges authorized such as Drugs?_____ Hospital?_____
                                     (Check)   (Check)

Code: O—Office; V—Home Visit; H—Hospital Visit; N—Night Visit; S—Operation; X—X-ray.

Month	1	2	3	4	5	6	7	8	9	10	11	12	13	14	15	16	17	18	19	20	21	22	23	24	25	26	27	28	29	30	31

TOTALS

First aid treatment (describe)_____ $_____

Office Visits_____ $_____
Home Visits_____ $_____
Hospital Visits_____ $_____
Operations_____ $_____
MATERIAL (Itemize at cost)_____ $_____
_____
_____
_____

Any charges shown above which are in excess of the scheduled fee must
be explained regarding nature of such services, indicating the date rendered.   **TOTAL** $_____

Make check payable to:

Doctor_____ Signature_____

Address_____ Zip_____ Date_____
          (Street)

_____
         (City)

LEAVE BLANK	
APPROVED	
BY_____	
(Dollars) (Cents)	DATE_____

IMPORTANT.—
Bills Must Be Submitted in Duplicate

FORM 60— 55420-218 8-71 35M △ OSP

STATE
FUND

14156 MAGNOLIA BOULEVARD
TORRES, XY 12349

SAMPLE

Case No.:
Injured:
Injury date:

DOCTOR'S SUPPLEMENTAL REPORT

The information requested in this report is necessary to establish eligibility for further benefits.
You may make your notations on this form (including reverse side if more space required) or, if more convenient, forward
a brief report containing the necessary information.

1. Have you discharged patient?_____If so, when?_____
   (if answer to above is yes and you expect *no* permanent residuals, you may disregard remainder of form, sign and
   return)

2. Date of last examination_____

3. Present condition and prognosis (indicate if diagnosis changed since last report)_____
   _____
   _____
   _____
   _____

4. Treatment required by injury in question (type, length and frequency)_____
   _____
   _____
   _____
   _____

5. Date injured was or will be able to return to work_____
6. When do you expect full recovery from injury in question?_____
   _____

_____   _____
          (Doctor's Signature)   **(Date)**

> If you wish to discuss this case in greater detail, please contact our Claims Department at the above
> address. Arrangements can be made for discussion with our Medical Department if you so desire.

FORM C-9

Chapter 11:
Dental Insurance

ASSIGNMENT 28

1. Complete the *Dental Insurance Form* on Mr. Ellis P. Alehouse and date it June 10. Treatment is not for orthodontic purposes and is not the result of an accident. No x-rays are to be enclosed with the insurance claim on this particular patient. Refer to Mr. Alehouse's Patient Record and ledger card for information.

2. In order to properly code the professional services rendered by the dentist, refer to the text on pages 279–280 to ascertain the three-digit code numbers that should be used for this particular claim.

3. Record on the ledger card the proper information when you have billed the dental insurance company.

Abbreviations pertinent to this record:

Refer to pages 295–300 at the end of Chapter 11 to learn the meanings of these dental abbreviations.

CDS_____ pt _____

DDS_____ re ch_____

mm _____ Retn_____

neg _____ Rx _____

path _____ wk _____

PO _____

ASSIGNMENT 29

1. Complete the *Denti-Cal Form* for authorization on October 18, showing only the first three itemizations for that date and fees. Assuming that this is then authorized by Denti-Cal and that the form is returned to the dentist's office, continue to complete the authorization for the next six itemizations, also listing the fees. Treatment is not the result of an accident. You will be enclosing three x-rays for the Denti-Cal authorization. Attach the proper Denti-Cal (Medi-Cal) labels and identify whether the label should be MEDI or POE. Indicate year and date, showing eligibility for the month(s) in question. You will be resubmitting the Denti-Cal form for payment after November 10. Refer to the Patient Record and ledger card to ascertain the proper information.

2. In order to properly code the professional services rendered by the dentist, refer to the text on pages 279–280 to ascertain the three-digit code numbers that can be used for this particular claim.

3. On December 7, Denti-Cal sends the dentist a check for $143. Complete the ledger, showing this payment. The check number is 307524.

Abbreviations pertinent to this record:

Refer to pages 295–300 at the end of Chapter 11 to learn the meanings of these dental abbreviations.

amal _____	N_2 _____
D̄ _____	MO _____
Ē _____	MOD _____
C̄ _____	MOFD _____
Ē _____	Prophy _____
C̄ _____	Pmt _____
D̄ _____	SC _____
F _____	W/Fl_2 _____

PATIENT RECORD

Alehouse,	Ellis	P.	03-03-42	M	013/678-9908
LAST NAME	FIRST NAME	MIDDLE NAME	BIRTH DATE	SEX	HOME PHONE

2435 Blakely Way,	Merck,		XY	12346
ADDRESS	CITY		STATE	ZIP CODE

truck driver   Standard Trucking Company
PATIENT'S OCCUPATION   NAME OF COMPANY
1108 Cantlay Street,   Dorland, XY 12347   013/653-0980
ADDRESS OF EMPLOYER   PHONE

Jane P. Ellis   Housewife
SPOUSE OR PARENT   OCCUPATION

EMPLOYER   ADDRESS   PHONE
California Dental Service   Ellis P. Alehouse
NAME OF INSURANCE GROUP   SUBSCRIBER
Standard Trucking Co. Plan,   Group 3100, Location #473
BLUE SHIELD OR BLUE CROSS CERT. NO.   GROUP NO.   CURRENT COVERAGE NO.   EFFECTIVE DATE
                                                    666-78-9090

MEDICARE NO.   MEDICAID NO.   EFFECTIVE DATE   SOC. SEC. NO.

Bert I. Strain (friend)
REFERRED BY:

NAME Alehouse, Ellis P.   ADDRESS 2435 Blakely Way, Merck, XY 12346 PHONE 013/678-9908

BILL TO_____ BUS. ADDRESS_____ BUS. PHONE_____

REFERRED BY_____ PHYSICIAN _____ BANK_____

| DATE | | | DESCRIPTION OF WORK | ACCOUNT RECORD | | |
MO.	DAY	YR.		CHARGE	PAID	BALANCE
6	2	77	Pt seen for persistent irritation of hard palate	35 —		
			Anesthetized hard palate, made 2 elliptical incisions			
			12 mm long, elevated & removed tissue island; undermined			
			the incision, placed 8 sutures to close incision. Sent			
			tissue to pathology. Rx for pain. Retn in 1 wk for PO			
			ch *A.O.Dont,D.D.S.*			
6	9	77	PO re ch, removed sutures, path report neg.	15 —		
			Arthur O. Dont, D.D.S			

RETAIN LAST COPY FOR YOUR FILES. MAIL ALL OTHER COPIES TO PLAN.

* IF PREDETERMINATION, PLAN WILL COMPLETE DATES FROM AND THRU IMMEDIATELY BELOW.
IF SERVICE WILL EXTEND BEYOND THRU DATE YOU MUST INQUIRE TO PLAN FOR CONFIRMATION OF CONTINUED ELIGIBILITY (SEE DENTISTS HANDBOOK.)

STAPLE X-RAYS (NOT REQUIRED FOR AMALGAMS, PLASTICS, SILICATES, EXCEPT FOR DENTI-CAL PATIENTS) TO TOP RIGHT CORNER OF FORMS.

TYPE OR PRINT YOU ARE PREPARING MULTIPLE COPIES

CHECK HERE IF DENTI-CAL CLAIM ☐
AFFIX BELOW A MEDI-CAL PROOF OF ELIGIBILITY LABEL FOR EACH MONTH SERVICES WERE PROVIDED

342352
SHADED AREA FOR CDS USE ONLY

ATTENDING DENTIST'S STATEMENT
SIGN BELOW
FOR PREDETERMINATION *
OR PAYMENT **

APPROVED BY
FROM
THRU

USE THIS NUMBER FOR INQUIRY

CALIFORNIA DENTAL SERVICE
P. O. BOX 7736
SAN FRANCISCO, CALIFORNIA 94120
A DELTA PLAN

1. PATIENT NAME
2. RELATIONSHIP TO EMPLOYEE — SELF | SPOUSE | CHILD | OTHER
3. SEX M | F
4. PATIENT BIRTHDATE MO. | DAY | YEAR
5. IF FULL TIME STUDENT SCHOOL — CITY

6. EMPLOYEE/SUBSCRIBER NAME — FIRST MIDDLE LAST
7. EMPLOYEE SOCIAL SECURITY NUMBER
9. NAME OF GROUP DENTAL PROGRAM

JAN.	FEB.	JAN.	FEB.
MAR.	APR.	MAR.	APR.
MAY	JUN.	MAY	JUN.
JUL.	AUG.	JUL.	AUG.
SEP.	OCT.	SEP.	OCT.
NOV.	DEC.	NOV.	DEC.

8. EMPLOYEE MAILING ADDRESS
CITY, STATE, ZIP
10. EMPLOYER (COMPANY) NAME AND ADDRESS

11. GROUP NUMBER
12. LOCATION (LOCAL)
13. ARE OTHER FAMILY MEMBERS EMPLOYED? EMPLOYEE NAME SOC. SEC. NO.
14. NAME AND ADDRESS OF EMPLOYER, ITEM 13

15. IS PATIENT COVERED BY ANOTHER DENTAL PLAN?
DENTAL PLAN NAME UNION LOCAL GROUP NO NAME AND ADDRESS OF CARRIER

16. DENTIST NAME — LICENSE NUMBER
24. IS TREATMENT RESULT OF OCCUPATIONAL ILLNESS OR INJURY? NO YES IF YES, ENTER BRIEF DESCRIPTION AND DATES
17. MAILING ADDRESS
25. IS TREATMENT RESULT OF AUTO ACCIDENT?
CITY, STATE, ZIP
26. OTHER ACCIDENT?
27. ARE ANY SERVICES COVERED BY ANOTHER PLAN?
18. DENTIST SOC. SEC. NO. OR T.I.N.
19. DENTIST LICENSE NO.
20. DENTIST PHONE NO.
28. IF PROSTHESIS, IS THIS INITIAL PLACEMENT? IF NO, ENTER REASON FOR REPLACEMENT.
29. DATE OF PRIOR PLACEMENT

21. FIRST VISIT DATE CURRENT SERIES
22. PLACE OF TREATMENT OFFICE | HOSP | ECF | OTHER
23. RADIOGRAPHS OR MODELS ENCLOSED? NO | YES HOW MANY?
30. IS TREATMENT FOR ORTHODONTICS? NO YES IF SERVICES ALREADY COMMENCED ENTER → DATE APPLIANCES PLACED MOS. TREATMENT REMAINING

IDENTIFY MISSING TEETH WITH "X"
FACIAL
RIGHT LEFT
LINGUAL
FACIAL

32. REMARKS FOR UNUSUAL SERVICES

31. EXAMINATION AND TREATMENT RECORD - LIST IN ORDER FROM TOOTH NO. 1 THROUGH TOOTH NO. 32. USE CHARTING SYSTEM SHOWN

TOOTH # OR LETTER	SURFACES	DESCRIPTION OF SERVICE (INCLUDING X-RAYS, PROPHYLAXIS, MATERIALS USED, ETC.)	DATE SERVICE PERFORMED MO. DAY YEAR	PROCEDURE NUMBER	FEE

USUAL AND CUSTOMARY ALLOWANCE

SAMPLE

I ACCEPT THIS ATTENDING DENTIST'S STATEMENT AND AUTHORIZE RELEASE OF INFORMATION RELATING HERETO. I CERTIFY THE TRUTH OF ALL PERSONAL INFORMATION CONTAINED ABOVE. I AGREE TO BE RESPONSIBLE FOR PAYMENT FOR SERVICES PROVIDED DURING ANY INELIGIBLE PERIOD.

PATIENT (PARENT OR EMPLOYEE) SIGNATURE X _____

! IMPORTANT !
WE HAVE REVIEWED AND APPROVED THIS ATTENDING DENTIST'S STATEMENT, THE COMPUTATIONS AND ANY ADJUSTMENTS MADE BY C.D.S.

X _____
PATIENT (EMPLOYEE) DENTIST

TOTAL FEE CHARGED
PATIENT PAYS
PLAN PAYS
AMOUNT APPLIED TO DEDUCTIBLE

* (PREDETERMINATION OF COST)
THE TREATMENT LISTED IS NECESSARY IN MY PROFESSIONAL JUDGMENT AND I REQUEST AUTHORIZATION IN ACCORDANCE WITH C.D.S. PARTICIPATING DENTIST RULES AND/OR DENTI-CAL RULES (See Reverse side of Page 4)

** (TREATMENT COMPLETED - PAYMENT REQUESTED)
THE TREATMENT LISTED WAS COMPLETED AND WAS NECESSARY IN MY PROFESSIONAL JUDGMENT. I REQUEST PAYMENT IN ACCORDANCE WITH C.D.S. PARTICIPATING DENTIST RULES AND/OR DENTI-CAL RULES (See Reverse Side of Page 4)

DENTIST SIGNATURE DATE
DENTIST SIGNATURE DATE

PAYMENT OF ABOVE BALANCE SUBJECT TO PERCENT WITHHOLD AS APPROVED BY PLAN BOARD OF DIRECTORS.

MARKED NUMBERS BELOW REFER TO ADJUSTMENTS AS EXPLAINED ON REVERSE SIDE OF PAGES 1, 2 & 3.

1 2 3 4 5 6 7 8 9 10 11 12 13 14 15 16 17 18 19 20 21 22 23 24 25 26 27 28 29 30 31 32 33 34 35
36 37 38 39 40 41 42 43 44 45 46 47 48 49 50 51 52 53 54 55 56 57 58 59 60 61 62 63 64 65 66 67 68 69 70

1. (SUBMIT TO CDS) - WHITE
2. (SUBMIT TO CDS) - GREEN
3. (SUBMIT TO CDS) - YELLOW
4. (RETAIN FOR YOUR FILES) - GOLDENROD

A SEPARATE FORM (CDS-505) LISTS DENTI-CAL PROCESSING POLICIES. CDS AND DENTI-CAL PARTICIPATION RULES ARE ON REVERSE SIDE OF PAGE 4 OF THIS FORM (CDS-105).

CDS 105 Rev. 9/75 FORM APPROVED BY THE COUNCIL ON DENTAL CARE PROGRAMS OF THE A.D.A. 1975

1

IMPORTANT - WHEN PAYMENT IS MADE BY CDS, THE PATIENT WILL RECEIVE THIS FORM AS A NOTICE OF PAYMENT.

PATIENT RECORD

Carter,	Jaime	H.	11-28-67	M	013/488-0696
LAST NAME	FIRST NAME	MIDDLE NAME	BIRTH DATE	SEX	HOME PHONE

112 Max Street,	Woodland Hills,	XY	12345
ADDRESS	CITY	STATE	ZIP CODE

child
PATIENT'S OCCUPATION   NAME OF COMPANY

ADDRESS OF EMPLOYER   PHONE

Mary O. Carter	housewife
SPOUSE OR PARENT	OCCUPATION

EMPLOYER   ADDRESS   PHONE

Denti-Cal
NAME OF INSURANCE GROUP   SUBSCRIBER

BLUE SHIELD OR BLUE CROSS CERT. NO.	GROUP NO.	CURRENT COVERAGE NO.	EFFECTIVE DATE
	19-35-7768092-1-03		none
MEDICARE NO.	MEDICAID NO.	EFFECTIVE DATE	SOC. SEC. NO.

Mrs. Hazel Plunkett (friend)
REFERRED BY:

NAME Carter, Jaime H.   ADDRESS 112 Max St.,Woodland Hills,XY PHONE 013/488-0696

BILL TO Denti-Cal   BUS. ADDRESS   BUS. PHONE

REFERRED BY   PHYSICIAN   BANK

ESTIMATE

REMARKS:

Exam #6
Prophy w/Fl₂ $15
Panorex w/Bw's $20

$14
$10 $14
$14 $25 $25

	DATE		DESCRIPTION OF WORK	ACCOUNT RECORD		
MO.	DAY	YR.		CHARGE	PAID	BALANCE
10	18	77	EXAM PANOREX w/BWS PROPHY w/Fl₂	41 —		
			DENTI-CAL FORM for AUTHORIZATION #143	—		
11	2	77	E|ᵐᵒ Amal D|ᵐᵒᴰ SC C|ᵐᵒFᴰ SC N₂	64 —		
11	10	77	E|ᵐᵒ Amal LC^F Amal LD^ᴰᴼ Amal N₂	38 —		
			DENTI-CAL FORM for pmt #143	—		
			Dennis Drill, DDS			

RETAIN LAST COPY FOR YOUR FILES. MAIL ALL OTHER COPIES TO PLAN.

✱ IF PREDETERMINATION, PLAN WILL COMPLETE DATES FROM AND THRU IMMEDIATELY BELOW.
IF SERVICE WILL EXTEND BEYOND THRU DATE YOU MUST INQUIRE TO PLAN FOR CONFIRMATION OF CONTINUED ELIGIBILITY (SEE DENTISTS HANDBOOK.)

STAPLE X-RAYS (NOT REQUIRED FOR AMALGAMS, PLASTICS, SILICATES, EXCEPT FOR DENTI-CAL PATIENTS) TO TOP RIGHT CORNER OF FORMS.

TYPE OR PRINT
YOU ARE PREPARING
MULTIPLE COPIES

CHECK HERE IF DENTI-CAL CLAIM ☐
AFFIX BELOW A MEDI-CAL PROOF OF ELIGIBILITY LABEL FOR EACH MONTH SERVICES WERE PROVIDED.

342353
SHADED AREA FOR CDS USE ONLY.

ATTENDING DENTIST'S STATEMENT
SIGN BELOW
FOR PREDETERMINATION ✱
OR PAYMENT ✱✱

APPROVED BY
FROM
THRU

USE THIS NUMBER FOR INQUIRY

CALIFORNIA DENTAL SERVICE
P. O. BOX 7736
SAN FRANCISCO, CALIFORNIA 94120
A DELTA PLAN

1. PATIENT NAME
2. RELATIONSHIP TO EMPLOYEE — SELF | SPOUSE | CHILD | OTHER
3. SEX — M | F
4. PATIENT BIRTHDATE — MO. | DAY | YEAR
5. IF FULL TIME STUDENT — SCHOOL — CITY

6. EMPLOYEE/SUBSCRIBER NAME — FIRST MIDDLE LAST
7. EMPLOYEE SOCIAL SECURITY NUMBER
9. NAME OF GROUP DENTAL PROGRAM

JAN.	FEB.	JAN.	FEB.
MAR.	APR.	MAR.	APR.
MAY	JUN.	MAY	JUN.
JUL.	AUG.	JUL.	AUG.
SEP.	OCT.	SEP.	OCT.
NOV.	DEC.	NOV.	DEC.

8. EMPLOYEE MAILING ADDRESS
CITY, STATE, ZIP
10. EMPLOYER (COMPANY) NAME AND ADDRESS

11. GROUP NUMBER
12. LOCATION (LOCAL)
13. ARE OTHER FAMILY MEMBERS EMPLOYED? EMPLOYEE NAME SOC. SEC. NO.
14. NAME AND ADDRESS OF EMPLOYER, ITEM 13

15. IS PATIENT COVERED BY ANOTHER DENTAL PLAN?
DENTAL PLAN NAME
UNION LOCAL
GROUP NO.
NAME AND ADDRESS OF CARRIER

16. DENTIST NAME
LICENSE NUMBER
24. IS TREATMENT RESULT OF OCCUPATIONAL ILLNESS OR INJURY? — NO YES — IF YES, ENTER BRIEF DESCRIPTION AND DATES

17. MAILING ADDRESS
PHONE NO.
25. IS TREATMENT RESULT OF AUTO ACCIDENT?

CITY, STATE, ZIP
26. OTHER ACCIDENT?
27. ARE ANY SERVICES COVERED BY ANOTHER PLAN?

18. DENTIST SOC. SEC. NO. OR T.I.N.
19. DENTIST LICENSE NO.
20. DENTIST PHONE NO.
28. IF PROSTHESIS, IS THIS INITIAL PLACEMENT? IF NO, ENTER REASON FOR REPLACEMENT.
29. DATE OF PRIOR PLACEMENT

21. FIRST VISIT DATE CURRENT SERIES
22. PLACE OF TREATMENT — OFFICE HOSP ECF OTHER
23. RADIOGRAPHS OR MODELS ENCLOSED? — NO ☐ YES ☐ — HOW MANY?
30. IS TREATMENT FOR ORTHODONTICS? — NO YES — IF SERVICES ALREADY COMMENCED ENTER ➡ DATE APPLIANCES PLACED — MOS. TREATMENT REMAINING

IDENTIFY MISSING TEETH WITH "X"

FACIAL
LINGUAL
RIGHT LEFT
LINGUAL
FACIAL

31. EXAMINATION AND TREATMENT RECORD - LIST IN ORDER FROM TOOTH NO. 1 THROUGH TOOTH NO. 32. USE CHARTING SYSTEM SHOWN.

TOOTH # OR LETTER	SURFACES	DESCRIPTION OF SERVICE (INCLUDING X-RAYS, PROPHYLAXIS, MATERIALS USED, ETC.)	DATE SERVICE PERFORMED MO. DAY YEAR	PROCEDURE NUMBER	FEE

USUAL AND CUSTOMARY
ALLOWANCE

32. REMARKS FOR UNUSUAL SERVICES

SAMPLE

(vertical left margin) IMPORTANT - WHEN PAYMENT IS MADE BY CDS, THE PATIENT WILL RECEIVE THIS FORM AS A NOTICE OF PAYMENT.

I ACCEPT THIS ATTENDING DENTIST'S STATEMENT AND AUTHORIZE RELEASE OF INFORMATION RELATING HERETO. I CERTIFY THE TRUTH OF ALL PERSONAL INFORMATION CONTAINED ABOVE. I AGREE TO BE RESPONSIBLE FOR PAYMENT FOR SERVICES PROVIDED DURING ANY INELIGIBLE PERIOD.

PATIENT (PARENT OR EMPLOYEE) SIGNATURE X

! IMPORTANT !
WE HAVE REVIEWED AND APPROVED THIS ATTENDING DENTIST'S STATEMENT. THE COMPUTATIONS AND ANY ADJUSTMENTS MADE BY C.D.S.

X
PATIENT (EMPLOYEE) DENTIST

TOTAL FEE CHARGED
PATIENT PAYS
PLAN PAYS

✱ (PREDETERMINATION OF COST)
THE TREATMENT LISTED IS NECESSARY IN MY PROFESSIONAL JUDGMENT AND I REQUEST AUTHORIZATION IN ACCORDANCE WITH C.D.S. PARTICIPATING DENTIST RULES AND/OR DENTI-CAL RULES (See Reverse side of Page 4)
DENTIST SIGNATURE DATE

✱✱ (TREATMENT COMPLETED - PAYMENT REQUESTED)
THE TREATMENT LISTED WAS COMPLETED AND WAS NECESSARY IN MY PROFESSIONAL JUDGMENT. I REQUEST PAYMENT IN ACCORDANCE WITH C.D.S. PARTICIPATING DENTIST RULES AND/OR DENTI-CAL RULES (See Reverse Side of Page 4)
DENTIST SIGNATURE DATE

AMOUNT APPLIED TO DEDUCTIBLE
PAYMENT OF ABOVE BALANCE SUBJECT TO PERCENT WITHHOLD AS APPROVED BY PLAN BOARD OF DIRECTORS.

MARKED NUMBERS BELOW REFER TO ADJUSTMENTS AS EXPLAINED ON REVERSE SIDE OF PAGES 1 & 3.

| 1 | 2 | 3 | 4 | 5 | 6 | 7 | 8 | 9 | 10 | 11 | 12 | 13 | 14 | 15 | 16 | 17 | 18 | 19 | 20 | 21 | 22 | 23 | 24 | 25 | 26 | 27 | 28 | 29 | 30 | 31 | 32 | 33 | 34 | 35 |
| 36 | 37 | 38 | 39 | 40 | 41 | 42 | 43 | 44 | 45 | 46 | 47 | 48 | 49 | 50 | 51 | 52 | 53 | 54 | 55 | 56 | 57 | 58 | 59 | 60 | 61 | 62 | 63 | 64 | 65 | 66 | 67 | 68 | 69 | 70 |

1. (SUBMIT TO CDS) - WHITE
2. (SUBMIT TO CDS) - GREEN
3. (SUBMIT TO CDS) - YELLOW
4. (RETAIN FOR YOUR FILES) - GOLDENROD

A SEPARATE FORM (CDS-505) LISTS DENTI-CAL PROCESSING POLICIES. CDS AND DENTI-CAL PARTICIPATION RULES ARE ON REVERSE SIDE OF PAGE 4 OF THIS FORM (CDS-105).

CDS 105 Rev. 9/75
FORM APPROVED BY THE COUNCIL ON DENTAL CARE PROGRAMS OF THE A.D.A. 1975

1

Chapter 12:
Computerized Billing and Insurance

ASSIGNMENT 30

1. Complete a *Family Master Card* for Mr. Brad E. Diehl for his first office visit on January 5. Mr. Diehl has one child, Meg L. Diehl, born on March 1, 1975. Mr. Diehl's computer account number will be 002781 and the type of insurance is Type I for Private Carrier. Dr. Input's group number is 987 and his doctor number is 04. Refer to Mr. Diehl's Patient Record to complete the assignment.

2. Complete separate *Patient Visit Slips* for Mr. Diehl's three visits made during the month of January. Following is additional information needed to complete the Patient Visit Slips:

   a. On January 5 Mr. Diehl comes in for an intermediate office visit, an EKG with interpretation and report which was done in the physician's office, AP and lat chest x-rays taken in the doctor's office, and an interpretation of a bone marrow aspiration ($10) Mr. Diehl pays the full amount by personal check.

   b. On January 14 a glucose tolerance test is performed ($35) and is sent to an outside laboratory. Dr. Input is billing for the outside laboratory. He is charging $10 for collection and handling of the specimen. Mr. Diehl pays $35 in cash on his account.

   c. On January 20 Mr. Diehl is seen in the office for a limited examination; a complete blood count is done in the office and an oral cholecystography is also performed ($60). Dr. Input is billing for these procedures. The patient pays $60 by personal check.

Abbreviations pertinent to this record:

abt _____	lat _____
Adv _____	mo _____
AP _____	neg _____
BP _____	Pt _____
CBC _____	WBC _____
cm _____	WNL _____
Dx, DX _____	wk _____
EKG _____	c̄ _____
hr _____	

PATIENT RECORD

Diehl,	Brad	E.	09/21/46	M	013/222-0123
LAST NAME	FIRST NAME	MIDDLE NAME	BIRTH DATE	SEX	HOME PHONE

3975 Hills Road,	Woodland Hills,	XY	12345
ADDRESS	CITY	STATE	ZIP CODE

radio advertising salesman	KACY Radio
PATIENT'S OCCUPATION	NAME OF COMPANY

4071 Mills Road, Woodland Hills, XY 12345	013/201-6666
ADDRESS OF EMPLOYER	PHONE

Tak E. Diehl (birthdate 2-7-45)	legal secretary
SPOUSE	OCCUPATION

Attys. Dilman, Forewise, and Gilson 12 W. Dix St., Woodland Hills, XY 12345	013/222-6432
EMPLOYER	ADDRESS	PHONE

Aetna Insurance Co. 2412 Main Street, Woodland Hills, XY 12345	Brad E. Diehl
NAME OF INSURANCE GROUP	SUBSCRIBER

Policy # 403119			
BLUE SHIELD OR BLUE CROSS CERT. NO.	GROUP NO.	CURRENT COVERAGE NO.	EFFECTIVE DATE

			561-02-1501
MEDICARE NO.	MEDICAID NO.	EFFECTIVE DATE	SOC. SEC. NO.

Raymond Skelton, M. D.
REFERRED BY:

DATE	PROGRESS
1-5-77	Pt. comes in complaining of coughing & sneezing. Some difficulty in breathing. Dizziness occasionally & stomach pain c̄ cramping of 6 mo duration. EKG essentially neg. AP & lat chest x-rays neg. Pt brought in bone marrow aspiration done by Dr. Skelton for interpretation only. BP 180/110. Adv to have glucose tolerance test in abt 1 wk. Dx: suspicion of irritable colon (diagnosis ICDA code no. 5639) and hypertension (diagnosis ICDA code no. 4031). No disability at this time. *Gaston Input, MD*
1-14-77	Glucose tolerance 3 hr test done on 5 specimens. Pt to return in 5 or 6 days for cholecystography & CBC. *G Input, MD*
1-20-77	Glucose tolerance test WNL. Oral cholecystography reveals a single 1.5 cm in maximal diameter radiolucent calculus within the cholecyst. WBC 10,000 DX: cholecystitis with cholelithiasis (diagnosis ICDA code no. 5749). Adv. cholecystectomy as soon as possible. *Gaston Input, MD*

MEDCOBILL SYSTEM — **FAMILY MASTER** — InTELLECTron InTErnaTional, IncorporaTED

GRP. NO.	ACCOUNT NO.	1 TYPE	2 LAST	NAME OF RESPONSIBLE PARTY	3 FIRST	4 M.I.	5 AREA	HOME PHONE NUMBER

60 CYCLE BILLING	6	NUMBER AND STREET	7	CITY AND STATE

DATE	9	8

PATIENT INFORMATION

FAMILY MEMBER NUMBER	FIRST NAME	M.I.	(LAST, IF DIFFERENT)	SEX	BIRTHDATE MO.	DAY	YR.	EMP. BY	OCCUPATION	INSURANCE CARRIER AUTO 1	AUTO 2	AUTO 3	1	2	3	P.N.
1																
2																
3																
4																
5																
6																
0																
	12	13	14	15	16			17	18	20	21	22	25	26	27	30

EMPLOYER NO. 1

EMPLOYER NO. 2

AGENCY OR INSURANCE INFORMATION

31 CARRIER **1**		CARRIER **2**		CARRIER **3**	
32 GROUP NO.		GROUP NO.		GROUP NO.	
33 MEMBER NO.		MEMBER NO.		MEMBER NO.	
34 SUBSCRIB. NO.	1 2 3 4 5 6 7 8 0	SUBSCRIB. NO.	1 2 3 4 5 6 7 8 0	SUBSCRIB. NO.	1 2 3 4 5 6 7 8 0

© 1975 InTELLECTron InTErnaTional, IncorporaTED

11-873

MED 0040

43776

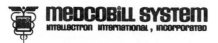

MEDCOBILL SYSTEM
INTELLECTRON INTERNATIONAL, INCORPORATED

GROUP NO.	DR. NO.	DATE	ACCOUNT NO.	ACCOUNT LAST NAME
FAMILY MEM. NO.		PATIENT FIRST NAME		PATIENT LAST NAME (IF DIFF. FROM ABOVE)

IF NOT OFFICE, INDICATE PLACE OF SERVICE: 1 - IN-PATIENT HOSPITAL   2 - OUT-PATIENT HOSPITAL
4 - PATIENT'S HOME   6 - ECF   8 - NURSING HOME   9 - OTHER

SERVICE	RVS		MOD	FEE		SERVICE	RVS		MOD	FEE	
NEW						**INJECTION**					
Initial Brief	90000	01		18	00	Penicillin	90705	22		10	00
Init. Limited	90010	02		27	00	B12	90705	23		10	00
Init. Intermed.	90015	03		45	00		90705				
Init. Comprehen.	90020	04		63	00	**IMMUNIZATION**				10	00
ESTABLISHED						Polio	90700	24		10	00
Minimum O.V.	90030	05		7	00	Dip Tet	90700	25			
Brief Exam	90040	06		11	00						
Limited Exam	90050	07		14	00	**SURGERY**					
Intermed. Exam	90060	08		18	00	I & D Abscess	10060	26		44	00
Extended Re-Exam	90070	09		27	00	Laceration Repair	12000	27		44	00
HOSPITAL											
Initial Brief	90200	10		27	00						
Init. Intermed.	90215	11		45	00	**PATHOLOGY**					
Init. Comprehen.	90220	12		63	00	Blood Type, RH	86100	28		4	00
Brief Exam	90240	13		11	00	CBC	85010	29		8	00
Limited Exam	90250	14		18	00	Pap Smear	88105	30		14	00
Intermed. Exam	90260	15		27	00	Rh Titre	86025	31		7	00
Extended Re-Exam	90270	16		36	00	Urinalysis	81000	32		4	00
MEDICINE						Pregnancy Test	83160	33		12	00
EKG	93000	17		27	00						
EKG –Trace	93005	18		18	00						
Surgical Tray	99070	19		5	00						
	99070					Collect & Handling	99000	34		5	00
	99070					**RADIOLOGY**					
Physiotherapy	97000	20		11	00	Chest, 1 View	71010	35		16	00
Physio-2 Mod.	97050	21		12	00	Chest, 2 Views	71020	36		24	00
						Foot, Complete	73630	37		22	00
						Pelvis, Limited	72170	38		28	00
						Skull, Complete	70260	39		48	00
						Spine, Complete	72050	40		53	00

4 RECALL	NEXT APPOINTMENT	**TODAY'S TOTAL CHARGES**		
8— —	DAY:			
4 DIAGNOSIS	DATE:	COURTESY DISC.	00060	5
1._____ 6._____	TIME: AM/PM	CASH PAYMENT	00010	7
	L-1 INS. NOW L-4 INS. MO. END	PERSONAL CHECK	00030	7
2._____ 7._____	MEMO:			

3._____ 8._____	CONDITION CAUSED BY	COMMENCEMENT DATE OF	INJURY ☐ ILLNESS ☐ PREGNANCY ☐	MO.	DAY	YR.
4._____ 9._____	1 ☐ INJURY 2 ☐ ILLNESS 3 ☐ PREGNANCY					
5._____		☐ NEW ILLNESS ☐ CONDITION DUE TO INJURY OR SICKNESS ARISING OUT OF PATIENT'S EMPLOYMENT ☐ NEW PATIENT				

IF INJURY, INDICATE HOW SUSTAINED
1 ☐ AUTO ACCIDENT   2 ☐ HOME   3 ☐ OTHER

MEDCOBILL COPY

MEDCOBILL SYSTEM
© COPYRIGHT 1975 INTELLECTRON INTERNATIONAL, INCORPORATED

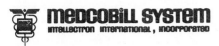

MEDCOBILL SYSTEM
Intellectron International, Incorporated

GROUP NO.	DR. NO.	DATE		ACCOUNT NO.		ACCOUNT LAST NAME	
FAMILY MEM. NO.		PATIENT FIRST NAME				PATIENT LAST NAME (IF DIFF. FROM ABOVE)	

IF NOT OFFICE, INDICATE PLACE OF SERVICE: 1 - IN-PATIENT HOSPITAL   2 - OUT-PATIENT HOSPITAL
4 - PATIENT'S HOME   6 - ECF   8 - NURSING HOME   9 - OTHER

SERVICE	RVS	MOD	FEE		SERVICE	RVS	MOD	FEE	
NEW					**INJECTION**				
Initial Brief	90000	01	18	00	Penicillin	90705	22	10	00
Init. Limited	90010	02	27	00	B12	90705	23	10	00
Init. Intermed.	90015	03	45	00		90705			
Init. Comprehen.	90020	04	63	00	**IMMUNIZATION**			10	00
ESTABLISHED					Polio	90700	24	10	00
Minimum O.V.	90030	05	7	00	Dip Tet	90700	25		
Brief Exam	90040	06	11	00					
Limited Exam	90050	07	14	00	**SURGERY**				
Intermed. Exam	90060	08	18	00	I & D Abscess	10060	26	44	00
Extended Re-Exam	90070	09	27	00	Laceration Repair	12000	27	44	00
HOSPITAL									
Initial Brief	90200	10	27	00					
Init. Intermed.	90215	11	45	00	**PATHOLOGY**				
Init. Comprehen.	90220	12	63	00	Blood Type, RH	86100	28	4	00
Brief Exam	90240	13	11	00	CBC	85010	29	8	00
Limited Exam	90250	14	18	00	Pap Smear	88105	30	14	00
Intermed. Exam	90260	15	27	00	Rh Titre	86025	31	7	00
Extended Re-Exam	90270	16	36	00	Urinalysis	81000	32	4	00
MEDICINE					Pregnancy Test	83160	33	12	00
EKG	93000	17	27	00					
EKG –Trace	93005	18	18	00					
Surgical Tray	99070	19	5	00					
	99070				Collect & Handling	99000	34	5	00
	99070				**RADIOLOGY**				
Physiotherapy	97000	20	11	00	Chest, 1 View	71010	35	16	00
Physio-2 Mod.	97050	21	12	00	Chest, 2 Views	71020	36	24	00
					Foot, Complete	73630	37	22	00
					Pelvis, Limited	72170	38	28	00
					Skull, Complete	70260	39	48	00
					Spine, Complete	72050	40	53	00

4 RECALL	NEXT APPOINTMENT		**TODAY'S TOTAL CHARGES**		
8— —	DAY:				
4 DIAGNOSIS	DATE:		COURTESY DISC.	00060	5
	TIME:	AM/PM	CASH PAYMENT	00010	7
1._____ 6._____	L-1 INS. NOW L-4 INS. MO. END		PERSONAL CHECK	00030	7
2._____ 7._____	MEMO:				

3._____ 8._____
4._____ 9._____
5._____

CONDITION CAUSED BY				MO.	DAY	YR.
1 ☐ INJURY 2 ☐ ILLNESS 3 ☐ PREGNANCY	COMMENCEMENT DATE OF	INJURY ☐ ILLNESS ☐ PREGNANCY ☐				

IF INJURY, INDICATE HOW SUSTAINED
1 ☐ AUTO ACCIDENT   2 ☐ HOME   3 ☐ OTHER

☐ NEW ILLNESS   CONDITION DUE TO INJURY OR SICKNESS ARISING OUT OF PATIENT'S EMPLOYMENT   ☐ NEW PATIENT

MEDCOBILL COPY

MEDCOBILL SYSTEM

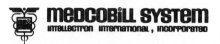

MEDCOBILL SYSTEM
INTELLECTRON INTERNATIONAL, INCORPORATED

GROUP NO.	DR. NO.	DATE	ACCOUNT NO.	ACCOUNT LAST NAME
FAMILY MEM. NO.		PATIENT FIRST NAME		PATIENT LAST NAME (IF DIFF. FROM ABOVE)

IF NOT OFFICE, INDICATE PLACE OF SERVICE: 1 - IN-PATIENT HOSPITAL 2 - OUT-PATIENT HOSPITAL
4 - PATIENT'S HOME 6 - ECF 8 - NURSING HOME 9 - OTHER

SERVICE	RVS		MOD	FEE		SERVICE	RVS		MOD	FEE	
NEW						**INJECTION**					
Initial Brief	90000	01		18	00	Penicillin	90705	22		10	00
Init. Limited	90010	02		27	00	B12	90705	23		10	00
Init. Intermed.	90015	03		45	00		90705				
Init. Comprehen.	90020	04		63	00	**IMMUNIZATION**				10	00
ESTABLISHED						Polio	90700	24		10	00
Minimum O.V.	90030	05		7	00	Dip Tet	90700	25			
Brief Exam	90040	06		11	00						
Limited Exam	90050	07		14	00	**SURGERY**					
Intermed. Exam	90060	08		18	00	I & D Abscess	10060	26		44	00
Extended Re-Exam	90070	09		27	00	Laceration Repair	12000	27		44	00
HOSPITAL											
Initial Brief	90200	10		27	00						
Init. Intermed.	90215	11		45	00	**PATHOLOGY**					
Init. Comprehen.	90220	12		63	00	Blood Type, RH	86100	28		4	00
Brief Exam	90240	13		11	00	CBC	85010	29		8	00
Limited Exam	90250	14		18	00	Pap Smear	88105	30		14	00
Intermed. Exam	90260	15		27	00	Rh Titre	86025	31		7	00
Extended Re-Exam	90270	16		36	00	Urinalysis	81000	32		4	00
MEDICINE						Pregnancy Test	83160	33		12	00
EKG	93000	17		27	00						
EKG – Trace	93005	18		18	00						
Surgical Tray	99070	19		5	00						
	99070					Collect & Handling	99000	34		5	00
	99070					**RADIOLOGY**					
Physiotherapy	97000	20		11	00	Chest, 1 View	71010	35		16	00
Physio-2 Mod.	97050	21		12	00	Chest, 2 Views	71020	36		24	00
						Foot, Complete	73630	37		22	00
						Pelvis, Limited	72170	38		28	00
						Skull, Complete	70260	39		48	00
						Spine, Complete	72050	40		53	00

4 RECALL	NEXT APPOINTMENT		**TODAY'S TOTAL CHARGES**			
8– –	DAY:					
4 DIAGNOSIS	DATE:		COURTESY DISC.	00060	5	
1._____ 6._____	TIME: AM/PM		CASH PAYMENT	00010	7	
2._____ 7._____	L-1 INS. NOW L-4 INS. MO. END		PERSONAL CHECK	00030	7	
3._____ 8._____	MEMO:					

				MO.	DAY	YR.
4._____ 9._____	CONDITION CAUSED BY	COMMENCEMENT DATE OF	INJURY ☐ ILLNESS ☐ PREGNANCY ☐			
5._____	1 ☐ INJURY 2 ☐ ILLNESS 3 ☐ PREGNANCY	☐ NEW ILLNESS	CONDITION DUE TO INJURY ☐ OR SICKNESS ARISING OUT OF PATIENT'S EMPLOYMENT	☐ NEW PATIENT		

IF INJURY, INDICATE HOW SUSTAINED
1 ☐ AUTO ACCIDENT 2 ☐ HOME 3 ☐ OTHER

MEDCOBILL COPY

MEDCOBILL SYSTEM
© COPYRIGHT 1975 INTELLECTRON INTERNATIONAL, INCORPORATED

ASSIGNMENT 31

On the following pages are three different insurance forms as output from the computer. See if you can locate the areas on each form that need completion before submission to the insurance company. In regard to Brad E. Diehl, refer to his Patient Record in Assignment 30. In regard to the other two patients, refer to their Patient Records if you need any pertinent information for the insurance claims. In regard to

Mr. Evert I. Strain, was any form fed out in error?_____. If not, what would Blue Cross

cover? _____ . What would Blue Shield

cover? _____ . Mr. Strain did not pay
anything on his account.

Abbreviations pertinent to the record of Evert I. Strain:

Adv _____	Hosp_____
ASHD_____	ltd _____
BP _____	PE _____
DC _____	pt _____
DX _____	SGOT* _____
Est _____	

_____

*See RVS pathology abbreviations on page 39.

PATIENT RECORD

Strain,	Evert	I.	09-11-16	M	013/678-0211
LAST NAME	FIRST NAME	MIDDLE NAME	BIRTH DATE	SEX	HOME PHONE

7650 None Such Road,	Woodland Hills,	XY	12345
ADDRESS	CITY	STATE	ZIP CODE

mechanical engineer	R and R Company
PATIENT'S OCCUPATION	NAME OF COMPANY

2400 Davon Road, Woodland Hills, XY 12345	013/520-8977
ADDRESS OF EMPLOYER	PHONE

Esther I. Strain (wife)	Administrative Assistant
SPOUSE OR PARENT	OCCUPATION

University College	4021 Book Road, Woodland Hills, XY 12345	013/450-9908
EMPLOYER	ADDRESS	PHONE

Blue Cross/Blue Shield	Evert I. Strain
NAME OF INSURANCE GROUP	SUBSCRIBER

453-32-4739	96476A		1-1-75
BLUE SHIELD OR BLUE CROSS CERT. NO.	GROUP NO.	CURRENT COVERAGE NO.	EFFECTIVE DATE

			453-32-4739
MEDICARE NO.	MEDICAID NO.	EFFECTIVE DATE	SOC. SEC. NO.

Gerald C. Jones, M. D. 1403 Haven St., Woodland Hills, XY 12345
REFERRED BY:

DATE	PROGRESS
1-8-77	Est.pt comes in complaining of frequency in urination, headaches, polyphagia, unable to remember current events. These problems have been present for almost a year. PE: BP 160/110. Ordered lab work SGOT, cholesterol, blood sugar glucose. DX: diabetes mellitus, (ICDA Code No. 2503) hypertension, ASHD. (ICDA Code No. 4031 and 4129) Adv hospitalization at College Hosp. on 1-9. Disability 1-9 thru 1-31-77. *Gerald Practon MD*
1-9-77	Hosp. visit ltd. Pt doing well on special diet *G Practon MD*
1-10-77	Hosp. visit ltd. Pt to remain in hosp for one more day. Continues to do well. BP 130/85. *G Practon MD*
1-11-77	DC from hosp. Pt to be seen in one month. *G Practon MD*

HEALTH INSURANCE
CLAIM FORM

READ INSTRUCTIONS BEFORE COMPLETING OR SIGNING THIS FORM

TYPE OR PRINT   ☐ MEDICARE   ☐ MEDICAID   ☐ CHAMPUS   ☒ OTHER

PATIENT & INSURED (SUBSCRIBER) INFORMATION

1. PATIENT'S NAME *(First name, middle initial, last name)* BRAD E. DIEHL	2. PATIENT'S DATE OF BIRTH 09 | 21 | 46	3. INSURED'S NAME *(First name, middle initial, last name)* BRAD E. DIEHL
4. PATIENT'S ADDRESS *(Street, city, state, ZIP code)* 3975 HILLS ROAD WOODLAND HILLS, XY 12345	5. PATIENT'S SEX MALE ☐ FEMALE ☐	6. INSURED'S I.D. No. or **MEDICARE No.** *(include any letters)*
	7. PATIENT'S RELATIONSHIP TO INSURED SELF SPOUSE CHILD OTHER	8. INSURED'S GROUP NO. *(Or Group Name)* 403119
9. OTHER HEALTH INSURANCE COVERAGE - Enter Name of Policyholder and Plan Name and Address and Policy or Medical Assistance Number NONE	10. WAS CONDITION RELATED TO: A. PATIENT'S EMPLOYMENT YES ☐ X NO B. AN AUTO ACCIDENT YES ☐ X NO	11. INSURED'S ADDRESS *(Street, city, state, ZIP code)* 3975 HILLS ROAD WOODLAND HILLS, XY 12345
12. PATIENT'S OR AUTHORIZED PERSON'S SIGNATURE *(Read back before signing)* I Authorize the Release of any Medical Information Necessary to Process this Claim and Request Payment of MEDICARE/CHAMPUS Benefits Either to Myself or to the Party Who Accepts Assignment Below SIGNED DATE		13. I AUTHORIZE PAYMENT OF MEDICAL BENEFITS TO UNDERSIGNED PHYSICIAN OR SUPPLIER FOR SERVICE DESCRIBED BELOW SIGNED (Insured or Authorized Person)

PHYSICIAN OR SUPPLIER INFORMATION

14. DATE OF: ILLNESS (FIRST SYMPTOM) OR INJURY (ACCIDENT) OR PREGNANCY (LMP)	15. DATE FIRST CONSULTED YOU FOR THIS CONDITION	16. HAS PATIENT EVER HAD SAME OR SIMILAR SYMPTOMS? YES ☐ NO
17 DATE PATIENT ABLE TO RETURN TO WORK	18. DATES OF TOTAL DISABILITY FROM THROUGH	DATES OF PARTIAL DISABILITY FROM THROUGH
19. NAME OF REFERRING PHYSICIAN		20. FOR SERVICES RELATED TO HOSPITALIZATION GIVE HOSPITALIZATION DATES ADMITTED DISCHARGED
21. NAME & ADDRESS OF FACILITY WHERE SERVICES RENDERED *(If other than home or office)*		22. WAS LABORATORY WORK PERFORMED OUTSIDE YOUR OFFICE? YES ☐ NO CHARGES:

23. DIAGNOSIS OR NATURE OF ILLNESS OR INJURY, RELATE DIAGNOSIS TO PROCEDURE IN COLUMN D BY REFERENCE TO NUMBERS 1, 2, 3, ETC. OR DX CODE

1.
2.
3.
4.

24. A DATE OF SERVICE	B* PLACE OF SERVICE	C FULLY DESCRIBE PROCEDURES, MEDICAL SERVICES OR SUPPLIES FURNISHED FOR EACH DATE GIVEN PROCEDURE CODE (IDENTIFY:) *(EXPLAIN UNUSUAL SERVICES OR CIRCUMSTANCES)*	D DIAGNOSIS CODE	E CHARGES	F
01-05-77	3	90015 OFFICE VISIT, INTERMEDIATE		45 | 00	
01-05-77	3	93005 EKG WITH INTERPRET. AND REPORT		27 | 00	
01-05-77	3	71020 AP AND LAT CHEST X-RAYS		24 | 00	
01-05-77	3	BONE MARROW, INTERPRETATION		10 | 00	
01-14-77	3	GLUCOSE TOLERANCE TEST 3 SPEC.			
01-14-77	3	GLUCOSE TOLERANCE TEST 2 SPEC.		35 | 00	
01-14-77	3	99000 COLLECTION AND HANDLING SPEC.		5 | 00	
01-20-77	3	90050 OFFICE VISIT, LIMITED		14 | 00	
01-20-77	3	85010 COMPLETE BLOOD COUNT		8 | 00	
01-20-77	3	ORAL CHOLECYSTOGRAPHY		60 | 00	

25. SIGNATURE OF PHYSICIAN OR SUPPLIER *(Read back before signing)*	26. ACCEPT ASSIGNMENT (GOVERNMENT CLAIMS ONLY) (SEE BACK) YES ☐ NO ☐	27. TOTAL CHARGE	28. AMOUNT PAID 201 | 00	29. BALANCE DUE
SIGNED DATE 01-25-77	30. YOUR SOCIAL SECURITY NO.	31. PHYSICIAN'S OR SUPPLIER'S NAME, ADDRESS, ZIP CODE & TELEPHONE NO.		
32. YOUR PATIENT'S ACCOUNT NO.	33. YOUR EMPLOYER I.D. NO.	GASTON INPUT, M. D. 4567 BROAD AVENUE WOODLAND HILLS, XY 12345 I.D. NO.		

*PLACE OF SERVICE CODES

1—(IH) —INPATIENT HOSPITAL	4—(H)—PATIENT'S HOME	7—(NH) —NURSING HOME	O—(OL)—OTHER LOCATIONS
2—(OH)—OUTPATIENT HOSPITAL	5— DAY CARE FACILITY (PSY)	8—(SNF)—SKILLED NURSING FACILITY	A—(IL) —INDEPENDENT LABORATORY
3—(O) —DOCTOR'S OFFICE	6— NIGHT CARE FACILITY (PSY)	9— AMBULANCE	B— OTHER MEDICAL/SURGICAL FACILITY

2331 5/75

APPROVED BY AMA COUNCIL ON MEDICAL SERVICE 6-74

SERVICE REPORT
MC 163 (REV. 9-70)

PATIENT'S NAME LAST	FIRST	MIDDLE INITIAL
STRAIN	EVERT	I

PATIENT'S ADDRESS

7650 NONE SUCH ROAD

CITY WOODLAND HILLS STATE XY ZIP CODE 12345

SUBSCRIBER'S NAME (IF PATIENT IS A DEPENDENT) LAST	FIRST	MIDDLE INITIAL

SUBSCRIBER'S EMPLOYER

COMPLETE FOR GOVERNMENT PROGRAM

CALIFORNIA MEDICAL ASSISTANCE PROGRAM
PATIENT'S IDENTIFICATION NUMBER.

CO. | AID | CASE NO. | FBU | PERS. NO.

FEDERAL MEDICARE NUMBER

PATIENT'S BIRTHDATE MONTH DAY YR AGE

COMPANY

GROUP NO. 96476 A   SECTION NO.

MEMBERSHIP NO. 453 32 4739

PATIENT'S RELATIONSHIP TO SUBSCRIBER
[ ] SELF [ ] SPOUSE [ ] CHILD

PATIENT'S SEX
[ ] MALE [ ] FEMALE

FOR PROVIDER'S USE ONLY

CONDITION CAUSED BY: [ ] INJURY [X] ILLNESS [ ] PREGNANCY

IF INJURY: INDICATE DATE, HOW AND WHERE SUSTAINED
[ ] AUTO ACCIDENT
[ ] HOME
[ ] OTHER
DATE OF INJURY MO DAY YR

IF PREGNANCY, DATE OF COMMENCEMENT

IS THIS A NEW ILLNESS? [ ] NO [X] YES

IS CONDITION DUE TO INJURY OR SICKNESS ARISING OUT OF PATIENT'S EMPLOYMENT?
[X] NO [ ] YES   IS THIS A NEW PATIENT? [ ] NO [ ] YES

IF PATIENT WAS REFERRED INDICATE: [X] FROM GERALD C. JONES, M. D. [ ] TO DOCTOR

IF TREATED IN HOSPITAL OR NURSING HOME-I.P. OR O.P. INDICATE NAME AND LOCATION
COLLEGE HOSPITAL
WOODLAND HILLS, XY 12345

ADMISSION DATE MO 01 DAY 09 YR 77
DISCHARGE DATE MO 01 DAY 11 YR 77

OTHER GROUP HOSPITAL, MEDICAL COVERAGE INCLUDING MEDICARE. [ ] NO [ ] YES
NAME OF COMPANY OR PLAN   HEALTH INSURANCE CLAIM NO.   LETTER

DIAGNOSIS AND CONCURRENT CONDITIONS

REMARKS

NAME AND ADDRESS OF PROVIDER OF SERVICE   PROVIDER NO.

ZZZ12345Z

GERALD PRACTON, M. D.
4567 BROAD AVENUE
WOODLAND HILLS, XY 12345

19 28 21

DATE THIS FORM WAS PREPARED ▶ 1-25-77

WAS LABORATORY WORK PERFORMED IN YOUR OFFICE?
[X] NO (IF NO, ENTER NAME AND ADDRESS OF LABORATORY BELOW) [ ] YES

#1 AUTOMATED LAB SERVICES
22030 SHERMAN WAY
WOODLAND HILLS, XY 12345

AMOUNT CHARGED TO PHYSICIAN BY LABORATORY
$ 22.00

THIS IS TO CERTIFY THAT THE FOREGOING INFORMATION IS TRUE, ACCURATE AND COMPLETE. I UNDERSTAND THAT PAYMENT AND SATISFACTION OF THIS CLAIM WILL BE FROM FEDERAL AND STATE FUNDS, AND THAT ANY FALSE CLAIMS, STATEMENTS, OR DOCUMENTS OR CONCEALMENT OF A MATERIAL FACT, MAY BE PROSECUTED UNDER APPLICABLE FEDERAL OR STATE LAWS.

SIGNATURE OF PROVIDER OF SERVICE REQUIRED FOR MEDI-CAL PROGRAM ▶

COMPLETE THIS SECTION ONLY IF CLAIM IS BEING MADE FOR DISABILITY PAYMENTS THE PT. HAS BEEN UNABLE TO PERFORM HIS REGULAR OR CUSTOMARY WORK
FROM   THROUGH

IF UNABLE TO PERFORM HIS REGULAR OR CUSTOMARY WORK WHEN SHOULD PT. BE ABLE TO RESUME

PLACE OF SERVICE CODES

1=IN-PATIENT HOSPITAL 2=OUT-PATIENT HOSPITAL 3=OFFICE 4=PATIENT'S HOME 8=NURSING HOME 9=OTHER

FOR COMPANY USE ONLY	DATE OF SERVICE MO DAY YR	PROCEDURE NUMBER RVS NUMBER / SMA NUMBER UNIT MODIFIER	DESCRIBE EACH SERVICE OR APPLIANCE SEPARATELY	FOR COMPANY USE ONLY	YOUR FEE	PLACE OF SERV CODE	FOR COMPANY USE ONLY
	01-08-77	90080	OFF VISIT COMPR REEXAM		50.00	3	
	01-08-77	93000	ECG W INTERP AND REPORT		27.00	3	
	01-08-77	82465 90	CHOLESTEROL BLOOD		6.00	9	
	01-08-77	84330 90	SUGAR GLUCOSE BLOOD		6.00	9	
	01-08-77	84450 90	TRANSAMINASE SGOT		10.00	9	
			REFERENCE LAB #1				
	01-09-77	90250	HOSP LIMITED EXAM		18.00	1	
	01-10-77	90250	HOSP LIMITED EXAM		18.00	1	
	01-11-77	90250	HOSP LIMITED EXAM		18.00	1	
			TOTAL		153.00		

SPECIAL PAYEE NAME

SPECIAL PAYEE NO. AND STREET   SPECIAL PAYEE CITY, STATE   ZIP CODE

CN | CD | CLM | MSG. | DIAG.

TYPE OF SERVICE | UNITS | LOC | MSG

TOTAL

CLAIM TYPE	PAY CODE	CPC	MDE	FEE	PROF.	HOSP.	MISC.	QUAL.	REL	PERS.	ORIG. EFF. DATE	EXPL	DATE OF CHG. OR CX
1	2	3	4	5	6	7	8	9	10				

HEALTH INSURANCE
CLAIM FORM

READ INSTRUCTIONS BEFORE COMPLETING OR SIGNING THIS FORM

TYPE OR PRINT   ☐ MEDICARE   ☐ MEDICAID   ☐ CHAMPUS   ☒ OTHER

Blue Cross of Southern California

Box 60465, Terminal Annex
Los Angeles, California 90060

PATIENT & INSURED (SUBSCRIBER) INFORMATION

1. PATIENT'S NAME (First name, middle initial, last name)	2. PATIENT'S DATE OF BIRTH	3. INSURED'S NAME (First name, middle initial, last name)
EVERT I STRAIN		EVERT I STRAIN

4. PATIENT'S ADDRESS (Street, city, state, ZIP code)	5. PATIENT'S SEX	6. INSURED'S I.D. No. or **MEDICARE No.** (include any letters)
7650 NONE SUCH ROAD WOODLAND HILLS, XY 12345	MALE ☐ FEMALE ☐	453 32 4739

7. PATIENT'S RELATIONSHIP TO INSURED
SELF   SPOUSE   CHILD   OTHER

8. INSURED'S GROUP NO. (Or Group Name)
96476 A

9. OTHER HEALTH INSURANCE COVERAGE - Enter Name of Policyholder and Plan Name and Address and Policy or Medical Assistance Number

10. WAS CONDITION RELATED TO:
A. PATIENT'S EMPLOYMENT   YES ☐   X   NO
B. AN AUTO ACCIDENT   YES ☐   X   NO

11. INSURED'S ADDRESS (Street, city, state, ZIP code)
7650 NONE SUCH ROAD
WOODLAND HILLS, XY 12345

12. PATIENT'S OR AUTHORIZED PERSON'S SIGNATURE (Read back before signing)
I Authorize the Release of any Medical Information Necessary to Process this Claim and Request Payment of MEDICARE/CHAMPUS Benefits Either to Myself or to the Party Who Accepts Assignment Below

SIGNED _____ DATE _____

13. I AUTHORIZE PAYMENT OF MEDICAL BENEFITS TO UNDERSIGNED PHYSICIAN OR SUPPLIER FOR SERVICE DESCRIBED BELOW

SIGNED (Insured or Authorized Person) _____

PHYSICIAN OR SUPPLIER INFORMATION

14. DATE OF: 06-76	ILLNESS (FIRST SYMPTOM) OR INJURY (ACCIDENT) OR PREGNANCY (LMP)	15. DATE FIRST CONSULTED YOU FOR THIS CONDITION 01-08-77	16. HAS PATIENT EVER HAD SAME OR SIMILAR SYMPTOMS? YES ☐ NO ☐

17. DATE PATIENT ABLE TO RETURN TO WORK

18. DATES OF TOTAL DISABILITY
FROM _____ THROUGH _____

DATES OF PARTIAL DISABILITY
FROM _____ THROUGH _____

19. NAME OF REFERRING PHYSICIAN
GERALD C. JONES, M. D.

20. FOR SERVICES RELATED TO HOSPITALIZATION GIVE HOSPITALIZATION DATES
ADMITTED 01-09-77   DISCHARGED 01-11-77

21. NAME & ADDRESS OF FACILITY WHERE SERVICES RENDERED (If other than home or office)
COLLEGE HOSP. 4500 BROAD AVE., WOODLAND HILLS, XY 12345

22. WAS LABORATORY WORK PERFORMED OUTSIDE YOUR OFFICE?
YES X   NO ☐   CHARGES: 22.00

23. DIAGNOSIS OR NATURE OF ILLNESS OR INJURY, RELATE DIAGNOSIS TO PROCEDURE IN COLUMN D BY REFERENCE TO NUMBERS 1, 2, 3, ETC. OR DX CODE

1.
2.
3.
4.

24. A DATE OF SERVICE	B* PLACE OF SERVICE	C FULLY DESCRIBE PROCEDURES, MEDICAL SERVICES OR SUPPLIES FURNISHED FOR EACH DATE GIVEN PROCEDURE CODE (IDENTIFY:)	(EXPLAIN UNUSUAL SERVICES OR CIRCUMSTANCES)	D DIAGNOSIS CODE	E CHARGES	F
01-08-77	3	90080	OFF VISIT COMPR REEXAM		50 00	
01-08-77	3	93000	ECG W INTERP AND REPORT		27 00	
01-08-77	A	82465 90	CHOLESTEROL BLOOD		6 00	
01-08-77	A	84330 90	SUGAR GLUCOSE BLOOD		6 00	
01-08-77	A	84450 90	TRANSAMINASE SGOT		10 00	
01-09-77	1	90250	HOSP LIMITED EXAM		18 00	
01-10-77	1	90250	HOSP LIMITED EXAM		18 00	
01-11-77	1	90250	HOSP LIMITED EXAM		18 00	

25. SIGNATURE OF PHYSICIAN OR SUPPLIER (Read back before signing)

SIGNED _____ DATE 1-25-77

26. ACCEPT ASSIGNMENT (GOVERNMENT CLAIMS ONLY) (SEE BACK)
YES ☐   NO ☐

30. YOUR SOCIAL SECURITY NO.
123-45-6789

27. TOTAL CHARGE
153 00

28. AMOUNT PAID   29. BALANCE DUE

31. PHYSICIAN'S OR SUPPLIER'S NAME, ADDRESS, ZIP CODE & TELEPHONE NO.
GERALD PRACTON, M. D.
4567 BROAD AVENUE
WOODLAND HILLS, XY 12345
I.D. NO. C 14021   013/486-9002

32. YOUR PATIENT'S ACCOUNT NO.

33. YOUR EMPLOYER I.D. NO.
95-3664021

*PLACE OF SERVICE CODES

1–(IH) –INPATIENT HOSPITAL	4–(H)–PATIENT'S HOME	7–(NH) –NURSING HOME
2–(OH)–OUTPATIENT HOSPITAL	5– DAY CARE FACILITY (PSY)	8–(SNF)–SKILLED NURSING FACILITY
3–(O) –DOCTOR'S OFFICE	6– NIGHT CARE FACILITY (PSY)	9– AMBULANCE

O–(OL)–OTHER LOCATIONS
A–(IL) –INDEPENDENT LABORATORY
B– OTHER MEDICAL/SURGICAL FACILITY

2331 5/75

APPROVED BY AMA COUNCIL ON MEDICAL SERVICE 6-74

Chapter 13:
Credit and Collection

ASSIGNMENT 32

Preparing Receipts

The following patients paid cash and amount in full at the time of their last visit. Check the fee chart on page 623 and then make out receipts for the total amount they paid. Begin your receipt numbers with 101.

12/7/77	Peter Barton	Office consultation	$_____
12/8/77	Mary Ellen Davidson	Allergy injection	$_____
12/8/77	Mrs. Erma O. Hamlyn	IUD insertion	$_____
12/9/77	Mrs. Marian O. Miller	CBC	$_____

ASSIGNMENT 33

Composing Letters

a. At the request of Mrs. Must U. (May I.) Deliver, 2390 Jeffers Avenue, Woodland Hills, XY 12345, send her a letter quoting fees of $2,000, $1,500, and $1,000 for delivery and prenatal care, including one postnatal office visit. The amount of the fee depends on the type of accommodation selected at the hospital—private, semi-private, or ward, respectively. Write this letter for Dr. Practon's signature and date it when you type it. Type this in block style (all lines beginning at the left hand margin; see Fig. 13–17). Type a number 10 envelope (see Fig. 13–8).

b. In checking through your records, you find that Mr. Bill Owen, of 5860 James Drive, Woodland Hills, XY 12345, has not paid his bill for three months. Write a letter over your own signature requesting payment. Type this letter in modified block (each paragraph indented). Date the letter March 20, 1978. Type a number 10 envelope (see Fig. 13–8). The professional services rendered were:

12-12-77	Office visit, complete checkup	$ 25.00
12-15-77	Appendectomy	275.00
12-22-77	Follow-up office visit	NC

ASSIGNMENT 34

Prepare a cover letter for the doctor's signature and an itemized statement for Mr. Peter F. Donlon, who expired from a cardiovascular accident (CVA) on July 10, 1977. Refer to Assignment 12 for information from his Patient Record and ledger card. Also refer to Table 13–2 on page 361 to ascertain where to file the claim in your state. See page 378 in Chapter 13 under the paragraph "Estate Claims" for further information. Date the letter July 30, 1977. Type the letter in block style as shown in Figure 13–17. Type a number 10 envelope by referring to Figure 13–8.

Dr. Practon's fee schedule is as follows:

Office visit (new pt first visit, complete checkup, or consult)	$ 25.00
Office visit (established pt - limited)	12.00
Office visit (established pt - brief)	8.00
House Call	20.00
Hospital Admission,History & Physical	35.00
Hospital visit	10.00
EKG	35.00
Total OB care	350.00
Circumcision	25.00
IUD insertion	40.00
Vasectomy	150.00

Injections

Flu vaccine	6.00
Rubella	8.00
Measles	8.00
MMR (measles, mumps and rubella)	15.00
Small Pox	5.00
Allergy	3.00
All other injections	5.00

Laboratory

CBC	8.00
UA (urinalysis)	4.00
Serology	8.00
Premarital male (VDRL)	7.00
Premarital female (VDRL and Rubella)	17.00
Pap Smear	20.00

No. _____   No. _____
                                                    _____ 19 ___
To _____
                       Received from _____
Date _____
                       _____ *Dollars*
For _____
                       FOR _____
Amount _____
                       $ _____   _____
_____

No. _____   No. _____
                                                    _____ 19 ___
To _____
                       Received from _____
Date _____
                       _____ *Dollars*
For _____
                       FOR _____
Amount _____
                       $ _____   _____
_____

No. _____   No. _____
                                                    _____ 19 ___
To _____
                       Received from _____
Date _____
                       _____ *Dollars*
For _____
                       FOR _____
Amount _____
                       $ _____   _____
_____

No. _____   No. _____
                                                    _____ 19 ___
To _____
                       Received from _____
Date _____
                       _____ *Dollars*
For _____
                       FOR _____
Amount _____
                       $ _____   _____
_____

Chapter 14:
Medical Ethics and Medical
Professional Liability

ASSIGNMENT 35

1. Mrs. Merry M. McLean is negligent about following Dr. Ulibarri's advice after she received surgery. Write an appropriate letter to Mrs. McLean advising her of the doctor's withdrawal from the case. Dr. Ulibarri will sign the letter. Use a typewritten letterhead and modified block style as shown in Figure 14–5. Refer to Assignment 1 for information from the Patient Record. Type a number 10 envelope by referring to Figure 13–8. Send the letter by Certified Mail with return receipt requested.

2. Mr. Walter J. Stone telephones on June 3, sounding extremely upset and irrational. He says that he is unable to return to work on June 22 and that he does not want to be seen by Dr. Input again. Write a letter to confirm this discharge by the patient. Suggest that he contact the local medical society for the names of three internists for further care. Refer to Assignment 3 for information from the Patient Record. Use a typewritten letterhead and modified block style as shown in Figure 14–6. Type a number 10 envelope referring to Figure 13–8. Send the letter by Certified Mail with return receipt requested.

3. Mrs. Virginia B. Drake calls on June 1 and makes an appointment for Stephen M. Drake to be seen at 3:00 p.m. on June 5, 1977. The patient does not show (DNS). Write a letter to Mrs. Drake about her son's failure to keep his appointment. Refer to Assignment 9 for information from the Patient Record. Use a typewritten letterhead and modified block style as shown in Figure 14–8. Type a number 10 envelope by referring to Figure 13–8.

Remember that all of these letters must be prepared for the physician's signature, as they are legal documents.

Chapter 15:
The Physician's Personal Insurance

ASSIGNMENT 36

1. If you, your husband, or your parents subscribe to a health insurance plan or work for or belong to a club, lodge, or similar organization that has a health insurance plan, make up two different *Pertinent Data Cards*. Call the insurance agent if all the information is not listed on the policies. This assignment could also be done on mortgage insurance or disability insurance. The card would then become a useful asset for future reference to the student.

2. If you are currently working for a medical office, the Pertinent Data Cards could be completed by filling in the proper information for the physician on the various forms of insurance held.

PERTINENT DATA CARD

Physician's Name _____

Name of Policy _____ Policy #_____

Type of Coverage _____

Insurance Company _____ Insurance Agent_____

Address_____ Phone No._____

Value of Policy $_____

Effective Date _____ Expiration Date_____

Annual Premium _____ Renewal Date _____
(quarterly, annual, every 3 yrs)

Dates of Each Premium Payment_____ Amount $ _____

_____ $ _____

Dr's age when policy was issued (if pertinent)_____

Beneficiary_____

Other Information_____

_____

PERTINENT DATA CARD

Physician's Name _____

Name of Policy _____   Policy #_____

Type of Coverage _____

Insurance Company _____   Insurance Agent_____

Address_____   Phone No._____

Value of Policy $_____

Effective Date _____   Expiration Date_____

Annual Premium _____   Renewal Date _____
   (quarterly, annual, every 3 yrs)

Dates of Each Premium Payment_____   Amount $ _____

_____ $ _____

Dr's age when policy was issued (if pertinent)_____

Beneficiary_____

Other Information_____

Chapter 16:
Canadian Medical Office Accounting and Insurance Form Processing

See exercises on pages 490–495.

INDEX

Italics denotes illustrations, t denotes tables.